MEDICAL NANOTECHNOLOGY AND NANOMEDICINE

PERSPECTIVES IN NANOTECHNOLOGY

Series Editor
Gabor L. Hornyak

MEDICAL NANOTECHNOLOGY AND NANOMEDICINE

Harry F. Tibbals

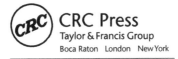

CRC Press
Taylor & Francis Group
Boca Raton   London   New York

CRC Press is an imprint of the
Taylor & Francis Group, an **informa** business

CRC Press
Taylor & Francis Group
6000 Broken Sound Parkway NW, Suite 300
Boca Raton, FL 33487-2742

International Standard Book Number: 978-1-4398-0874-0 (Paperback)

Library of Congress Cataloging-in-Publication Data

Tibbals, Harry F.
   Medical nanotechnology and nanomedicine / Harry F. Tibbals.
      p. ; cm. -- (Perspectives in nanotechnology)
   Includes bibliographical references and index.
   Summary: "This book is an introduction to nanoscience and nanotechnology as applied to medicine, written for doctors and patients, caregivers and laypersons, and all those who advise and make decisions on, or have an interest in, health care. The summary attempts to be comprehensive without being too detailed or technical. References and sources are given for those who wish to pursue an in-depth study on techniques, instruments, and practices. The book provides a comprehensive coverage of all areas in which nanotechnology may impact medicine and health-care management and delivery. It also provides a broad overview of the history, current global status, and potential prospects of nanotechnology and its impact on medicine and health in the broadest sense"--Provided by publisher.
   ISBN 978-1-4398-0874-0 (pbk. : alk. paper)
   1. Nanomedicine. 2. Nanotechnology. I. Title. II. Series: Perspectives in nanotechnology.
   [DNLM: 1. Nanomedicine--methods. 2. Nanostructures--therapeutic use. QT 36.5]

R857.N34T53 2011
610.28--dc22   2010030229

Visit the Taylor & Francis Web site at
http://www.taylorandfrancis.com

and the CRC Press Web site at
http://www.crcpress.com

Contents

Part II Beginnings of Medical Nanotechnology

Foreword

This book, *Medical Nanotechnology and Nanomedicine*, is an introduction to nanoscience and nanotechnology for those with medical backgrounds and interests. It is an overview and guide, with references and keywords for further pursuit into the rapidly growing fields of medical nanotechnology and nanomedicine. It is meant for the layperson, in the sense of both the non-medical specialist and the nontechnical healthcare professional.

The currently available literature as well as various media sources on nanotechnology contain a number of differing views of the impact of nanotechnology on the future of medicine. This book gives an overview of the many alternative and sometimes conflicting concepts proposed for the application of nanotechnology to medicine, along with a review of some recent research and development, illustrating the accomplishments and possibilities for the application of nanoscience to medicine.

Just as with nanotechnology in general, popularized presentations of nanomedicine have included a variety of viewpoints, from futuristic and speculative visions to rather straightforward applications of existing techniques on a limited scale. But nanomedicine and medical nanotechnology are taking an interesting and promising direction. The terms "nanomedicine" and "medical nanotechnology" have been formally established since their adoption into major program initiatives by the National Institutes of Health and other leading medical bodies worldwide. Leading pharmaceutical and medical device companies have set up their own departments focused on nanomedicine and have been joined by a number of start-up enterprises, backed, in some cases, by investment groups focused on medical nanotechnology ventures.

In an environment full of news about nanotechnology, the general reader (including the medical professional not particularly familiar with nanotechnology) will do well to get started with an introduction to nanomedicine and its evolving organizational infrastructure, both available and proposed. An exhaustive, technical coverage of nanotechnology applied to biomedical areas does not serve the purpose as an introduction, nor do futuristic projections that have little to do with actual medical practice. This book intends to provide a practical guide about nanomedicine for the interested, curious, or perplexed individual. It is intended for laypersons, patients, and medical practitioners and professionals who are looking for a clear understanding of the rapidly developing nanotechnology revolution impacting their field of work. Medical professionals are used to rapid and sometimes transformational advances in technology and practices. Planning, investment, and continuing medical education are directed at constantly moving targets. Although conservative and skeptical of new claims, the medical profession is constantly seeking to evaluate new possibilities for breakthroughs.

Content and Intended Audience

The content covered will be of interest for members of the public concerned about their health and healthcare options in the future; patients and potential patients who increasingly want to be involved and make informed decisions about their medical care; medical professionals, including doctors, physicians, surgeons, specialists, nurses, assistants, allied healthcare professionals, and medical and clinical technology specialists; managers and planners for healthcare organizations, hospitals, clinics, and research organizations; managers of healthcare-oriented businesses; investors; planners; leaders in government and social services; journalists; and members of the general public with an interest in healthcare policy and advances in medical science.

This book is intended to be a readable and affordable resource that is designed to fit into the tight schedules of busy people. It offers the reader a sense of the *status quo* with regard to nanomedicine and a base of information for planning and decision making. It has been written in a free-flowing style, and concise but informative examples and case summaries have been provided. Graphical illustrations have been used where they enhance concepts without digressing from the flow of the narrative. Prominent leaders in the field have been identified and their works have been concisely described. In the Perspectives in Nanotechnology Series, this book fills the niche of a readable perspective on the medical aspects of nanotechnology, current and future, and the developing infrastructure that surrounds it.

Organization of the Material

The content organization follows the precedent of the series—it is divided into three parts: a historical perspective, current status, and future prospects. Part I gives a historical background and introduction (including definitions of nanomedicine and related terms) and a broad overview of recent trends and forces. Part II investigates the current status of nanotechnology and how it is being applied to medicine and related biomedical sciences, including a survey of major initiatives and leading labs and innovators. The landscape of nanomedicine encompassing government, academia, and the private sector is also outlined. Part III looks at some projected future directions and capabilities, their champions and detractors, and some of the choices facing us in the application of nanotechnology and technology, in general, to medical care. This final section concludes with a brief discussion of issues of sustainability and equity.

This book is part of the Perspectives in Nanotechnology Series, centered broadly on the societal implications of nanoscience and nanotechnology. This book can be a stand-alone reference and guide but also fits into the broader landscape of the series. Although technological topics are presented and discussed in lay terms, the focus of the book is on the societal implications of this exciting and rapidly expanding field.

Summary

This book on applications and impacts of nanotechnology on medicine offers laypersons an informed overview of the emerging influence of nanoscience on healthcare. Rather than a comprehensive detailed report on nanomedicine, it is written to enhance awareness, providing a foundation from which decisions and planning can be made. It attempts to provide a critical, balanced, and realistic evaluation of nanomedicine developments and prospects. It complements the treatment of societal implications of nanotechnology covered in the Perspectives in Nanotechnology Series, which provides an integrated perspective of nanotechnology over a range of topics.

Preface

Medicine as a profession is as much art as science, in which concern, care, and respect for life and well-being are the sworn principles. So it is with humility that a non-practitioner presumes to present an overview of new technology for the practice of medicine. As a toolmaker for physicians and surgeons, I have made a career of adapting new technology to the needs of medical caregivers and researchers, developing medical computer, electrochemical and imaging instruments, and devices to augment and extend the perceptions and powers of the skilled practitioner. So in this small book, I offer an introduction to medical nanotechnology to physicians and to the public, covering the latest techniques to observe, manipulate, and transform our bodies and environment.

This book is an introduction to nanoscience and nanotechnology as applied to medicine, written for doctors and patients, caregivers and laypersons, and all those who advise and make decisions on, or have an interest in, healthcare. The summary attempts to be comprehensive without being too detailed or technical. References and sources are given for those who wish to pursue an in-depth study on techniques, instruments, and practices. The book provides a comprehensive coverage of all areas in which nanotechnology may impact medicine and healthcare management and delivery. It also provides a broad overview of the history, current global status, and potential prospects of nanotechnology and its impact on medicine and health in the broadest sense.

Parts I through III cover the background, and provide a description and projection of the state of nanoscience's applications and impacts on medicine. From a historical perspective (Part I), we find that medicine and biomedical science were the forces that led to the current rapid expansion in nanoscience. Medicine and nanoscience are natural partners because of the size scale of macromolecular machinery at the basis of life. This is being realized worldwide, with many new programs and initiatives to develop useful applications of new nanotechnologies in medicine. In Part II, we survey these applications, starting from the simplest nanomaterials developed for medical imaging and treatment to complex medical systems that are enabled by new nanotechnologies. In Part III, we discuss some evident future directions for the development of nanotechnologies that are fully integrated into medicine, as well as some implications of increasing capabilities to alter and monitor our lives at the biomolecular level.

Nanoscience and nanotechnology are undergoing rapid exponential growth. Many of the applications that will result are not yet evident. This brief introduction hopefully suggests opportunities to pursue further study, leading to new possibilities and cures.

Acknowledgments

I would first like to acknowledge Dr. G. Louis Hornyak for suggesting this work and editing the series; for being a source of research expertise and leadership on nanotechnology, especially carbon nanotubes; and for being a good friend and coworker. I would also like to thank coworkers and mentors at the University of Texas Southwestern, Dallas, Texas—Profs. Robert Eberhart, Ann Word, Ralph Mason, Daniel Scott, Shou Tang, and Mario Romero-Ortega; Profs. Austin Cunningham, Bruce Gnade, Roy Chaney, Robert Moore, Andrew Blanchard, J.-B. Lee, and Ray Baughman at the University of Texas Dallas; Profs. J. C. Chiao, J. Hao, R. Meletis, Patricia Holcombe, and Carolyn Cochrane at the University of Texas at Arlington; and to Prof. Robert Fossum, for discussions and encouragement. Thanks also to those acknowledged throughout the book for giving us permission to use their work, and to all those who spared their valuable time in providing advice and guidance. Special thanks go to the University of Texas Southwestern vice president for technology development, Denis Stone MD, and associate vice president, James Watson, for encouragement and support. A special note of thanks goes to James von Ehr and John Randall of Zyvex, Stephen Buerger of Sandia, and Adrian Denvir and Gareth Hughes of Lynntech. Thanks also to Dennis Harding, David Rhind, and Earl Saxon for encouragement to write, and to many others, kind and wise, not mentioned here. Sincere thanks to the staff of Taylor & Francis, CRC Press, especially Nora Konopka and Jill Jurgensen, for their excellent and professional editorial work, and to Brittany Gilbert, Rachael Panthier, Sathyanarayanamoorthy Sridharan, and the other members of the editorial and production staff who were invaluable. Finally, I am very grateful to Cindy Gillean and my family for their patience and helpfulness during the preparation and writing of this book.

Author

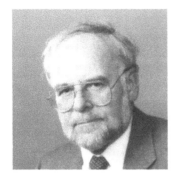

Harry F. Tibbals is director of the Bioinstrumentation Resource Center at the University of Texas Southwestern (UTSW) Medical Center at Dallas, Texas, providing basic science and engineering support to clinical and biomedical science research, and leading a number of research and development projects, including the development of sensors for medical applications, testing and evaluation of life support systems for use in space flight and extra-vehicular activity by NASA, and the development of test instrumentation for Alcon Research Ltd., Fort Worth, Texas, for the diagnosis of eye diseases. His work involves consultation and guidance on a wide variety of analytical, materials, and systems technology, and advising on risks and cost benefits for technology decisions.

Prior to joining UTSW in 1997, Tibbals was involved in the development of biomedical, environmental, and analytical instrumentation, as president and cofounder of Biodigital Technologies, Inc., Dallas, Texas, and as product line manager for digital cardiology imaging for Jamieson Kodak. He also served as a consultant and manager for Rockwell International, United Technologies Mostek, Martingale Research Corporation, Inmos, and SGS Thompson for developing instrumentation for anesthesiology; identification of bacterial and viral disease agents; monitoring, analyzing, and reducing environmental hazards; and a number of systems involving enhancement and augmentation of skilled tasks and communications by application of advanced sensors and signal processing. Biodigital's clients included NEC, Teledyne, Marathon Energy Systems, Coors, Bank One, Shelby Technologies, Innovative Systems SA, Optical Publishing Inc., and Colorado Medical Physics among others. He also worked as a consultant for the development of a production and distribution control system for the world's largest nitrogen fertilizer complex at BASF Ludwigshafen.

During the 1970s, Tibbals served as an academic and research staff member at Glasgow and Durham Universities in the United Kingdom, where he worked with the Edinburgh Regional Computing Centre, the Digital Cartography Unit, and the Glycoprotein Research Laboratory. He also taught at the Open University and at Jordanhill College, and held visiting research and teaching positions at Bogazici University and at the University of North Texas.

Tibbals received his PhD in physical and analytical chemistry at the University of Houston, Houston, Texas, and his BS with majors in chemistry and mathematics from Baylor University, Waco, Texas. He was the recipient of a Science Research Council (SRC) Postdoctoral Fellowship in 1970, pursuing research on silicon chemistry and on applications of computing to science, medicine, and engineering at the University of Leicester, the University of Glasgow, and Durham University. He has served as a visiting faculty member in chemistry at the University of North Texas, as an adjunct professor at the University of Texas at Dallas School of Human Development, as a guest lecturer in materials science at the University of Texas at Arlington, and on the Biomedical Engineering faculty at UTSW. He has lived, traveled, and worked in Europe, the Near East, Japan, Brazil, Canada, and Mexico in universities, research institutes, and in industry.

Tibbals along with G. Louis Hornyak and others is a coauthor of titles published by CRC Press on nanoscience and nanotechnology, with contributions in analytical and physical chemistry, biomolecular nanoscience, natural nanomaterials, nanobiotechnology, biomimicry, and medical nanotechnology. Their text *Fundamentals of Nanotechnology* was awarded an American Library Association Outstanding Title Choice in 2010.

Part I

Perspectives

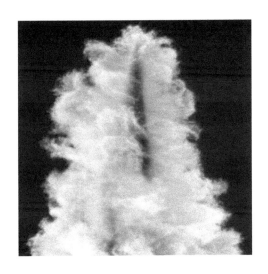

1

Nanomedicine: Scientific Basis and Societal Implications

How does nanomedicine separate itself from other traditional research fields? Is it really different from research that scientists conducted a decade or more ago?

Thomas J. Webster, Division of Engineering and Orthopedics, Brown University [1]

1.1 Introduction

To understand the place and significance of nanomedicine, one must first understand both medicine and nanotechnology.

The English word *medicine* has its roots in the Greek μέδομαι—the verb (medome), meaning "to care for." In both Greek and English usage, the word for *care* also holds the meaning of "to think deeply." It also means "to execute artfully," which for us should emphasize that medicine is as much an art as a technology.

The modern word *nanotechnology* was derived from the term nano, which is the prefix used in the International System of Units (SI) for one billionth of a meter, or 10^{-9} m. The prefix nano, like milli-(one thousandth) and micro-(one millionth), was adopted by the SI standard from Greek and Latin root words [2]. Nano comes ultimately from the Greek word for dwarf, and is also related to the Spanish word niño (feminine: niña)—"young child." The term was coined by Professor N. Taniguchi in 1974, who defined nanotechnology as "the processing of separation, consolidation and deformation of materials by one atom or one molecule," thus providing a conceptual focus for a number of technological trends that were emerging with increasing importance [3].

1.2 Medicine

Medicine is the knowledge and practice of maintaining and restoring health. Health is the state of a person, an organism, or an organ in which its systems are able to perform their functions without failure in the face of external threats and internal complications. Living systems are constantly meeting challenges such as stress, injury, malformation in development, genetic errors, invasions by viral, bacterial, and parasitic agents, cancer, degeneration, and challenging normal life events such as pregnancy and delivery, puberty, menopause, aging, and death. It is the goal of medicine to support, maintain, and restore productive functioning of life while minimizing suffering and doing no harm. The roots of medicine lie in our empathy for our fellow creatures, starting with our fellow human beings. Medicine is essentially a human art, which is supported by observation, evidence, recording, and passing on of knowledge and experience, training, and standards. "There is no one division of medicine by which we know and another by which we act" [4]. Medical science is inseparable from medical practice, as the ultimate significant observation is the outcome for a patient.

Medical science is the application of scientific methods to the study of living systems with the goal of improving medical practice. Medical science is based on any scientific or technological discipline that can contribute knowledge and techniques that advance the practice and understanding of medicine. These have historically included anatomy, physiology, chemistry, physics, engineering, and other disciplines. The development of medical science is inextricably involved with other sciences. The student who aspires to work in medical practice or research must be prepared with a solid base in multiple disciplines relevant to human health. Increasingly, these disciplines will include aspects of nanoscience and nanotechnology as applications to medicine emerge.

Modern understanding of health is based on the concept of regulation of metabolism by a complex network of molecular-based communication mechanisms known as cell signaling that governs basic cellular activities and coordinates cell actions. Cells in the body perform their life cycle functions in part by genetic programming, but also by responding to molecular signals generated within the cell and received through receptors on the cell membranes. These networks respond to, are controlled by, and can be disrupted by processes that take place on the electrical, molecular, macromolecular, and supramolecular scales. The latter are the domain of nanotechnology, where current advances are offering applications for medicine.

Healthy organisms tend to maintain homeostasis, from the Greek words meaning "like or same" and "still or static." Homeostasis is defined as the stable state controlled by a system of feedback: the system reacts to changes sensed in its state and/or environment to counter influences that tend to destabilize it or divert its development from the normal path. For example, body temperature, blood pressure, levels of carbon dioxide in the lungs and tissues, and the osmotic pressure within cells are homeostatically regulated. Living organisms and systems as a whole are not static: they undergo growth, development, and death in their normal life cycle. Health must be considered as a dynamic rather than a static process, by which a healthy cell or organism responds appropriately to environmental and developmental challenges. Medical science advances the understanding of how these responses are regulated through a complex network of molecular and supramolecular interactions.

Medical science draws upon engineering concepts and methods to create its own unique models for understanding biological networks as not only chemical but also physical and structural—as complex machinery with subtle control systems acting through specific detailed interactions at the macromolecular and nanoscale level. This approach underlies medical nanoscience, a perspective that gives us a framework to model, understand, and intervene in living processes at the level of supramolecular machinery with selectivity and precision [5].

1.3 Nanotechnology

Nanotechnology is a new way of looking at how we manipulate and utilize matter on a very small scale—the nanoscale, or 10^{-9} m. Nanoscale dimensions lie between the size of atoms and small molecules (measured in angstroms = 10^{-10} m), and familiar microscopic and submicroscopic entities such as biological cells and the features fabricated on electronic microchips, whose dimensions range from hundreds of microns to fractions of a micron (=10^{-6} m).

The application of nanoscale entities and phenomena is not especially new. Artisians, technologists, and scientists have utilized nanoscale particles and filters for many purposes for centuries. Physics and chemistry have dealt with matter on extremely small scales for more than 200 years. What makes nanotechnology new is the scientific investigation and technical exploitation of properties that depend uniquely on the nanoscale. And what is enabling the revolutionary impact of nanotechnology is the new capability for precise observation, measurement, and manipulation of individual nanoscale units of matter, opening a new frontier of human knowledge and resources for all kinds of applications.

Over the past 25 years, due to the development of new techniques and tools, precisely controlled manipulation of matter at the nanoscale has become possible for the first time. The emergence of nanotechnology has impacted the traditional domains of chemistry, biology, and medicine. Nanotechnology is now an exponentially growing focus of research and development.

The scientific basis of this interdisciplinary field is being conceptualized into a study of nanoscience: the science of the surprisingly unique and peculiar phenomena describing the behavior of matter on the nanoscale, as feature and particle sizes approach the dimensions of a few tens to a few thousands of atoms. These phenomena emerge from the high surface-to-volume ratios of nanoparticles, the predominance of surface energy interactions over bulk and chemical energetics which results, the interaction of nanoparticles with light of nanoscale wavelengths, and the interactions between particles—dependent primarily on surface, steric, and entropic factors determined by the shapes and surface properties of the particles and their absorbed layers of solutes and ligands—especially in water. These surface interactions can even produce surprising effects in macroscale objects when their interfaces possess nanoscale features.

Each advance in understanding phenomenon on the nanoscale leads to new opportunities for exploitation with new tools, materials, techniques of assembly (and controlled self-assembly), and devices such as sensors and nano-actuators. It is hardly an exaggeration to say that nanoscience and nanotechnology open an entire new world for exploration and exploitation, possibly launching a new age of economic, scientific, and social development.

The new opportunities opened by nanoscience are especially significant in the biological and life sciences, because, as we are beginning to understand, so many of the critical, intriguing, and uniquely powerful properties of living systems depend on nanoscale phenomena. Hence, it is already evident that nanoscience and nanotechnology will be particularly important to medicine, yielding new understandings and capabilities.

1.4 What Is Nanoscience and Where Does It Fit in the Sciences?

1.4.1 Definition and Scientific Basis

Nanoscience is the science of the phenomena peculiar to matter on the scale from 1 to several hundred nanometers (10^{-9} m). Individual atoms are on the order of 10^{-10} m ($=1$ Å). Down to a few tenths of a micrometer (10^{-6} m = the micro scale), the properties of matter are not much different from those familiar at the macroscopic scale ($>10^{-4}$ m). At the macroscopic scale, the bulk properties of matter predominate over the surface properties, but at the nanoscale, new phenomena emerge.

Bulk macroscopic material presents a sharp interface to its environment, when it comes to interactions with other material and energy, whether solids, liquids, gases, or electromagnetic radiation, including light. This is the domain of classical physics. On the other extreme, interactions at the atomic scale are characterized by quantum physics and chemistry, which govern the behavior of chemical bonds, atomic and molecular spectra, photochemistry, and chemical reactions.

Nanoscience is the science of matter and energy in the transitional scale between the atomic and macroscopic states of aggregation of atoms. Some unique properties of matter emerge when features are on the nanoscale. Understanding and appreciation of these properties open new opportunities, which have been ignored or poorly understood until the past few decades because the technology was not available to explore and manipulate matter at the nanoscale.

By the middle of the twentieth century, the science of matter on the atomic and subatomic scale—chemistry and physics—had advanced by brilliant and intricate experiments and deductions based on observations of interactions at the macroscale (large numbers of atoms and molecules undergoing chemical reactions, and interactions between matter and energy—heat, light, and radiation). Micro- and cell biology and genetics were giving life scientists tantalizing glimpses and suggestions of the intricate precision of macromolecular mechanisms that must be the basis for life. But the tools were not available to observe and manipulate particles and features on the nanoscale until relatively recently, and the range and power of such nanotools are still being rapidly developed and improved.

As chemists worked out an understanding of the behavior of matter, the description and modeling of isolated pairs of atoms or molecules came first, and was then generalized with statistical mechanics and kinetics to theories that successfully described the bulk behavior of very large numbers of molecules, all acting in similar ways in an averaged environment. Having to take into account the specifics of atomic and molecular arrangements on the nanoscale gets one into formidable complexity, except where the arrangements are repetitive and highly regular, as in crystals, polymers, and minerals such as zeolites. The physical and theoretical tools for dealing with this complexity come from mathematics, computer science, physics, chemistry, and biology. Elements of all of these disciplines are essential foundations for understanding nanoscale phenomena. For the sake of coherence in communicating and educating, the interdisciplinary study of nanoscale phenomena needs to be properly integrated into a focused discipline of nanoscience.

Nanoscience derives its scientific content from physics, chemistry, and biology. The physics of nanoscience deals with the interaction of coherent light with nanoscale particles and features, the relationship between surface energies and internal energies in finely divided matter, and the effects of polarization and electromagnetic fields on particles of nanoscale size where small induced forces become significant relative to the inertial mass of the particles. From chemistry, nanoscience obtains understanding of the behavior of colloids, proteins, macromolecules, catalysts, and surface phenomena. The life sciences have provided a motivating force for understanding nanoscale phenomena presenting innumerable examples of natural nanomachinery as proofs of existence and challenges to be understood. The techniques and disciplines for dealing with the nanoscale in life sciences are a major challenge at the core of the intellectual content of nanoscience.

1.4.2 Nanotools: The Tools, Techniques, and Methodologies of Nanoscience

Some of the first tools for dealing with matter on the nanoscale come from biology. The ceramic filters first used in the nineteenth century to separate viruses from cellular life are an application of nanoscale porosity. The patch clamp technique developed in the 1940s uses nanoscale capillary probes to examine individual cell surface receptors, which are active nanoscale molecular structures. The electron microscope and x-ray crystallography enabled observation of nanostructure in fixed preparations of biological materials and macromolecules.

As early as the 1940s, field emission microscopy enabled the observation of individual atoms on surfaces, but only under severe conditions not suitable for delicate macromolecules. By the 1980s, the scanning tunneling microscope (STM) and atomic force microscope (AFM) provided the ability to measure and manipulate nanoscale structures, even down to atomic scales. The scanning probe microscope (SPM) extended the capability to observe and manipulate individual atoms on solid surfaces.

Low energy atomic and ion beams, nanoscale mechanical probes, and macromolecular fiber probes allowed probing and building of nanoscale surface layers with precision. Optical trapping and dielectrophoresis techniques provided the ability to manipulate micro- and nanoscale particles with precise control in 3D suspension.

By the end of the twentieth century, electron microscopy was being extended to image wet biological nanostructures, and near-field and confocal microscopy combined with fluorescent and chemiluminescent probes were being refined to approach imaging of nanoscale structures.

Nuclear magnetic resonance (NMR) techniques were being developed to unravel macromolecular structure on the nanoscale, using pulsed techniques to produce 2D Fourier transform NMR spectra. The interaction of nuclear spins on different parts of a macromolecule and on adjacent molecules could be mapped to generate an indication of the 3D structure of macromolecules such as proteins.

The control and execution of the multiple sequences of pulses and scans, and the gathering and analysis of the massive amounts of data involved in structural NMR experiments, as well as techniques such as SPM, electromagnetic trapping, and advanced microscopy depended on advances in computer technology, which was advanced by accelerating refinements in microfabrication technology, supporting the microelectronics for powerful computers running large and complex software programs.

In addition to driving the powerful nanotools used to capture, gather, and organize information at nanoscale resolutions, computers and software enabled the complex theoretical calculations and simulations of matter and energy interactions on the nanoscale, which interpreted, guided, and inspired experimentation.

1.5 Origins of Nanotechnology

In a rationally ordered world, science develops first, followed by the application of scientific knowledge to technology. In actuality, there is complex and subtle interplay between theory and practice. Often scientific knowledge progresses by trying to understand new phenomena revealed by manipulating the world with new tools. In the same way that

> Science owes more to the steam engine than the steam engine owes to Science.
>
> **L. J. Henderson (1917)**

nanoscience could not have developed without nanotechnology.

Nanotechnology, like space flight, arose first in the imagination of scientific visionaries. Only later did a series of developments begin to make possible something like the original dreams—but also in practice much different.

Although early pioneers such as H. W. Herwald at Westinghouse and Forrest L. Carter at the U. S. Naval Research Laboratories contributed to significant development of technology such as molecular electronic circuits, widespread awareness of the concept of nanotechnology, and political and economic support within government, business, educational, and scientific institutions, did not quickly follow.

Nanotechnology as a concept that widely captured the imagination and energies of inventors and engineers dates to the charismatic, imaginative, playful, and iconoclastic leadership of Richard Feynman. His "plenty of room at the bottom" lecture in 1958 led to the challenge of the first Feynman prizes—for a motor less than half a millimeter on a side, and for condensation of readable text to less than 1/25,000 the size of a normal book page (Figure 1.1).

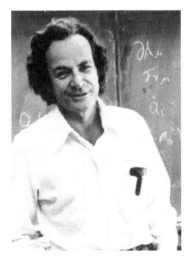

FIGURE 1.1

Richard Feynman inspired the concept of nanotechnology by showing that there were no physical barriers to manipulating individual atoms and molecules. (Photo by Floyd Clark; Courtesy of Caltech Archives, Pasadena, CA.)

Following the talk, Feynman was regularly contacted by a series of inventors who claimed to have built a motor to meet the prize specifications, to no avail. In 1960, engineer William McLellan brought a large grocery carton into Feynman's office at Cal Tech. As soon as he saw the box, Feynman thought it was yet another waste of time; the box was absurdly too big for a device small enough to win the prize. But when McLellan put the box down and opened it, he took out not a motor but a microscope. Feynman's skepticism turned to interest; nobody else had brought a microscope before. He spent the rest of the day with McLellan putting the motor through its paces while observing through the microscope, and subsequently wrote a check for the prize.

It turned out that making a micromachine small enough to win the first Feynman prize did not involve molecular manipulation—the very thin gauge wire and the tiny armature were fabricated painstakingly with conventional tools including sharpened toothpicks and a jeweler's lathe. It was a fine piece of microfabrication handiwork, but nowhere near the atomic level nanotechnology envisioned in the speech that had inspired it.

In the succeeding years, microfabrication continued to advance, driven by the demands for microelectronics. Invention of the transistor at Bell Labs had spurred the shrinking of electronic circuits. In the 1950s, Geoffrey W. A. Dummer in the United Kingdom, Jack St. Clair Kilby at Texas Instruments, and Robert Noyce at Fairchild Semiconductor independently developed the concept and techniques for integrating large numbers of transistors onto a single piece of silicon (Figure 1.2). Thenceforth, solid-state electronics progressed steadily from the micron to submicron levels, entering the nano-region, using microphotolithography, which eventually met the second challenge posed by the Feynman prize. The first nano-manipulation of atoms was demonstrated at IBM laboratories in the 1980s. New developments in optics and electronics such as AFM, optical tweezers, and dielectrophoresis of colloidal particles provided techniques for manipulating matter on the submicron to nanoscale.

In the 1990s, an enthusiastic champion for the idea of atomic and molecular nanomachinery arose from MIT—Richard Drexler—who effectively promoted and evangelized the idea of nanoscale machinery with energy and passion. Drexler's eloquent persuasiveness led to support from political, military, and entrepreneurial circles, as well as interest

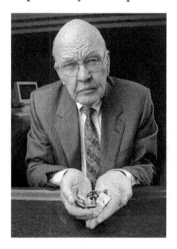

FIGURE 1.2
Jack St. Clair Kilby, one of the pioneers of solid-state electronics integration, which led to the fabrication of submicron (nanoscale) electronic devices. Such devices are one of the key factors enabling nanotechnology and nanomedicine. (Courtesy of Texas Instruments, Dallas, TX.)

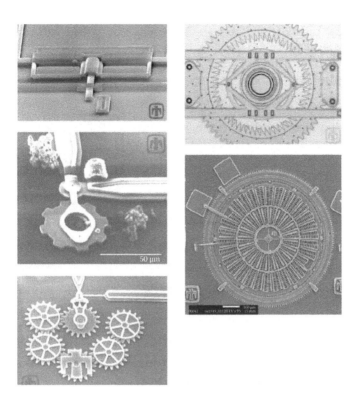

FIGURE 1.3
Nanomachinery: Drexler and others developed the concepts of nanomachines built from assemblies of atoms and molecules. (Courtesy of Sandia National Laboratories, SUMMiT(TM) Technologies, Albuquerque, NM, www.mems.sandia.gov.)

from scientific and engineering establishments, especially once it was seen that funding was forthcoming from governmental and military development agencies (Figure 1.3).

In the meantime, nanotechnology based on the science of chemistry produced a breakthrough that in its elegance, beauty, and simplicity captured public and scientific imagination equally with the idea of nanoscale robotics. Richard Smalley, Robert Curl, Harry Kroto, and graduate students James R. Heath and Sean C. O'Brien at Rice University worked out a structure for the carbon-60 entity that had become a familiar peak of known stability in physical organic mass spectrometry for many years. Their structure was elegant and beautiful, a masterpiece of symmetry with the geometric facets of a gem, and they proved it existed as a chemical reality, despite skeptics who seemed to have a stereotypical hard-nosed prejudice against such elegance, much less beauty in the businesslike and down to earth world of hydrocarbons. Besides, it seemed to be of no possible practical use; its only relevance was apparently for the exotic world of instellar space chemistry.

Perhaps, it did not help that the structure was the dodecahedron, adapted by the iconoclastic counterculture hero Buckminster Fuller in engineering and architecture, and a structure shared by the icon of the European—even French and Brazilian—sport: soccer, which they irritatingly insisted on calling football. It helped even less that the "Buckyball"—in the form of the geodesic dome—had been adopted by back-to-nature advocates; and Smalley enthusiastically called the structure the "buckyball," formally naming it buckminsterfullerene (Figure 1.4).

It was an achievement of creative discovery akin to the discovery of the structure of DNA (or at least of the Alpha helix or benzene ring)—the discovery in nature of familiar, comprehensible, and beautiful geometry hidden in the invisible depths of molecules too small to see—but nevertheless revealed by the power of reason, imagination, and lots of hard experimental work in the laboratory.

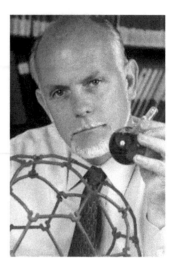

FIGURE 1.4
Richard Smalley elucidated the structure of the nanoscale carbon macromolecule buckminsterfullerene, which led to appreciation of carbon structures from a nanoscience perspective. (Courtesy of Brookhaven National Laboratory News, September 15, 2004, BNL Media & Communications Office, New York, http://www.bnl.gov/bnlweb/pubaf/pr/photos/2004/smalley-300.jpg. With permission from Rice University Office of Media Relations.)

The elucidation of the 60-carbon buckyball structure created great interest in other nanoscale molecular structures, including carbon nanotubes. The unique properties of carbon nanotubes suggested many potential applications. These included structural fibers with many times the strength-to-weight ratios of other materials, molecular-scale probes, high surface area electrodes, and nanoscale molecular electronic circuit components, as well as sensors based on functionalized nanotubes.

1.6 Molecular and Cell Biology and Protein Bioscience: A Model of Life as Organic Nanomachinery

A major reason for increased interest in nanoscience and nanotechnology is that life science researchers are discovering structures and mechanisms whose description involves more than traditional biochemistry or even macromolecular protein chemistry.

Over the past half century, molecular and cell biology and protein bioscience exploited technical and scientific advances that gave unprecedented access to subcellular structures. The intricate and beautiful structures of membranes, cytoplasmic endoskeletons, mirochrondia, chloroplasts, and the awesome ordered complexity of cellular machinery began to be unraveled. It became no longer possible to think of cells and vesicles as microscopic chemical test tubes—instead a model of life as organic molecular nanomachinery took hold.

1.6.1 Bionanotechnology

In molecular biology, the new field of bionanotechnology worked out descriptions of how protein-based cellular machinery functioned, and synthetic analogs and modifications of natural cellular nanodevices were created. Artificial organic nanoengines were built, inspired by the construction methods and starting materials of molecular biology. These ranged from rotary engines to nanowalkers, to computing circuits based on DNA.

1.6.2 Biological and Biomimetic Nanostructures

Another area in which biology dramatically impacted the development of nanotechnology was in the unraveling of biological mechanisms based purely on surface nanostructure—dependent on nanoscale geometry and surface properties rather than molecular biology. Examples are the nanostructures and hydrophobic materials that give lotus leaves their water repellent and self-cleaning properties, and with slight variations give certain spider webs and insect carapaces water harvesting and absorbing properties.

Other examples are the photonic properties of butterfly wings, feathers, and iridescent beetles and flies created by photon resonance effects dependent on the nanostructure rather than the material or chemical pigmentation. A particularly dramatic effect is the ability of gecko feet to adhere to smooth surfaces, which was shown to be due to the nanostructure of the finest details of the foot, without the aid of sticky glues, suction cups, or micromechanical hooks or grappling devices.

These fields produced practical results—in some cases with large returns on investment. The "lotus effect" was copyrighted and artificial lotus effect surfaces were patented for applications in fabrics, windscreens, deicing, reduction of friction in water transport, improving flow in medical devices, and other areas. The reverse lotus effect was utilized in agriculture, adhesives, and other applications. Sensitive opto-chemical sensors were designed using the butterfly wing effect, and surgical attachments and other devices were designed based on the functions of the gecko foot.

1.6.3 Functional Biological Nanomaterials and Nanoengines

As biology advanced using new nanotools to understand macromolecules, awareness grew of nanoscale phenomena in both biomaterial structure and cellular function. The nanoscale hierarchical organization of materials such as shell, bone, chitin, hair, plant fibers, spider silks, silica scaffolds, and other natural structures became models for nanotechnology.

The nanoscale structure of collagens and the cell adhesion structures formed by the interplay of actins and cadherins revealed the complex nanoscale interactions involved in the construction of multicellular organisms. The nanoscale mechanisms of action of potassium ion channels, proton pumps, and other transmembrane pores and receptors were found to involve an orchestration of electronic, chemical, steric, and conformational interactions on the nanoscale.

Likewise, the repair of DNA by enzymes and the synthesis of proteins by ribosomes, the transport of organelles along microtubules within cells by kinesins, and the coordinated movement between myosin and actin filaments to produce muscle movement are all examples of organic nanomachinery, in which macromolecules interact to perform work on the nanoscale.

One of the most striking and most accessible examples of biological nanomachinery is the bacteriophage T4. Details of how this and other viral mechanisms work have been painstakingly elucidated, revealing a complex interplay of interacting molecular components. The T4 base attaches to specific bacterial cell walls and positions an enzyme to cut a nano-sized hole in the wall. The arms around the base lock into position, and at the same time their change in conformation triggers the contraction of the tube, forcing viral DNA through the nanopore into the bacteria where it can take over the production of and replication of vital proteins (Figure 1.5).

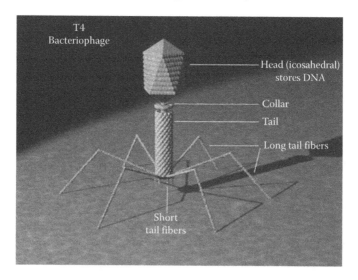

FIGURE 1.5
Bacteriophages use protein nanomachinery to insert DNA in host bacteria. (From Hornyak, G. L. et al., *Introduction to Nanoscience and Nanotechnology*, CRC Press, Boca Raton, FL. With permission.)

Equally intricate is the nanoscale functionality of SNARE complexes whose details are still being unraveled. SNARE is a complex of protein nanomachinery that acts to pull neuronal synaptic vesicles to the inner surface of the neuron cell membrane prior to neurotransmitter release. To do so, it must overcome the repulsive forces of the cellular and vesicle membranes for each other.

Another area in which nanoscale structure and features have been shown to be important is immunology, not only in antibody–antigen recognition, but also in the inflammatory response interaction of leukocytes with endothelial cells, in which adaptable adhesive proteins (selectins) interact with integrins in the cell membranes.

1.6.4 Need for Nanoscience in Description of Life

In molecular biology, life science researchers work with structures and mechanisms whose description involves phenomena that are unique to the nanoscale. The molecular mechanisms of life are multilevel. Just as the structural description of macromolecules such as proteins have expanded beyond the chemical bonding to require tertiary and quaternary levels, their biological functions also require electronic, chemical, steric, and mechanochemical levels of description.

Biological science is being drawn into considerations of protein robotics. Molecular biologists may not necessarily be equipped or trained like engineers to deal with the theory and design of nanoengines. But they are prepared to look carefully at the subtle and complex effects of solvents, surface effects, and inter- and intramolecular interactions that govern the operation of organic nanomachinery.

These are effects that engineers seeking to design nanoengines from scratch must learn to take into account as well. Thus, all disciplines have a great deal to learn from each other. And new generations of scientists, engineers, and medical researchers need an outlook encompassing a set of knowledge and skills that crosses many current disciplinary boundaries.

1.7 Nanotechnology Leads to a Fundamentally New Approach to Engineering Design

When engineers and scientists are able to work with nanoscale quantities and dimensions, it opens new possibilities for design. What happens is much more than simply applying traditional and conventional engineering design approaches to smaller scales—the process itself is altered in a radical manner.

To see why this is so, it helps to look at another new frontier of technology that is rapidly opening—the field of biomimetics—and some deep relationships between biomimetics and nanotechnology.

Studies analyzing engineering designs compared to natural systems have shown that traditional engineering methodology approaches problems in a fundamentally different manner from the way that natural biological evolution has solved similar problems. The TRIZ design studies systematically compared hundreds of natural and engineered systems and found that on the macroscale, engineered and natural systems differed much less than on the nanoscale in materials and energy utilization.

Human inventors may have started dreaming about, say, heavier than air flight by considering birds and flying insects—but as they applied the tools, materials, and power sources available during the previous industrial eras, they ended up with solutions that in many ways (such as power and speed) far outstripped the natural capabilities of birds and insects. But in subtle features like maneuverability, soft landings, hovering, and efficient use of recyclable energy and materials (all of which have become much higher priorities in a more crowded and resource short world), the natural systems are far superior.

Similar contrasts are seen when we compare computing and communication and control systems to organic brains and nervous and sensory systems, power generation, storage and utilization systems with photosynthesis, ATP, and muscle, engineered materials for architecture and armor with wood, chitin, and shell, and many other man-made versus natural systems. In all these cases, the man-made solutions are more powerful by far, but lack subtly in use of energy and materials, and are therefore less sustainable.

The challenge posed by biomimetics is whether and to what extent we can improve the sustainability of our man-made built environment by learning lessons from nature. Nanotechnology makes the response to this challenge possible on the nanoscale: the scale at which nature works to achieve its efficiency, sustainability, and sometimes surprising capabilities that would seem to be impossible to duplicate in man-made systems. This challenge cannot be dismissed when we find that so many natural nanoscale phenomena have profound effects observable at the macroscale.

These "proofs of existence" include, for example, the Lotus Effect, butterfly photonics, and gecko adhesion, and significantly, the profound effects of small amounts of low molecular weight substances on large and complex organisms—drugs like aspirin, hormones, neurotransmitters, and regulators like ethylene and nitric oxide. Observations of these effects of the angstrom scale on the macroscale have been the pathway to understanding many significant mechanisms and phenomena on the nanoscale in biological systems.

Biology is the arena where we see the effects and power of nanoscale phenomena all around us. Before we recognized the importance and uniqueness of the nanoscale, these phenomena remained mysterious and inaccessible.

Difficult and complicated to study, they were often ignored in favor of low hanging fruit in science and technology.

Nanoscience—knowledge of how things work on the nanoscale—gives us the ability to work at the same scale as biological systems for the first time. Previously, we could influence the outcomes of nanoscale processes in subtle and indirect ways by applying heat, light, catalysts, and taking advantage of the statistics of large assemblages of molecules and subtle knowledge of how they interact (chemistry, materials science), and by harnessing natural biological processes (biology, agricultural science, biotechnology).

With nanotools, we can manipulate matter on the nanoscale directly and with deliberation, even with power and elegance (those most admired and sought after properties of scientific and technological work). This was up to now a privilege denied to us, as Feynman put it, "because we are too big."

1.8 Societal and Economic Impacts

For some time in the early development of nanotechnology, the nanomechanical, nanorobotic, nanochemistry, and nanobiology fields were developing independently, in a competitive way. Public debates ran on between leading researchers in nanochemistry and advocates of atom-by-atom fabrication of inorganic nanorobots. The tone of these debates is summed up by the comment of one eminent chemist: "Nanotechnology just means that engineers have discovered chemistry." Others, perhaps unappreciative of the uniqueness of the nanoscale, wondered "I have been working with atoms and molecules for years—why should chemistry and physics be called nanotechnology?" A published debate between Drexler and Smalley appeared in *Chemical and Engineering News* in 2003.

As research and development in all fields progressed, it became apparent that progress in understanding phenomena on the nanoscale, and exploitation of the benefits to be derived, were best served if the diverse multidisciplinary efforts could be unified in a new discipline for purposes of education, communication of research efforts, and for seeking public support from government and investors. Development, educational, and advocacy groups, which originally focused on different aspects of nanotechnology, have widened their scopes to varying extents. Professional and technical bodies have created study groups, divisions, and publications in nanoscale aspects of chemistry, biology, physics, materials science, and electronics. Academic institutions have begun to offer courses in nanotechnology, which incorporate an integrated approach to these multidisciplinary areas.

The potential benefits of nanotechnology have spurred governments to invest, starting with the leading edge research programs focused on national defense and industrial competitiveness. A wave of private investment is well underway, from research labs of large corporations such as IBM, Hewlett-Packard, and firms in electronics, materials, engineering, biomedicine, and other fields. Many states and countries have organized nanotechnology development initiatives, hoping to share in economic growth and job creation that is predicted to come with novel nanotechnology applications and products.

Economic forecasts made in the past 10 years have to be considered in light of the financial recession of 2008–2009, but there is no doubt that nanotechnology will grow in economic importance. Nanotechnology is emerging at a time of economic recovery when increased needs for energy efficiency, environmental sustainability, and new approaches to healthcare need to be met. Nanotechnology opens new approaches to use of energy and materials to meet these needs. In addition, nanotechnology is creating many new types of products and applications, which will fuel economic growth as they are adopted and integrated into the marketplace.

Estimates for the economic impact of nanotechnology have been prepared by the U.S. National Academy of Science, by the Nanotech Institute, the European Union, Japan, China, Russia, and elsewhere, including many U.S. state nanotechnology initiatives. The estimates range up to many billions of dollars in economic impact per year in the next decades. Since the implementation of the U.S. National Nanotechnology Initiative with initial funding of over US$400 million in 2000, annual spending in nanotechnology as of 2006 had reached US$750 million in Japan, US$710 million in the Unites States, US$335 million in Europe, and US$551 million in China, Korea, and Taiwan together [6,7].

The economic impact of nanotechnology is great because it opens breakthrough paths around technological bottlenecks and impasses faced by key technologies underlying development. Some of the first and most important areas to be affected are energy efficiency, green energy production, and elimination of carbon emissions through nanotechnology innovations in tribology, catalysts, energy conversion, photovoltaics, artificial photosynthesis, photoelectric hydrogen generation, hydrogen storage, battery electrodes, hypercapacitors, lightweight smart materials for vehicles and motor components, artificial muscles, and high efficiency improvement to conventional motor designs.

Nanotechnology innovations support efficiency of materials usage, for higher productivity, extension, or avoidance of scarce resource utilization, and elimination of by-products, waste, and pollutants. Nanotechnology is showing ways to go beyond the projected limits of circuit, energy, and information storage densities in future miniaturization of electronics for controls and computing.

Significantly, nanotechnology is leading already to tangible advances in medicine with enhanced imaging, drug delivery and targeting systems, tissue scaffolding, and advances in interfaces for neuroprosthetics and brain–machine interfaces. Indirectly but significantly, nanotechnology and nanoscience make major contributions to the understanding of disease processes and the design of drugs and therapeutics by providing powerful new tools and techniques for research and applications.

1.9 Impact of Nanotechnology on Medicine

Nanotechnology is directly relevant to medicine because of the importance of nanoscale phenomena to cellular signaling, enzyme action, and the cell cycle. Nanotechnology provides tools for analyzing the structure of tissue on the most important scale between the atomic and the cellular levels, and for designing and making synthetic biomaterials on the nanoscale for therapies and replacements. Nanotechnology provides a means to address biological pathways with precisely targeted nanodrugs that are designed to fit the protein and nucleic acid sites associated with disease and disorders. Nanotechnology also provides the tools and techniques to deliver delicate organic macromolecules and peptides to their effective sites of action, protected from degradation, immune attack, and shielded to pass through barriers that would normally block passage of large molecules.

The impact of nanotechnology has been the subject of much hyperbole, but real and serious applications are emerging with support from the NIH, private foundations, major pharmaceutical companies, medical device makers, and entrepreneurs.

1.10 The Grand Challenge of Nanotechnology

Nanotechnology can be thought of as the response to the challenge of the nanoscale by the engineering, scientific, and medical communities—the grand challenge opened up by new tools that extend our vision and reach into the nanoscale. This challenge has evoked many different responses in the biomedical community: some aggressively visionary and radically ambitious proposals, some conservatively incremental and gradual, and some cautious (just like the responses to the challenge of the possibility of space travel). What is significant, and has raised nanotechnology to the level of attention that it now receives, is that a major new frontier is opening, with groundbreaking prospects for progress in sustainable and powerful technology.

1.11 Some Definitions and Nanomedical Areas of Emphasis

Thus far in this introductory chapter we have reviewed the basic definitions and background of nanoscience and nanotechnology and their potential impacts. In Sections 1.11.1 and 1.11.2, we focus on medical nanotechnology and nanomedicine, starting with some definitions and terminology.

A number of terms are used in the public discourse and scientific literature, with no clear standardization of definitions, so we will give some working definitions here.

Taking the definition of nanotechnology to be any technology based on the nanoscale, *biotechnology* can be considered the nanoengineering of DNA and RNA, the genetic material of cells. *Bionanotechnology* has emerged as the term for protein nanoengineering, the manipulation and exploitation of the natural nanoengines of biological systems.

Biomolecular nanotechnology is the term generally used to describe the use of biological macromolecules as the starting point for fabrication of nanoscale devices, independent of whether they are intended for use in biomedical applications. Biomolecular nanotechnology includes using DNA as a template for molecular-scale computational engines, adapting muscle and flagella mechanisms to make artificial nano-actuators, etc.; it involves application of nanofabrication, biotechnology, biophysics, biochemistry, nanoelectronics, and materials engineering to design novel and useful devices and materials.

Biomedical nanotechnology is the term that has been generally used for the application of nanotechnology to biomedical devices for diagnosis, high-throughput screening, drug delivery, biomaterials, tissue engineering, and enhancement materials for medical imaging. Another term that has been used with some overlap is *nanobiotechnology*, defined as the application of nanotechnology to biological materials to design devices that exploit uniquely nanoscale properties.

Two terms for application of nanotechnology in medicine are *nanomedicine* and *medical nanotechnology*. They have come to be used in slightly different meanings: *Nanomecidine* refers to programs for application of newly emerging nanotechnologies to molecular processes at the cellular level. *Medical nanotechnology* is a broader term, which includes a wide array of nanoscale technologies directly and indirectly applied to medicine, many of which predate the new paradigm and recent popularization of nanotechnology.

1.11.1 Medical Nanotechnology

While one may visualize future nanobots traveling through the body performing surgeries and therapies, there are less dramatic but equally revolutionary ways in which nanotechnology will change medicine. Medical nanotechnology can make broad incremental contributions to lowering costs and improving effectiveness of existing drugs, diagnostics, implant materials, prosthetics, patient monitoring, and personal healthcare maintenance. The actual near-term impacts of nanotechnology are likely to be in the following areas [8,9].

1.11.1.1 Advanced Medical Instrumentation

Nanotechnology is an enabling technology that contributes to easily and inexpensively extracting information from the body and transmitting it to patients and caregivers: Nanotechnology enables extreme miniaturization of diagnostic devices, requiring minute amounts of tissue samples, or even single cells, for measurement and diagnosis. All kinds of medical devices profit from the miniaturization of electronic components as they move beyond micro to nano. This affects diagnostic tools, pacemakers, "cameras in a pill," and other devices for healthcare delivery through smaller, more powerful, less costly point-of-care monitoring and treatment.

1.11.1.2 Powering Systems Biology and Theranostics

Nanotechnology is enabling the design of research and clinical instruments that can measure large numbers of cells and biological molecules rapidly, precisely, and cheaply: With the capability of monitoring large numbers of physiological, biochemical, genetic, and cellular systems simultaneously, the human body can be studied as a dynamic network of molecular biological processes. This opens the possibility of treating disease with specific strategies targeted at altering and controlling molecular pathways in the network. This is leading to the concept of theranosis (or theragnosis)—the tailoring of medicines to the individual's genomic and physiological state based on rapid detailed individualized testing.

1.11.1.3 Enabling Distributed Personalized Care

Because nanotechnology enables acquisition and analysis of biological information more quickly, accurately, and cheaply, nanotechnology opens possibilities for more predictive and preventative medicine: medicine that is more personalized, with more individual participation in maintaining one's own health. Nanotechnology allows self-monitoring and speedy diagnosis with portable testing kits, personal monitoring, and therapy devices. Digital health monitors are envisaged based on expanded versions of today's personal digital assistant devices or smart cell phones. Such devices could have a variety of functions from measuring activity level, blood pressure, heart rate, glucose levels, and other vital data to suggesting exercises and diet choices. They could remind us to take medications or even trigger the release of medications from implanted or inserted microdevices. Although the devices themselves would be on the macro- or microscale, their design and implementation with full functionality will depend on nanoscale technologies.

1.11.1.4 Medical Materials

Medical nanotechnology contributes to improvements in artificial bone and joint implants through nanoengineered materials. Nanostructured surfaces can serve as scaffolding for controlled tissue growth in wound healing and reconstructive surgery. Nanoengineered adhesives are being developed for use in surgery. Nanoengineered surfaces and materials contribute to improved stents and valve implants in cardiology and vascular surgery, to artificial ocular lenses, cochlear implants, and nerve growth guides for neurosurgery.

1.11.1.5 Nanoparticles for Image Enhancement

Nanoparticle synthesis is creating new contrast agents and visualization tools to provide more sensitive and selective medical imaging and yield a closer look at cellular processes. These are based on quantum resonance, dendrimer molecules, and magnetic or radio-opaque nanoparticles functionalized with antibodies and other molecular recognition coatings.

1.11.1.6 Drug Delivery

Nanotechnology is being applied to improve drug delivery in a number of ways. Nanosized particles are optimized for absorption of drugs through inhalation therapy. Nanoparticles are especially adaptable for delivery of non-soluble and hydrophobic drugs. The size domain of particles between 10 and 100 nm lies between the sizes of materials that are extracted from the blood by the microtubule filtration in the kidneys, and the sizes that are trapped by the liver, gall bladder, and liver, or that block capillaries in the lungs or other organs to cause emboli.

Nanosized particles and capsules can deliver drugs in novel ways. Encapsulation strategies include polymers with absorbed drugs, dendritic molecules or coordination compounds with drugs bonded covalently or weakly attached, and artificial or natural micelles or liposome vesicles containing nano-doses of insoluble or toxic drugs which can be selectively released on targets. Release can be controlled by pH, exploiting the fact that pH levels in tumors are lower than in normal tissue. Another strategy for triggering release is functionalizing the surfaces of nanoparticles with antibodies to localize the particles in tumors or other targeted tissue, then stimulating release of drugs, or heating up the particles by application of electromagnetic radiation or light. Even the body's own blood cells can be adapted to carry nanomedicines: nanoparticulate steroids have been introduced into red blood cells; as the cells die their natural deaths, the steroids are released into the body in very small doses, thus minimizing side effects.

1.11.1.7 Overcoming Natural Barriers to Drug Delivery

Nanoparticulate pharmaceutical agents can penetrate cell membranes effectively as well as being able to cross the blood–brain barrier. Nanopharmacology uses a variety of Trojan horse techniques to pass the defensive gates of the blood–brain barrier and other barriers within the body.

1.11.1.8　Protecting Implants from the Immune System

Nanoencapsulation has been employed to protect medically implanted cells from rejection by the host immune system. This usage has promise for regeneration of insulin-producing cells and other vital endocrine tissues.

1.11.1.9　Advanced Prosthetics

Nanotechnology is enabling new advances in lightweight motor, neuro-, and sensory prosthetic devices with advanced distributed controls and feedback for natural movement and interaction with the user's body and nervous system. Nanotechnology is allowing smaller assist devices such as cardiac pacemakers with lower power requirements and better interfaces to tissue. Nanotechnology is improving neurostimulation and monitoring devices, including brain–machine interfaces. Nanotechnology is increasing the functional power while reducing size and energy consumption of cochlear implants, and making new types of vision prostheses possible. Nanosurface developments are improving the performance and longevity of stimulation electrodes for prostheses while giving improved resistance to biofilm growth.

1.11.1.10　Advanced Biosensors and Therapeutic Implants

Nanotechnology is a key input for new generations of tiny implantable sensors for pressure, pH, temperature, glucose, and other physiological parameters, which can report data wirelessly without the need of implanted batteries or other power sources. These sensors are being used in research to understand normal physiological function and disease processes, and in some cases are contributing to medical diagnosis and monitoring of chronic diseases. Active implants to deliver insulin or other therapies are being considered as nanotechnology makes them more feasible and cost effective.

1.11.1.11　Guarding against Spread of Disease

Nanotechnology is contributing to detection and filtration of pathogens from air, water, and food supplies. Antibacterial surfaces incorporating photocatalytic or biocidal nanoparticles are being developed to reduce the spread of infection in medical facilities and public buildings and transport.

1.11.1.12　Medical Nanotechnology: A Broad Base for Medical Innovation

In the above examples, we focused on the broad incremental contributions made to medicine by advances in nanotechnology. Some are quite impressive and could be considered revolutionary. We discuss some examples of these ongoing developments in Part II. We also look at the closely related and overlapping area more commonly referred to as nanomedicine.

1.11.2 Nanomedicine

While *medical nanotechnology* was driving improvements to a wide range of medical resources and practice, the concept of *nanomedicine* was taking shape as an ambitious enterprise with a more visionary program. In contrast to the diffuse but pervasive impact of medical nanotechnology on the science and technology underlying modern medicine, nanomedicine was born as a focused movement applying nanotechnology with intensity to a set of formidable medical challenges.

The term "nanomedicine" originated with conceptions of how the Drexler vision of nanomechanical robotics could be applied to medicine. The word first appeared in the 1991 book "Unbounding the Future" by Eric Drexler, Christine Petersen, and Gayle Pergamint. Robert A. Freitas published a pioneering paper in 1998 expanding on these ideas, followed a year later by the first of a series of books on nanomedicine, filled with ingenious ideas of how nanomachinery might be applied to medicine, and exhaustively surveying applications of nanoparticles and other applications of medical nanotechnology. In the same year, the term nanomedicine began to appear in the technical literature. Since then a number of nanomedicine journals, societies, and government initiatives have been launched.

The field has grown rapidly and in many directions, overlapping in part with the areas of medical nanotechnology described earlier as it matured. But a distinction has developed between nanomedicine and medical nanotechnology, set forth in a number of reviews and reports on the field. Nanomedicine has a set of goals for breakthrough applications of nanotechnology, and has thus been the focus of much attention.

Nanomedicine has been defined in many ways in the literature and popular writings, some broad enough to include all areas of medical nanotechnology, but most emphasize direct control and manipulation of cellular-level processes on the nanoscale, applied for diagnostics and healing. As is typical for a new and rapidly evolving field, there are many definitions and not all are in agreement. Observing the popular literature, typified by a recent article in Salon, one gets the impression that nanomedicine is defined less by a formal specification than by a visionary spirit aiming for spectacular and bold goals to be achieved by revolutionary breakthroughs in medical technology.

But nanomedicine is a serious undertaking, backed by major initiatives from governments, industries, and academies. Some of their defining statements give the scope of the field.

The NIH roadmap for nanomedicine research starts out with a visionary statement for the possibilities of nanomedicine:

> What if doctors could search out and destroy the very first cancer cells that would otherwise have caused a tumor to develop in the body? What if a broken part of a cell could be removed and replaced with a minia-ture biological machine? What if pumps the size of molecules could be implanted to deliver life-saving medicines precisely when and where they are needed?

The roadmap introduction then goes on to state that these are long-term goals and gives a concise definition:

> Nanomedicine, an offshoot of nanotechnology, refers to highly specific medical intervention at the molecular scale for curing disease or repair-ing damaged tissues, such as bone, muscle, or nerve.

The online technology dictionary, Whatis?com [10], gives a definition con-sistent with the early expositions of Drexler and Freitas and much current discussion:

> Nanomedicine is the application of nanotechnology (the engineering of tiny machines) to the prevention and treatment of disease in the human body. This evolving discipline has the potential to dramatically change medical science.

This is expanded by the editorial definition given in the *International Journal of Nanomedicine* [11], taken in part from the Foresight Institute's definition:

> Nanomedicine may be defined as the monitoring, repair, construction, and control of human biological systems using engineered nanodevices and nanostructures at the molecular level. ... this definition is founded on the design, synthesis, and evaluation of nanomaterials in medicine. Basic nanostructured materials, engineered enzymes, and the many products of biotechnology will be enormously useful in near-term medical applications ... One part of nanomedicine is the development of precisely controlled or programmable medical nanomachines and nanorobots.

The European Science Foundation defined nanomedicine in 2004 as

> the science and technology of diagnosing, treating, and preventing disease and traumatic injury, of relieving pain, and of preserving and improving human health, using molecular tools and molecular knowl-edge of the human body [9].

In its 2006 Forward Look on Nanomedicine, the European Science Foundation distinguished between *scientific nanomedicine* and a more general definition of *medical nanotechnology*. Nanomedicine was described as medicine based on molecular knowledge of the human body, using nanoscale molecular tools for the diagnosis and treatment of disease. Medical nanotechnology would by default cover all the other ways in which nanotechnology affects healthcare, including miniaturization of devices and their integration into diagnostic and therapeutic uses along with communication and information processing technologies [8].

Discussions involving nanomedicine, with their emphasis on direct medical intervention at the nanoscale, have tended to focus on a relatively few areas from within the field of medical nanotechnology: biomaterials, imaging enhancement, drug delivery, diagnostic nanodevices, active implants, and nanodrugs such as gene delivery nanoprobes.

These areas form a subset of the broader field of medical nanotechnology discussed above; thus, in many useful and authoritative books with titles such as "Nanotechnology in Biology and Medicine," "Nanotechnology in Therapeutics," and "BioMEMS Technologies and Application," for example, one may not find the term nanomedicine in the preface, introduction, index, or section headings. The NIH National Cancer Institute's Alliance for Nanotechnology in Cancer has a Cancer Nanotechnology Plan, but does not use the term nanomedicine in its outline statements [12].

Nanomedicine has been readily adopted by the pharmaceutical field to refer to drug delivery by means of encapsulation or incorporation into nanoparticles, and many formulations are now referred to as "nanomedicines." Nanomedicine is also frequently used to refer to the use of nanoparticles to enhance imaging.

An area on which nanomedicine is especially focused is the concept of *theranostics*—the combination of diagnostic and therapeutic functionality in one device, enabling presymptomatic treatment (the term theragnostics is also sometimes used with a very similar meaning). Theranostics is often used to describe nanoparticles that have been engineered for both imaging and drug delivery, for example, particles that selectively attach to cancer cells to enhance imaging, and can be induced to release energy or drug molecules once localized in the diseased tissue.

Nanomedicine is also associated with *polymer therapeutics* (meaning the rational design of nanomedicines), *targeted drug delivery* (meaning individualized medicine tailored in response to a genomic profile, especially of a malignancy), and *regenerative medicine* (cell repair by nanoengineered insertion of genetic or therapeutic materials). These medical nanotechnologies are showing significant near-term promise for more effective, individualized, dose reduced, and affordable therapies [5].

In Part II, we will discuss some examples of these nanomedicine developments. Many nanomedical advances are moving from the lab to clinical trials, where they are producing promising results. These include imaging enhancement nanoparticles, theranostic nanoparticle and encapsulation formulations for cancer treatment, and nanoengineered delivery of drugs for targeted drug delivery. But first we look at the question of the relevance of nanomedicine and medical nanotechnology to current healthcare needs and priorities.

1.12 Healthcare Crisis: How Can Nanotechnology Contribute to a Solution?

Societies are constantly seeking ways to improve healthcare provision—in cost, coverage, effectiveness, and meeting challenges of emerging diseases and shifting demographics. Nanotechnology is being examined critically to determine how the new capabilities it represents can best be applied to current healthcare needs.

In examining the relevance of nanotechnology to healthcare needs, a distinction has been drawn by a number of observers between the potential offered by nanomedicine and medical technology as more broadly defined. For example, we noted earlier a division between scientific nanomedicine and medical nanotechnology. The latter, by covering integration of nanodevices into communications and information processing systems, also encompasses personal and remote health monitoring with the potential to radically alter traditional hospitals and doctor–patient relationships.

In a recent European Commission nanobiotechnology report, nanomedicne is characterized as disease centered, aiming to improve traditional medical approaches of diagnostics and therapeutics by taking them to the cellular and molecular level with nanotechnology [8]. "Because it is disease centered, nanomedicine leaves to medical nanotechnologies the more general and perhaps more profound transformations of healthcare: these concern public health monitoring, the integration of medical practices into daily patterns of work and leisure, the redefinition of the physiological body as a body of data, and the reorganisation of the therapeutic context with its medical experts, insurance companies, state interests, and healthcare institutions."

Because nanomedicine inherits its focus on certain diseases from current ongoing medical research, its primary aims have been toward noninfectious diseases, especially cancer, and on the degenerative diseases characterizing the increasingly sedentary and aging populations of the wealthiest countries that lead in medical research and medical expenditures. In an example given in the nanobiotechnology report cited above, the European Technology Platform includes a focus on nanomedicine for treatment of arthritic joints. In the wider context, nanomedical alleviation of painful arthritic joints would be part of an integrated treatment and prevention approach that would include nutrition, mobility, and the management of obesity, along with medical nanotechnologies for monitoring and feedback, physical therapy, as well as geriatric sociopsyschological, economic, and political incentive approaches.

Leaving aside for the moment the European and developing nations contexts, nanomedicine and medical nanotechnology, in particular, present universal opportunities for transforming efficiencies in healthcare.

1.12.1 The Wired World

Ever-present wireless communications are transforming the way business and leisure are conducted. The ubiquity and power of wireless coverage, and unobtrusive personal instruments for its access and use, are made possible largely by advances in electronics, with increased speed and processing capabilities, superior power requirements, lower costs, and smaller and lighter physical profiles. These advances are the outcome of the ability to fabricate circuits in dimensions that are shrinking to the nanoscale. This is another pervasive impact of nanotechnology, which is also ready to change healthcare.

The application of nanotechnology-based wireless technology starts in the hospital, with wireless patient monitoring, RFID tracking, automated data collection in the OR and ICU, and other adoptions of wireless sensors and monitors to improve quality and efficiency of patient care. Wireless technology is also improving communication among caregivers and access to patient records and test results, important factors in quality of care.

Wireless technologies are taking healthcare from the hospitals and doctors' offices to accompany the patient. Low-cost ubiquitous monitoring and feedback to both patient and caregivers can integrate healthcare into daily lifestyles at home, work, and leisure.

The Internet has increased patient knowledge and awareness, leading to greater participation in healthcare decisions and alerting patients to treatment alternatives. Access to inexpensive genotyping and widespread imaging services can lead to increased knowledge of individual biological makeup and risks on the part of patients, relatives, and caregivers. Access to more data does not necessarily equate to better informed patients and public. This puts more demands on caregivers for communication with patients and families and participation in the wireless information networks.

Easier access to information and communication between caregivers is especially important in supporting the distribution of healthcare tasks over a range of skill and responsibility levels, and more effective specialization. Thus, the wired world can contribute to efficiencies and quality of care by teams of health professionals that include general practitioners, physician assistants, nursing specialists, therapists, counselors, clinical specialists, and others.

Widespread medical wireless devices have the potential to facilitate tailored healthcare, with monitoring, prevention, and early intervention. Tailored healthcare is also enabled by genome awareness, as well as knowledge of proteome, immunome, health history, and environmental and other stress exposures—all of which can be the focus of information gathering by personal healthcare devices tied to a healthcare database and communication network. The personalization of digital wireless technology is already spreading rapidly over the whole world. It is a relatively small extension to add healthcare monitoring and communication to ever more advanced personal digital devices that provide voice data communication, track location, manage schedules, entertain, and perform an increasing list of functions in daily life.

With greatly increased information available about each individual, the likely costs associated with future care become more predictable, and thus risks are reduced. This changes the paradigm for insurance, which is a concept based on pooling resources to share against unknown risks. If the risks are known, costs and rewards for assuming risks can be less, and planning for assumption of risks can be made on a more rational basis. Once risks are known, it is a decision for society to make on how to pay for the costs, and how to couple those costs with employment, other forms of contribution and participation in society, and access to and distribution of resources in general.

1.12.2 Human Augmentation

Nanotechnology, in the form of electronics and distributed sensors and actuators for communication and control, makes possible the extension of self into new types of augmentation—prosthetics, brain–computer interfaces, and avatars. In a sense, we already augment our memories with digital electronic storage, our eyes and voices with telecommunications, and our hands with remote devices of all kinds. Nanotechnology will continue to accelerate the possibilities, including those with direct applications to care and maintenance of health.

Nanotechnology is a key enabler for robotic-assisted surgery, personal helper and companion robots, and in automated lifeplace systems in homes, work, and transportation. These can impact health in negative as well as positive ways, for example, in leading to more sedentary lifestyles.

1.12.3 Environmental Impacts

Environmental impacts of nanotechnology may result from effects of exposure to nanoparticles in clothing, food, water, dust, and aerosols, for both humans and ecosystems. A major impact, either positive or negative, will be the effect of nanotechnology on consumption of energy and materials. Effects of increased exposure to all kinds of nanomaterials and their fates in the body and environment will need to be analyzed, assessed, and measured. Environmental and public health will need to respond to the challenges and opportunities posed by nanotechnology. Among the opportunities will be improved and more effective water purification and air filtration systems.

1.13 Conclusion

Thus, nanotechnology is positioned to have a major influence on issues that are at the forefront of concerns about the future direction of healthcare. It is therefore important for everyone with an interest in healthcare to gain awareness and knowledge of nanomedicine and medical nanotechnology and their promises and implications.

References

1. T. J. Webster, Nanomedicine: what's in a definition?, *International Journal of Nanomedicine*, 1, 115–116 (2006).
2. B. N. Taylor (ed.), *The International System of Units (SI)*, NIST Special Publication 330, 2001 edn., United States Department of Commerce National Institute of Standards and Technology, Washington, DC, 2001.
3. A. Sandhu, Who invented nano? *Nature Nanotechnology*, 1, 87 (2006).
4. H. J. Cook, What stays constant at the heart of medicine, *British Medical Journal*, 333, 1281–1282 (2006).
5. G. L. Hornyak, H. F. Tibbals, J. Dutta, and J. J. Moore, *Introduction to Nanoscience and Nanotechnology*, CRC Press, Boca Raton, FL, 2009.
6. J. Venugopal, M. P. Prabhakaran, S. Low, A. T. Choon, Y. Z. Zhang, G. Deepika, and S. Ramakrishna, Nanotechnology for nanomedicine and delivery of drugs, *Current Pharmaceutical Design*, 14, 2184–2200 (2008).
7. National Materials Advisory Board (NMAB), *A Matter of Size: Triennial Review of the National Nanotechnology Initiative*, The National Academies Press, Washington, DC, 2006, http://books.nap.edu/openbook.php?record_id=11752&page=63 (accessed April 21, 2008).
8. European Science Foundation, Nanomedicine, An ESF-European Medical Research Councils (EMRC) Forward Look Report, ESF, Strasbourg, France, 2004.
9. National Institutes of Health, National Institute of Health Roadmap for Medical Research: Nanomedicine (2006), URL: http://nihroadmap.nih.gov/nanomedicine/ (accessed April 21, 2008).
10. Whatis?com, website at URL: http://whatis.techtarget.com/definition/0,,sid9_gci512908,00.html (accessed July 30, 2009).
11. T. J Webster, IJN's second year is now a part of nanomedicine history!, *International Journal of Nanomedicine*, 2, 1–2 (2007).
12. U. S. NIH National Cancer Institute, URL: http://nano.cancer.gov/about_alliance/mission.asp (accessed July 30, 2009).

2

Historical Perspectives and Technological Breakthroughs

> I do anatomize and cut up these poor beasts, he said to Hippocrates, to see the cause of these distempers, vanities, and follies, which are the burden of all creatures.
>
> **—Democritus, from The History of Melancholy**

2.1 Introduction

In this chapter, we look at how we got to this point in the development of medical nanotechnology. In a new field with many changes occurring rapidly and simultaneously, with competing models for conceptualization and organization, it can be useful to have a brief historical perspective.

2.2 Brief Highlights of Nanomedicine History

Nanomedicine, as we mentioned in Chapter 1, was coined as a terminology by Drexler and colleagues in the 1980s, but nanoscale techniques were being used in medical research and applied in diagnostics long before the term "nanotechnology" was introduced by Professor Norio Taniguchi in 1974, and even before Feynman introduced the concept in 1959.

The new field of nanoscience is essentially a new way of looking at science and technology, with the perspectives of new possibilities opened by vastly more powerful tools for examination and manipulation of matter on the submicron scale. This new paradigm is rapidly opening new possibilities in medical research and practice. In this respect, the impact of nanoscience parallels the impacts made on medicine by microscopy, chemistry, physics, electronics, and computing, which led to new theories of disease, more effective approaches to treatment, and powerful new imaging and surgical tools.

2.2.1 Nanoscience Streams of Development

Various streams of scientific and technical work on the nanoscale have arisen independently, developed divergently, sometimes collided and clashed, and finally are beginning to merge into a unified body of knowledge. There have been complications on the way; this is not new or unusual for the social activity we call science, much less technology.

Medicine has been a key motivation in creating the scientific knowledge that is the basis of our civilization. As noted before, it was curiosity about the mysterious processes of life that led Priestley and Lavoisier to the discovery of oxygen and the stoichiometry of combustion, and thus to atomic and molecular theory, leading to the science of chemistry. And it was dissection of frog legs to unravel the structures of nerve and muscle that surprised Galvani with the discovery of electric current and led to Volta's capture of electrons in storage jars from static electricity sources, leading eventually to the science and technology of electromagnetism that together with chemistry has transformed our world.

Without the boldness to investigate the sacrosanct origins and pillars of life, science could never have advanced beyond elegant speculations and beautiful models of the order of the heavens, though nothing would have prevented the practical advancement of firearms, wind and water turbines, and heat engines. But the key technologies based on chemistry and electromagnetism needed hints from the internal mechanisms of living creatures to overcome confusion, inertia, and resistance. And again today, medicine and biology are serving as the impetus and key to open the gates on a continent of scientific knowledge and technical capability—the nanoworld.

Once chemistry and electromagnetic physics were unleashed, their progression from macroscales to micro and beyond was inevitable. This progression took place via a number of independent but interleaving courses.

One stream started with electron beam and thin film deposition and etching to make layers a few atoms thick: microfabrication. Another line of research was biological: ceramic nanopore filters for viruses and nanoscale capillaries for cell membrane electrode measurements (cell patch technique). Another was microscopic: pushing the limits of imaging further and further through electron microscopy, x-ray diffraction, field emission microscopy, and atomic force microscopy.

Another was supramolecular chemistry: colloids, membranes, molecular sieves, dendrimers and chelation complexes, clathrates, etc. Another was biochemical: protein chemistry, DNA, RNA, cellular polymer microtubules, cell membranes, ion gates, mechanisms of neurotransmission, photosynthesis, cell division, etc.

Another was carbon nanochemistry: carbon nanotubes, buckminsterfullerenes, diamondoids, and graphenes. Another was materials science, including natural materials—micro and nanoencapsulation, quantum dots, and quantum resonance surfaces including butterfly wings, lotus effect surfaces, and gecko feet. These disparate fields were brought together as the unified focal point of attention by the visionary proposals of the nanotechnologists, inspired by the ideas of Feynman. Some were brought in kicking and screaming, but a unified field of nanoscience and technology is emerging. And in this field the proposals of Freitas formed the visionary and provocative thesis of nanomedicine that demanded a response, thereby pulling together the disparate efforts that are becoming known as nanomedicine and medical nanotechnology.

The drive to understand the basis of life has propelled science toward smaller and smaller units of organization from organs to cells to molecules to atoms, electrons, and subatomic particles. Penetrating deep into the molecular and subatomic scale, chemistry and physics bypassed the nanoscale, which turns out to be highly significant in the organization of living cells. This was partly because neither physics nor chemistry nor biology had a language or tools with which to deal with the middle ground between molecular genetics and cell biology [1]. Now we are catching up, coming back to study and understand more fully the intricate interactions that are possible between small assemblages of molecules, and between light and matter divided into nanoscale particles. It appears that we rushed to grasp the outer reaches of the universe and the inner depths of subatomic matter before coming back to the middle ground to attempt to understand the processes of life that lie halfway between the knowable extremes of size and energy scales. But only by this route did we gain the tools, both physical and conceptual, to comprehend the middle kingdom of living things.

2.2.2 Interrelationship between Nanotech Development and Medical Development

There is an inseparable relationship between advances in science and technology and advances in medicine. Understanding the mechanisms of charge transfer in the process of photosynthesis and energetics of cellular metabolism led to breakthroughs in photoelectric engineering and solar power generation. The study of human speech and hearing development had impacts on computer speech synthesis and recognition. Investigation of the world based on nanotechnology generates new tools for application in medical practice, resulting in new understanding of health and disease. Many nanoscale technology and science developments were the result of biological experiments, and nanotechnology has always been readily applied to the investigation of biological phenomena.

Chemistry advanced by reacting Avagradro's numbers of molecules, whereas Feynman conceived of building by assembly of one molecule or atom at a time. This was a challenge that produced a response, first by the Drexler school of bottom-up constructionists, and then a counterresponse by Smalley and the carbon-based self-assembly school. The former have tended to start with physics and engineering of atoms and inorganic materials; the latter have emphasized the self-assembly possibilities inherent in carbon and organic molecules such as carbon nanotubes and dendrimers. In the meantime, biologists have explored and elucidated the nanoscale processes taking place with the macromolecular structures of cell membranes, antibodies, proteins, and DNA.

Over time, a synthesis is emerging to combine the best aspects of these disparate approaches. Out of this synthesis, we can find many applications of nanoscience to medicine, from nanoencapsulation of drugs to biosensors that rely on nanoscale effects.

2.3 Medical Milestones

There are numerous resources available in print and on the internet that chart the milestones of development of nanotechnology and nanomedicine. A selection is listed at the end of this chapter [2,3]. Here, we will list a set of medical milestones taken from a millennial article in the *New England Journal of Medicine*. The journal chose the most important discoveries and developments in medicine in the past 500 years.

Besides such major advances in practice such as anesthesia and rigorous statistical clinical trials, the scientific breakthroughs included a series of trends toward understanding of life science on a broadly smaller scale, from the gross to the submicroscopic.

Elucidation of Human Anatomy and Physiology, beginning in the sixteenth century

Accurate anatomies, circulation, pulse, blood pressure, electrical nerve stimulus, and control of muscle by nerves.

Discovery of Cells and their Substructures, from the sixteenth through the twentieth centuries

Microscope, discovery of bacteria and protozoa, complex inner structures of plant and animal tissues, plant cells, animal cells, cell division, nucleus, etc., electron microscope, isolation of mitochondria.

Development of Biochemistry, from the seventeenth through the twentieth centuries

Concept of active "fermet" replaces idea of passive "humors"; discovery of oxygen, other gases, development of organic and physical chemistry, enzyme chemistry, pathways of metabolism, Krebs cycle, role of calcium, sodium, potassium, magnesium, etc., chlorophyll, hemoglobin, hormones, neurotransmitters, cell signaling.

Discovery of the Relation of Microbes to Disease, beginning in the nineteenth century

Displacement of spontaneous generation theory of microbial life by continuous inheritance principal, association of microbes with diseases, discovery of viruses, pasteurization, vaccination with weakened microbes and viruses, isolation of bacteria in pure culture, antiseptics, recognition of importance of sanitation and sterilization, disease vectors.

Elucidation of Inheritance and Genetics, beginning in the nineteenth century
   Mendelian laws of inheritance, inheritance of errors of metabolism, genes, chromosomes, mapping of genes on chromosomes, specification of enzymes by genes, identification of DNA as genetic material, base pairing rules in DNA, isolation and x-ray diffraction of DNA molecules, identification of double helix structure of DNA, role of RNA in transcription of proteins coded in DNA, messenger RNA, methodology for decoding sequences of bases in DNA, discovery of reverse transcriptase which converts RNA into DNA, polymerase chain reaction method for DNA amplification, establishment of a relationship between a molecular mutation and a specific disease, "molecular disease" concept.

Knowledge of the Immune System: Discovery of first-known antibodies (in diphtheria antitoxin), identification of role of phagocytes engulfing foreign bodies, cellular theory of immunity, major advances in vaccines, killed virus vaccines, and first vaccine produced by DNA technology (hepatitis B).

Medical Imaging and Biomarkers for Diagnosis and Research: Discovery of x-rays, use to image bone and hard tissue structure, radioactive tracers for imaging, ultrasound, development of contrast agents; use of power of electronic controls and digital computation to generate detailed multilayer and dimensional images of organs and vessel structure: magnetic resonance imaging, computed tomography, Doppler ultrasound, functional magnetic resonance imaging, image enhancement agents, radiotracers for metabolic and cellular pathways, photochromic markers, bioluminescent markers of molecular activity within cells; use of medical imaging to guide surgery and minimally invasive procedures; and use of antibodies labeled with photonic and magnetic targets to identify cancer cells.

Discovery and Development of Antimicrobial Agents: First antibiotic compound—salvarsan, discovery of antibiotic activity of dyes, Prontosil for strep infections, sulfa drugs, penicillin, discovery of antibiotics in soil organisms, development of streptomycin, and understanding of ability of microbes to develop resistance to antibiotics.

Development of Molecular Pharmacotherapy: Concept of chemotherapy, extension of pharmaceutic application from microbes to cancer cells, removal or deactivation of hormone-producing glands (ovaries, testes, etc.) to treat cancer of organs regulated by hormones (breast cancer, prostate cancer, etc.), treatment of lymphomas by nitrogen mustard, methotrexate for leukemia, cis-platinum for cancer, beta-blockers; design of drugs for specific molecular targets, explanation of genetic-based variability of drug response.

   When we review the above list of medical advances, there is a trend from treatment of bodies and organs to specific focus on detailed molecular mechanisms in both diagnosis and treatment. Advances in science and engineering went hand in hand with advances in medicine to apply therapy more precisely and efficiently. Advances in technology led to new tools, which applied in the life sciences resulted in advances in medical understanding and practice.

2.3.1 Some Medical Nanotechnology Milestones

A number of historical developments presage and underpin the modern development of nanotechnology and nanomedicine. Perhaps, the most fundamental was the atomic theory: the idea that matter existed in the form of discrete particles with definitive properties and extremely small sizes rather than as fluids, spirits, or humors. This world view of matter allows for the idea that one might be able to manipulate the fundamental particles explicitly and mechanistically rather than shape matter by spells, heat, interactions with other fluids, or other influences.

The opposing concepts of matter as fluid versus particles have risen and fallen since at least the classical Greek period. The theory based on "elements" of fire, earth, air, and water, corresponding to the humors of black bile, blood, yellow bile, and phlegm, was especially attractive for its simplicity and unity. Human states of health and mind were linked to astronomy/astrology, alchemy, the seasons and weather, foods, and other aspects of everyday experience in an easily grasped model. Today's concept of homeostasis— a balanced equilibrium between bodily functions—echoes in a general way this concept from early medicine.

The replacement of the humors and phlogiston models by atomic theory made possible the development of chemistry. The vision of matter as composed of discrete building blocks made it easier to conceive of living creature as composed of cells. The intellectual framework of atomic theory made possible the concept of the electron and the development of electromagnetic theory, even though fields and waves were invoked to explain electromagnetic force. More recently, quantum mechanics and relativity have blurred the distinction between particle and wave models of matter, but the idea of discrete atoms still made possible the concept of manipulation of atoms and molecules that underlies nanotechnology.

On the practical side, artisans and technologists were making and using nanoparticle materials since at least early classical times, as in the use of finely dispersed gold (nanoparticles) to produce unique effects in glass. As noted previously, ceramic filters with nanoscale pore sizes made possible the demonstration of the existence of viruses with their infectious ability to propagate at sizes smaller than any cell. And nanoscale capillaries made possible the study of cell membrane receptors and gates by the cell patch clamp technique.

But the conceptual side of nanomedicine has roots in the idea of chemotherapy, which was given a major breakthrough by Paul Ehrlich with his concept of "magic bullet" drugs to target specific bacteria and pathogens. Ehrlich, a brilliant bacteriologist, was familiar with the highly specific absorption of dyes by bacteria, and reasoned that if he could combine lethality with stains, he could target pathogens. His successful formulation of salvarsan in 1908 was the first instance of targeted chemotherapy design, setting the pattern for a century of drug development [2].

The magic bullet chemotherapy idea was based on the specificity of dye stains used to make bacteria visible under the microscope, and to classify different classes of microbes according to stain affinities. Underlying this specificity was the concept of a "lock and key" mechanism guiding specific interactions between molecules, a concept that was arising out of studies of enzymes and antibodies. The lock-and-key concept of molecular recognition developed as enzymes, antibodies, and macromolecular catalysts were studied and understood in the mid-twentieth century.

About the same time, how structural macromolecular biopolymers fit together to form stable structures began to be understood, using new tools such as x-ray diffraction and the electron microscope, applied to natural biomaterials such as wool and cartilage. During the same period, based on the earlier understanding of thin films, micelles, and polymers by Langmuir and others, the structure and function of cell membranes began to be understood, most notably and first with the elucidation of the mechanism of transport of nerve impulses [2,3].

The study of cell membrane ion gating channels, made possible by the cell patch clamp technique, further showed how cellular processes act like nanoscale machinery with precisely controlled molecular mechanisms rather than random reactions between freely flowing biomolecules. Mapping of the role of ion channels and membrane receptors in the life of cells further advanced the understanding of the body's network of signaling pathways, controlling and regulating the balance of metabolic functions. This in turn gave a new model for disease and treatment for many metabolic and degenerative disorders, by targeting cell receptors to modify cellular signals.

In the 1950s and 1960s, the structure and function of DNA and RNA was worked out, with the major breakthrough made by Watson, Crick, and colleagues in establishing a structure for DNA. The revelation of the genetic encoding of life by a macromolecular mechanism placed an intricate and precise nanomachinery at the very heart of the most vital life processes. The further understanding of the genetic code and its practical application in biotechnology would follow along with breakthroughs in reverse transcriptase and gene amplification.

The immune system plays an important role in medical nanotechnology as well as biotechnology. Phagocytes presage nanorobots, patrolling the body-fighting invaders and repairing damage, but antibodies provided the immediate means to fabricate highly specific molecular targeting for a variety of tasks. The development of monoclonal antibodies by Köhler and Milstein in the 1970s coupled with the discovery of reverse transcriptase by H. Temin and D. Baltimore was a double breakthrough that opened the possibilities for genetically engineering cells to produce large quantities of peptides including antibodies [2].

Antibodies can be generated by exposure of mammalian immune systems to any number of antigens. Like DNA and RNA, antibodies can be used as macromolecular templates to recognize and bind to other selected molecules. Antibodies or DNA segments can be fixed onto biochip substrates and used to search for matching complimentary molecules with sensitivity, specificity, and discrimination, even in complex mixtures of similar molecules. Readout of the biochip can be with optical, electronic, or chemical indicators.

Another area of development, protein bioscience, was at the same time moving from consideration of proteins as chemicals toward an understanding of their functions as mechanical structures and even as machinery in the functions of the cell. The function of the protein coat in the macrophage was striking as an example of molecular machinery, as was the mechanism of muscle contraction, flagella rotation, actin transport, and many other cellular processes. The more the cellular mechanisms were elucidated, the more the cell began to resemble a factory equipped with intricate molecular machinery [3].

Drugmakers had been quick to apply methods of polymer microencapsulation to medication delivery, and diagnostic and clinical analysis device developers were even more quick in applying the possibilities of enzyme and nucleotide recognition to make microsensors and microchips for rapid inexpensive testing, DNA analysis, disease diagnosis, and high throughput biomedical screening. These developments were made possible by concurrent advances in design and fabrication for microelectronics, microfluidics, and materials and polymer science.

All of the above developments in biology, cell biology, molecular biology, enzymology, molecular diagnostics, genetics, and biotechnology, along with many others in biomaterials, cell scaffolds, and mechanisms of muscle and nerve action were taking place pretty much independent of the development of nanotechnology as a program for assembly of atomic machines by physical or engineering methods, as well as the development of carbon nanotube chemistry, until the proposals to apply nanotechnology to medicine by the Drexler school, notably Freitas and others, starting in the 1990s. There is a historical parallel: During the development of colloid science, many biologists working with proteins and enzymes continued their work with macromolecules with minimal involvement in the colloid–macromolecule controversy.

Advances in exploiting the unique properties of the nanoscale for medical purposes would depend on merging an understanding of the truly unique properties that emerge with division of matter into nanoscale features, with a fluent understanding of the biomolecular and cellular context in which nanoscale effects would operate; in other words, developing an integrated approach to medical nanotechnology. Only then would the possibilities for application of nanostructures and nanoeffects to medicine can be realized.

2.3.2 Some Cautionary Notes for a New Field

The history of new and rapidly developing fields of science and technology are marked by many false starts before a coherent body of knowledge is established. An established field has a core body of facts and rules based on well tested and verified experimentation and trial. Mature fields have a few societies that meet, review advances in the knowledge of the field, publish and educate, recognize achievement, maintain standards of discipline, and serve as a gateway for interaction with government and business.

New fields typically have difficulty gaining recognition from established societies and academies; this is a useful and necessary function of knowledge gatekeepers to validate novelty and put a brake on the fragmentation of knowledge. Pioneers who create, discover, or have insights into new paradigms or truly new fields of enquiry may wander in the wilderness until the new field is proven to have merit, after which it is either accepted as a new specialization in an old field or more rarely, achieves an independent niche.

New fields may evolve quietly, or may be led by charismatic visionaries, whose imagination and energy blaze new trails. Such persons or groups inevitably meet strong resistance; sometimes the merits of the new field get lost in personality conflicts. Where there is a basis in factual reality for new knowledge, the situation eventually sorts itself out in a relatively short time.

In science, examples of this process are the replacement of phlogiston theory by atomic theory of combustion, the replacement of the ether model by relativity, and the acceptance of continental drift and plate tectonics in geology. In medicine, examples are the acceptance of germ theory (especially the value of sterilization in surgery), the acceptance of laproscopic surgery, and the existence of disease germs, viruses, and prions.

During the early stage of development of a field, there is a vulnerability to exploitation of the field by those tempted to self-promotion or worse. It is more difficult to verify claims in a new field where a substantial body of fact and procedure are yet to be developed. The vacuum created by the need for avenues of publication and validation may be filled by those most eager to promote their own interests rather than the propagation of knowledge. There have been examples of new academies and societies that spring up prematurely with inadequate backing and vetting. Such instances tend to retard the advancement of the field of knowledge, but only temporarily. Where the field has merit, facts eventually assert themselves.

An example particularly relevant to nanotechnology in its molecular subject comes from the history of colloidal science. At the beginning of the twentieth century, chemists were used to working with well-behaved compounds, which could be purified and analyzed, with molecular weights of at most a few hundred. The existence of compounds with molecular weights in the thousands or hundreds of thousands was strongly doubted by the leading organic chemists of the day. Instead, substances such as proteins, polysaccharides, and rubber were held to be poorly defined clusters of much smaller "true" molecules. Studies of inorganic colloids such as colloidal gold and hydrated silica have shown them to be aggregates, with variable size and composition depending on environment and conditions of formation. It seemed incredible and unreasonable that compounds with molecular weights larger than several hundred could exist as actual molecules. After all, the best organic synthetic efforts had not been able to create molecules larger than the size of an 18-member peptide chain. Besides, intellectual and tangible results were more forthcoming from work on simple, well-behaved compounds than on messy goo.

The colloidal/macromolecule debate was quite intense up until the 1930s when macromolecular chemistry became established as an independent field of science. Until then, dominant colloid chemists held fast to the dogma that what might appear to be macromolecules were merely loose aggregates of smaller true molecules. Some historians of science have referred to this period as "the dark age of biocolloidology," which retarded the biological sciences. This is true despite the fact that protein scientists had long recognized on the basis of elemental analysis that hemoglobin and other "albumin-like substances" were molecules with regular compositions and molecular weights much larger than ordinary organic compounds [4].

Nevertheless, the controversy between the champions of a new way of looking at colloids as macromolecules and the staunch upholders of established dogma became a long, acrimonious battle. At its height it involved famous and great scientists such as W. Ostwald, A. A. Noyes, S. P. L. Sorensen, T. Svedberg, and many others. In the end, the truth won out, culminating with the belated award of the Nobel Prize in 1953 to Hermann Staudinger, the champion of the macromolecular concept.

The resistance to new ideas during the colloid controversy was in part fueled by instances of overenthusiasm and even outright chicanery. During the 1930s, Dorothy Wrinch aggressively promoted a theoretically elegant but chemically impossible proposal for protein structure, gaining a hearing around the world and attracting the support of Langmuir and others.

Walter Bancroft, professor at Cornell University and founder of the *Journal of Physical Chemistry*, proposed colloid theories of anesthesia, poisoning, drug addiction, and insanity during the 1930s. He attributed all nervous disorders to precipitation of proteins in nerve fibers and believed that they could be cured by injection of salts that were known to dissolve proteins in the laboratory. This discredited him in scientific circles and raised the wrath of the medical profession, especially as the theories were spread by newspaper stories. Some "colloid healers" had previously become celebrated and wealthy practicing their art, inspired by the writings of A. Lumiere and others who claimed that all maladies were the result of colloid imbalances. The dream of a magical healing philosopher's stone is ageless, as is the temptation to seize on every new discovery and concept as the universal key to medical miracles [4].

Nanotechnology, as a new concept and a rapidly developing field, has not been exempt from similar controversies and even instances of exploitation and misrepresentation. Caution must always be observed; even Nobel laureates in other well-established fields and institutions have been touched by scandals involving falsification of research results. The temptations and pressures are great, but nanotechnology is in no way uniquely vulnerable.

2.3.3 A Positive Look Forward

Medical doctors are conservative in their approach to adopting new technologies. Guided by the admonition to "first, do no harm," and rigorously trained through mentorship, the medical profession sets high standards which any new proposed technique or device must pass. This is supported not only by the culture of the medical profession and community, but also embodied in the legal framework of medical regulation by the FDA and similar bodies. Such conservatism toward innovation is laudable, and works to ensure safety and efficacy in an age that rushes to adopt innovations that are developed ever more rapidly by a continuous revolution of advancing science and technology. Modern evidence–based medicine welcomes innovation to meet growing needs brought about by constantly evolving pathogens, new chronic and environmental diseases and disorders, and growing and aging populations. But medicine remains fundamentally about human care, in which technology is only a means to an end. Any new technology has the power to do good and harm. I have full confidence that in the hands of our medical fraternity, it will be used for good.

References

1. A. Kornberg, We must try to bridge the gap between biological and chemical sciences, *The Scientist*, 2, 15 (1988).
2. G. L. Hornyak, H. F. Tibbals, J. Dutta, and J. J. Moore, *Introduction to Nanoscience and Nanotechnology*, CRC Press, Boca Raton, FL, 2009.
3. A. Y. Grosberg and A. R. Khokhlov, *Giant Molecules*, Academic Press, San Diego, 1997.
4. C. Tanford and J. Reynolds, *Nature's Robots: A History of Proteins*, Oxford University Press, Oxford, U.K., 2001.

3

Emerging National and Global Nanomedicine Initiatives

> Nanosciences and nanotechnology are transforming a wide variety of products and services that have the potential to enhance the practice of medicine and improve public health. But there are a number of health, safety, and environmental issues to be addressed.
>
> **B. Walker and C. P. Mouton, *JAMA* (2007)**

Medical nanotechnology and nanomedicine are beginning to have practical applications in healthcare as well as medical research. Nanomedicine and medical nanotechnology are now important components of research and development all over the world, in all sectors of public and private endeavor: governments, national laboratories, universities, corporations, nonprofit groups, and organizations concerned with social, economic, environmental, legal, and ethical impacts. Governments and industry are responding with initiatives providing support and investment to realize the potential health and economic benefits.

3.1 Some Developments in Nanomedicine

The nanomedicine field is growing rapidly, so this survey will cover the highlights of a moving target. The lists and citations in the following sections are a sampling, with many omissions. As an introduction, they are meant to convey the direction of developments. Pursuit of the keywords and sources sampled here will lead to many other examples in the various special fields represented.

3.2 Current Examples of Nanomedicine in Practice and Research

Nanoscience and nanotechnology are influencing thinking and practice in medicine. The nano-perspective thinks in terms of precisely controlled manipulation of structures at the scale of nanometers. This is the scale of the macromolecular machinery of cells and life. Traditional science and medicine have dealt in terms of bulk macroscale drugs and physical treatments and interventions. Initiatives are underway in the United States and globally to develop medical breakthroughs based on nanotechnology. Some research initiatives, publications, organizations, and meetings that indicate the growing activity in nanomedicine are listed below [1–4]:

- The U.S. NIH *Nanomedicine Initiative* is a major program in *NIH Roadmap* for medical research, including research centers in major universities and medical and engineering schools.
- Nanomedicine is a major part of the European Community's CORDIS Nanotechnology Action Plan.
- The Canadian Regenerative Medicine and Nanomedicine Enterprise (CARMENE) will apply nanotechnology to develop biomaterials and scaffolding for cartilage and bone regeneration.
- Nanomedicine awareness and initiatives have been started at major pharmaceutical and biomedical device and instrumentation companies, including Pfizer, GSK, Astra Zeneca, Genentech, Merck, Weyth, and others.
- A large number of international conferences on nanomedicine are being organized by the NIH, NCI, European Commission, European Science Foundation, Case Western Reserve University, and others.
- New companies are starting based on nanomedicine devices and technologies (see chapters on specific technical applications).
- Increased interest and popular attention are given to nanomedicine and nanomedical devices in the media, radio, TV, interviews, and cover stories.

3.2.1 Books

Books on nanomedicine topics include

- Nanomedicine book series by Robert A. Freitas Jr., *Nanomedicine, Volume I: Basic Capabilities*, Landes, Austin, TX, 1999.
- Robert A. Freitas Jr., *Nanomedicine, Volume IIA: Biocompatibility*, Landes, Austin, TX, 2003.
- A. Elaissari (Ed.), *Colloidal Biomolecules, Biomaterials, and Biomedical Applications*, CRC Press, Boca Raton, FL, 2003.
- Robert A. Freitas Jr., *Kinematic Self-Replicating Machines*, Landes, Austin, TX, 2009.

- *2006 Guide to Nanomedicine Technology—Medical Research, Healthcare, NIH and NCI Research, Nanoscale Materials, Nanobots, Nanobiotech, Nanotubes, Biosensors* (CD-ROM) by U.S. Government, 2006.
- T. Vo-Dinh (Ed.), *Nanotechnology in Biology and Medicine: Methods, Devices and Applications*, CRC Press, Boca Raton, FL, 2006.
- N. H. Malsch (Ed.), *Biomedical Nanotechnology*, CRC Press, Boca Raton, FL, 2005.
- R. Shetty MD, *Nanotechnology: The Future in Medicine*, Mezocore Technologies, Inc., Quebec, Ontario, Canada, 2006.
- K. K. Jain (Ed.), *The Handbook of Nanomedicine*, Springer—Humana, Totowa, NJ, 2008.
- I. Majoros and J. Baker Jr., (Eds.), *Dendrimer Based Nanomedicine*, Pan Stanford Publishing, Singapore—c/o World Scientific Publishing, Hackensack, NJ, 2008.
- C. Wei, *Nanomedicine*, An issue of *Medical Clinics*, 91–5, Elsevier—Saunders, 2007.
- T. Chang and S. Ming, *Artificial Cells: Biotechnology, Nanomedicine, Regenerative Medicine, Blood Substitutes, Bioencapsulation, and Cell/Stem Cell Therapy*, Lavoisier, 2007.
- K. Gonsalves, C. Halberstadt, C. T. Laurencin and L. Nair (eds.), *Biomedical Nanostructures*, John Wiley & Sons, Inc., New York, 2007.
- V. Torchilin and M. Amiji, *Handbook of Materials for Nanomedicine*, Pan Stanford Publishing, Singapore, 2009.
- S. Ramakrishna, M. Ramalingam, T. S. S. Kumar and W. O. Soboyejo, *Biomaterials: A Nano Approach*, CRC Press, Boca Raton, FL, 2010.
- A. Sasson, *Recent Progress in Medical Biotechnology and Nanomedicine: Achievements, Prospects and Perceptions*, United Nations University Press, Tokyo, Japan, 2008.

Examples of books with an emphasis on biotechnology, biochemistry, and protein chemistry rather than medicine include

- D. E. Reisner, *Bionanotechnology: Global Prospects*, CRC Press, Boca Raton, FL, 2008.
- D. S. Goodsell, *Bionanotechnology: Lessons from Nature*, Wiley-Liss, New York, 2004.
- E. Masayoshi, I. Keizo, O. Noriaki, O. Noriko, S. Masaaki, and T. Yamaguchi (eds.), Future medical engineering based on bionanotechnology, in *Proceedings of the Final Symposium of the Tohoku University 21st Century Center of Excellence Program,... International Center*, Japan 7–9 January, Imperial College Press, London, U.K., 2006.

- D. S. Goodsell, *The Machinery of Life* (Paperback), Springer, New York, 1997.
- D. S. Goodsell, *Our Molecular Nature: The Body's Motors, Machines and Messages*, Springer, New York, 1996.
- R. S. Greco, F. B. Prinz, and R. L. Smith (eds.), *Nanoscale Technology in Biological Systems*, CRC Press, Boca Raton, FL, 2004.
- C. M. Niemeyer and C. A. Mirkin (eds.), *Nanobiotechnology: Concepts, Applications and Perspectives*, Wiley-VCH, Weinheim, Germany, 2004.
- C. M. Niemeyer and C. A. Mirkin (eds.), *Nanobiotechnology II: More Concepts and Applications*, Wiley-VCH, Weinheim, Germany, 2007.
- G. K. Knopf and A. S. Bassi (eds.), *Smart Biosensor Technology*, CRC Press, Boca Raton, FL, 2006.
- J. P. Fisher, A. G. Mikos, and J. D. Bronzino, *Tissue Engineering*, CRC Press, Boca Raton, FL, 2007.

In addition, a number of general books on nanotechnology futures, textbooks, and introductions to nanotechnology contain short chapters or sections on nanotechnology in medicine. The term "nanomedicine" has practically become a franchise of Freitas and the Foresight Institute. Therefore, terms like "medical nanotechnology" are used more generally. The NIH used the term "nanomedicine technology" to distinguish its CD-ROM from "nanomedicine."

3.2.2 Journals

Several journals are now published devoted exclusively to nanomedicine, in addition to the many nanotechnology journals that also cover nanomedicine and medical nanotechnology. The table below gives a few examples and is not meant to be exhaustive. Many more journals with nanomedicine and medical nanotechnology coverage can be found in the list of references accompanying each of the chapters in this book. Nanomedicine articles now appear in the *Journal of the American Medical Association*, the *Proceedings of the American Academy of Sciences, Science*, and other general and specialist science and medical journals.

Journals

Nanomedicine: Nanotechnology, Biology and Medicine (Elsevier)
http://www.nanomedjournal.com/
An international, peer-reviewed journal publishing basic, clinical, and engineering research in the innovative field of nanomedicine.

International Journal of Nanomedicine (Dove Press)
http://www.dovepress.com/international-journal-of-nanomedicine-journal
An international, peer-reviewed journal focusing on the application of nanotechnology in diagnostics, therapeutics, and drug delivery systems.

Nature Nanotechnology
http://www.nature.com/nnano/index.html
The nanotechnology specialist journal in the Nature family of scientific publications; it carries many nanomedicine articles and maintains a nanomedicine index and archive.

ACS Nano
http://pubs.acs.org/journal/ancac3
The nanoscience journal of *the American Chemical Society*; includes coverage of nanobiotechnology, self- and directed-assembly and related subjects.

Nanoscale
http://www.rsc.org/Publishing/Journals/NR/index.asp
Publication of *the Royal Society of Chemistry* with coverage of nanoscience and nanotechnology, including nanomedicine.

3.2.3 Web Sites

A large number of Web sites and Web journals with an emphasis on nanomedicine have appeared. The table below includes a few examples. New nanomedicine-related sites, blogs, and newsletters are appearing regularly on the Web.

Web sites

http://www.nanomedicinecenter.com/
NanomedicineCenter.com is a Web site founded in March 2008. It is dedicated to nanomedicine and bionanotechnology, very exciting subfields on nanotechnology. The site is maintained by five students from all around the world (United States, Austria, Australia, Bosnia and Herzegovina, and India).

http://www.foresight.org/nanomedicine/NanomedResearch.html
This site has extensive information on nanotechnology/nanomedicine including information on nanomedicine researchers (biographies), information on nanotechnology (from general to technical), and a thorough list of nanomedicine research, governmental, and commercial organizations.

---

http://nanotechnology.zunia.org/tag/nanomedicine/
This site covers nanotechnology for development, emphasizing opportunities and applications of nanoscience to aid and accelerate developing countries.

http://www.futuremedicine.com
A publishing site for articles on medical advances including nanomedicine.

http://www.nanoscienceworks.org/
NanoScienceWorks.org is a not-for-profit community portal for the nanoscience research community supported by Taylor & Francis Group, LLC—the publisher of this book. It is maintained and updated with articles and links on nanoscience and nanomedicine from many sources.

http://www.nano-biology.net/
A Web portal covering medicine on the nanoscale at a popular level.

http://www.library.ualberta.ca/subject/nanomedicine/index.cfm
The University of Alberta Libraries maintain a *Resource Guide for Nanomedicine* with a comprehensive list of links to nanomedicine Web sites and other resources, similar to those maintained at many libraries serving institutions active in nanoscience. It is a source for updated links to nanomedicine resources.

3.2.4 National Initiatives and Institutes

Governments and nonprofit bodies have commissioned centers and initiatives to develop nanoscience. A few among many with particular emphasis on nanomedicine and nanotechnology are listed in the table below.

National Initiatives

Canada:
Canadian Regenerative Medicine and Nanomedicine Enterprise (CARMENE)
(Canadian National Institute for Nanotechnology of the National Research Council of Canada)
Canadian Institutes of Health Research (CIHR) (http://www.cihr-irsc.gc.ca)
Canadian NanoBusiness Alliance (CNBA, http://www.nanobusiness.ca/)

China:
National Center for Nanoscience and Technology of China
www.nanoctr.cn/english/
See also:
http://cancerres.aacrjournals.org/cgi/content/full/69/13/5294

Europe:
European Technology Platform NANOMEDICINE http://cordis.europa.eu/nanotechnology/nanomedicine.htm
(See also the many initiatives of the individual European countries)

India:
Nano Science and Technology Mission (Nano Mission)
http://203.200.89.92/dst/scientific-programme/ser-nsti.htm
(Ministry of Science and Technology)
http://203.200.89.92/dst/admin_finance/rs_209/un_sq2832.htm
Agharkar Research Institute, Pune
http://203.200.89.92/dst/about_us/ar07-08/dst-inst-app.htm
See also:
http://203.200.89.92/dst/whats_new/press-release06/california-university.htm
http://203.200.89.92/dst/admin_finance/un-sq-r-2531.htm

Japan:
National Institute of Health Sciences (NIHS)
http://www.nihs.go.jp/english/index.html
www.nihs.go.jp/mhlw/chemical/nano/nanoindex.html

Korea:
Nano System Institute (NSI)
http://www.nsi.snu.ac.kr

Russia:
RusNano
http://www.rusnanoforum.com/Home.aspx

Singapore:
Institute of Bioengineering and Nanotechnology
http://www.ibn.a-star.edu.sg/

South Africa:
South African Nanotechnology Initiative (SANI)
http://www.sani.org.za/

Taiwan:
The Center for Nanomedicine Research (C-NMR) at NHRI
http://cnmr.nhri.org.tw/popout.php

Thailand:
NANOTEC National Nanotechnology Development Center
http://www.nanotec.or.th/en/index.php

United States:
US NIH Nano Task Force
http://www.nih.gov/science/nanotechnology/

Other Examples of Nanoscience and Nanomedicine Initiatives in all Parts of the World Include
ACTION-GRID: a consortium for medical technology and nanomedicine among countries of the European Union, Latin America, the Western Balkans, and North Africa.
http://www.action-grid.eu/

See also:

Worldwide Development and Commercialization of Nanomedicine
Chapter in: *The Handbook of Nanomedicine*
Kewal K. Jain, Editor
Publisher: Humana Press
DOI 10.1007/978-1-60327-319-0
2008

In addition, there are many state and local nanoscience initiatives within countries, many of which emphasize medical nanoscience applications. An example is the Alliance for NanoHealth (ANH), established in 2005, comprising eight leading research universities and institutions within the Texas Medical Center and the Greater Houston Region.

The ANH is a multidisciplinary collaborative research endeavor to develop nanotechnology-based solutions to unresolved problems in medicine, by bridging the gaps between medicine, biology, materials science, computer technology, and public policy. Its principal goal is to provide new clinical approaches to saving lives through better diagnosis, treatment, and prevention. (see: http://www.nanohealthalliance.org/about-us)

For many other similar examples of nanotech alliances and initiatives, see http://www.google.com/Top/Science/Technology/Nanotechnology/

3.2.5 Societies

A number of societies and associations have been formed with various degrees of backing and support from the medical profession and technical community. Among the more substantial are the following:

Nanomedicine Professional Societies
America–Japan Nanomedicine Society (AJNS)
Nanomedicine: Nanotechnology, Biology and Medicine, 2(4), 297–298
T. Urisu, C. Wei

American Society for Nanomedicine (ASNM) (www.amsocnanomed. org)

ASNM is a professional nonprofit, medical society that promotes worldwide research activities in nanomedicine and explores the applications of nanotechnology in the pharmaceutical, device and biotechnology industries. Members also discuss issues such as ethics, toxicity, patents, and commercialization. They are drawn from diverse and overlapping fields such as biotechnology, engineering, medicine, policy, and law. Members enjoy numerous benefits, including reduced rates to attend ASNM conferences and discounted rates to ASNM-affiliated journals.

Contacts: Dr. Esther Chang, Acting President, American Society for Nanomedicine, Professor of Oncology, Georgetown University Medical Center, Washington, DC, USA; Phone: +202 687 8418 esther.chang9@ gmail.com

The European Society of Nanomedicine promotes research into nanomedicine application and implications for humanity and environment, keeping always in view the welfare of individuals and society. ESNAM represents the clinical nanomedical community to governmental and international boards, associations, and industry oriented networks. *Contact*: European Society for Nanomedicine®
c/o European Foundation for Clinical Nanomedicine
Alemannengasse 12
CH-4016 Basel
Phone +41 61 695 93 95
Fax +41 61 695 93 90

Japan Nanomedicine Society
http://nanomedicine.ims.ac.jp/

3.2.6 Publications, Patents, and Product Development

Since 1990, the number of nanomedicine papers in the technical and scientific literature has increased steadily, accelerating since 2001. The number of patents has grown with even more acceleration since 2000. In 2006, a review by V. Wagner et al. published in *Nature Biotechnology* gave figures for growth in nanomedicine papers, patents, companies, products, and research projects (Figure 3.1).

The article contains graphs and tables with data up until 2005, including sectors such as image enhancement, drug delivery, diagnostics, biomaterials, and implants. More than 200 companies were listed with nanomedicine products sales estimated totaling $6.8 billions. In addition to development taking place within major companies, a number of partnerships were in place between small start-up companies and large pharmaceutical and

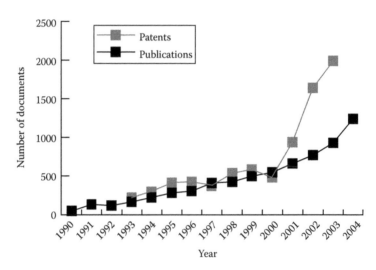

FIGURE 3.1
Growth of published papers and patents in nanomedicine (1990–2004). (From Wagner, V. et al., *Nat. Biotechnol.*, 24, 1211, 2006. With permission.)

medical device companies. Since 2006, the growth in nanomedicine and medical nanotechnology has continued its acceleration.

3.3 NIH Nanomedicine Initiative

In this section, we take a quick look at one of the most far-reaching and comprehensive programs for the development of nanomedicine, that of the United States National Institutes of Health (NIH). The spirit behind this program is summed up in the following quotation from the NIH Roadmap for Medical Research:

> What if doctors could search out and destroy the very first cancer cells that would otherwise have caused a tumor to develop in the body? What if a broken part of a cell could be removed and replaced with a miniature biological machine? What if pumps the size of molecules could be implanted to deliver life-saving medicines precisely when and where they are needed? These scenarios may sound unbelievable, but they are the long-term goals of the NIH Roadmap's Nanomedicine initiative that we anticipate will yield medical benefits as early as 10 years from now.

The NIH defines nanomedicine as the highly specific application of nanotechnology to medical intervention at the molecular scale for curing disease or repairing damaged tissues, such as bone, muscle, or nerve. The nanometer-size scale—about 100 nm or less—is the scale on which biological molecules and structures inside living cells operate.

Nanotechnology involves the creation and use of materials and devices at the level of molecules and atoms. It is essential to understand the physical and chemical properties of molecules or complexes of molecules in order to control them. The same holds true for the molecules and structures inside living tissues.

Medical science has powerful tools to examine the parts of cells in detail down to the molecular level. It is the goal of nanomedicine to understand further how intracellular structures operate, in order to build "nano" structures or "nano" machines that are compatible with living tissues and can safely operate inside the body. The ultimate goal is to design diagnostic tools and engineer structures for highly specific and precise treatments of disease and repair of tissues.

3.3.1 Nanomedicine Research Programs

Under the leadership of the NIH, nanoscience is being developed in conjunction with advanced medical science for further precision in diagnosis and treatment. Multidisciplinary biomedical scientific teams including biologists, physicians, mathematicians, engineers, and computer scientists are working to gather information about the physical properties of intracellular structures upon which biology's molecular machines are built. New emphasis is being given to moving medical science from the laboratory to the bedside and the community.

As researchers gain knowledge of the interactions between molecules and larger structures, patterns will emerge, and we will have a greater understanding of the intricate operations of processes and networks inside living cells. Mapping these networks and understanding how they change over time will, in turn, enable researchers to use this information to correct biological defects in unhealthy cells. New tools that will work at the nanoscale and allow scientists to build synthetic biological devices such as nanosensors to scan for the presence of infectious agents, or metabolic imbalances that could spell trouble for the body, and miniature devices to destroy infectious agents or fix the "broken" parts in cells are being developed.

3.3.2 The NIH Nanomedicine Roadmap

The NIH has developed a series of roadmaps planning research to develop new means to intervene at the nanoscale or molecular level. These include the *National Technology Centers for Networks and Pathways*, a network of centers that will create new tools to describe the dynamics of protein interactions. The Centers will develop instruments, methods, and reagents for quantitative measurements at subcellular resolution and very short timescales. In addition, the NIH is creating *Nanomedicine Development Centers* [**see boxes**] that will focus on the engineering of new tools for medical interventions and diagnosis at the nanoscale or molecular level. The Nanomedicine Centers' research will support the development of synthetic biological devices, such as miniature, implantable pumps for drug delivery, or implantable or mobile sensors to scan for signs of infectious agents, metabolic imbalances, or other biomarkers to detect disease [2].

Some of the areas in which emerging medical nanoscience is targeted to impact are the following:

1. New medical materials for cell growth scaffolding and tissue repair
2. Enhancement of diagnosis and imaging
3. Enhancement of drug delivery
4. Understanding and control over biomolecular mechanisms
5. Discovery of properties and medical effects of smaller units of life and nanoparticles

Areas of medical care that will benefit from the above nanoscience advances are as follows:

1. Plastic surgery and wound healing using nanogels and nanoengineered scaffolding materials.
2. Repair of cut nerves using nanofabricated growth channels with cell growth coating patterns.
3. Improved healing and fusion of bone fractures using nanopatterned porous implants.
4. Selective image enhancement of diseased cells with antibody-coated nanoparticles.
5. Reduction of MRI interaction with surgical and sensor probes by nanoengineering coatings.
6. Targeted drug delivery with surface modified and coated nanoparticles.
7. Drug delivery across the blood–brain barrier with "smart" nanoparticles.
8. Custom-designed molecular enzymes to selectively switch cell functions on or off.
9. Custom-designed phage-like molecular machines to deliver drugs or kill cancer cells.
10. Custom-designed molecular enzyme machines to diagnose and repair subcellular structures.
11. A suite of molecular enzyme machines to selectively initiate cell death in cancer cells.
12. Artificial molecular agents to engulf and deactivate prions, attack viruses, and digest refractory plaques.

The First Eight NIH Nanomedicine Centers and Their Research Areas

Summary of the work at the Nanomedicine Development Centers funded to date (2006) through the National Eye Institute and their goals for diseases and medical research. Each of the centers is highly multi-disciplinary and involves multiple institutions such as schools of bio-medical science, medicine, engineering, and hospitals. For a guide and links to further information, see the NIH Web site.
Source: http://nihroadmap.nih.gov/nanomedicine/fundedresearch.asp (Accessed May 2007)

1. Nanomedicine Center for Mechanical Biology
   Columbia University leading partnership of six institutions
   Research on the roles of force, rigidity, and form in regulating cell functions signaling pathways and gene expression, and their influence on diseases such as cancers, immune disorders, genetic malformations, and neuropathies, using tools of nanotechnology and modern cell biology.

2. UCSF/UCB Center for Engineering Cellular Control Systems
   University of California San Francisco and University of California Berkley
   Work on engineering "grand challenges" to develop modified cells or cell-like molecular assemblies that perform intelligently guided precision therapeutic functions, such as tissue repair or "search and deliver" treatment of microscopic tumors or cardiovascular lesions by focusing on reengineering cell guidance, cell force generation, and cell motility systems.

3. National Center for Design of Biomimetic Nanoconductors
   University of Illinois Urbana-Champaign
   Research to design synthetic arrays of ion transport channels based on biological ion channels and other ion transport proteins, inserted in arrays of pores on substrates to study cell signaling, energy transport, and generation of osmotic pressures and flows, in order to gain insight into biological processes and disease targeting, and to develop practical applications such as biosensors, osmotic pumps, and power generation.

4. Center for Protein Folding Machinery
   Baylor College of Medicine with Stanford University
   An interdisciplinary program to define the basic chemical and physical principles used by molecular chaperones in the folding of proteins in order to engineer protein machines to assist the folding of any protein of interest, as well as develop strategies to alleviative or prevent protein misfolding associated with a number of human diseases.

5. Nanomedicine Development Center for the Optical Control of Biological Function
   University of California Lawrence Berkeley National Laboratory
   Developing methods for rapidly turning select proteins in cells on and off with light, developing chemical and molecular toolkits for integration of optical control into proteins, viral delivery of photo-switchable proteins into cells, and light delivery systems to address these nanodevices in vivo, with the aim of treating retinal and cardiac pathologies by gaining optical control over the signaling and enzymatic activity of cells.

6. The Center for Systemic Control of Cyto-Networks
   University of California Los Angeles
   The goal for this center is to use engineering principles to develop global system control methods to investigate and manipulate the complex cell signaling network governing homeostasis of cells in order to control and correct perturbations in the network by invading organisms, accumulation of pathologic substances, and uncontrolled cell growth that are the hallmarks of most morbid and mortal illness, especially conditions like cancers, infectious diseases, and stem cell–related disorders.

7. Nanomotor Drug Delivery Center
   Purdue University
   Creation of biocompatible membranes and arrays with embedded phi29 in vitro viral packaging biomotors for DNA insertion applications in medicine by reverse engineering the phi29 motor, incorporating the active nanomotor into lipid bilayers, and developing active nanomotor arrays that enable drug delivery and diagnostics.

8. Nanomedicine Center for Nucleoprotein Machines
   Georgia Tech with Emory University and Medical College of Georgia
   Using nanotechnology and biomolecular approaches, elucidate the structure–function relationships within and among DNA repair nanomachines, for precise modification of DNA and RNA, leading to therapeutic strategies for a wide range of diseases.

3.3.3 Center for Nucleoprotein Machines

For example, the NIH-funded National Nanomedicine Center for Nucleoprotein Machines based at Georgia Tech, in collaboration with Emory University and the Medical College of Georgia, will take a biomedical engineering design approach to the repair of DNA, focusing on a model nanomachine that carries out nonhomologous end joining (NHEJ) of DNA double strand breaks. This and other DNA repair machines have relatively simple structures (<20 components) and significant biological and clinical relevance, and thus are promising as feasible models for nanoscience engineering approaches. DNA repair is vitally important to human health, as both normal metabolic activities and environmental factors can cause DNA damage, resulting in as many as 100,000 individual molecular lesions per cell per day. If allowed to accumulate without repair, these lesions interfere with gene transcription and replication, leading to premature aging, apoptosis, or unregulated cell division. The nucleoprotein machine engineering approach is as follows:

1. Develop protein tags and fluorescence probes including quantum dot bioconjugates for nanomachine targeting.
2. Decipher structure–function relationship for the NHEJ reaction.
3. Characterize the dynamics of nanomachine assembly and disassembly in the repair process.
4. Determine the dimensions and structure of repair foci at high resolution in fixed cells.
5. Establish engineering design principles for DNA double-strand break repair.

The Georgia Nucleoprotein Machines Center will complement the other NDCs that focus on filaments, membranes, and protein-folding enzymes. The probes, tools, and methodologies developed in these centers will be useful as tools for biological and disease research, and may ultimately provide genetic cures for common human diseases based on the ability to manipulate the somatic human genome using nanomedicine.

To match the NIH nanomedicine initiative, many of the institutes comprising the NIH that focus on specific medical specializations and diseases are proposing supporting programs to provide medical areas of application as motivation for the new tools being developed at the nanomedicine centers. These programs are aimed at improving diagnosis and treatment with nanotechnology-based techniques and materials in the areas of cancer, radiology, and others. For example, the National Cancer Institute (NCI) has a Nanotechnology Plan that is distinct from, but complementary to, the NIH Nanomedicine Roadmap. The NCI plan "focuses on using knowledge from basic research discoveries and translating that into clinical oncology applications. The endpoints of this effort will be technology platforms in the context of diagnostics and therapeutics." [3]

The goals of nanomedicine are extrapolations of advances that have been made in the past by application of new science and technology to medicine. Not all will be successful in their application. Many will be controversial, which is not new in the history of medicine.

3.4 Putting Medical Nanoscience into Practice: Medical Nanotechnology and Nanomedicine

In the remaining chapters, we explore how nanoscience is being applied to medicine in many areas: radiology, oncology, endocrinology, neurology, orthopedics, cardiology, otology, ophthalmology, emergency care, obstetrics and gynecology, gastroenterology, surgery, and others. These include nanoparticles, nanoencapsulation, biomolecular nanotechnology, and nanodevices such as microfluidic biochips, diagnostic lab-on-a-chip devices, nanodroplet dispensers, cell manipulation and separation chips and micromanipulators, and DNA/RNA nanotechnology, with applications in pathology, diagnostics, cytology, genetics, forensic medicine, etc. Clinical nanotechnology applications are being applied to enhance or enable new diagnostic and therapeutic methods, including

1. Enhancement agents for medical imaging
2. Finding and destroying cancer cells
3. Delivering drugs deep into tumors (cancer)
4. Delivering insulin through novel routes (diabetes)
5. Delivering drugs through the blood–brain barrier (Alzheimer's, Parkinson's, etc.)
6. Guiding and stimulating nerve regeneration (spinal cord injury, paralysis)
7. Improving neural stimulation (cardiac pacemakers, neuroprosthetics)
8. Noninvasive, sensitive detection of nerve activity (ECG, Brain–Machine Prosthetics)
9. Less invasive hearing and vision prosthetics (hearing and vision loss)
10. Improved remote medical monitoring (preventive, postoperative, recuperative, etc.)
11. Wearable and minimally invasive wireless physiological sensors (GI, Ob-Gyn, etc.)
12. New tissue scaffolds and artificial tissues and organs (surgery, wound care, etc.)
13. Advanced minimally invasive and effective surgical tools and techniques

Ultimately medical technologies will merge across the micro, nano, and molecular scales into an integrated medical science supporting more powerful and effective medical practice, made more accessible and cost effective by the availability of tools that operate on the scale of the machinery of the cell.

References

1. V. Wagner, A. Dullaart, A.-K. Bock, and A. Zweck, The emerging nanomedicine landscape, *Nature Biotechnology*, 24, 1211–1217 (2006).
2. NIH Roadmap Web page at http://nihroadmap.nih.gov/initiatives.asp (2008).
3. NCI Nanotechnology Plan Web page at http://www.cancer.gov/researchfunding/NIHRoadmapFAQs (2008).
4. H. Fenniri, The Canadian Regenerative Medicine and Nanomedicine Enterprise (CARMENE), *International Journal of Nanomedicine*, 1, 225–227 (2006) PMCID: PMC2426808.

Part II

Beginnings of Medical Nanotechnology

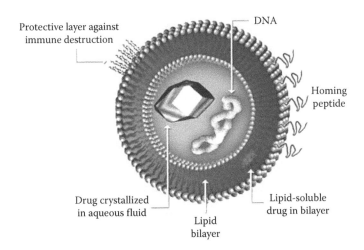

Liposome for drug delivery

4

Nanomedicine: Proposals and Promise

> Nanomedicine, the application of nanotechnology in healthcare, offers numerous very promising possibilities to significantly improve medical diagnosis and therapy, leading to an affordable higher quality of life for everyone.
>
> **Nanomedicine, European Technology Platform, November, 2006**

4.1 Introduction and Overview

Part II is an overview of the nanotechnology-based developments that are impacting medicine.

This chapter gives a brief overview of the main influences driving nanotechnology impacts on medicine, and some of the current directions of those impacts, which will be covered in Chapters 5 through 9.

The theme of Chapter 5 is *medication*: how nanotechnology helps to deliver drugs and therapies by identifying and reaching targets. We begin our overview of nanotechnology in medicine with a look at the simplest nanoscale level: the role of nanoparticles and nanotechnology in imaging and targeting for delivery of molecular drugs, thermal energy, radiation, and other therapies.

The theme of Chapter 6 is *intervention*: how nanotechnology and nanotechnology-based tools extend the reach and capacities of surgery. In this chapter, we deal with nanotechnology at the macrolevel: nanotechnology impacts on surgical techniques such as endoscopy, robotic surgery, and other advanced technologies to salvage, repair, and reconstruct tissues and organs.

The theme of Chapter 7 is *regeneration*: how nanotechnology is used to support and guide cell and tissue growth. Here, we look at regenerative tissue engineering and how nanotechnology is used with cellular engineering to guide the growth of regenerated tissues to modify the DNA of cells and to reprogram cells and create stem cells for tissue renewal.

The theme of Chapter 8 is *restoration*: how nanotechnology helps to restore and/or replace missing and disabled functions and organs. In Chapter 8, we look at nanomaterials for implants and for tissue and organ replacement, and the nanotechnology impact on prosthetics, including how nanotechnology enables the creation of dynamic functional motor prostheses and neurosensory prostheses.

The theme of Chapter 9 is *diagnosis*: how nanotechnologies improve capabilities for detection, analysis, and monitoring of health and disease. In this chapter, we conclude Part II with a look at how nanotechnology makes feasible and affordable sensors for single molecule detection, monitoring of disease, personal monitoring, personal DNA analysis, and new capabilities for diagnosis and clinical analysis.

4.2 Impacts of Nanotechnology on Medicine

The application of nanotechnology to medicine is advancing in many different areas. In the development of nanomedicine, three trends are discernable: a subtle evolutionary and incremental development path, a radical and revolutionary program proposal, and an indirect and less deliberate but inevitable impact of nanotechnologies affecting broad areas of society and economy. These developments are converging to fill a long-acknowledged gap between the science and technology of the chemical scale and what has been accessible on the biological scale.

The first impact of nanoscience on medicine is evolutionary: naturally arising from research that has progressed from the micro- to the nanoscale in cell biology and from the molecular scale back up to the nanoscale in biochemistry and molecular biology. This long-term and natural development arose from the discovery and appreciation of the role of the nanoscale in the macromolecular basis of life.

A second development is explicit and revolutionary, emphasizing great advances to be gained by radical new nanotechnology approaches (most notably the enthusiastic programs of nanoengineering and carbon nanotube applications). This group of initiatives and proposals has attracted much attention and support, and has led to a coalescing of thought and organization around formal programs such as the NIH nanomedicine initiatives.

A third source of nanotechnology impact on medicine is indirect through the development and application of ever-improving nanotools and devices based on smaller and more precise technologies. These technologies impact research, diagnostics, and therapeutics, and have been developed in most cases outside the context of any nanomedicine program. Nevertheless, the capabilities of such instruments are being expanded, driven by advances in nanotechnology. Less direct, but equally important, nanotechnology is beginning to impact medicine by the way it is enhancing and transforming computing, communications, and information storage and retrieval.

4.2.1 The Natural Evolution of Nanomedicine from Physics, Chemistry, and Biology

The evolutionary growth for nanomedicine arose from research that progressed from the micro- to the nanoscale (in the case of microbiology, cell biology, and histology), and from the molecular scale back up to the nanoscale (in the case of molecular biology, biophysics, biochemistry, and pharmacology). This evolution has culminated by the embracing of nanoscience language and concepts by many molecular biologists in describing mechanisms and structures of DNA, RNA, proteins, membranes, and cell signaling. This has been a long term and natural development as tools and techniques revealed the nanoscale features and mechanisms involved in the macromolecular basis of life. These developments have proceeded incrementally and quietly in research laboratories, attracting relatively little attention as a unified trend. Their successes and accomplishments have been divided among the many different traditional academic disciplines and biomedical specializations. These developments have only lately come to be thought of as a unified advance within the context of nanoscience.

4.2.2 Revolutionary Program Proposals

The second development, characterized as explicit and revolutionary, is an outgrowth of the nanotechnology movement, emphasizing great advances to be gained by radical new nanotechnology approaches (most notably the enthusiastic programs of nanoengineering and carbon nanotube applications). It is this arena that is sometimes thought of as exclusively constituting nanomedicine, thereby drawing attention away from the broader parallel developments. The nanotechnology proposals have even tended to eclipse earlier nanoscale work in molecular electronics and biological nanomanipulation. This group of initiatives and proposals has attracted much attention and support, and has led to a coalescing of thought and organization around formal programs such as the DoD, NSF, and NIH nanomedicine initiatives. The latter has sought to bring various threads of the first two areas under one umbrella. As with most revolutions, the more radical elements tend to be co-opted over time and their energies harnessed into the mainstream.

4.2.3 Inevitable Indirect Impacts of Nanotechnology

The third nanotechnology impact on medicine was simply the development and application of ever-improving nanotools such as electron microscopy, atomic force microscopy, dielectrophoresis, optical tweezers, membrane patch techniques, nanoscale probes and sensors, and sub-micro devices and tools for image enhancement, diagnostics, therapeutics, and prosthetics. These techniques and tools have been developed in some cases by biomedical researchers to meet challenges embodied in biology, but in other cases they have been adopted from instruments originally developed for physical and material applications. In both instances, they have resulted in bringing new developments in physics, chemistry, electronics, and engineering to bear on biological research. Thus, they are a less direct trend than the intrinsic and more recognized growth of biological and cellular nanoscience, for which they serve as tools in aid of discovery and analysis.

Even less directly, but equally important, nanotechnology is posed to have profound impacts on medicine by enhancing and transforming computing, communications, and information storage and retrieval. The spread of electronic intelligence, sensing, and interaction into every aspect of social and economic life will impact medicine just as every other activity and experience.

4.2.4 Effect of Technology on Skilled Practice

For a picture of how technology could impact the highly skilled practitioner in medicine, examine for a moment the impact that technology has had across the board on professions that depend on a high level of individual and team performance by skilled individuals. Take for example, performance art. Entertainment often leads in the adoption of new technologies into lifestyle in disruptive ways. In part, this is simply because entertainment is by far the largest economic sector, encompassing music, art, theatre, cinema, sports, leisure reading, tourism, gambling, games, and outdoor recreational activities such as hiking, hunting, fishing, gardening, collecting, crafts, and many other activities, some of which disguise themselves as political, business, and religious.

Performance was once a poor cousin to more participatory sectors of the entertainment economy such as grand tours, jousts, hunts, and pilgrimages. Musical and acting troupes were practically synonymous with beggars and itinerant hucksters. But technology vastly magnified the productivity of musicians, first by standardizing performance with written music, permitting repeatable and larger scale performances that could reach larger and broader audiences, then by recording the performances, so that an initial performance investment could be resold and rebroadcast manifold.

As late as the 1960s, it was seriously stated that technology and mass production could not affect music, because the product was the performance itself. But a revolution had already occurred, starting late in the nineteenth century, as recordings, radio, motion pictures, and television took primacy over live performances. In the process, music and drama became much more widely accessible and affordable. The same process concentrated production by an enormous factor, creating huge wealth for those who leveraged the magnifying power of the new electronic media.

Eventually, the ubiquity and cheapness of these media shifted control of artistic content toward the masses in an ever-widening and lowering wave. Paradoxically, performance of singing, music, dance, and sport became less and less participatory and more and more became passive consumption of performances delivered effortlessly via the media. Even live performances took on more and more electronic media special effects, with productions replacing performances. Are there implications in this history for the future development of medicine?

Today, medicine is one of the last bastions of the highly skilled guild crafts. All of the other most worthy and worshipful crafts have succumbed to technology and capital, with the possible exceptions of the politician, the lawyer, the lobbyist, and the financial CEO. Technology works change, and especially nanotechnology, because it addresses the core content of the medical craft—biology on the nanoscale. But technology does not eliminate the premium placed on human management skills, creativity, responsiveness, and dedication: airline pilots are still skilled and valuable in spite of cockpit controls and autopilot systems.

Technologies such as mass-produced pharmaceuticals and diagnostic tests have tended toward commoditization of much of medical care. Consumers of healthcare are becoming more knowledgeable and participating more in healthcare decisions (or at least more opinionated—with much the same effect). Major decisions are being removed from control of the individual practitioner as care becomes more highly technical and specialized. Laboratory tests and reviews by specialists who never actually see the patient become key factors in medical decision making, not to mention rules and guidelines exercised by insurance and healthcare organization coordinators. Care is becoming more automated and instrumented. Precision drugs, devices, and therapies are prescribed by the physician, but also proscribed in time and form of usage by codes and conventions of practice. Automated monitoring and response are systematized and extend care out of the physicians' clinic and hospital to the patient's home, workplace, and living space.

Characterization of the patient's individual genotype and physiology are made possible and economically feasible by the nanotechnology which has shrunk the time and cost of gene sequencing as well as by the ability to gather, store, and process the vast amounts of information that results, and to enable that information to be communicated and carried wherever the patient goes. The very concept of a patient—who comes to the doctor with a complaint to be treated—has been replaced increasingly by the concept of a member of a health maintenance community—whose health condition is to be monitored, guided, and even predicted based on knowledge of genotype, phenotype, work, and lifestyle.

What do these changes have to do with nanotechnology? Nanotechnology is the driving enabler for smaller, faster, cheaper, more powerful, electronic, photonic, and wireless devices and systems, which are becoming more ubiquitous, saturated, and integrated into our lives. Nanotechnology, in essence, is no different than microtechnology, angstrom-technology (chemistry), or macrotechnology—it is unique in many aspects and phenomena that are found only in matter at the nanoscale—but it differs from earlier technologies only in being less explored, and in that it opens vast new possibilities that are being exploited at exponential rates. The majority of even the most avid advocates of the nanotechnology future admit that the boundaries are arbitrary. It is technology that is driving and embodying change—and nanotechnology being very small, has an inversely proportional very large possibility for exploration and innovation, with the use of proportionally small expense of energy and materials.

Medicine has already undergone a major repositioning in its role in society over the past half century. Huge amounts of medical effort were once devoted to the treatment and prevention of infectious disease. With the conquest of disease pathogens by antibiotics, effort was redirected to manage, control, prevent, and treat the symptoms of chronic diseases such as arteriosclerosis, heart failure, stenosis, gastric ulcers, osteoporosis, and diseases such as diabetes and sickle cell anemia. But also increasingly medicine has served less life-threatening medical needs, and in some cases, elective choices about patient's bodies and health—contraceptive pills, erectile function, infertility, plastic and cosmetic surgery—the line is blurred between an illness to be remedied and a shortcoming to be enhanced. Medicine is not the first place that technology removed or displaced or postponed stark moral dilemmas and choices.

Nanotechnology, along with wireless technology, photonics, chemistry, electronics, computing, physics, and biology is making possible the distribution of individualized custom medicine throughout every aspect of life—work, leisure, rest, entertainment. Medicine may be integrated into lifestyle and implemented on the individual level in personalized devices, which communicate with a broad network for monitoring, treatment, and prevention.

These concepts are already becoming a reality. At the Mary Crawford Cancer Center in Dallas, for example, the first step in treatment is to perform a genetic analysis. Only after analysis of the genetic testing is a treatment prescribed—specific to the patient's genetic makeup. Companies like Vertex are developing drugs for disorders like cystic fibrosis with a genetic component—drugs that target a specific genetic modification for any one of the multiple genetic defects that contribute to the manifestation of the disease. These drugs are targeted to influence specific steps in the folding of a key protein that is an essential part of chloride gates in cell membranes. The design and delivery of such drugs depends on detailed and specific knowledge of protein and membrane processes at the nanoscale.

The instruments necessary to decipher such processes and to perform massive screening and selection for effective targeted drugs are products of nanotechnology in the broad sense, meaning the technology for analyzing and manipulating with precision at the nanoscale. Such a strategy of drug targeting and development would not have been possible with classical biochemistry and pharmacology.

4.2.5 The Integrated Effect of Three Trends

The simultaneous interaction of all three trends—incremental, radical, and incidental—combines to develop a new paradigm of individual personalized medicine delivered over a multilevel network of medical, economic, and social organization. This organization is based on nanoscale knowledge of biological processes and materials gained through (1) continually advancing biomedical research, (2) focused programs to apply new nanoscale technologies to medicine, and (3) the rapidly growing capabilities of multiple technologies being expanded at the nanoscale to provide new molecular sensor probes, high-capacity adaptable communications networks, and powerful distributed information processing capabilities.

There is no doubt that nanotechnology will make contributions to medicine, but real progress will come about only when the technology is integrated and subordinated to the needs of medicine.

4.3 An Overview of the Architecture of Medical Nanotechnology and Nanomedicine

In the remainder of Part II (Chapters 5 through 9), we describe some of the interesting areas where nanotechnology is being applied to medicine, and how its impacts are being felt. We start with an overview of the new medical nanotechnologies, how they are natural outgrowths of historical trends in the development of medicine, and where they have the promise of making the most effective progress.

Figure 4.1 is a schematic representation of the different types of sub-nano-, nano-, micro-, and macrotechnology applications in medicine, laid out on an x–y planar graph. The lower left origin of the diagram represents the smallest and simplest units available to apply as therapeutics—heat, light, elementary particles, atoms, and small molecules. When we expand the development of medical technology in the direction of geometric extension in space (structural dimensionality), we start to build complex molecules, macromolecules, nanofibers, nanotubing, and 2D and 3D scaffolding and structures with nanoscale features in their geometry. When we move in the direction of more complexity, along the horizontal axis, we stay with nanoparticles, but we start to build increasing functionality, with mechanical, electrical, optical, and chemical actions on the nanoscale. When we develop along both directions together, we obtain nanodevices, smart materials, bioactive wound dressings, implants and scaffolds, MEMS, artificial organs, and prostheses (Figure 4.1).

Medical technology can supply therapies for application over a wide range of these size and complexity domains. Therapies start at the lowest size

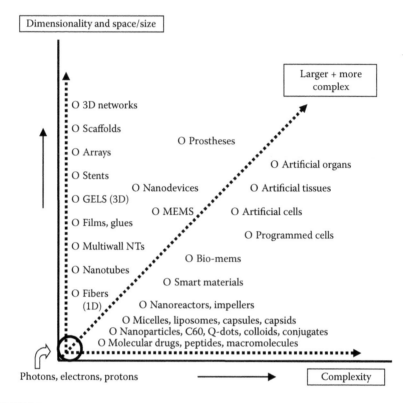

FIGURE 4.1
Architecture of medical nanotechnologies.

and increase in scale: from heat and light to x-rays, protons, and neutrons, to atoms, to small molecules, large molecules, and macromolecules. From the high end, therapies range from whole body treatments (iron lung, compression chambers, isolation units, ICUs) down through limb and sensory prostheses and assistive devices, to artificial organs, replacement valves and lenses, stents, artificial cells, stem cells, etc. Complexity can vary more or less independent of the size scale, once we expand above the molecular level. Medical nanotechnology occupies the domain connecting the molecular scale and below to the microscale and above.

On the chart, the technologies and therapeutics on the upper left side of the diagonal line are in general more derived from chemical, materials, electronic, and device engineering; those on the lower right side of the line tend to be more heavily derived from biochemistry, pharmacology, polymer and protein science, and molecular, cell, and genetic biology. But in the nano-region, the central part of the chart, these distinctions break down, as nanotechnologies involve the integrated application of all of these disciplines.

On the chart in Figure 4.1, we could also have irregular shaped and overlapping areas representing the different disciplines that address these domains: biochemistry, physiology, biophysics, molecular genetics, molecular biology, biotechnology, cell biology, tissue engineering, etc. The Venn diagram would have to be of Byzantine complexity to represent the weird and wonderful divisions of academic and technical specialities.

As it stands, the placement of categories on the diagram is very approximate: they would be more accurately represented by overlapping areas with fuzzy boundaries. Medical nanobots as generally portrayed in popular depictions would fall somewhere in a fuzzy area around MEMS, nanodevices, impellers, and artificial cells (perhaps on the imaginary axis). Another dimension not represented on the chart in Figure 4.1 is time—as in pharmacodynamics, time release and biodegradable capsules, adaptive bioactive scaffolds, therapy schedules, etc.

It has been realized for a long time that there is a gap in biology and medicine between the microscale and the chemical scale. Biochemistry, physiology, and molecular biology can offer insights and therapies up to a point. Cell biology and microbiology approach from the opposite size scale, but there is a substantial gap remaining in the domain of large subcellular structures and mechanisms—precisely in the size domain of nanoscience. This gap is being rapidly filled by research and development, which may or may not go by the names of nanoscience and nanotechnology. Those terms have become recognized in recent years as a useful and integrative way to describe this highly complex and interdisciplinary area.

In Chapter 5, *Medication*, we start along the nanoparticle axis, from relatively simple nanoparticles used for medical imaging to more complex therapeutics including photothermal and drug delivery particles. In discussing examples of how these nanomedicine particles are applied to some specific diseases such as cancer and diabetes, we explore tentatively into the upper middle of the chart, with encapsulation, nanodevices, micropumps, smart materials, and other nanoengineered devices for targeted drug delivery and multipurpose therapies. We conclude Chapter 5 with an introduction to theranostics. We return to an overview discussion of these latter areas in the final chapters.

Chapter 6, *Intervention*, continues with discussion of the materials, engineering, and nanotechnology aspects of surgical therapy. In Chapter 6, we follow the vertical axis—the "nanostructures" axis—and discuss surgical materials, then move toward the center of the chart to discuss endoscopic technologies and surgical robotics.

Chapter 7, *Regeneration*, is devoted to the nanobiological aspects that come into play with tissue engineering and truly restorative therapy as opposed to tissue repair or replacement. The application of these technologies focuses especially on the challenge of restoring and regenerating neural tissues, but there are other applications as well. Regenerative nanomedicine takes us into a discussion of scaffolding and support for encapsulated and implanted stem cells, and into the new area of epigenetic cell reprogramming to create induced plutipotent stem cells, and their medical implications.

In Chapter 8, *Restoration*, we discuss applications of nanoengineered particles, fibers, films, scaffolding, and other nanomaterials for tissue restoration and prostheses, including smart materials, MEMs, NEMS, and other active nanodevices. We discuss wound healing therapies for soft tissues and bones to give specific examples of how these nanotechnologies are being applied. We discuss the nanotechnologies that contribute to the design and fabrication of artificial organs, and we survey prostheses for neurostimulation, sensory organ replacement, and motor prosthetics. Nanotechnology has an indirect but vital contribution to these macroscale devices, with nanoengineered materials, energy storage, electronics, sensors, and actuators benefiting the design of smaller and more powerful microdevices for use in prostheses.

Chapter 9, *Diagnosis*, concludes Part II with nanotechnology impacts on biomedical sensors, medical monitoring, and DNA sequencing and gene screening, which brings us to a discussion of personalized medicine and targeted theranostics based on genetic profiles.

In Part III, the final three chapters cover a summary of how all the technologies discussed previously are being integrated, how these new technologies are changing medical practice, and their societal impacts.

The chapters in Part II contain summaries of technology backgrounds and recent research and development, at the level of reviews, with ample reference sources for readers interested in pursuing each subject in more detail. Part III returns to a less technical level for readers more interested in the economic and societal impacts of new nanomedical developments.

4.4 Nanoscience: Bridging the Gap between Biochemistry and Cell Biology

In the technology review chapters of Part II, the choice of topics is drawn from the areas on the graph that lie between chemistry and cell biology. A central goal of nanoscience is to fill the widely recognized gap in knowledge and technology between the science of life on the biochemical scale and the science of cells and organisms [1–5]. A focus on this area under the unifying theme of nanotechnology can help to redress the tendency to specialize only in aspects of the biochemistry, the genome, or cell biology, as was famously pointed out by Kornberg [1]. And, as Olson observed, following the 2003 Cold Spring Harbor Symposium on the human genome (CSHSQB LXVIII) [6]:

> At the end of his Nobel Lecture in 1955, Hugo Theorell referred to the "yawning gulf" between biochemistry and morphology. At the end of CSHSQB LXVIII, in the darkness of Grace Auditorium, we were looking out at the still larger gulf between the genome and organismal biology.

That the gap persists and is being filled by nanotechnology is acknowledged as recently as 2007 in the synopsis of a conference on single molecule detection and manipulation [7]:

> It is widely recognized that there is a considerable "Nano-Gap" in biology and medicine: Biochemistry provides a wealth of insight into interactions between small molecules up to the size of proteins, and cellular biology sheds light on the function of entire living cells. But a substantial gap remains in our understanding of the function of large sub-cellular structures. The gap in medicine is even larger: there are hardly any therapeutic measures on the scale between drugs and surgery.
>
> The reason for this gap is twofold: the inaccessibility of sub-cellular structures to experimental interrogation in vivo, and the complexity of models, as the tight coupling to the molecular and cellular scale requires sophisticated multiscale modeling. Nanotechnology can help bridge this gap by engineering structures that can interact with biological entities on the nanoscale to interrogate, manipulate, or simulate these biological systems.

In his acceptance speech for the 1974 Nobel Prize in physiology or medicine, Christian de Duve had this to say about the gap, following a reference to the earlier Nobel lecture by Theorell [8]:

> The gulf still yawns today. But it is a particular pleasure for me to be able to tell my old friend Theo that it yawns a little less. In our efforts to narrow it, my coworkers and I have been privileged to contemplate many marvelous aspects of the structural and functional organization of living cells. In addition, we have the deep satisfaction of seeing that our findings do not simply enrich knowledge, but may also help to conquer disease.

Hopefully, current researchers and practitioners who are applying nanotechnology to medicine will share that deep satisfaction for the same reasons. And hopefully, the review that follows will be useful in that endeavor.

References

1. A. Kornberg, We must try to bridge the gap between biological and chemical sciences, *The Scientist*, 2, 15 (1988).
2. P. Schuster, Extended molecular evolutionary biology: Artificial life bridging the gap between chemistry and biology, in C. G. Langton (ed.), *Artificial Life: An Overview (Complex Adaptive Systems)*, The MIT Press, Cambridge, MA, 1997.
3. C. Ahlberg, Visual exploration of HTS databases: Bridging the gap between chemistry and biology, *Drug Discovery Today*, 4, 370–376 (1999).

4. M. Barbieri, *The Organic Codes—An Introduction to Semantic Biology*, Cambridge University Press, Cambridge, U.K., 2003, reviewed in: *Genetics and Molecular Biology*, 26, 1, 105–106 (2003).
5. O. Schärer and C. Schultz, Closing the gap between chemistry and biology, *ChemBioChem*, 6, 3–5 (2005).
6. M. V. Olson, The new quantitative biology, in B. Stillman and D. Steward (eds.), *The Genome of Homo sapiens* (*Symposia on Quantitative Biology Series LXVIII*), Cold Spring Harbor Laboratory Press, Cold Spring Harbor, NY, 2004, p. 495.
7. N. Walter, J.-C. Meiners, E. Meyhofer, R. R. Neubig, R. K. Sunahara, N. C. Perkins, D. G. Steel, and J. A. Swanson, Under the microscope: Single molecule symposium at the University of Michigan, 2006, Session 4—Single molecule bionanotechnology, *Biopolymers*, 85, 106–114 (2007).
8. C. de Duve, Exploring cells with a centrifuge (Nobel Lecture, Nobel Prize for Medicine or Physiology 1974), *Science*, 189, 187–193 (1975).

5

Medication: Nanoparticles for Imaging and Drug Delivery

I think that what is exciting about working in the nanoscale is that you are in the exact perfect size to be interacting in the most effective ways with biological systems. So from the single cell level—well, even smaller, from proteins and peptides, nucleic acids—to tissues and whole organs for biomedical research. There is a natural affinity in many ways in length scale between nanotech and biotech.

Naomi Halas, Rice University [1]

5.1 Introduction: The Emergence of Nanotechnology Applications in Medicine

In Chapter 4, we surveyed some global nanomedicine initiatives. In the remaining Chapters 5 through 9 of Part II, we look at some innovations being stimulated by these and other developments. Significant results are emerging from initiatives like those of the United States Department of Health and Human Services, where the National Institutes of Health (NIH) is currently investing several hundred million dollars each year in biomedical nanotechnology research. This investment is generating advances in understanding fundamental properties of nanomaterials, development of new materials for ultrasensitive identification and detection of significant molecules for disease, and in new nanomaterials that deliver medicines to diseased or damaged cells and tissues. Many other investments around the world are directed toward improved manufacture of nanomaterials, understanding of their actions in the body, and devising of new diagnostic methods and treatments that exploit the properties of nanostructures.

From these investments, new techniques are emerging to help doctors accelerate the healing process and protect health: medicine-coated nanoparticles, nanoscale diagnostic and therapeutic devices, nanoprobes for monitoring subtle changes in the body, nanofibers for repair and regeneration of tissue, and nanoelectrodes for managing pain and regaining lost neural capabilities. These techniques are producing results in the treatment of asthma, cancer, arterial and heart disease, bone and tooth repair, prosthetics for motor and nerve function, and many other areas of medicine.

Nanoscience and nanotechnology research are also being applied to health issues such as water purification and monitoring, preservation and improvement of food, and investigation of potential health and safety issues of nanomaterials as they interact with the human body and our environment.

5.1.1 Medical Applications of Nanoparticles

As examples of the medical applications being produced by nanomedicine research initiatives, we start with the simplest type of nanomaterials— nanoparticles. Nanoparticles made of metal, carbon nanotubes, polymers, or other materials can be used in a variety of medical applications, especially when combined with antigen-specific coatings or functional groups on their surfaces (Figure 5.1). In this section, we look at some examples.

The terms "nanomedicines" and "nanomedical particles" are customarily applied to structures from 1 to 1000 nm in size. This usage is justified from a practical point of view because the synthesis or fabrication of materials in this size range generally involves nanoscale control, and produces features that result from nanoscale phenomena. Making and using molecular assemblies in this size range results in new medical effects and also requires novel, scientifically demanding chemistry and engineering. Traditional small-molecule drugs are not specifically engineered on the nanoscale, but many of

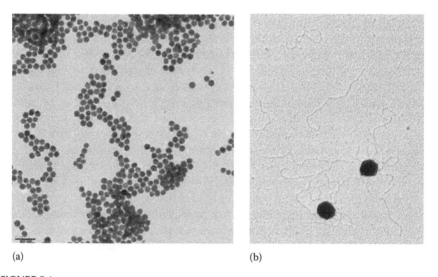

(a)   (b)

FIGURE 5.1
(a) Gold nanospheres, 15 nm diameter and (b) gold nanospheres coated with protein, with DNA strands attached. (Images courtesy of Nanopartz, Inc., Loveland, CO, http://www.nanopartz. com/Images.htm)

their therapeutic effects involve subtle interactions with proteins and other biological macromolecular structures, which may involve catalyzed changes in nanoscale conformations. Thus, there is by no means a sharp dividing line between nanobiology, molecular biology, and cell biology [2,3].

The therapeutic and diagnostic usefulness of nanoparticles depends on their size and physical properties in addition to their chemical composition. They must be small enough to circulate through the blood stream and tissues without becoming lodged in capillaries or other microanatomies. But they must be larger than atomic size in order to lend enhancement to images or perform some of their unique nanoscale functions.

Particles in the size ranging from 10 to 100 nm are in a fortuitous zone for medical applications. They are small enough not to become entrapped in the microstructures of the lungs, capillaries, kidneys, and liver, and thereby cause blockages, while they are large enough that their clearance time in tissues and organs is long in relation to small molecules. Thus, they are useful where we need to enhance imaging long enough to obtain useful diagnostic information and where we want to release therapeutic agents over time.

Nanoparticles have another useful property solely due to their size. Infections and cancerous tumors typically cause inflammation in the surrounding tissues and linings of the associated blood vessels, and with severe inflammation, the junctions between the cells lining the walls of the vessels are dilated. This results in preferential delivery of nanosized particles through the linings of capillaries and small vessels into the inflamed areas. Thus, imaging of a targeted diseased area can be enhanced. In addition, nanoparticles can be functionalized with antibodies to target selected tissues, making enhancement particularly selective [4–10].

5.1.2 General Requirements for Use of Nanoparticles

Nanoparticles used for medical applications in the body must be biodegradable or clearable, but agents used in cell culture or microscopy of biopsy samples need not be so. Agents used in the body must degrade over time with minimal toxic by-products. In addition, the particles must degrade in size and not aggregate or precipitate in tissues, to facilitate clearance from the body. There must be minimal risk of release of toxic compounds from encapsulated or embedded agents in nanoparticles. The nanoparticles should be colloidally stable in aqueous media and remain stable when mixed with physiological buffer solutions.

Nanoparticles for medical imaging applications should be stable in aqueous media and possess strong absorbance or fluorescence in the required wavelengths relative to tissue; they should have stronger optical activity than alternative fluorescent or bioluminescent agents. In general, nanoparticles are not subject to optical quenching, and are thus superior to organic dyes and contrast agents in this regard.

It is increasingly desirable for biodegradable nanoparticles and other agents to be manufactured by "green" chemical and physical processes. Manufacturing steps should be free of toxic materials, which may leave residues in or on the final product.

The surface coating of nanoparticles that are considered candidates for medical imaging or therapies should be readily functionalized for custom targeting.

Within these constraints, there are multiple metal, organic, ceramic, and polymer routes to the fabrication and synthesis of nanoparticles for medical imaging and therapy delivery, with many yet to be explored.

5.2 Nanoparticles for Medical Imaging

One of the most straightforward applications of nanoparticles is enhancing medical images. Nanoparticles have been used to capture and enhance images since the development of silver halide photography, but the new nanoscience has developed much more powerful and selective particles, which exploit the unique optical features found at the nanoscale. Nanoparticles are being used to enhance medical imaging for diagnosis with many modalities including x-ray, computed tomography (CT), magnetic resonance (MRI), optical coherence tomography (OCT), confocal reflectance, wide-field optical, photoacoustic, fluorescent microscopy, infrared (IR), and ultrasound imaging.

Contrast enhancement of images is important in the diagnosis of soft tissue disorders and diseases. Thus, it is particularly useful in cardiovascular medicine and in the diagnosis of cancer and neurological diseases. In addition to contrast enhancement, nanoparticles can be functionalized to target specific cells, thus highlighting tumors, inflammation, endocrine disorders, and other types of diseases. In this respect, nanoparticles can be used in a manner similar to nuclear medicine's pharmaceutical agents, but without the disadvantages of radioactivity.

Nanoparticle contrast agents provide several advantages over traditional compounds. They can incorporate a higher density of the contrast-generating species, thereby greatly increasing sensitivity and detectability. Nanoparticles can easily be functionalized to bind to specific cells and be retained in targeted tissues. Multiple properties may be easily combined within one nanoparticle for detection with several imaging techniques or for delivery of drugs or therapeutic actions. Integrating different imaging enhancement capabilities in nanoparticles enhances the use of imaging modalities that are complementary to each other, such as MRI and optical imaging.

5.2.1 Enhancement for X-Ray and Tomography Imaging

Nanoparticles are used as contrast enhancement and image intensification agents for x-ray imaging and CT. Conventional x-ray and tomography imaging agents are molecular iodine compounds such as iodinated benzoic acid derivatives. In addition to having risk factors associated with intravenous iodine injection, such low molecular weight chemical imaging agents clear from the human body relatively rapidly, making it difficult to target disease sites.

Iodinated molecules can be encapsulated into liposomes, but stability of the liposome membrane is a concern because of possible leakage and iodine toxicity. Nanoparticles of iodine compounds (sized from 200 to 400 nm diameter) can be encapsulated in a polymer coating, but this approach also involves risk of iodine toxicity should the coating break down [11–14].

Conjugation compounds containing gadolinium (Gd) and radioisotopes in a dendritic molecular structure have been developed for CT imaging. However, in such systems, only a relatively small number of heavy atoms may be delivered to the vicinity of the target tissues. Such approaches deliver, at most, a couple of hundred heavy atoms (i.e., iodine or gadolinium).

Nanoparticle contrast agents offer an alternative to the drawbacks of chemical agents, even those encapsulated in liposomes or polymers. In order to enhance an x-ray image, an agent must deliver a detectable number of heavy atoms into the imaged tissue without toxic effects. Nanoparticles of elemental heavy metals have high density (number of heavy metal atoms/ volume), but they must be biologically inert and stable. Nanoparticles of inert metals such as gold are not very cost effective. This issue can be overcome using nanoparticles made of heavy metal compounds encapsulated in gold shells, or even using hollow gold nanoparticles.

Gold-coated nanoparticles can be made by vapor or electrodeposition onto nanoparticles; gold can also be deposited into nanoscale mold templates of silicon, carbon, alumina, or other material with nanosize pores or wells. In the case of silicon, the wells can be created artificially in a silicon wafer using nanofabrication techniques. In the case of carbon nanotubes or alumina, the templates are made by controlling the synthesis or electrodeposition of the material. Hollow gold nanospheres have been fabricated electrochemically by sacrificial galvanic replacement of cobalt nanoparticles, and by a process in conjunction with the generation of hydrogen at an electrode, and are being evaluated as image enhancement agents [15–17].

Organic compounds with sulfide (–S–H) groups (thiols) can be used to coat gold particles with uniform organic monolayers. The sulfide group attaches to the metal surface leaving the remaining portion of the molecules exposed as an organic layer. By functionalizing proteins with thiol groups, gold particles can be coated with selectively binding antigens, antibodies, or target compounds for receptors on the surfaces of cells. By targeting receptors unique to certain types of cancer cells, gold nanoparticles can be made to enhance an x-ray image to increase the ability to detect the cancer cells by many orders of magnitude [18–21].

5.2.2 Enhancements with MRI Imaging

MRI imaging can be intensified by solutions or dispersions of dendritic macromolecules designed for biocompatibility, or by chelating paramagnetic (gadolinium) or supermagnetic (iron or manganese) ions [22]. Metal and silicon nanoparticles made of magnetic materials can also be used to enhance MRI imaging [23–26]. Large chelate complexes and nanoparticles are too large to pass through the blood–brain barrier, and are thus useful in imaging vasculature. Concern over possible toxic exposure to gadolinium and other heavy metals has led to the development of nanoparticle contrast agents enclosed in polymer coatings [27,28].

Silicon particles fabricated into shapes and coated with conductive layers can have enhanced magnetic resonance interactions with an imaging field. Such specially fabricated nanoparticles are being developed and evaluated at Johns Hopkins and elsewhere [29]. Coatings and RF filters made from nanoparticles engineered for electromagnetic susceptibility can reduce image artifacts and enhance the visibility of many biomedical devices, both implantable and interventional, that today are difficult to image due to eddy currents and other problems that interfere with MRI fields. Special coatings can also improve the ability to image guidewires and devices used in many surgical procedures.

Thin-film nanomagnetic particle coatings are being developed with the goal of shielding conductive wires and surgical instruments from radiofrequency-induced fields in MRI instruments. The high magnetic fields used for MRI, in addition to the radiofrequency signals, normally prevent use of conductors inside the field space. This is a problem for pacemaker wires and other devices. Safety problems can involve device heating and, in some cases, induced voltages that can cause very rapid heartbeats.

Specially engineered magnetic nanoparticle coatings might enable devices contraindicated for MRI due to safety concerns—devices such as pacemakers, defibrillators, neurostimulators, guidewires, endoscopes, etc.—to be used in the MRI. These developments could open the way to increased and simplified use of MRI for guiding surgical procedures. Magnetic resonator nanocoatings have been demonstrated to mitigate the Faraday cage effect produced by cardiac stents in blood vessels. The nanofabricated coatings eliminate the magnetic susceptibility artifacts caused by the stent material, enabling MRI imaging of clots and restenosis (re-narrowing of blood vessels) inside the stents [30].

5.2.3 Nanodots and Quantum Resonant Nanoparticles

The exploitation of quantum resonance effects on the nanoscale is a logical extension of the use of contrast agents for x-ray and signal intensification agents for MRI imaging. Quantum nanodots are powerful and versatile in a wide range of modalities from x-ray to ultraviolet fluorescence, visible, and infrared imaging [31,32].

Nanoshell particles with optical resonances in the infrared have been functionalized and used to enhance imaging of cancer cells. Metal nanoshells are composite spherical nanoparticles consisting of a dielectric core covered by a thin metallic shell, typically gold. By varying the relative dimensions of the core and the shell, the optical resonance of nanosized particles can be tuned from the near-UV to the mid-infrared. Work on this type of nanoshell for cancer treatment is being carried out by research groups at a number of centers [33–39].

5.2.4 Nanoparticles in the Enhancement of IR, Visible, and UV Imaging

Nanoparticles that have strong optical sensitivity (absorption and scattering) in the near infrared (NIR) and visible region (500–800 nm) can be used for contrast enhancement for many optical biomedical imaging techniques important in cellular imaging and diagnosis, including photoacoustic imaging (PA, also optoacoustic imaging, optoacoustic tomography (OAT), and laser optoacoustic imaging system (LOIS)), optical coherence tomography (OCT), dark field microscopy, confocal microscopy, and fluorescence microscopy.

5.2.5 Nanoparticles with Visible and UV Resonance for Cellular Probes

In addition to diagnostic tools and innovative therapies, nanoparticle imaging agents are being used as probes to understand biological processes at the molecular level. Nanoparticles with UV and visible resonance have been synthesized for use as imaging agents to study cell signaling pathways, by biofunctionalization of metal, semiconductor, ceramic, and dye-doped silica nanoparticles. These particles can be applied as imaging probes to detect signaling pathway components and cellular responses to signals (apoptosis and degranulation) in inflammatory and cancer cells [40].

Imaging agents such as fluorescent dye-doped silica nanoparticles, quantum dots, and gold nanoparticles overcome many of the limitations of conventional contrast agents (organic dyes) such as poor photostability, low quantum yield, and low in vitro and in vivo stability. For these reasons, nanoparticles with resonance in the visible and ultraviolet are a viable alternative to fluorescent dyes for cellular imaging for diagnosis of cancer [41,42]. In one study, 30 nm gold nanoparticles conjugated with cancer antibodies were compared to the same antibodies with fluorescent dye reporters. The emission intensity of the gold nanoparticles was about 10 times stronger than that of the autofluorescence of the Karpas-299 line of cancer cells at the same excitation power, and was significantly stronger than that for fluorescent dyes. The nanoparticles also had higher photostability than the dyes [43].

Nanoparticles with absorbance and emission in the NIR enable real time and deep tissue imaging via new optical methods such as OCT and PA. Multimodal nanoparticles with both optical and MRI activity have been developed to enhance deep tissue imaging with those preexisting technologies. The design of contrast agents such as dye-doped silica nanoparticles, quantum dots, and gold nanoparticles with improved properties for noninvasive bioimaging with new modalities is a very active and rapidly progressing area [44,45].

5.2.6 Nanoparticle Image Enhancement for Ultrasound and Optoacoustic Imaging

Nanoparticles are strong contrast agents for ultrasound imaging [46], and for OAT. OAT is a novel medical imaging method that uses laser optical illumination and ultrasonic detection to produce deep tissue images based on ultrasound effects produced by light absorption. Although the principle of the optoacoustic effect has been known since the time of Edison, only recently have advances in powerful integrated and precisely timed laser pulsing, sensing and computing microelectronics made its exploitation possible for medical imaging [47–51].

OAT has been of interest as a technique to image tumors, based on differential blood content from normal tissue. Abnormal angiogenesis in advanced tumors increases the blood content of the tumor, yielding an endogenous image contrast factor that can be detected by OAT. In addition, the blood in aggressively growing malignant tumors is hypoxic relative to benign tumors; Therefore, imaging using four laser wavelengths matching the absorption peaks in oxy- and deoxyhemoglobin, water, and lipids provides a means for quantitative diagnosis of breast cancer. Just two wavelengths are sufficient for qualitative differentiation. A difference in intensity of image feature brightness of up to twofold has been reported between tumor and normal vascularized tissue, with resolution of sub-millimeter features.

In early stages, however, angiogenesis may not be sufficient to differentiate a tumor from normal tissue. Thus an exogenous contrast agent may be needed to improve the reliability of this technique for detection of early tumors. Contrast agents composed of gold nanoparticles conjugated to monoclonal antibodies have been developed to improve OAT imaging for potential use in detecting deep tumors in early stages of cancer or metastatic lesions [52].

Gold nanorods have been shown to produce a uniquely strong optoacoustic contrast effect. The optical absorption in gold nanorods is over 1000 times stronger than that of organic molecules. Average near-IR absorption of cancerous tissue loaded with nanorods in concentration of only 10 nanorods per cell provides additional contrast of delta-mu about 0.5/cm relative to normal tissue. Furthermore, the laser-induced acoustic signal from gold nanorods was found to be an order of magnitude stronger than an optoacoustic signal from a dye solution with equal absorbance [53].

Synthetic gold nanorods with scattering and absorption bands that span the wavelength regime between 675–850 nm are of particular usefulness to optical medical imaging modalities such as OAT. This band is in the most important part of the "optical imaging window" where light penetration in tissue is high due to reduced scattering and absorption coefficients. Optical imaging techniques that rely on scattering and/or absorption contrast to detect pathological tissue can benefit from the use of such nanoparticles with or without targeting capability [54].

5.3 Nanoparticles for Targeted Imaging and Delivery of Energy

In addition to imaging, nanoparticles can be used to deliver targeted energy to kill pathological cells. With functionalized nanoparticles, radiation can be delivered to a tumor or to individual cells selected by interaction with antibodies or other ligands attached to the nanoparticle (photothermal or photodynamic therapy). The optical radiation absorbed by quantum resonant nanoparticles is converted into heat in the surrounding microenvironment. This local heat can be exploited for killing cancer cells and for remotely releasing drugs from the nanoparticle.

5.3.1 Photothermal and Photodynamic Therapies

Nanoshells and similar quantum resonance nanoparticles can destroy attached cells by absorbing heat on irradiation with infrared light at a frequency that is not absorbed by tissue. The plasmon resonance absorption heats the particles and destroys any cells selectively bound to the nanoshell particle. The nanoshells typically consist of a dielectric core and a gold shell, whose core–shell ratio determines their optically resonant frequency. Thus the nanoparticles can be fabricated with specific absorption characteristics, depending on composition, size, and shell thickness. Nanoparticles with intense absorption, light scattering, and emission properties in the "water window" of the NIR (800–1300 nm) are optimally suited for bioimaging and biosensing applications [55,56].

The growing interest in application of thermodynamic therapy and thermally initiated drug release has led to detailed theoretical studies of the effects produced by heating of nanoparticles on the surrounding microenvironment. These studies use computed finite element analysis to investigate the process of heating of a spherical gold nanoparticle by nanosecond laser pulses and of heat transfer between the particle and the surrounding medium. The theoretical simulations include thermal conductivity changes, vapor formation, and changes of the dielectric properties as a function of temperature, assuming no mass transfer from the nanoparticles.

These studies can provide useful insights for the development of molecular targeting of gold nanoparticles for applications such as remotely triggered drug release of therapeutics and photothermal cancer therapy. For maximum efficacy, it is believed that the gold nanoparticles should be engineered to specifically target cancer cells and enter the cell through endocytosis [57].

Gold nanorods have optical properties that make them especially attractive for photothermal therapy [58]. The gold surface is biocompatible and readily functionalized for conjugation to a wide variety of biological molecules for targeting or probes. With suitable coatings, they have long circulation times of several hours in vivo. Gold nanorods have minimal cytotoxicity—unlike gold nanospheres, they do not fit into the molecular template of DNA and RNA.

Most distinctively, gold nanorods have absorption and scattering cross sections that are up to 2 orders of magnitude per micron greater than nanoshells. They can be fabricated with intense absorption and scattering bands in the NIR, orders of magnitude greater than spherical gold nanoparticles or quantum dots, at biologically useful wavelengths not available to either. Their two-photon fluorescence is equal to that of quantum dots, with a high photothermal conversion rate, for photothermal therapy (Figure 5.2).

Quantum nanoshells and nanorods have a photonic resonance due to their size and structure, but nanoparticles can also be useful in photodynamic therapy as delivery vehicles for optically sensitized dyes. Photodynamic therapy is a minimally invasive cancer treatment approach that is particularly useful for treating local tumors. In molecular photodynamic therapy, a photosensitizer dye is administered and then activated by locally directed

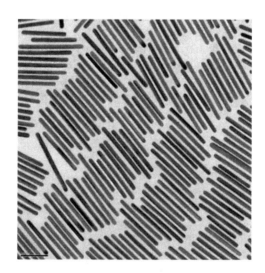

FIGURE 5.2
Gold nanorods. (Images courtesy of Nanopartz, Inc., Loveland, CO, http://www.nanopartz.com/Images.htm)

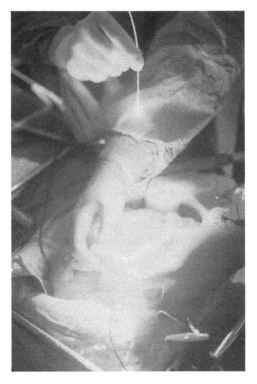

FIGURE 5.3
Photodynamic therapy uses molecular agents or functionalized nanoparticles, which are activated by light. (Image courtesy of National Cancer Institute, Bethesda, MD, John Crawford (photographer), http://visualsonline.cancer.gov/details.cfm?imageid=2340)

light (Figure 5.3). The light is selected in a specific wavelength that interacts with the dye to release reactive oxygen species (singlet oxygen free radicals, $^1O_2$). The elevated formation of reactive oxygen can lead to the destruction of tumor tissues.

Coated biocompatible gold nanoparticles have been used as a vehicle to deliver photosensitizer to tumors. The use of gold nanoparticles functionalized to carry dyes can significantly increase the accumulation of photosensitizer in tumor cells and result in a high efficiency for their destruction.

Some dyes with the best combination of good photochemical properties and ready absorption into cells have biological disadvantages: prolonged skin sensitivity that requires patients to avoid sunlight for many weeks, lack of tumor selectivity, poor light penetration into the tissue due to relatively short light wavelengths for activation, and difficulty in synthesizing and maintaining pure, easily characterized, and quantifiable preparations.

On the other hand, attractive alternatives that have been found without these disadvantages have generally been hydrophilic compounds that do not readily absorb into cells or cross tissue barriers. By conjugating these more attractive photosynthesizers onto positively charged gold nanoparticles using electrostatic interaction, researchers were able to enhance uptake of the dye by cells and increase specificity for tumor cells.

The size of the nanoparticles was favorable for cell permeability, and the high surface-to-volume ratio delivered a significant concentration of dye. As a result, an effective and specific destruction of tumor cells was achieved with minimal damage to healthy cells. In addition, the gold nanoparticles have an intrinsic activity for surface-enhanced Raman scattering (SERS), which allows for Raman imaging of intracellular activities during the photo-dynamic treatment [59].

Rare earth nanoemitters, which are brightly luminescent rare earth ions incorporated into a silica nanoparticle matrix, have also been fabricated and applied to photodynamic and biological sensor applications [60].

The use of polymer nanoparticles to contain the dyes for photodynamic therapy can circumvent the chemical toxicity of the photosensitizer dyes, a factor which has limited the use of this type of therapy in the past. Encapsulation of a toxic but efficient sensitizer dye into a biocompatible nanoparticle matrix has been used to demonstrate effective phototoxicity for glioma cells, while controls exposed to the nanoparticles in the absence of light showed no toxic effects. This demonstrated that the nanoparticle encapsulation could protect cells in non-targeted tissue from the chemical toxicity of the dye, while allowing controlled and effective lethal application of phototherapy [61]. Other researchers have used novel liposome formulations in a similar manner, by incorporating lipophilic photosensitizer molecules into the lipid bilayer of the liposomes. The nanoscale liposomes (<0.1 μm) are readily taken up by cells, and release the antitumor drugs upon activation by photolysis [62].

5.3.2 Combined Radiation and Photodynamic Therapy

Nanoparticles are attracting great interest because they can combine imaging with therapy, or combine several therapies in one delivery vehicle. An example is a new nanoparticle-based cancer treatment with a combination of radiation and photodynamic therapies. The goal is to lower the dose of radiation needed to kill cancer cells by supplementing conventional radiation therapy with photodynamic therapy. This was carried out by using nanoparticles with attached photosensitizers such as porphyrins, which produced scintillation or persistent luminescence when subjected to ionizing radiation. The resultant luminescence activates the photosensitizers, producing singlet oxygen ($^1O_2$), which is known to be effective in killing cancer cells. The advantage of in vivo luminescent nanoparticles is that an external light source is not required. Application of the therapy can be more localized and the potential of damage to healthy cells is reduced, lower doses of ionizing radiation are needed, and the costs and complexity of lasers or other external light delivery systems are eliminated [63].

5.3.3 Magnetic Nanoparticles for Targeting Cancer Cells

Ferromagnetic micro- and nanoparticles can be functionalized with antibodies, allowing cancer cells to be separated out of tissue samples such as blood and concentrated manyfold for diagnostic analysis. This is an important promising technique because cancer cells are released into the blood stream in large numbers by microscopic tumors too small to be detectable by imaging modalities. If the circulating cancer cells can be concentrated and detected from a blood test, it would provide a means for early detection of cancer, with greatly improved prognosis for treatment versus detection after the tumor has grown to a size detectable by imaging. This technique is being developed and evaluated in a number of research centers and is being introduced into therapeutic use by more than one medical device company [64–68].

In principle, a similar technique could be based on mass enhancement rather than magnetic susceptibility enhancement, with separations based on centrifugation. Similarly, combinations of nanoparticle with electrically polarizable or charged functionalities could be used for electrophoretic separations. In practice, separation by strong permanent magnets is simpler and less elaborate. In some cases, separation and concentration is enhanced by a combination of techniques, as in magnetic separation followed by concentration from suspensions by centrifugation. A system has been developed which uses 20 nm diameter luminescent/magnetic nanocomposite particles composed of superparamagnetic particle cores coated with CdSe/ZnS quantum dot shells, for ease of quantitative measurement of separated cells [69]. Other systems have been devised to enhance x-ray and MRI imaging of cancer with nanoparticles combining antibodies with magnetic components.

Nanomagnetic particles or ferrofluids can be used for magnetically controlled drug targeting. This technology is based on binding established anticancer drugs with ferrofluids that concentrate the drug in the area of interest (tumor site) by means of magnetic fields. Then, the drug desorbs from the ferrofluid and acts against the tumor. Nanoparticles are one option along with magnetic liquids for magnetically controlled anticancer chemotherapy [70–72]. Magnetic particle separations can also be used to separate cancer cells from bone marrow and other tissues, and for the isolation, identification, and genetic analysis of specific DNA sequences [73,74].

5.4 Nanoparticles for Delivery of Drugs

In the previous sections, we described how nanoparticles can be coated with selective compounds to adhere to cancer cells for imaging and for delivering killing blows of energy, and how nanoparticles can be used in conjunction with phototherapy and magnetism. Nanoparticles can be loaded with absorbed or encapsulated drugs for delivery to cancer cells or disease agents in a variety of ways [75–80].

5.4.1 Direct Application of Nanoparticles for Therapy

The most direct way of using nanoparticles to attack cancer is to embed the particles directly into tumors or other sites of diseased tissue. This approach has some advantages over simply circulating the drug through the body, because it concentrates the drug release on the site of the tumor, with minimal effect on healthy cells. It has been used for cancer and for ocular diseases, cases where disease is often localized to special cell types in locations that are difficult to reach by other therapies [81–83]. This technology approach merges over into tissue scaffolding, a topic which is discussed in Chapter 8.

Drug-laden nanoparticles can be injected into tumors with minimally invasive procedures. Their effect can be enhanced by using drugs that are further activated by radiation that can be directed onto the tumor. Drugs can be infused into the tumor which may be very potent, but difficult to deliver selectively through the circulatory system because of toxicity, insolubility, or reaction with enzymes or other compounds [84,85]. Drug release can also be triggered by heat or changes in pH, taking advantage of the difference in pH and metabolism rate between tumors and healthy tissue [86].

5.4.2 Targeted Drug Delivery

Nanoparticles can be targeted for drug delivery just as for imaging and photothermal therapy. Targeting a cell type involves adding a molecular recognition function to the particle so that it preferentially binds to or enters selected cells. To do this, we use the same type of molecular lock and key mechanisms that characterize the body's immune system—antibodies. Alternatively, we can utilize RNA and DNA templates to target the genetic material in cells, or utilize other chemical affinities and ligands to selectively bind to diseased cells or protect healthy cells. We can take advantage of unusual chemical and physiological environments associated with diseased tissue: abnormal pH, temperature, or oxygen levels. We can also look for special metabolic characteristics like higher or lower metabolic rate and higher cell division rate—all is fair in the fight against disease—or any marker that will address the cell or tissue to be targeted. We are limited only by knowledge and creativity. One of the active goals in targeting nanoparticles is to find alternatives to antibodies because of the expense and difficulty of obtaining purely selective antibody preparations. Another challenge is to find effective targeting drugs that can avoid immunogenic and nonspecific interactions which the body uses to clear away foreign particles.

The better we understand the special properties of matter on the nanoscale, the more we will be able to exploit constructs of this size range in a beneficial way, and to avoid undesirable side effects. Nanosize materials behave differently from smaller molecular weight drugs. Their surfaces and volumes interact in different ways with cellular anatomy and physiology, with membranes, cytosomes, and DNA, for example. A practical and reasonably complete understanding of the physiology, biodistribution, and toxicity of nanoparticles is being developed, including understanding of how particles interact with the biological conditions of the local physiological environment [87–89].

Functionalized nanoparticles are being used in new therapies for cancer and infectious diseases. In this section, we take some examples that show the directions and possibilities among the many new applications in this rapidly advancing field. We see how targeted functionalized nanotechnology is leading to a combination of imaging with genetic and cellular-level diagnostics and individually targeted therapeutic agents [78,90–92].

5.4.3 A Historical Note on Targeted and Nanoparticle Drug Delivery

The germ of the idea for drugs formulated as particles that would target disease can be traced to Paul Ehrlich and his concept of the "magic bullet" in the first decade of the twentieth century. Anecdotally, Ehrlich got the idea after attending a performance of the opera *Der Freischütz*, in which a devilish magic bullet plays a central role. Undoubtedly, Ehrlich's earlier work with bacterial stains and their specificity for certain types of bacteria also lay behind the idea, which led to the famous "magic bullet" drug formulations and set the model for drug discovery and targeting for more than a century (Figure 5.4).

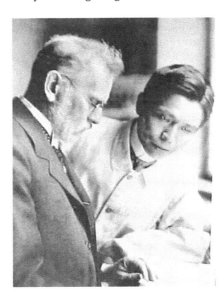

FIGURE 5.4
Paul Ehrlich in his laboratory with his colleague Sachahiro Hata, working on the "magic bullet" (testing candidate compounds synthesized by Alfred Bertheim to find success on the 606th trial).

What has been somewhat less well appreciated outside of pharmaceutical circles, in the past few years of excitement over the new advances in nanotechnology and nanomedicine, is that pharmaceutical scientists working at ETH Zürich in the late 1960s and early 1970s were pioneering the use of nanoparticles for controlled drug release, delivery across the blood–brain barrier, and prolonged blood circulation time for improved pharmacokinetics. The early work of Ursula Scheffel, followed by the advances made by Prof. Peter Speiser and his students, miniaturized drug delivery systems that reached true nanoparticulate size and functionality. They developed the first nanoparticles in the late 1960s for drug delivery and for vaccines, before the term "nanoparticle" came into use.

Methods were developed at ETH for preparation of polymerized micelle nanoparticles and their use in drug delivery and immunology, using emulsion polymerization or heterogeneous polymerization. One of Professor Speiser's students, Dr. Jörg Kreuter, has written a short and readable history of these developments [93]. It is worth noting that even disruptive developments have their roots in past accomplishments. In every era, people seem drawn to enlist the latest technology as a metaphor in the war against disease—bullets in the nineteenth century and "smart bombs," "guided missiles," "stealth vehicles" and "nano-robots" in the twentieth century and beyond.

The essential elements of the "magic bullet" drug model are appealing and durable. The challenges remain the same whether using small molecules, nanoparticles, or microcapsules: identify a target that is on a critical path for the disease, find a drug that effectively knocks out the target, and deliver the drug in a stable and efficacious form while avoiding biological barriers, clearance mechanisms, and harmful side effects [94–96].

5.4.4 Advantages of Nanoparticles for Drug Delivery

Two requirements for the effectiveness of a therapeutic drug are delivery, that is, getting the right amount in the right form to the right place (pharmacokinetics), and actions once it reaches its target (pharmacodynamics). Use of nanoparticles can change the process of delivery from free-flowing circulation to targeted release in a chosen controlled environment.

Targeted and timed release of drugs can be achieved in a number of ways: drug conjugates with antibodies and other macromolecules, microencapsulation, and nanoparticles. But nanoparticles (including many larger drug-polymer conjugated particles) have particular advantages over use of smaller (molecular scale) or larger (micro scale) delivery carriers [97].

In general, drug delivery with nanoparticles provides capabilities not attainable by other therapies. Nanoscale carriers can deliver drugs selectively to targets in concentrated local dosages, can penetrate and evade biological barriers and clearance routes, and prevent exposure of non-targeted tissues to toxic or other undesirable effects of the drug on normal cells. Some of these advantages are shared with conjugated systems, and not all nanoparticle delivery systems possess all of these advantages. The advantages of targeted nanoparticle drug delivery are generally as follows:

1. *Control of pharmacokinetics*: Nanoparticles can be tuned by varying their size and surface properties to provide long or short residence times in the body and tissues. Particles can be made in a range of sizes for differing cell uptake and circulatory clearance effects. (For example, as noted earlier, 10–100 nm is a range that is not cleared from the body by the kidneys but does not risk blockages.) The surface properties can be formulated to control the degree of nonspecific interaction with cells and proteins. (The surface can be functionalized for interaction with specific cell types, and the surface charges can be made negative to minimize nonspecific interactions with proteins and cell membranes.) This combination of size, surface properties, and functionalization provides a set of parameters that can be varied to produce particles to target cells and generate therapeutic effects more selectively than with conventional drugs, or even with drug–antibody conjugates.

2. *Separation of pharmacokinetics from therapeutic activity*: With nanoparticles, the active drug molecules can be sealed within the particle and released at the target so that the pharmacokinetics and biodistribution can be controlled independently of the type of therapeutics used. In conventional drugs and molecular conjugates, the pharmacokinetics cannot be separated from the end-point therapeutic activity—a single chemistry must perform both tasks.

3. *Payload capacity*: Nanoparticles are about one to several hundred times larger than individual drug molecules. A nanoparticle can aggregate a large number of drug or siRNA molecules in a highly concentrated package for delivery to a cell. For example, a 70 nm nanoparticle can carry 2000 siRNA drug molecules, whereas antibody conjugate drugs can typically contain less than 10. The same considerations apply to image enhancement molecules and atoms carried by nanoparticles.

4. *Multiple affinity effects*: Since nanoparticles are roughly 1–2 orders of magnitude larger than the ligands and cell-surface receptors that govern binding to the cells, a single nanoparticle can be built to contain multiple targeting ligands that provide for multivalent binding to cell membranes. The designer of nanoparticle drugs has two parameters for tuning the strength of binding to targeted cells: affinity (binding strength of each type of ligand) and density (number of targeting ligands per particle). These multivalency effects can yield very high effective affinities even when only low-affinity ligands are available. Thus, the repertoire of molecules and receptor sites that can be used for targeting is greatly expanded.

5. *Combination of therapy effects*: Nanoparticles are large enough to carry multiple types of imaging and drug molecules. Multiple imaging and therapeutic interventions can be simultaneously applied with a single type of nanoparticle in a controlled manner.

6. *Trojan horse effects*: Nanoparticles can carry vulnerable drugs through biological barriers. They can also bypass multidrug resistance mechanisms that involve cell membrane transport because they enter cells via endocytosis or in stealth packages. This is important for treating bacterial and cancer cells, which can readily develop drug resistance.

All of the above characteristics of nanoparticles open new opportunities for development of more effective drugs, able to overcome many prior obstacles, and avoid many side effects. This is a very active area for new therapies, which is beginning to produce results in the form of clinical trials and emergence of new approved therapies into healthcare practice.

5.4.5 Nanotoxicology

The emergence of any new medical technology raises concerns about efficacy as well as safety. Just as with any material, a long list of preclinical and clinical risk assessments and tests must be performed for any nanoparticles which are to be introduced into the human body. Critical issues include biodistribution, circulation, immune response, toxicity, sedimentation, and clearance. Nanoparticle drug carriers should disintegrate slowly in aqueous solution and thereby be cleared from an organism, but be stable enough to ensure that the particles do not prematurely decompose and release their valuable (and perhaps dangerous) contents on the way to the targeted tissue. On the other hand, too high a stability can be a problem, as solid particles can accumulate in tissues, leading to other complications over time.

Nanoparticles raise concerns even more than novel chemicals, because the interactions with living cells at extremely small dimensions could have unexpected effects. One cannot assume nanomaterials will have the same properties as their parent bulk materials, and exposure to nanoparticles could have unique toxicological consequences. The new field of nanotoxicology can draw from a long-established body of knowledge based on experience with the toxicology of fibers, mineral particles, and the interaction of viruses with cells. Nanoscale particles in the natural and built environment, such as silica and asbestos, have been extensively studied, providing useful lessons for the potential risks of exposures to newly engineered nanoparticles [98].

In toxicology, identification of nanoscale specific effects of particles due to small sizes and large surface areas date from the early parts of the twentieth century, but the emergence of nanoscience has led to further understanding of the mechanisms of action and kinetics of nanoparticle effects. The ability of nanoparticles to cross biological barriers, enter cells, and disrupt subcellular structures was in many cases first discovered through toxicology studies, as well as the induction of oxidative stress as a major mechanism of nanoparticle effects. Thus, in addition to providing warnings of risks and setting boundaries, nanotoxicology research can provide useful insights for the design of nanotherapeutics. Uncovering the impacts and physicochemical roles of nanomaterials that can initiate effects in organisms and the environment will continue to be an important area for research [99,100].

5.4.6 Few Examples of Cellular Nanomachinery Targeted by Nanodrugs

Before surveying the types of nanodrugs, it will be good to take a brief look at some examples of the cellular nanomachinery which will be targeted, bypassed, or disabled by some typical nanoparticles and the drugs that they carry.

5.4.6.1 Aspirin: Targeting in the Inflammatory Response Pathway

Aspirin (acetlysalicylic acid) is a notable example of a simple molecular drug that acts by subtle interaction with a large complex of cellular nanomachinery. Aspirin is originally derived from the plant material salicin, a natural product that gives the same basic therapeutic benefits of aspirin, but which had severe side effects. There are many other examples of drugs acting on human regulatory pathways, derived from compounds found naturally occurring in plants: *digitalis* acts specifically on heart muscle; *coumarins* act on blood clotting mechanisms. Today more than 120 important and widely used medicines derive directly from plant precursors, and many others derive from fungi and marine organisms. Most of the natural product precursors of these drugs have problems if used directly in their natural forms: toxicity, insolubility, side effects, etc. A vast amount of effort goes into analyzing their structure and synthesizing derivatives to find molecules that preserve the beneficial activity without the side effects when the drugs are administered systematically. Nanoparticles provide a potentially shorter route to beneficial therapeutic use of many natural products.

Aspirin's therapeutic uses, as well as its success as an over the counter remedy, generated much research seeking improvements and alternatives, but for many years the mechanism of action of aspirin was not fully understood. Eventually, aspirin was found to inhibit the *arachidonic acid pathway* that leads to the synthesis of *eicosanoids*, potent mediators of pain and inflammation. In 1971, researchers led by the British pharmacologist John Robert Vane, at the Royal College of Surgeons in London, showed that aspirin suppresses the production of the prostaglandins and thromboxanes involved in inflammation. This discovery led to major breakthroughs in understanding molecular signaling pathways between cells. The Nobel Prize for Medicine for 1982 was awarded to Professors Bengt Samuelsson, John Vane, and Sune Bergstrom for this discovery.

Aspirin was the model for the class of pharmaceutical agents known as nonsteroidal anti-inflammatory drugs (NSAIDs). Many but not all NSAIDs are derivatives of salicylates; all have similar effects—most act by nonselective inhibition of the enzyme cyclooxygenase, needed to synthesize prostaglandin and thromboxane. *Prostaglandins* are local (*paracrine*) hormones whose diverse effects include transmission of pain information to the brain, modulation of the hypothalamic thermostat, and regulating inflammation. Thromboxanes are involved in aggregation of platelets that form blood clots. Aspirin can irreversibly block the formation of thromboxane A2 in platelets, producing an inhibitory effect on platelet aggregation. This is the mechanism of aspirin's anticoagulant effects used to reduce the incidence and severity of heart attacks. A side effect is a general reduction in the ability of the blood to clot, which may result in excessive bleeding with the use of aspirin.

Aspirin suppresses the production of prostaglandins and thromboxanes by its *irreversible* inactivation of the cyclooxygenase (COX) enzyme, which is required for prostaglandin and thromboxane synthesis (Figure 5.5). Aspirin acts as an acetylating agent, covalently bonding an acetyl group to a serine residue in the active site of the COX enzyme. This *irreversible* mode of action is different from other NSAIDs (such as diclofenac and ibuprofen), which are *reversible* inhibitors. Recently, reversible blocking of COX-2 by synthetic NSAID drugs has been found to lead to harmful effects, showing that we still have some lessons to learn from the subtle mode of action of the natural product.

In addition to inactivation of prostaglandin and thromboxane production, aspirin has two additional modes of action, contributing further to its strong analgesic, antipyretic, and anti-inflammatory effects. Aspirin buffers and transports protons across membranes involved in energy release by ATP in

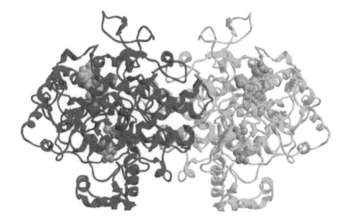

FIGURE 5.5
Action of aspirin on the structure of COX-2 (prostaglandin H synthase). The COX-2 molecule is a dimer; the light and dark halves are identical. In each monomer, the active *serine* site has been acetylated by aspirin, inactivating it. (Image by Jeff Dahl.)

the mitochondria where it uncouples oxidative phosphorylation and disrupts energy release. As a weak acid, aspirin can carry protons, diffusing from the inner cell membrane space into the mitochondrial matrix, where it ionizes to release protons. Aspirin stimulates the formation of NO-radicals that enable the body's white blood cells (leukocytes) to fight infections more effectively. Dr. Derek W. Gilroy was awarded Bayer's International Aspirin Award in 2005 for his research revealing the effects of aspirin on NO production.

The study of aspirin has contributed to our understanding of inflammation and the mechanisms of proton transport across membranes and the role of NO-radicals in cell metabolism. Salicylic acid and its derivatives have been found to modulate signaling through a number of transcription factor complexes that play central roles in many biological processes, including inflammation. Inflammation involves many mechanisms that protect us against tissue injury and promote the restoration of tissue after damage: our well-being and survival depends upon its efficiency and carefully balanced control [101,102].

The story of aspirin and the NSAID drugs illustrates how a small molecule drug works, and how it must be delivered deep into the right target in the cellular nanomachinery in order to execute its effects. Aspirin and the NSAIDs represent an achievement of this delivery through pharmaceutical biochemistry. Once the NSAIDs are safely delivered into the cell, they can target the transcription factor complexes, the COX enzyme, and mitochondrial proton pumps.

5.4.6.2 P-Glycoproteins: Circumventing the Nanomachinery of the Cell Membrane

To get a further appreciation for how cellular nanomachinery can be effectively targeted by nanoparticle delivery as an alternative to conventional drugs, let us look at a cell membrane proton pump, the P-glycoprotein (Pgp) (Figure 5.6). In the introduction to this chapter, we mentioned that nanoparticles can carry vulnerable drugs through biological barriers, and can bypass multidrug resistance mechanisms that involve cell membrane transport.

An important example of cell surface transport nanomachinery is the P-glycoprotein, (Pgp). This glycoprotein transmembrane proton pump plays an important part in many cell surface transport mechanisms. It is one of a family of proteins that transports various molecules across extra- and intracellular membranes. Pgp is an ATP-binding cassette (ABC) transporter, which is involved in tumor resistance, bacterial multidrug resistance, cystic fibrosis, and a number of other inherited human diseases [103]. Pgp also functions as a transporter in the intestinal epithelium, and the blood–brain and the blood–testis barriers.

Pgp and other ABC membrane–associated proteins act as ATP-driven cellular efflux pumps. They expel a wide range of xenobiotic compounds, which are not recognized as being part of the normal cell metabolism, out through the membrane. Among their normal functions are the removal of

Extracellular   Cytoplasmic
face   face

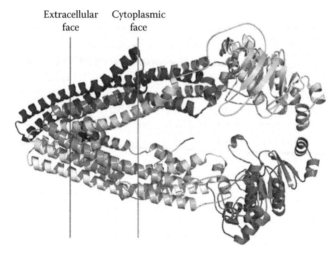

FIGURE 5.6
Structural representation of a mouse P-glycoprotein. The approximate positioning of the protein in the cell membrane is indicated by the left (extracellular face) and right (cytoplasmic face) lines. (Image from Wikipedia, released to public domain 2009; A donation has been made to Wikipedia in acknowledgement by the author. http://en.wikipedia.org/wiki/File:MDR3-3g 5u.png.)

toxic metabolites and xenobiotics from cells into urine, bile, and the intestinal lumen, and transport of compounds out of the brain across the blood–brain barrier. Thus they counteract drug accumulation in cells, and their active expression is associated with the development of resistance to drugs (Figure 5.7). This is especially important in bacterial and cancer cells, which can readily develop drug resistance.

Nanoparticle drug delivery can overcome this type of drug resistance by a number of strategies:

1. Appropriately surface-treated nanoparticles can enter cells via endocytosis, thus bypassing the cell transport mechanism and releasing an overwhelming concentrated drug cargo deep within the cytoplasm or nucleus.

2. Nanoparticles can be formed by encapsulating or conjugating drugs with coatings which disguise their xenobiotic cargoes from the recognition mechanisms used by the barrier and expelling pump mechanisms.

3. Nanoparticles can display a recognizable xenobiotic template, but be combined with moieties which poison or block the Pgp pumps (This mechanism is not unique to nanoparticles—it can also be employed as a strategy for molecular drugs).

In any case, these examples show how nanoparticles act at the cellular level. While drug carrying nanoparticles are much larger and more complex than

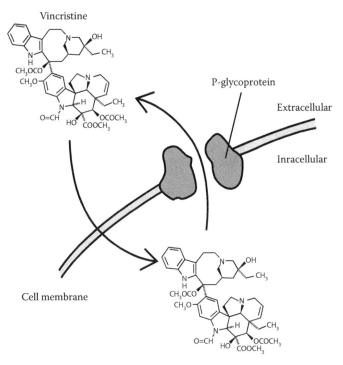

FIGURE 5.7
P-glycoproteins (Pgp) pump anticancer drugs out of the cell through the membrane, and can contribute to anticancer drug resistance and development of multidrug resistance in bacteria. (Image from Wikipedia, released to public domain 2009; A donation has been made to Wikipedia in acknowledgement by the author. http://commons.wikimedia.org/wiki/File:Function_of_P_glycoprotein.png)

molecular drugs, they are still in general very simple and small in relation to the complex, intricate, and large-scale nanomachinery of the cells that they regulate.

5.4.6.3 Taxol: Disabling the Cell Division Nanomachinery (Tubulin)

In this section, we look at an example of a drug whose action would have been extremely difficult to predict had it not been discovered as a natural product; it works not by modulating a signaling or transport pathway, but by blocking a fundamental nanoscale process involved in cell replication. The therapy associated with this class of drugs is an important example of the usefulness of nanoparticle delivery in dealing with toxic and insoluble but very potent anticancer drugs.

From the 1960s, the NIH sponsored research screening thousands of natural product extracts for potential use as cancer drugs. By the 1980s, tests of extracts from bark of the Pacific yew tree yielded promising results on cancer-prone mice strains. Further tests found that a compound in the Pacific yew

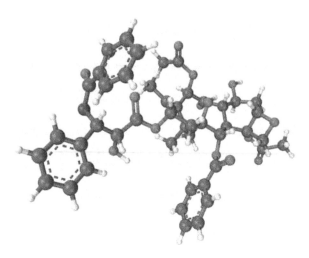

FIGURE 5.8
Taxol molecule chemical structure. (Courtesy of U.S. NIH government image, presented to Congress, Bethesda, MD.)

extract, taxol, was especially effective in halting the growth of certain types of human breast cancer, which were resistant to other treatments. The structure and mechanism of taxol were elucidated by further research sponsored by the NIH and pharmaceutical companies (Figure 5.8). It was found that taxol disrupted the functioning of the microtubules involved in guiding chromosomes as they separated in mitosis during cell division. Rapidly growing tumor cells were preferentially affected compared to normal cells, as they were blocked from reproducing by the action of taxol. Taxol, also known by the generic name paclitaxel, has been found effective in treatment of lung, ovarian, breast cancer, head and neck cancer, and advanced stages of Kaposi's sarcoma, and is used for the prevention of *restenosis* in patients with blocked blood vessels.

Taxol is an especially interesting drug from the nano perspective, because it acts by absorbing on specific sites in the microtubule structures that act as scaffolding and guideways in the separation of chromosomes during cell division. Taxol stabilizes these structures, making them rigid and unable to function—it "gums up the works." It acts in the domain between the chemical and the mechanical—the nanoworld. It is one of the most important and effective drugs against many kinds of cancers [106,107].

The action of taxol is at the nanoscale level of microtubules formed in mitosis; thus it lies between the domains of biochemistry and cellular biology (Figure 5.9). Taxol-derived drugs are examples of discovery of drug design and action by observations from nature. Taxol is also a cautionary tale of the costs of ignoring the importance of preserving the irreplaceable information contained in ancient biodiverse ecological systems [108].

Taxol is typical of many highly potent anticancer drugs derived from natural plant products in being insoluble, hydrophobic, toxic, and difficult to

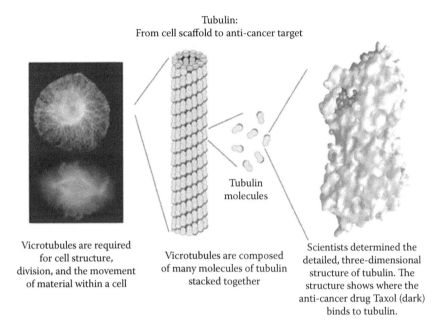

Tubulin:
From cell scaffold to anti-cancer target

Tubulin molecules

Vicrotubules are required for cell structure, division, and the movement of material within a cell

Vicrotubules are composed of many molecules of tubulin stacked together

Scientists determined the detailed, three-dimensional structure of tubulin. The structure shows where the anti-cancer drug Taxol (dark) binds to tubulin.

FIGURE 5.9
Taxol stabilizes the tubulin network, inhibiting cell division. Taxol must be delivered selectively to cancer cells to minimize toxic effects on other parts of the body. Nanoparticles offer a route to targeted delivery. (Courtesy of U.S. NIH government image, presented to Congress, Bethesda, MD.)

deliver through biological barriers to the sites of tumors. Nanoparticulate strategies are being increasingly used for delivery of these types of drugs.

5.4.7 Nanoparticles: Their Materials and Fabrication for Drug Delivery

A large number of therapeutics with nanoscale dimensions and properties have been developed, and have come to be referred to generally as nanomedicines. The development of new types of nanoparticles, nanostructures, and nanoformulations for therapeutics is a very large and active area. Many types of materials and strategies for attachment, entrainment, bonding, and encapsulation are used for nanoparticle drug delivery, including multifunctional targeting that combines imaging and diagnosis with therapy. We describe a few examples in this section.

5.4.7.1 Some Materials and Geometries of Drug Delivery Nanoparticles

Nanoparticles for drug delivery have been fabricated from many types of materials, from inorganics to polymers to bacterial cell walls and viral capsids [109–112]. The use of nanotechnology for drug delivery is a highly developed and very active field, using a wide variety of formulation approaches [113–117]. Some formulations used are listed below. This list is given roughly in increasing order of complexity (from crystals to solid particles, conjugates, emulsions, micelles, liposomes, nanocapsules, and to macromolecular nanomachinery). It is an enumeration rather than a classification: there is considerable overlap in the physical structures of particles that go by different names, for example, colloids, emulsions, and gels. Examples are given in the following sections with details of structures, formulations, and applications.

- Nanocrystals (Examples: oral drugs Rapamune® and Emend®)
- Albumin-based particles (Example: Abraxane®)
- Colloids (polymers, lipids, etc.)
- Emulsions (polymers, solid lipids, etc.)
- Gels
- Nanodiamonds
- Fibers
- Nanotubes
- Dendrimers (Example: PAMAM)
- Polymer-based particles (Examples: drugs XYOTAX™, IT-101, CT-2106, AP5346)
- Polymer conjugates
- Polymeric micelles (Examples: Genexol-PM, SP1049C, NK911, NK012)
- Liposomes (Examples: DaunoXome, Doxil®)
- Polymersomes
- Nanocapsules
- Viral capsids
- Nanocapsules with active elements

(See also Figure 5.10 for some examples.)

5.4.7.2 Some Nanoparticle Drug Delivery Systems

Nanoscale therapeutics that could now be classified as nanoparticles existed for some time before the emergence of nanotechnology as a discipline and area of special focus. A number of materials and formulations have been used for drug delivery since the 1960s. The advent of newer nanomaterials is creating many new options for drug delivery.

Nanocrystals of drug molecules were formulated and approved for oral administration; however, these drugs dissolve rather than reaching their site of action in nanoparticle form. Examples are Rapamune (Wyeth), a formulation of rapamycin (or sirolimus), an immunosuppressant first discovered in

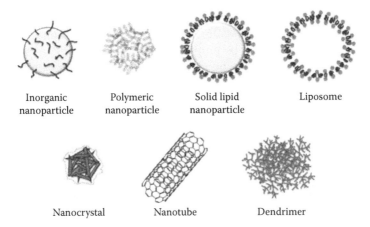

FIGURE 5.10
Some types of nanoparticles: inorganic, polymeric, solid lipid, liposome, nanocrystal, nanotube, and dendrimer. (Reprinted from Farajia, A.H. and Wipf, P., *Bioorg. Med. Chem.*, 17, 2950, 2009. With permission.)

a bacterium from a soil sample from Easter Island, and Emend (Wyeth), an antinausea drug (aprepitant) [118–120].

Albumin-based nanoparticles (for example, Abraxane, a solvent-free albumin formulation of paclitaxel from Abraxis BioScience, LLC, Los Angeles, CA) also dissolve upon administration into the circulatory system, and thus are not true nanoparticle therapeutics, but many formulations of albumin nanoparticles have found use in pharmacology [121].

Colloids, emulsions, and gels: In describing nanoscale drug formulations, three terms are frequently used which refer not to the composition or structure of the particles, but to their physical state in relation to the medium in which they are transported [122].

Colloidal is a general term describing any material mixture where particles of one substance (the colloid) are dispersed evenly throughout a medium composed of a different substance (the dispersant). The colloid particles are not in solution, retaining their own intermolecular structure, but they are small enough (generally between 0.1 and 1000 nm in diameter) to remain suspended in liquid and gas phases. At the lower end of this size range, particles making up colloidal suspensions can consist of individual macromolecules, such as proteins, which are too large to be solubilized. In physical behavior, colloids can be distinguished from solutions in that colloids can be separated from their dispersing medium by physical means, such as centrifugation or ultrafiltration, unlike solutes. Colloidal particles in a suspension may have the same composition but a range of sizes and weights, or may be uniform in size. Many nanoparticle drug delivery formulations are colloidal suspensions, prepared, for example, to aid delivery of insoluble drugs [123,124].

Emulsions are colloidal suspensions of liquid globules or droplets of colloidal size. Generally, an emulsion consists of two immiscible liquid phases, such as oil and water. Emulsions can be prepared by vigorous mixing, as with sonication [125]. Emulsification can be aided by the participation of a surfactant (or emulsifier), which helps form a boundary between the two phases [126]. Micelles and liposomes are particular kinds of emulsions in which the suspended globules are surrounded by an organized emulsification layer or layers.

Gels are semirigid colloidal dispersions of a solid within a fluid (liquid or gas), generally formed by cooling or evaporation of an emulsion. By removing more of the fluid phase, solid gels can be formed with nanoscale or microscale voids or tunnels, which can be used for drug delivery or tissue scaffolding [127,128].

Nanodiamonds have been investigated as a promising nanomaterial for drug delivery, owing to their exceptional biocompatibility and unique surface properties. Insoluble drugs for cancer therapy have been formulated as water-dispersed complexes with nanodiamonds. Nanodiamonds have also found use for localized drug-release coatings in wound healing and surgical implants [129].

Fibers of nanoscale dimensions are being used for delivery of drugs, as nanosensor probes, and as delivery vehicles for genetic modification. Biodegradable nanofibers for drug release can be fabricated by electrospinning, a simple and cost-effective technique capable of producing continuous fibers of various materials from polymers to ceramics. The electrospinning technique is well known in polymer science, and can be used for the preparation of porous biodegradable scaffolds for drug delivery and tissue engineering. Characteristics such as porosity, pore diameters, topology, and mechanical properties can be varied with this and other fabrication techniques [130–132].

Nanotubes, including carbon nanotubes, polymer, and ceramic fabrications, are also being explored for drug delivery and other therapies, including genetic modification of cells [133,134].

Alumina nanotube films can be used as drug delivery vehicles and scaffolding, or can form template molds for fabrication of drug-embedded rods of polymer and other materials [135,136].

Dendrimers (or *dendrons*) are repeatedly branched, typically highly symmetric compounds (named from the Greek *dendron*, meaning "tree"). Unlike most polymers, which are formed by undirected additions of monomer unit building blocks, a dendrimer of any given chemical composition consists of distinct molecules of uniform structure and molecular weight. High molecular weight dendrimer macromolecules may be considered a very special case of polymers; they are also variously referred to as highly branched polymers, hyperbranched polymers, brush polymers, dendrimer star polymers, and dendrimer-like polymers. The importance of dendrimers for medical imaging and drug delivery is that the repeated branches provide multiple uniform and tunable sites for amplification of imaging enhancement and/ or drug delivery functionality. Also, their controllable uniform macro- molecular size gives uniform dispersion rates for drug delivery kinetics (monodispersivity) [137–139]. A widely used dendrimer for drug delivery is poly(amidoamine), abbreviated as PAMAM [140].

5.4.7.3 Polymers and Polymer Conjugates as Drug Delivery Vehicles

Polymers used in fabrication of nanoparticles for drug delivery are generally chosen to be biodegradable, with nontoxic and readily cleared degradation by-products. Examples include polysaccharides, polylactides, and polygly- colides, and their copolymers. Techniques used to load the particles with drugs include absorption on the particle surface; swelling of the particles in a solvent containing the drug, with passive diffusion into the interior of the particle as a result; pressure-enhanced incorporation of the drug into particles; inclusion of the drug into the particle during the polymerization process; and dissolving or mixing the drug into a polymer melt or polymer solution, followed by spray drying/cooling [141]. Different combinations of polymer chemistry and loading methods are used to select the timing and rate of release for delivery into different parts of the body [142]. Polymers with useful functionality such as ion-exchange resins may be used to give added control and selectivity over drug release [143].

Polymer conjugates utilize chemical bonding instead of physical absorption or inclusion to load drugs onto water-soluble polymer nanoparticles. Polymer conjugates can be larger than antibodies or other single biological macromol- ecules used as drug conjugates. In addition, antibodies and other functional units used for site-specific selection can be conjugated onto the polymer along with the drug. Examples of nanoparticle polymer-formulated drugs are XYOTAX (paclitaxel poliglumex, a polymer–drug conjugate of paclitaxel and poly-L-glutamic acid); IT-101 (an experimental nanoparticle therapeutic that consists of the anticancer drug camptothecin (CPT) conjugated to a cyclodex- trin polymer); CT-2106 (a camptothecin conjugate with polyglutamate), and AP5346 (diaminocyclohexane–platinum conjugate) [141,144–147].

Polymer conjugates are showing promise in cancer therapy, both in the form of polymer–protein conjugates (the first type to become available as approved drugs), and polymer conjugates with nonprotein drugs (in devel- opment). Conjugation of proteins with polyethyleneglycol (PEG) is used to reduce immunogenicity, prolong residence time in plasma, and enhance protein stability. Polymer–drug conjugation promotes tumor targeting by enhancing permeation and retention and by lysosomotropic delivery into cells. Polymer conjugates can enter through the cell membrane by mecha- nisms such as receptor-mediated endocytosis. Inside the cell, they can be taken up by lysosomes and interact with the molecular biology of the cytoplasm where the drug release can be most effective. Polymer-drug linkers cleaved by lysosomal thiol-dependent proteases and the reduced pH of endosomes and lysosomes have been exploited to facilitate drug liberation. Improved anticancer activity with conjugates has been observed in chemotherapy refractory patients, and some conjugated formulations have demonstrated a marked reduction in drug toxicity [148–150].

Recently the term "polymer therapeutics" has been used to describe therapies based on polymeric particles, of polymer–drug conjugates, polymer–protein conjugates, polymeric micelles (to which a drug is covalently bound), and multicomponent polymer complexes being developed as nonviral vectors for gene delivery into cells [151]. These nanoscale medicines are being designed to improve drug, protein, and gene delivery, based on a combination of advanced polymer chemistry and precision nanoscale molecular engineering, together with knowledge of the pathophysiology of normal and diseased cells. As pharmaceuticals, these nanomedicines act to deliver therapeutic effects targeted precisely to known targets in the network of the molecular processes of the cellular machinery. In this respect, they go beyond conventional drug delivery systems or formulations, which simply entrap, solubilize, or control drug release. This is the path through which the full therapeutic potential of the postgenomics era will be realized.

The polymer therapeutics approach designs conjugates to deliver specific individual drug payloads (protein, low-molecular-mass drug, gene therapy) to each molecular pharmacological target. Polymer conjugates are tailor-made using a basic tripartite structure (Table 5.1) consisting of (1) a water-soluble polymer, (2) a linker, and (3) the bioactive agent. The molecular mass and physicochemical properties of the polymer are frequently the most important factors governing biodistribution, elimination, and metabolism of the conjugate; hence the choice of polymer is critical. The water-soluble polymer carrier must be nontoxic, non-immunogenic, and suitable for repeated administration. In clinical tests, the most widely used polymers are PEG, N-(2-hydroxypropylmethacrylamide) (HPMA) copolymers, and poly(glutamic acid) (PGA). Of these three, only PGA is biodegradable; consequently, the molecular masses of PEG and HPMA copolymers have been limited to <40 kDa to ensure renal elimination. In the case of nondegradable polymers, the release of the drug depends on the polymer–drug or polymer–protein linker. The ideal polymer–drug linker is chosen so as to be stable during transport to the targeted tumor, but able to release drug at an optimum rate on arrival.

5.4.7.3.1 Polymer–Protein Conjugates

Although the number of peptide-, protein-, and antibody-based drugs entering clinical use is growing rapidly, the limitations of these often include a short plasma half-life, poor stability, and, in the case of proteins, immunogenicity. Conjugates of therapeutic proteins with polymer nano-carriers provide an improved means of delivery [151].

TABLE 5.1

Tripartate Design Components of Polymer Conjugate Nanomedicines

Compound	Polymer	M Mass (g/mol)	Linker	Drug (Loading)	Cleavage Conditions
Polymer–Protein Conjugates					
SMANCS	Styrene–maleic anhydride (SMA) copolymer	15,000	Amine	Neocarzinostatin	Non-biodegradable
Oncaspar®	m-PEG	5,000	Amide	L-asparaginase	Non-biodegradable
Neulasta™	m-PEG	20,000	Amide	G-CSF	Non-biodegradable
PEG-Asys®	Branched m-PEG	40,000	Amide	IFNα-2a	Non-biodegradable
PEG-intron™	m-PEG	12,000	Carbamate	IFNα-2b	β-Lactamase or basic hydrolysis
Polymer–Drug Conjugates					
XYOTAX™	Poly-L-glutamic acid (PGA)	40,000	Ester	Paclitaxel (37 wt%)	PGA degraded by cathepsin B and ester linker by esterases or acid hydrolysis
PK1	HPMA copolymer	30,000	Amide	Doxorubicin (8.5 wt%)	Thiol protease cathepsin B
PK2	HPMA copolymer	25,000	Amide	Doxorubicin (7.5 wt%) and galactosamine (1.5–2.5 mol%)	Thiol protease cathepsin B
AP5280; AP5346	HPMA copolymer	25,000	Malonate; Malonate-DACH	Pt (7 wt%)	Hydrolysis
CT-2106	Poly-L-glutamic acid (PGA)	40,000	Ester	Camptothecin (33–35 wt%)	PGA degraded by cathepsin B and ester linker by esterases or acid hydrolysis
PROTHECAN™	PEG	40,000	Ester	Camptothecin (1.7 wt%)	

Source: Reprinted from Vicent, M.J. and Duncan, R., *Trends Biotechnol.*, 24(1), 40, January 2006. With permission.

SMANCS (Zinostatin stimalamer®), a polymer conjugate of neocarzinostatin (NCS) (derived from *Streptomyces macromomyceticus*) was developed for liver cancer therapy in Japan in the 1990s, and was the first polymer–protein conjugate to be brought to market [152]. NCS has been effective in a number of patients; it has been used synergistically with lipidiol, an iodine-lipid contrast agent that is adhesive to blood vessels in tumors [153]. The conjugate reduces side effects and increases plasma half-life. It consists of two polymer chains of styrene-co-maleic anhydride (SMA) covalently bound to the NCS antitumor protein.

PEG is one of the most widely and successfully used polymers for protein conjugation (PEGylation). Polymer conjugation increases protein solubility and stability, reduces protein immunogenicity, and prolongs plasma half-life through prevention of renal elimination and avoidance of receptor-mediated protein uptake by the reticuloendothelial system (RES). Consequently, polymer-conjugated therapeutics require less frequent dosing.

A PEG–enzyme conjugate, PEG-L-asparaginase (Oncaspar®) (Enzon) was the first antitumor PEGylated protein to be approved for clinical use. This conjugate contains multiple PEG chains (molecular mass 5000 g/mol) linked to the enzyme; it is used as a treatment for acute lymphoblastic leukemia (ALL). The unconjugated enzyme induces hypersensitivity reactions and has a relatively short plasma half-life, which necessitates daily administration for several weeks, whereas the PEG-L-asparaginase conjugate has a plasma half-life of 14 days and can, therefore, be administered by a relatively short infusion every 2 weeks. The reduced immunogenicity of the conjugate enables use in combination with chemotherapy to treat patients who are hypersensitive to the native enzyme.

A number of other PEGylated enzymes are undergoing clinical development, including PEG–recombinant arginine deiminase (rhArg) as a treatment for hepatocellular carcinoma both as a single agent, to deplete arginine, and also in combination with 5-fluorouracil (5-FU). A combination of PEGylated–glutaminase (PEG–glut) and the glutamine antimetabolite 6-diazo-5-oxo-l-norleucine (DON) is also being clinically evaluated, based on the hypothesis that DON will be more effective when glutamine levels are depleted.

PEG is also being used in the development of polymer–cytokine conjugates. PEG–granulocyte colony stimulating factor (PEG–GCSF) (Neulasta™/ PEG-filgrastim) (Amgen) is used to prevent severe cancer chemotherapy-induced neutropenia, reducing the dosing frequency and eliminating most allergic reactions seen with the native protein, although bone pain, another side effect, was not reduced by the conjugate.

Two PEG–interferon-α conjugates—PEG-Intron™ (Shering Plough) and PEGASYS® (Roche)—have been under investigation as antitumor agents. Interferon-α (IFN-α) is active in melanoma and renal cell carcinoma (RCC) patients, but the native protein has a short half-life (2.3 h) necessitating administration three times per week, and its side effects include mild-to-moderate nausea, anorexia, fatigue, and depression. Both of these PEG–IFN-α conjugates have prior approved usages to promote sustained viral response in the treatment of hepatitis C, and their usefulness as anticancer agents is currently being investigated.

A number of PEG–protein conjugates are on the market or under investigation and development, and this field is expected to continue rapid expansion.

5.4.7.3.2 Polymer–Drug Conjugates

Concurrently with the emergence of polymer–protein conjugates, polymer–drug conjugates have been developed with the aim of exploiting the endocytic pathway by means of "lysosomotropic drug delivery." The concept of this drug targeting model was originated by de Duve and coworkers in the course of his work to decipher the structure of cellular architecture, for which he was awarded the Nobel Prize in 1974. Lysosomotropism is the action of drugs that are partitioned selectively between the lysosomes and the cytosol of certain cell types, typically ionic and acidic compounds, or active oxidative species, which may be useful in chemotherapy for destruction of tumor cells [154]. The combination of the idea of lysosomotropism with the optimization of polymer structures for drug delivery [155] opened the way for the active development of many families of polymer–drug conjugates [156].

Conjugation of drugs to water-soluble polymers tends to limit uptake through the endocytic pathway of normal cells relative to tumor cells. This limits exposure of normal cells to the toxicity of chemotherapeutic chemicals, leading to tumor-specific targeting. Polymer conjugates also help to solubilize hydrophobic drugs such as doxorubicin and paclitaxel, facilitating intravenous delivery. Examples of polymer–drug conjugates in clinical development are listed in Table 5.1 from the review by Vicent and Duncan [151].

One of the factors allowing selective targeting of tumors by polymer conjugates and other nanoparticle medicines is the leakiness of blood vessels in tumors. In the normal state, the endothelium cells that line the interior walls of blood vessels are sealed, not allowing the passage of cells or particles. In an inflamed state, the endothelium is signaled to open, allowing the passage of white blood cells through the endothelium into the underlying subendothelial matrix, where they can fight the source of the inflammation. The blood vessels of tumors are in a heightened state of inflammation, allowing passage of cells and nanoparticles. This hyperpermeability can allow cancer cells to spread and metastasize, but it also allows nanoparticles to permeate from the vasculature into the tumor tissue.

In addition, tumor tissue typically lacks an effective organized lymphatic drainage, resulting in retention of fluids and accumulation of nanoparticles and drugs in the tumor. In cancer therapeutics, this factor, along with hyperpermeability, is collectively referred to as "passive enhancement," "passive targeting," or the "enhanced permeability and retention (EPR) effect." The EPR could potentially be enhanced further by signaling molecules that cause loosening of the junctions between endothelial cells, provided that receptors can be found that are unique or at least more common in tumor cells.

A number of potential candidates of this type have been investigated, using saccharides, antibodies, proteins, and peptides as targeting ligands, but so far none have proven effective without toxicity or other obstacles. For example, hepatocytes, the functional cells of the liver, display a unique asialoglycoprotein receptor (ASGPR), which could possibly be used to target liver cancer. A conjugate using N-(2-hydroxypropyl)methacrylamide (HPMA) copolymer in an HPMA–doxorubicin–galactosamine particle formulation (PK2, FCE28069) was investigated for effectiveness against hepatocellular carcinoma, but was discontinued after preliminary trials [157–159]. The galactose ligand was used to target the ASGPR that is expressed on hepatocytes, but it did not provide enough differentiation between tumor cells and healthy hepatocytes.

Many promising drug candidates never enter further development after initial tests. Failure of nanoparticle and other drug candidates in clinical development remains a critical issue for the pharmaceutical and biotechnology industries. Although a number of HPMA conjugates have achieved proof-of-concept status by showing antitumor activity with reduced toxicity, it is too early to tell whether any of these will be proven in all phases of required clinical trials. Lessons are learnt from each early phase clinical study, for example, the failure of HPMA conjugates of paclitaxel and camptothecin in phase I clinical trials underlines the importance of designing a polymer–drug linker that is stable in transit to the tumor [151]. Such negative outcomes are a part of the research and development process; against the extremely complex problem of cancer, we need every tool and creative approach possible.

An advanced anticancer drug conjugate tested in clinical trials is the PGA–paclitaxel conjugate XYOTAX. It has shown antitumor activity against several different cancers. Phase III trials showed that XYOTAX offered a less toxic and more convenient treatment option for non-small-cell lung cancer; in tests with ovarian cancer, patients' response rates were as high as 98%. XYOTAX has also been reported as a novel radiation sensitizer, eliciting a major tumor response in 81% of patients with esophageal or gastric cancer when given in combination with radiation therapy [151].

5.4.7.3.3 Other Developments in Polymer Conjugates

Drugs and proteins have been conjugated with special types of polymers. Dendrimers and dendronized polymers, with their well-defined monodisperse structures, are being explored for improved precision of therapy delivery over heterogeneous, random-coiled, polymeric carriers. Dendrimers, dendronized polymers, stars, hyperbranched polymers, and similar polymer structures can be synthesized with monodisperse nanoscale geometries and high functional group density. Dendrimers, with multiple sites for ligands on their outer surfaces, offer an especially attractive vector for targeting folate receptors, $P2Y_{14}$ receptors, and other G-protein-coupled receptors [160–164]. Other interesting polymer architectures being explored include chimeric block copolymers with amino acid sequences in the polymer, and other hybrid glyco- and peptide-derivatives [165,166].

The development of polymer conjugates remains an active field. New polymeric carriers (including carriers of unique architecture), innovative techniques for polymer–protein and peptide conjugation, and a number of polymer–antibody and targeted polymer–drug conjugates continue to provide new candidates for clinical development. Polymer–protein antitumor conjugates are becoming an established addition to the pharmaceutical armory and a number of polymer–drug conjugates continue to undergo clinical testing. However, there are still many challenges to address as well as opportunities for further research in this area.

5.4.7.3.4 Novel Combination of PEG–PAMAM Dendrimer Conjugates for Radiation and Phototherapy

Dendrimers, with their multiple attachment sites on a single well-defined macromolecule, are ideal for packaging photoactive or radioactive functional groups for concentrated delivery. Large numbers of paramagnetic or radioopaque ions can be attached in combination with a targeting ligand to a dendrimer such as polyamidoamine (PAMAM), to deliver an image enhancement agent to selected sites in the body [167]. Attachment of radioactive atoms to the dendrimer along with a targeting vector can be used in a similar manner to deliver radiotherapy to tumors. But single dendrimer macromolecules are small enough that they are eliminated by the body's hepatic system (and other RES) before they can reach their targets in significant concentration. And radioactive species can decay in route to their targets, lessening their specificity. Boron neutron capture therapy is a means of creating the radioactive particle-emitting species in place, by neutron bombardment activation of precursor boron ^{10}B nucleotides after they have been absorbed by the target tissue. In this case, the challenge is to deliver a sufficient number of boron atoms to the tumor cells prior to neutron activation. Researchers at Ohio State University, Columbus, Ohio have taken a creative approach to solve these obstacles. Using the fact that folate receptors are overexpressed in many types of cancer cells, they synthesized folic acid conjugates of boronated PEG containing PAMAM dendrimers [168]. The folic-conjugated dendrimers were further functionalized by covalent bonding with 12 to 15 decaborate clusters on each macromolecule. A number of PEG polymer units with varying chain lengths were linked to the boronated dendrimers, increasing the particle size to reduce hepatic uptake. Testing on mice with folate receptor–amplified sarcomas demonstrated selective tumor uptake of the dendrimers. Further development is continuing with variations of the PEG and folic acid content to improve the selectivity and pharmacodynamics and reduce hepatic and renal elimination of the conjugates [169].

5.4.8 Nanoencapsulation for Drug Delivery

While conjugation with the nanoparticle carrier material offers many delivery possibilities, an alternative is to enclose the drug inside a protective shell, giving a more complete separation between the delivery vehicle and the therapeutic agent (Figure 5.11).

5.4.8.1 Encapsulation Methods

With nanoencapsulation formulations, release of the drug can take place gradually through diffusion, dissolution, or biodegradation of the container material, or the nanocapsule can be engineered to deliver the drug to a selected environment in response to localized chemistry or enzyme action. Release can also be triggered thermally or photonically. The surface of the drug encapsulation material can be functionalized to selectively attach to

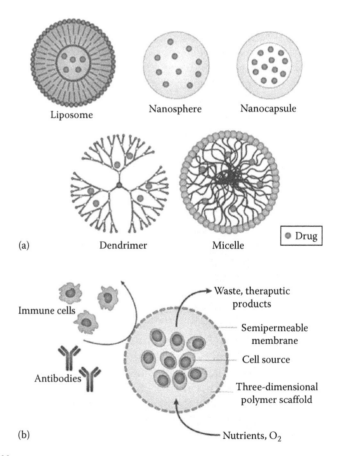

FIGURE 5.11
Some more examples of nanoparticles and nanoencapsulation types. (From Orive, G. et al., *Nat. Rev. Neurosci.*, 10, 682, September 2009. With permission.)

targeted cells, just as with polymer-conjugated delivery systems. A wide variety of methods may be employed to fabricate enclosing spheres, capsules, and containers of different forms and strengths [170–175].

5.4.8.1.1 Polymeric Micelles

Although insoluble drugs can be prepared for aqueous delivery by emulsification, more stable emulsions with drug-filled micelles can be created by use of polymers in the formation of the micelle wall. Stable nanosized micelles have been used in many drug formulations [176,177], including block copolymer micelles as carriers for chemotherapy [178]. Drugs can be incorporated in micelle carriers by covalent or ionic bonding to the micelle-forming material [179,180]. In this case, engineered delivery mechanisms may rely on cleavage of chemical bonds between the polymer and the drug by (a) hydrolysis, (b) enzymes that are located within and outside of cells (e.g., esterases), or (c) enzymes that are located only within cells (e.g., cathepsin B).

Particle size affects the pharmacokinetics, biodistribution, tumor accumulation, and tumor penetration of drug delivery. Polymeric micelles and other particles between 10 and 100 nm in diameter accumulate more readily in tumors than the larger liposomes [181,182]. Movement of a particle throughout a tumor is also size dependent. Therefore, careful control of particle size is important for optimal tumor penetration.

Micelles are notably useful as drug delivery systems for poorly soluble pharmaceuticals. An example is Genexol-PM (polymeric micelle formulated paclitaxel free of Cremophor® EL—a surfactant which has been associated with allergic reactions in some other paclitaxel emulsions) with clinical trials for ovarian and breast cancer (Phase III, 2009) and with carboplatin for advanced ovarian cancer (Phase I/II). Genexol-PM nanoparticles are formulated with paclitaxel entrapped in poly(ethylene glycol)–poly(D,L-lactide) copolymer micelles [183].

NK012 is another polymeric micelle drug formulation loaded with the irinotecan metabolite SN-38, with two Phase II clinical trials for breast and lung cancer (2009). SN-38 (7-ethyl-10-hydroxy-camptothecin) is a biologically active metabolite of the prodrug irinotecan (CPT-11), which binds to and inhibits topoisomerase I by stabilizing the cleavable complex between topoisomerase I and DNA, resulting in DNA breaks, inhibition of DNA replication, and apoptosis. SN-38 has been reported to exhibit up to 1000-fold more cytotoxic activity against various cancer cells in vitro than irinotecan. This SN-38-releasing nanodevice is constructed by covalently attaching SN-38 to the block copolymer PEG-PGlu, followed by self-assembly of amphiphilic block copolymers in an aqueous milieu. This formulation increases the water solubility of SN-38 and allows the delivery of higher doses of SN-38 than those achievable with SN-38 alone [183].

Other micelle drug formulations include NK911, a polymeric micelle carrier system for doxorubicin [184], and SP1049C, which has US FDA clearance and orphan drug status for treatment of gastric cancer [185]. SP1049C

(Supratek Pharma, Inc., Montreal, Quebec, Canada) is doxorubicin noncovalently incorporated into pluronic block copolymer micelles.

Polymer micelles have demonstrated some successes, especially with incorporation of block copolymers, to help evade elimination by the immune system. Some perceived disadvantages of micelles include low loading efficacy of the drug into the micelles, problems with controlling the release rate of the drug, micelle stability, and the use of organic solvents in their manufacture.

5.4.8.1.2 Doughnut Micelles for DNA Delivery

Targeted delivery of drugs to specific tissues requires that the delivery vehicles evade detection and elimination by cellular defenses. Micelle nanoparticles with a hydrophobic core of polylactic acid and a surface coating of hydrophilic PEG have been fabricated by researchers at the University of Nottingham, School of Pharmaceutical Sciences, Nottingham, England, and were shown to evade destruction by mononuclear phagocytes and reach target organs, probably because of the lack of adsorbed serum proteins on their hydrophilic surfaces. These researchers found that mixing a polymer with a net positive electrical charge with negatively charged DNA spontaneously creates a toroid, or doughnut-shape micelle. They are investigating the use of these doughnut micelles to deliver DNA to target tissues without attracting the attention of mononuclear phagocytes for possible use in gene therapy [186].

5.4.8.1.3 Liposomes

Liposomes are nanoparticles that differ from micelles in having a double layer membrane, like the membranes in cells, whereas micells have only a monolayer. Liposomes are vesicles consisting of a lipid bilayer surrounding an aqueous interior. Liposomes are generally made using phospholipids, providing a chain molecule with a hydrophilic head and hydrophobic tail, for assembly into the bilayer. Since natural cell membranes are composed on a base of phospholipid bilayers, liposomes assembled from this type of molecule have good biocompatibility and biodegradability.

Phospholipids are surfactants that self-assemble into planar bilayers in water. To make enclosed liposomes, the planar layer must be disrupted by application of energy or use of a catalyst. Liposomes can be made by a number of methods, including sonication with addition of electrolytes for stabilization, extrusion, spray drying, or decompression processes [187–193]. Liposomes can be unilameral or multilameral, with many layers like an onion.

Liposomes can solubilize drugs and extend circulation time and cell uptake, particularly if they are stabilized with polymers (e.g., PEG). The simplest liposome formulations provide no control or targeting for drug release. Liposomes generally do not provide intracellular delivery of drug molecules, and thus are not effective against drug-resistant disease. Unless protected, they are rapidly removed from the body by the RES (liver, spleen, and lymphatic tissues) [194].

If the liposome is stabilized and its surface is formulated to protect it from detection and destruction by the body's immune system (stealth liposomes), circulation times can be extended and they can be used effectively in therapy. Stealth liposomes are fabricated to present a layer of inert PEG on the outside of the membrane, which prevents recognition and elimination by the body's immune system. The inert PEG coating prevents immune recognition, but it also hinders binding of the liposome to the delivery sites on cell membranes. To counteract this, most PEG-coated liposomes also have one or more biological species attached to match receptors expressed at binding sites. Targeting ligands can be monoclonal antibodies (immunoliposomes), vitamins, or specific antigens to address particular cell types in the body [195,196].

Liposomes may be stabilized by coating with sugars such as hyaluronan, which also provide potential binding sites [197]. These binding sites can be used to conjugate ligands for targeted delivery. In addition to carrying drugs, liposomes can be used to entrap and deliver siRNA and viruses for gene therapy. Entrapment of large molecules is carried out by lyophilizing (freeze-drying) followed by resuspending them in a solution containing the molecules [198].

Liposomes with special properties can be made from artificial materials other than phospholipids. For example, biomimetic liposomes have been designed from waxy lipids for thermal drug release at relatively low temperatures in the treatment of solid tumors [170].

An example of a liposomal drug formulation is Doxil, generic name: doxorubicin liposomal, a formulation of doxorubicin in spherical liposomes. Doxorubicin is an antitumor antibiotic, a class of drugs produced by the soil fungus *Streptomyces*, which acts on specific phases of the cell growth and division cycle.

5.4.8.1.4 Polymer-Caged Liposomes (Matrix-Reinforced Liposomes)

One of the challenges in using liposomes for drug delivery is their lack of stability. Researchers at the Nanomaterials for Cancer Diagnostics and Therapeutics Center for Cancer Nanotechnology Excellence at Northwestern University, Chicago, Illinois have developed a method for stabilizing liposomes within a polymer which can fall apart and trigger drug release when taken into cells. The cage is constructed by inserting cholesterol-poly(acrylic acid) into the outer membrane of a liposome and then cross-linking the poly(acrylic acid) chains to form a polymer cage. The polymer-surrounded liposomes are stable in serum and with freeze-drying and rehydration, a process that destroys conventional liposomes. The polymer cage is unstable at pH levels found within tumor cells, enabling targeted release of drug contents [199].

5.4.8.1.5 Polymersomes

Polymersomes is a term coined for vesicles similar to liposomes, but made with synthetic amphiphilic block copolymers to form the vesicle membranes, rather than lipid or surfactant bilayers. In general, they can be prepared by the methods used in the preparation of liposomes.

Like liposomes, polymersomes are used to encapsulate and deliver drugs, proteins, and genetic material [200].

If comb or dendronized polymers are used to form the polymersome membrane, it has the same bilayer morphology as a liposome, with the hydrophobic blocks of the two layers in the interior of the membrane. More commonly, a linear diblock or triblock copolymer membrane is used, with one hydrophobic block adjacent to or between one or two hydrophilic blocks. The choice of block copolymers gives a wide range of options for properties such as stability, permeability, biodegradability, and control of release rates and targeting. The surfaces can be studded with peptides and other cell signaling ligands [201].

Polymersomes are being actively investigated for therapeutic targeting and delivery, and as a potential tool for cell tracking [202]. Polymersomes have also been used to fabricate nanoreactors that contain active enzymes with selective transport of substrates through the membrane, and are of great interest for the design of artificial cells and organelles containing, for example, hemoglobin [203].

5.4.8.2 New Designs and Applications for Therapeutic Nanoparticles and Nanocapsules

In this section, we review other types of functional nanoparticles and nanocapsules that do not fit easily into the previously discussed categories. These include some remarkably innovative and effective creations, some of which have been developed at the NIH nanomedicine centers or through other nanomedicine initiatives in recent years. They also include some new adaptations and enhancements to nanomaterials discussed earlier for imaging and photothermal applications (such as gold nanoparticles and quantum dots), which extend their usefulness into drug delivery and gene therapy. The addition of biomolecular functionality to nanoparticles enables combination of imaging, targeting, drug delivery, and other therapies in the same multifunctional nanodevice, bringing nanomedicine closer to the realization of nanoengineered molecular medicines. A number of excellent reviews are available in the scientific and medical literature on recent developments in these areas, which we briefly summarize here.

5.4.8.2.1 Functionalized Gold Nanoparticles

Gold nanoparticles and nanorods can be functionalized with polymers in a large number of ways to encapsulate the gold core with polymers, dendrimers, or biomolecules. In addition to the imaging and photothermal therapies discussed previously, functionalized gold nanoparticles can be used as the basis for sensors, drug carriers, and DNA/gene delivery. Examples are given in a recent review [204] of synthesis methods and applications in therapies for Alzheimer's, HIV, hepatitis, tuberculosis, arthritis, diabetes, and advanced imaging. The review also discusses toxicology and optical properties of functionalized gold nanospheres and nanorods. A wide range of sizes, shapes, and functionalizations have been synthesized and applied.

5.4.8.2.2 Quantum Dots

The same range of numerous surface functionalizations that apply to polymer and gold nanoparticles are applicable to quantum nanodots with many of the same potential medical applications. Quantum dots are especially attractive for multifunctional biomedical investigation because of their broad-range excitation, size-tunable narrow emission spectra, and high photostability. Because of their toxic metal content, nanodots are being explored most rapidly as research tools. Therapeutic uses are proceeding cautiously pending resolution of health and safety issues [205].

5.4.8.2.3 Fluorescent Nanodiamonds

One interesting alternative to conventional quantum dots is based on nanodiamonds, which offer a nontoxic analogue to quantum dots for imaging of cellular membranes and other hydrophobic components of biological systems. Hydrophobic blue fluorescent nanodiamond can be synthesized by covalent linking of octadecylamine to the surface of nanodiamond particles. The material is easily dispersible in hydrophobic solvents, forming a transparent colloidal solution, producing a bright blue fluorescence. Similar surface modification can be used for other carbon nanoparticles [206].

5.4.8.2.4 Solid Lipid Nanoparticles

Nanoparticles based on solid lipids have developed as modern nanofabricated extensions of early lipid emulsion drug formulations dating back to the 1960s. Early lipid emulsion drugs were successful in reducing drug side effects and extending release times, but the emulsions tended to be unstable, leading to agglomeration and breakup of the emulsions. Liposomes and polymeric nanoparticles eclipsed these early forms of lipid emulsions for a time, but work has continued to produce improvements. Three types of solid lipid nanoparticles have been developed for drug delivery and therapy: "solid lipid nanoparticles," "nanostructured lipid carriers" and "lipid drug conjugates" [207]. These nanodrugs have been formulated with the aim of overcoming some of the difficulties of liposomes: limited physical stability, leakage of drug, difficulty in cell targeting, and clearance by the immune system, while providing improved biocompatibility, low drug loading, and low selectivity in comparison with polymer conjugates [174,208].

5.4.8.2.5 Polymers, Nanopore Membranes, and Nanoporous Implants

Nanoscale polymer implants for drug release into tumors or wounds can be implanted directly for efficient drug release into the tissue. Work has been ongoing in a number of laboratories to develop many types of nanoporous plugs, membranes, and other implants for therapy delivery and tissue regeneration. We discuss tissue regeneration in Chapter 7. As imaging, drug delivery, and tissue engineering materials become more multifunctional, there is considerable overlap between nanoparticle drug carriers and tissue scaffolding functionalized to stimulate and guide growth and reduce infection.

Nanoporous membranes and other implants are designed to meet the needs for continuous release of therapeutic agents in a localized area over a long time period. Drug delivery with nanoporous implants can reduce systemic toxicity and improve efficacy for cancer and wound healing therapy. Implants are being developed in order to provide for ease and low frequency of administration, overcome problems of patient compliance, minimize the needed intervention of healthcare personnel, and decrease length of hospital stays [209,210]. Nanoporous materials are also being developed for use in stents and other surgical implants, which are discussed in Chapter 6.

5.4.8.2.6 Nanogels

Another method of encapsulating drugs in colloidal polymers is with nanogels, a unique type of nanoparticle formation. Nanogels are nanosized hydrogel particles composed of a network of flexible hydrophilic crosslinked polymer strands. The hydrophilic polymers can absorb large amounts of water, swelling the particles into a gel. Nano- and microgels have been found to be very useful in drug delivery and tissue regeneration because of their tissue compatibility, biodegradability, and versatility. Drugs are readily absorbed into the particles along with water or other solvents, and released upon biodegradation. Biocompatible nanogels can be readily made using polymers derived from natural materials such as polysaccharides (chitosan, hyaluronan, dextran, cellulose, pullulan, alginate, and chondroitin sulfate). By variation of their molecular composition, size, and morphology, nanogels can be designed to encapsulate diverse classes of bioactive molecules, and made to respond to environmental changes for controlled drug release [211–213].

Nanoparticle hydrogels can be prepared by emulsion or precipitation polymerization to form a stable colloidal dispersion. By use of free radical scavenging metals to slow the polymerization process, nanogel particles can be prepared with highly controlled uniform polymer chain lengths and crosslinkages, in a process called atom transfer radical polymerization (ATRP), also known as "living polymerization" because the polymerization chain reactions are not terminated as randomly as in an uncontrolled process [214,215]. Under special conditions, certain drugs with affinity for absorption onto the nanogel polymer chains can be loaded spontaneously into the nanogels, displacing absorbed water and resulting in the reduction of the solvent volume, leading to gel collapse and formation of dense drug-laden nanoparticles [216].

5.4.8.3 Encapsulation Techniques and Materials for Proteins and Peptides

A critical requirement for effectiveness of a therapeutic drug is delivery—getting the right amount in the right form to the right place. Proteins make up the nanomachinery of cells, and therefore proteins or peptides would make the ideal drug for many diseases, but proteins are broken down and modified by enzymes and blocked from passing through many barriers in the body. For much of medical history, successful pharmaceuticals have been based on small molecules, such as aspirin, which act to regulate complex biological networks, or larger molecules (but still small compared to proteins), which inhibit or disrupt a precise part of the cellular machinery. But driven by examples of therapeutic proteins such as insulin, research efforts have continued to advance the delivery of therapeutic peptides and proteins by increasingly effective, convenient, and less invasive means. Much of this recent progress is based on nanoparticle technologies like those discussed in the preceding sections. This work continues to advance with new materials and formulations focused in particular on peptide delivery.

5.4.8.3.1 Protein Nanoencapsulation with Polysaccharides

Nanoencapsulation with polymeric nanoparticles is offering new drug delivery routes for peptides and proteins. One useful encapsulation material is chitosan [217], a derivative of the chitin polysaccharide found in insect and arthropod shells [218]. Extensive research is taking place on many formulations for encapsulating insulin and other peptides, including detailed models of absorption and desorption rates [219].

One method developed for encapsulating nanoparticles with chitosan is the polyionic coacervation fabrication process, useful in particular for protein encapsulation and release. This process has been systematically manipulated and studied in a number of laboratories to improve pharmacokinetic predictability and effectiveness [220,221]. Bovine serum albumin (BSA) is used as a model protein, which is encapsulated using the polyanion tripolyphosphate (TPP) as the coacervation cross-link agent to form chitosan–BSA–TPP nanoparticles.

The BSA-loaded chitosan–TPP nanoparticles are characterized for particle size, morphology, zeta potential (colloidal electrokinetics), BSA encapsulation efficiency, and subsequent release kinetics. These properties have been found to be dependent on chitosan molecular weight, chitosan concentration, BSA loading concentration, and chitosan/TPP mass ratio. Protein-loaded nanoparticles can be prepared under varying conditions in the size range of 200–580 nm, with a high positive zeta potential. An advantage of chitosan over some other encapsulation materials is that later stage particle degradation and disintegration does not yield a substantial follow-on release, as the remaining protein molecules, with adaptable 3D conformation, seem to be tightly bound and entangled with the cationic chitosan chains.

The polyionic coacervation process for fabricating protein-loaded chitosan nanoparticles offers simple preparation conditions and a useful range for manipulation of physiochemical properties of the nanoparticles (e.g., size and surface charge). A weakness of chitosan nanoparticle encapsulation is typically with difficulties in controlling initial burst effects, which can release large quantities of protein molecules [172].

5.4.8.3.2 *Cyclodextrin Nanostructures in Drug Delivery*

The cyclodextrins are a family of cyclic oligosaccharides composed of α-(1,4) linked glucopyranose subunits. Cyclodextrins have generated intense interest because of their many useful properties for drug delivery, not least as enhancers of nanoparticle delivery. Cyclodextrin molecules are shaped like cones with a hydrophilic outer surface and a lipophilic central cavity presenting an environment comparable to an aqueous ethanol solution. They have a cage-like supramolecular structure, which is the same as the crown ethers, whose ring forms an open-ended cone shaped by six or more glucopyranose units, making them useful molecular chelating agents [222–224].

Cyclodextrin molecules are relatively large (molecular weight ranging from almost 1000 to over 1500), with a central cavity diameter on the order of a nanometer or more, giving room for a smaller molecule to form a host–guest complex, or inclusion compound, with high trapping efficiency. This form of chelation can be used to deliver drugs through membranes and protect them from enzymes, and protect the body from toxic and irritant effects of drugs [225,226].

Cyclodextrins act as penetration enhancers by a unique mechanism, increasing drug availability at the surface of biological membranes without modifying or disrupting the lipid layers of the biological barrier. The cyclodextrin ring has a hydrated outer surface, which normally presents a barrier to penetration of biological membranes. But cyclodextrins can keep hydrophobic drug molecules in solution and deliver them to the membrane surface, where they can partition into the lipophilic center. The relatively lipophilic membrane has a low affinity for the hydrophilic cyclodextrin molecules, which do not cross the membrane.

Cyclodextrins have also been incorporated into the nanostructure of semipermeable membranes as osmotic pumping agents for controlled delivery of poorly soluble drugs [227–232].

Cyclodextrins have unique structural, physical, chemical, and biological properties. They readily link both covalently and non-covalently as building blocks for nanoscale structures. The covalent conjugation of molecules with different properties provides a very attractive approach for building multifunctional particles for pharmaceutical applications. Cyclodextrin conjugates with amines, amino acids, peptides, and aromatic systems have been synthesized. Fascinating compounds including enzyme mimics, abiotic receptors, fluorescence indicators, and molecular actuators have been synthesized by exploiting the appropriate combination of the hydrophobic nature and the different sizes of the cavity with the specific features of the attached molecules.

Derivatives can vary the solubility and provide intermolecular linkages for assembly of nanostructures, for example, spontaneous association of hydrophobized dextran and poly-β cyclodextrin into nano-assemblies. Erythrocyte-like liposomes that could possibly serve as artificial red blood cells or drug vehicles have been prepared by means of amphiphilic cyclodextrin sulfates. Other interesting structures prepared include beta-cyclodextrin/ polyacrylic acid microspheres [233].

5.4.8.3.3 Polyelectrolyte Capsules

Researchers in Ghent University in Belgium have prepared polyelectrolyte capsules for delivery of DNA and a variety of other substances into cells, using a layer-by-layer adsorption of polymers onto sacrificial template particles. DNA can be precipitated onto template particles with spermidine, coated with electrolyte multilayers, and then released into the capsule interior upon dissolution of the core template particle. Capsules can also be fabricated by coating the sacrificial template particle with electrolyte, dissolving the core template, dehydrating the resulting capsules, and rehydrating in a solution containing the content to be loaded, such as DNA. Multifunctional delivery systems can be made by incorporating functional polyelectrolytes or other nanoparticles in between the layers formed during electrostatic self-assembly around the templates to yield particles with different properties such as controlled and triggered release in response to temperature, pH, and light. This technique can also be used to load the multilayers with magnetic nanoparticles to form drug delivery vehicles that can be manipulated and guided by magnetic fields [234].

5.4.8.3.4 Viral Capsids, Bacterial Shells, Ghost Cells

Viral capsids, composed of large polypeptide chains, have been recognized for some time as being applicable for use in encapsulation of drugs and other substances. Viruses form highly symmetrical monodisperse polymeric architectures, with multivalent display of surface ligands which they use to attach to cell membranes. They are thus ideal templates for nanoengineering the multifunctional encapsulation of inorganic and organic materials. For this reason, viral capsids have been studied in comparison to polymersomes, and are used to design biomimetic drug encapsulation and delivery systems [235–237].

In one example, the dendrimer plug from a bioengineered virus was adapted as a drug delivery capsule. Researchers used viral coat nanoparticles that incorporate receptors in their outer shells acting on biological effectors inside cells. The receptor and effector together act to detect a specific biochemical signal that then affects the viral capsid nanocontainer and its contents. The effects can include drug release or the generation of a diagnostic signal [238]. The viral nanocontainers are loaded with an enzyme that converts substrate molecules into a light-emitting fluorescent form. The substrate molecules are specifically transported by bacterial membrane pore proteins engineered into the viral nanocontainer, where they react to produce light that can be seen using fluorescence microscopy, demonstrating that the delivery capsule is working. This method could insert an enzyme that converts an inactive drug into its active form for release only inside a diseased cell.

A novel system for the packaging of drugs as well as vaccines is the use of bacterial cell walls. These "bacterial ghosts" are intact, non-denatured bacterial envelopes that are created by lysis of bacteria using phage enzymes under controlled conditions [239–241]. Diatom shells have also been studied as potential templates for drug encapsulation [242].

5.4.8.3.5 Trojan Horse Targeting for Tumors

Not only dead bacteria, but live cells as well can be used to deliver drugs. Tumor cells create inflammation signals, which attract white blood cells. In a very clever strategy, researchers have used the recruitment of monocytes into tumor tissue as "Trojan horses." First, the monocytes are induced to engulf specially coated gold nanoshells. These white blood cells are released to invade the tumor, then the phagocytized gold nanodots are heated by photoinduction. The monocytes become kamikaze cells, destroying the surrounding tumor cells [243].

5.4.8.3.6 Fatal Magnetic Sugar Bait for Cancer Cells

In another creative and innovative strategy, the tumor cells themselves have been induced to ingest and carry their own therapeutic instruments of self-destruction. Cancer cells in expanding tumors need much more energy to support their abnormally rapid growth rate. Their overcharged metabolism induces them to ingest special sugar-coated magnetic nanoparticles, unlike normal healthy cells, for which the ingestion rate is negligible in comparison. After an incubation period, the affected portion of the body is subjected to an oscillating magnetic field, which thermally agitates the nanoparticles and kills the cancer cells. This technology is being developed and tested for therapeutic use by MagForce Nanotechnologies AG in Germany [244].

5.4.8.3.7 Encapsulation with Alumina Nanotubes

Carefully controlled anodization of aluminum can produce arrays of aluminum oxide pores on the metal surface. This nanolayer array can be electrochemically detatched and electroformed into a robust array of nanoporous alumina capsules with highly uniform pores of 25–55 nm. Applications of these capsules for controlled drug delivery have been developed, demonstrating that molecular transport could be readily controlled by selection of capsule pore size. A branched membrane structure, with a stepwise change in pore size from large to small, was fabricated to provide small pore-sized membranes with sufficient mechanical strength for handling [245].

5.4.8.3.8 Therapeutic and Diagnostic Silicon Nanotechnology

Silicon-based devices have played a central role in the development of microelectronics, MEMS, and nanodevices. Silicon and other solid-state semiconductor materials served as the platforms for pioneering work that proved concepts and demonstrated implementations for nanoscale electronics, sensors, and mechanical devices. Thus far in this overview we have focused on quantum dots, polymers, and other materials, but now it is time to look at silicon and similar materials. There is an enormous wealth of technology and experience in solid-state semiconductor and thin-film fabrication, which holds potential for application to nanodevices for medical applications. Because of its unique electronic and chemical properties, silicon can be useful as the material for functional nanoparticles for diagnostic sensing and drug delivery, as well as a fabrication material for more elaborate devices.

As an example, the use of sacrificial layers that are dissolved or etched away to leave a desired pattern or structure is a classic technique in solid-state microfabrication. Sacrificial layers can also be used to release drugs along with other material in nanodevices and nanoparticles [246].

One issue with silicon and other inert inorganic nanoparticles, as opposed to polymers, is the need to be cleared from an organism. The high structural and chemical inertness of many inorganic nanoparticle materials can be an advantage, ensuring that the contents remain intact on the way to the targeted tissue, whereas leakage and instability is often encountered as a problem with organic nanoparticles. It is necessary, however, to reach a trade-off between stability and degradability, to ensure eventual delivery of the drug contents and avoid accumulation of particles in the body. This balance has been achieved in some cases by careful engineering design and functionalization of silicon-based nanoparticles.

One way in which silicon can be used for drug delivery is in the form of porous silicon nanoparticles. In development experiments, a number of different researchers have fabricated silica nanospheres permeated with a honeycomb-like network of pores. Porous silicon spheres with diameters of less than 400 nm can easily be taken up into cells. The pores can be filled with a content of "guest molecules" that can be released by diffusion.

To be most useful for drug delivery and imaging, silicon nanoparticles should have the ability to disintegrate slowly in aqueous solution and thereby be cleared from an organism. A research team based at the University of California San Diego's UCSD NanoTUMOR Center, San Diego, California has fabricated biodegradable porous silicon–based nanoparticles which were demonstrated in mice to degrade into renally cleared components in a relatively short period of time, with no evidence of toxicity.

The particles are made by electrochemically etching the surface of a silicon wafer to produce porous silicon, which is then broken down into nanoparticles by ultrasonication. Filtration yields particles less than 200 nm in size, which are then incubated in water to allow growth of a surface layer of silica (silicon dioxide, SiO_2). Nanoporous silicon particles thus treated have an intrinsic NIR photoluminescence that can be used for monitoring of accumulation and degradation of the particles in vivo. The luminescence in the nanoparticles is due to electron trapping in defects between the silicon and silica. These defects also act as reactive points for hydrolysis, leading to degradation of the particles. Thus, in contrast to most optically active nanomaterials (carbon nanotubes, gold nanoparticles, and quantum dots), these porous silicon nanoparticles self-destruct in the body into nontoxic, systemically eliminated products. The researchers have proposed that the degradation product is orthosilicic acid, which is known to be readily eliminated in urine [247].

The UCSD researchers loaded the silicon nanoparticles with the anticancer drug doxorubicin and demonstrated its slow release under physiological conditions in a culture of cancer cells. Coating the nanoparticles with dextran (a glucan polysaccharide) slowed their degradation and enhanced accumulation in tumors in mice. Work is continuing to refine control of the timing and degree of drug release [248].

In other sophisticated functional nanoparticle designs, pores in mesoporous silica are gated by nanovalves that are opened by pH or solvent interactions for controlled and selective release. In one nanoparticle system developed by a team at Northwestern University, a skewer-like bisammonium molecular stalk is attached at the entrance of each pore. The stalk protrudes from the sphere's surface, where it complexes with a doughnut-shaped molecule called cucurbituril, effectively plugging the pore. The electrostatic bonding between the bisammonium stalk and the cucurbituril plug is pH dependent, demonstrating a switchable release mechanism with potential for medical applications. Further work is exploring similar release control mechanisms that could be triggered by enzymes present only in diseased cells, and in devising pH controlled switches that operate in a range that discriminates between healthy and cancerous cells [249].

5.5 Some Therapeutic Application Areas for Nanoparticles

In the previous sections of this chapter, we have reviewed the different types of technologies and materials used for therapy delivery. Now we review some of the medical areas to which these nanotechnologies are being applied and see specific details of how they are being used to treat diseases. Nanotechnology for drug and therapy delivery have been used in many medical practice areas including dermatology for topical applications, ocular drug delivery, gastrointestinal, orthopedics, cardiology, pulmonology, radiology, surgery, and many other areas, for treatment of infectious, autoimmune, degenerative, and other diseases [250–252]. Perhaps the greatest impact of nanotechnology drug delivery is in cancer treatment. But first we show examples from some of the areas that have received less publicity.

5.5.1 Infectious Diseases

Nanotechnology drug delivery is as applicable to antibiotics as it is to anticancer drugs, with similar benefits. Nanoparticles can, in principle, be targeted to attack specific types of pathogens. Nanoparticles have the important additional benefit against both cancer cells and infectious agents that they can be engineered to overcome mechanisms of drug resistance. These attributes of nanoparticle delivery are likely to become increasingly more important for utilization against pathogens in the future [253,254].

For the present, nanoparticles are being investigated and tested for use against bacteria, particularly tuberculous and other mycobacteria [255,256]. Dendrimer nanoparticles have been formulated and tested as antibacterial drug carriers, using sulfamethoxazole as a model drug [257].

Nanoparticle therapy is also being used against viral infections. Nanoparticles based on pegylated interferon alpha-2a have been developed to treat chronic hepatitis-C to improve pharmacodynamics of the protein resulting in a more effective medication [258]. Nanoparticle techniques are also being explored in applications against other viruses, notably against herpes, HIV, and other sexually transmitted diseases. Nanoparticles can have novel modes of action against viruses, including attaching to form conjugates that are prevented from entering the cell membrane [259]. A dendrimer product, VivaGel (SPL7013, Starpharma), has passed two US FDA Phase I trials as an antiviral for prevention of HIV and genital herpes infections. VivaGel is a formulation of a lysine-based dendrimer with naphthalene disulphonic acid surface groups [260].

Nanotechnology is also being used to develop advanced vaccines and for vaccine delivery, including vaccines for topical application [261,262]. The nanoparticle formulations enable the vaccine to be transferred through the skin without injections.

As one example of the close relationship between biomimetic nanomachine concepts, macromolecules, and immunology, researchers in Texas and France have been developing biomimetic protein adhesive nanogrippers based on thioester proteins found in the immune systems of mosquitoes to attack and immobilize malaria parasites [263,264].

5.5.2 Degenerative and Autoimmune Diseases

Nanomedicines have potential for treatment of chronic and degenerative conditions because of their capability for sustained and targeted release, with the ability to deliver powerful drugs to specific tissues while minimizing side effects. These attributes have been used in nanoformulated drugs for treatment of Crohn's disease [265], rheumatoid arthritis [266], essential hypertension [267], and for neurodegenerative diseases such as Alzheimer's and Parkinson's [268,269]. The ability of nanoparticles to effect penetration of the blood–brain barrier is an important aspect of their effectiveness for neurodegenerative disorders and brain tumors, which we discuss in detail in the following sections and in Chapter 7.

5.5.3 Nanoparticle Drug Delivery in Cardiology and Vascular Disease

Besides their use in cardiac imaging enhancement [270–273], nanoparticles are being developed for drug delivery in atherosclerosis, ischemic heart disease, and heart failure, and for the targeted delivery of drugs to promote angiogenesis for the salvage of ischemic tissue. Nanomedicine is being developed to offer options for diagnostic and therapeutic challenges encountered in treating transient ischemic attacks and strokes. Antiangiogenic paramagnetic nanoparticles may be used to assess the severity of atherosclerotic disease in asymptomatic, high-risk patients by detecting the development of plaque neovasculature, which reflects the underlying lesion activity and vulnerability to rupture. Nanoparticles can also be used to deliver locally targeted antiangiogenic therapy to retard plaque progression and thereby enhance the effectiveness of statin therapy. Nanoparticles in an imaging modality can serve as quantitative markers to guide atherosclerotic management, which can be especially important for asymptomatic patients. Nanoscaffolds for cell growth and nanoparticle-coated stents are another application of nanotechnology to cardiovascular therapy, which we review in Chapters 6 and 7 [274–277].

5.5.4 Usefulness of Nanoparticles in Otolaryngology

Traditionally, otolaryngologists have embraced new technologies for their ability to improve precision of diagnostic accuracy and surgical intervention in the ear, nose, and throat. Nanomedicine provides new opportunities to help otolaryngologists meet the challenges of visualization and access in a complex and inaccessible part of the body [278,279].

5.5.5 Ocular Applications of Nanocarrier Drug Delivery

Nanocarriers were adopted early for external ocular drug delivery, where they were found to be useful to counteract the clearance mechanisms of the eye, and thus prolong residence time at the ocular surface after instillation [280–283]. This enables reduction in the administered dosage and instillation frequency. Nanoparticle drug carriers can also be used in intraocular drug delivery to control the release rate of the drug, reduce the number of injections required, and target the drug to the site of action, thus reducing the dose required and decreasing side effects. Nanocarriers have been found effective in targeting the posterior tissues of the eye, which otherwise present difficulties for access [83,284,285].

5.5.6 Nanoparticle Drug Delivery for Neuroinflammatory Diseases

Researchers at Wayne State University in Michigan have developed a den-drimer nanomedicine that targets drug release for maternal intrauterine inflammation of the type that has been implicated in the development of periventricular leukomalacia and cerebral palsy. Anti-inflammatory drugs that are currently available for neonatal and perinatal applications show high plasma binding, requiring high doses and producing side effects. PAMAM dendrimer-based nanodevices that deliver the drug in response to inflammation markers are being developed to help prevent these serious and incurable conditions [286]. This research could also address other neuro-inflammatory conditions associated with age-related macular degeneration, Alzheimer's, multiple sclerosis, amytrophic lateral sclerosis, and Parkinson's disease.

5.5.7 Nanotherapies for Insulin Delivery

Diabetes mellitus is a diseased state caused by failure of the production and regulation of insulin, a peptide hormone which regulates the metabolism of glucose. There are two forms of diabetes: Type I, or juvenile diabetes, is an autoimmune disease resulting from the loss of insulin production cells in the pancreas. Type II, or adult onset diabetes, is characterized by insulin resistance in the tissues and eventual insulin cell failure in many cases. In both types of diabetes, the body eventually fails to produce enough insulin and glucose can build up in the blood and lead to damage of tissues.

Diabetes is treated by insulin replacement therapy, which requires delivery of the peptide to the blood stream. Insulin was the first peptide to be used as a successful drug. Because insulin, like other peptides, is rapidly broken down by the digestive system, it is generally administered by incuta-neous injection with hypodermic needles [287,288].

The discovery of insulin and its therapeutic value for diabetes represented an enormous breakthrough for one of the oldest documented diseases. The main cause of type I (insulin-dependent) diabetes mellitus is degeneration of insulin-producing β cells in the islets of Langerhans, located in the pan-creas. Named after the German pathologist Paul Langerhans, who discov-ered them in 1869, the islets are clusters of specialized cells that produce a number of hormones in addition to insulin. The islets contain five types of cells: alpha cells that make glucagon, which raises the level of glucose in the blood; beta cells that make insulin, which lowers blood sugar and is needed by cells to metabolize it; delta cells that make somatostatin which inhibits the release of numerous other hormones in the body; and PP cells and D1 cells, about which much is still unknown.

Ever since the discovery of insulin, efforts have been underway to find an alternative to incutaneous injection with hypodermic needles. Besides the inconvenience and discomfort of injection, there are risks of improper dosage and rates of release. Insulin is released in controlled amounts by the pancreas in response to changes in blood sugar and other network stimuli, which are difficult to simulate by injections. And accidental injection of insulin directly into the bloodstream results in insulin shock, a dangerous and potentially fatal condition of hypoglycemia.

One approach to the insulin delivery problem is to synthesize or find compounds that have similar activity to insulin, but would survive modification in the digestive tract, passing into the blood stream in an active form. Other approaches seek injectable forms of insulin that have a more controlled release, and/or which are suitable for alternative forms of delivery, such as inhalation or intravenous or transcutaneous administration by micropumps. Progress has been slow on most fronts, but nanoparticles are providing new alternatives.

One approach using nanoparticles that has been explored is to encapsulate insulin in a protective coating that would allow its release after passing through the digestive system. An alternative release technique is to encapsulate insulin for injection into the soft tissues, in order to achieve a gradual, controlled rate of release into the blood stream for a basal level of insulin, which can be supplemented as needed by injections. Many methods of encapsulation for injection have been tried, including liposomes, which can be administered intravenously [289].

The encapsulation of insulin and other drugs into liposomes, microcapsules, and nanocapsules is an example of practical nanoengineering to which much effort has been devoted over many years with the goal of seeking improved treatments for diabetes. A related approach is to infuse insulin into porous or absorbent polymer particles for gradual release [290]. The greatest benefits would come from a non-injected delivery mechanism, so much effort has been directed toward usable oral insulin formulations [291–295].

In a typical method for preparing nanoparticles of insulin or other peptide, the peptide is dissolved in an aqueous solution; then a nonsolvent such as a low molecular weight (C_1 to C_6) alcohol is stirred in with the aqueous solution. The alcohol absorbs up to 100% of its weight of water, causing the peptide to precipitate out of solution, with particles having diameters in the range of about 100–200 nm. If the mixture contains a suitable polymer, the particles are spontaneously coated as they precipitate; the process is called phase inversion nanoencapsulation.

Zinc insulin is a slowly released form of insulin that has been encapsulated in various polyester and polyanhydride nanosphere formulations using phase inversion nanoencapsulation. The encapsulated insulin maintains its biological activity and is released from the nanospheres over a span of hours. Some formulations have been shown to be active orally. These formulations typically have about 10% of the efficacy of intraperitoneally delivered zinc insulin, but they are able to control plasma glucose levels when faced with a simultaneously administered glucose challenge. The key properties that make such formulations promising for oral administration are size of dosage, release kinetics, bioadhesiveness, and ability to traverse the gastrointestinal epithelium.

As colloidal and nanofabrication techniques have advanced, more sophisticated forms of encapsulation have been developed and tested, using new types of polymer and inorganic coatings and matrices. With the advent of genetic engineering and biotechnology on a large scale, numerous bioactive peptides besides insulin are available in large quantities. Administering these substances by the oral route remains a formidable challenge due to their insufficient stability in the gastrointestinal tract and their poor absorption pattern. This has given new impetus to investigating new approaches to improve their oral bioavailability. The use of polymeric microparticles and nanoparticles is an actively pursued concept. Encapsulating or incorporating peptides in particles should at least protect these substances against degradation and, in some cases, also enhance their absorption [296–299].

Some newer nanotechnologies that are being explored for insulin delivery include multilayer, asymmetric, polymeric devices to enhance penetration of drug from encapsulated material across the epithelial barrier [300]. These could be used as a patch on the skin or other epithelial location. Another new approach to nanoparticle insulin delivery is the use of nanodiamond–insulin complexes as drug carriers for pH-dependent peptide delivery [301].

Nanogels are being developed as an approach to oral insulin delivery: complexation hydrogels are being evaluated as delivery vehicles for insulin–transferrin conjugates [302,303]. These pH responsive matrices rely on nano-engineered mucoadhesive surface properties to protect the peptide drug in the digestive tract and deliver it through the intestinal epithelial barrier for absorption into the bloodstream [304,305].

Developments in nanotechnology have assisted the miniaturization of insulin pumps, especially in their transdermal delivery mechanisms. Some of the formulations for delivery through insulin micropumps could make use of nanoparticle formulations as the delivery agent, so nanocarrier technology will still be involved, even in the most successful insulin micropumps. Recently, great advances have been made in reducing the size, cost, power requirements, and intrusiveness of wearable insulin pumps, along with improvements in the power and sophistication of their computational control [306–311].

Two developments which could make nanoparticle delivery of insulin moot are the artificial pancreas (based on islet encapsulation or an entirely synthetic device) and advances in understanding of the biochemistry, molecular biology, and cell-signaling networks involved in glucose metabolism. It is generally acknowledged that there is currently insufficient knowledge about the structure and dynamics of the insulin hormone and glycemic control. But nanotools for research are helping to elicit this knowledge, using improved nanosensors for single molecule sensing, and in vivo targeted molecular imaging of cell signaling and metabolic pathways [312–314].

5.5.8 Nanoencapsulation for Immunoprotection

One of the key reasons that peptides and other large drug molecules benefit from encapsulation is protection from the action of the body's immune system. Whether by antibodies or engulfing or attaching white blood cells, foreign proteins run the risk of being identified as nonself and targeted for elimination from the body. Nanoencapsulation formulations may also be specifically designed to protect drugs from particular enzymes or harsh pH environments in parts of the body on the way to the drug delivery target. These formulations are useful for protecting insulin and other substances such as enzymes for therapeutic delivery. For example, the encapsulation of enzymes like urease for delivery to the lower intestine has been the subject of recent research toward a treatment for disorders where normal metabolic enzymes are absent [315].

Another area where nanotechnology is applied is encapsulation of living cells for implantation. One option for treatment of diabetes is transplantation of healthy pancreas beta cells to the patient, but rejection of the foreign cells by the host immune system is a major problem. For several decades medical researchers have tried various attempts to encapsulate or shield the transplanted tissue with barriers that would protect it from immune attack. Only in recent years, with advances in nanotechnology for fabricating nanostructured porous biocompatible materials, has this approach been brought closer to feasibility.

Microscale capsules have been fabricated to contain living cells. Nanoscale pores in the sides of the capsule cages allow small molecules such as nutrients, oxygen, and carbon dioxide to pass through, but can be sized to keep out antibodies and protect the enclosed cells from attack by macrophages. Assemblies of encapsulated cells, enclosed in silica gel [316], silicon [317–319], alumina [320,321], alginate [322], and other materials have been used. This type of encapsulation merges into bioengineering to make active tissue scaffold implants and bioartificial organs, which are being tested for effectiveness in various types of tissue implants ranging from pancreatic beta cells to bone marrow [323–327]. These larger scale forms of bioencapsulation and nano-bioengineering are discussed further in Chapters 7 and 8.

In one of the most striking examples of the transfer of silicon-based nanoengineering to biomedical use, a group at Johns Hopkins have developed self-assembling silicon nanocubes which can be used for cell encapsulation. Cells have been successfully enclosed in the containers as they fold from their flat silicon lithography state into closed cubes with windows in their walls for circulation [328].

Most work on transplanting encapsulated cells has been in the area of insulin-producing pancreatic beta cells. This line of research has included methods of closely coating individual cells, or even chemical attachment of functional groups to the cell membrane to avoid immune attack. After years of having experiments result in the implants being smothered by plaques and invaded by the immune system of the host, promising results are beginning to appear, using new nanoengineered encapsulation materials and techniques [329–331].

In a recent example of work in this field, researchers in Germany achieved the first successful transplantation of functioning microencapsulated islets of Langerhans. They used a novel alginate-based microencapsulation formulation to implant human islets into immunocompetent diabetic mice [332]. More recently, transplantation of alginate-encapsulated pig islets into primates (*Cynomolgus maccacus*) has been reported with 6 month survival [333]. These and perhaps other approaches, which must be subjected to many rigorous trials in animals and humans as they move toward clinical application, may soon lead to a treatment for diabetes that restores normal blood-sugar regulation [334–336].

5.5.9 Nanoparticles for Inhalation Therapy

Shortly after the discovery of insulin, researchers began to investigate the possibility of delivery by inhalation. The surface area of the interior of the lungs in an adult human is roughly the size of a tennis court, so if insulin could be delivered to the capillaries and alvedi of the lung, there is high potential for absorption directly into the blood stream, bypassing the problems of digestion (the pharmacological "first pass effect") and barriers to absorption in the gastrointestinal tract and avoiding the risks and inconvenience of injection. Nanoparticle formulations are key to pulmonary delivery, both for creating stable aerosols and facilitating passage through the lung tissue into the capillaries [98,337–340].

The long efforts to develop inhalation therapeutics for insulin bear testimony to the challenges of understanding the processes by which micro- and nanoparticles are processed by the cilia and alveoli in the lungs. The advantages of large surface area and relative lack of immunological responses and enzyme attack are offset by the protective biological barrier properties of the alveolar environment. Thus, inhalation therapy has been limited by low bioavailability of administered drugs, even with the best of modern aerosol formulation technologies. Targeted nanoparticles are of great interest in inhalation therapy because of their ability to overcome cellular barriers to absorption. They are being investigated for potential in escaping pulmonary clearance mechanisms and targeting specific cells within the lung [341,342].

Much work has been done on pulmonary diseases, airborne bacteria and virus infections, smoking, and air pollution, which provides insights that may be useful in formulating nanoparticles for inhalation therapies [98]. Nanotechnology has much to contribute in solving lung disease problems as well as finding new effective inhalation drug delivery methods. Inhalation routes to drug delivery are an important and growing area of biomedical research in many areas besides diabetes, and are likely to be an area where nanotechnology will make a large impact.

One additional reason that nanoparticles are of interest for nasal drug delivery is that inhalation therapy can offer a means of bypassing the blood–brain barrier [343].

5.5.10 Nanoencapsulation for Penetration of the Blood–Brain Barrier

Delivery of drugs across the blood–brain barrier is another important area where nanotechnology gives new routes of access. The existence of the blood–brain barrier was discovered in the nineteenth century when Paul Ehrlich and his student Edwin Goldman found that dyes used to stain tissues would not pass between the central nervous system and the other tissues of the body. In the central nervous system, the epithelial cells lining the walls of blood vessels overlap in tight junctions, unlike those in the rest of the body. This closes off easy transport of large molecules (greater than molecular weight around 500 Da) between the blood and the brain. In addition to this physical barrier, there are also enzymatic metabolic barriers. This combined barrier helps protect the sensitive and vital central nervous system from disturbance by chemicals and pathogens (for example, viruses) that are tolerated by the more robust tissues of the body.

The olfactory region in the nasal cavity is closely linked to the olfactory bulb of the brain. This is a route by which some drugs may bypass the blood–brain barrier and reach the cerebro-spinal fluid, which surrounds the brain and the actual brain tissue, directly from the nasal cavity, but this transport is highly dependent on the properties of the drug. There is much interest in the use of nanoparticles to facilitate drug delivery by this route [344].

The tight epithelial barrier surrounding the central nervous system is highly lipophilic. Small lipophilic molecules can cross by dissolving through the lipid bilayer (for instance, alcohol, caffeine, nicotine, and antidepressants). Other molecules needed for the brain to function make use of specific natural transport mechanisms in the cell membranes. Small polar molecules, such as glucose and amino acids, and larger proteins, like insulin and the iron-transporting protein transferrin, are transported through the blood brain chemical traffic by "gatekeeping" processes. Each of the required small molecules has its own transporter protein that carries it through the cell membranes—this process is called carrier-mediated transport. For proteins, specific cell membrane receptors bind the large molecules and pull them across the barrier in a mechanism called receptor-mediated transcytosis. In addition, some ionic proteins (e.g., cationic albumin) bind to and penetrate the blood–brain barrier using electrostatic interactions, in a process called absorptive-mediated transcytosis [344–346].

Many of the mechanisms that mediate transport across the blood–brain barrier are unknown; elucidating them is an active area of research in genomics, proteomics, and molecular biology. In the meantime, pharmaceutical research is seeking to exploit the pathways that are known. Some success has been made in modifying drugs, linking them to molecules that have transporter proteins, and thus hitching a ride across the barrier. For example, nipecotic acid, which has potential for treating Parkinson's disease, has been conjugated to ascorbic acid, which has access to ascorbate transporters, and has been delivered across the blood–brain barrier in rats, while the unconjugated nipecotic acid is barred. Other pathways have also been exploited using these "Trojan horse" and "chimeric peptide" techniques [144,347,348].

Potential drugs for treating Alzheimer's disease, Huntington's disease, stroke, and brain cancers often have molecular weights from 10,000 to 100,000 or even greater. Many new high molecular weight peptides are being identified with potential use for central nervous system therapy. It has been estimated that up to 98% of potential drugs for the brain are not usable because of the blood–brain barrier, but this area has until recently been underdeveloped in the neurosciences. One reason is the difficulty of identifying each transport mediator path and synthesizing a chimeric or Trojan horse version of each drug to match.

Nanotechnology is beginning to offer a possible alternative for transport through the blood–brain barrier that is more generally applicable to a wide range of drugs. Drugs can be encapsulated in biodegradable polymers to make artificial liposomes, which are coated with a polymer to which antibodies can be attached. The antibodies are recognized by the brain-capillary receptors, which mediate their passage through the blood–brain barrier. Once inside the central nervous system, the liposomes release their contents [349,350].

These biodegradable polymeric nanoparticles, with appropriate surface modifications that can deliver drugs of interest through the blood–brain barrier, are being formulated with various physicochemical properties. These nanocarriers can be made with safe materials, including synthetic biodegradable polymers, lipids, and polysaccharides. Different surfactant concentrations, stabilizers, and amyloid-affinity agents are being evaluated to determine how they influence the transport mechanism.

Recently, the radiolabeled Cu^{2+} or Fe^{3+} metal chelator clioquinol, which has a high affinity for amyloid plaques which are a factor in neurodegenerative disease, has been encapsulated within small, spherical, lipophilic drug carriers capable of crossing the blood–brain barrier [351].

Another nanoparticle-based platform that has been formulated to cross the blood–brain barrier is based on rod-shaped semiconductor nanocrystals (quantum rods) conjugated with transferrin [352]. The quantum resonance fluorescence of the nanoparticles gives a direct means of visualizing the transmigration of biomolecules into the brain. This imaging capability will facilitate the development of nanoprobes for early diagnosis and therapy of various disorders of the brain. Quantum rod and quantum dot bioconjugates are already used as targeted optical probes for two-photon fluorescence imaging of cancer cells [42]. More than one therapy can be monitored simultaneously, by exploiting the fact that quantum rods emit in different colors with a small change in size. These carefully functionalized quantum rods possess very low toxicity, are structurally robust, and are large enough, having the potential to conjugate and transport multiple agents. The multiple agents can be selected so that they function in a synergistic way in the brain and the efficiency of a therapeutic molecule can be monitored noninvasively in real time using their optical resonance as a diagnostic probe.

These and similar nanoencapsulation formulations have the potential to deliver many drugs to the central nervous system, opening new possibilities for therapy in brain cancer and other central nervous system diseases [353]. Laboratory studies and in vivo experiments with blood–brain barrier nano-carriers are showing potential ways to overcome other important biological boundaries, such as the mucosal intestinal, nasal, and ocular barriers. This may present a strategy for making cheaper and faster, more efficacious medicines for many other uses.

5.5.11 Nanoparticle Delivery for Cancer Therapy

Nanoparticle formulations are having a significant impact in diagnosis and treatment for neurodegenerative, infectious, degenerative, inflammatory, and other conditions in many areas of medicine. Many more examples can be found in the literature and on the Internet [354,355]. Perhaps the broadest and most intense application of nanotechnology has been in the treatment of cancer [356–359].

Cancer is a leading cause of mortality worldwide. Although advances have been made in cancer treatment, more effective therapies are needed. Treatments too often fail, leading to local recurrence of tumors, spread to lymph nodes, and general metastasis. Available treatments include surgery, chemotherapy, radiotherapy, immunotherapy, and hyperthermia.

Ways are being explored to apply nanotechnology to overcome limitations of conventional mainstream treatments. Surgery is limited to tumors that are accessible, and may not remove all cancerous cells. Conventional chemother-apy is associated with significant side effects and is subject to development of resistance by the tumor. Radiotherapy can cause damage to healthy tissue in the path of the radiation beam or neighborhood of implanted radioiso-topes. Immunotherapy is a promising treatment whose development is still in the nascent stage. Hyperthermia, the application of heat for tumor abla-tion, is a relatively new form of treatment. Its successful application requires controlled targeting to the tumor with minimal heating of surrounding tis-sue. Nanotechnology, especially nanoparticles for imaging and drug deliv-ery, can contribute to enhancement of all of these therapies, and in some cases can offer new and creative methodologies for more effective treatment.

Regardless of the treatment modalities, early detection greatly improves the prognosis for cancer. Much of the utility of nanoparticle image enhance-ment is for diagnosis of cancer, especially in complex and inaccessible anatomy. Nanoparticle image enhancement is especially useful in malignan-cies of organs or cells where special hormonal or other functionalities that facilitate targeting can be exploited. Nanoparticles can also be employed in selective targeting to separate and concentrate cancer cells circulating in the body, for earlier diagnosis and more effective application of therapy. Over the past 10 years there has been a steadily increasing volume of research with progress in applying nanotechnology for imaging, drug delivery, and therapy against cancer [360–364].

Every nanoparticle type and technique discussed so far in the previous sections of this chapter has been applied to cancer therapy, including targeting particles with ligands to deliver drugs selectively to cancer cells [365–368]. Types of targeted particles include dendrimers [369], conjugates [370], micelles [371,372], liposomes [373,374], and exosomes [375].

Exosomes are produced naturally from some cells as endosomes are released through the cell membrane, carrying proteins into their surroundings. Exosomes are normally secreted by hematopioetic bone marrow cells that develop into reticulocytes, platelets, B and T lymphocytes, and dendritic cells, through fusion of multivesicular endosomes with the cell's plasma membrane. Exosomes may mediate intercellular communications, by shipping messages through the transfer of a panel of proteins from one cell to another. This is believed to be a mechanism by which exosomes signal the antitumor action of immune cells, with their protein contents as a source of tumor antigens. By manipulating exosomes and their contents, researchers at Aix-Marseille Université in France have been able to induce apoptosis of pancreatic cancer cells. This could lead to a new type of cancer therapy [375].

Nanoparticles targeted on cancer cell signatures have been used to deliver photothermal therapy selectively to tumors with high-energy lasers [369], as well as chemotherapy and imaging agents [369–374]. Biodegradable polymersome nanoparticles have been formulated and shown to enhance delivery of insoluble drugs such as paclitaxel and doxorubicin, shrinking tumors with minimized side effects [376].

In a novel nanoassembly drug design, bioconjugation of gemcitabine (2′,2′-difluorodeoxyribofuranosylcytosine), an anticancer nucleoside analogue active against a wide variety of solid tumors, with squalene, a natural lipid, has been used to produce a conjugate that forms self-organizing nanoassemblies in water. Previously, gemcitabine administered by intravenous administration was found to be rapidly inactivated by enzymatic deamination, resulting in a short biological half-life and necessitating high doses, leading to undesirable side effects. The "squalenoylated" gemcitabine nanoassemblies resisted deamination, improving the therapeutic index, with significantly higher anticancer activity compared with the unconjugated drug [377].

5.5.12 Nanoparticle Delivery of Natural Product Therapies

Nanoparticles have been found especially useful as delivery agents for poorly soluble drugs [378]. A large percentage of new pharmacologically potent molecules show poor aqueous solubility, leading to their low effective concentration in biofluids and therefore poor bioavailability. Conventional means of increasing solubility include chemical modification of the candidate molecule, but this is likely to alter the action and safety as well as the solubility [379]. Another frequently used method to improve bioavailability is the solid-dispersion technique. This method simply dissolves the drug with an emulsifying agent in ethanol, evaporates the organic solvent, and dries the solid dispersion. It is difficult to control the drug release rate accurately through this method, and this type of preparation cannot always be used for injection. To overcome these difficulties, nanoparticle conjugation or encapsulation has found increasing application to aid delivery of insoluble drugs as more and more drug candidates are larger molecules, many derived from natural products. An example of a highly effective natural product–derived drug for which nanoparticle delivery has proven effective is simvastatin (Zocor), a statin cholesterol-lowering drug derived from a fermentation product of *Aspergillus terreus* [380].

A number of promising anticancer agents are found in compounds from plants and other natural sources. These new drug candidate compounds typically are large molecules with low solubility in the blood (simpler and smaller molecules having been screened long before). Their action may depend on highly specific macromolecular steric and binding interactions between the large molecule and nanoscale molecular machinery in the cell. In addition, they may be highly toxic to cells in general, with particular toxicity to certain cancer cell lines because of their rapid cell division or abnormal metabolism. Cancer cells spend an abnormally high percentage of their lifetimes in the prophase state, as they are undergoing rapid division. The challenge is to deliver the agent to the cancer cells without harming normal cells on the way, and to keep it from being transported rapidly away from the target before it can have time to act.

Nanoencapsulation and conjugation have been used in many cases to improve delivery of doxorubicin, an anthracycline drug derived from *Streptomyces* bacteria. The anthracyclines are some of the most effective anticancer treatments ever developed and are effective against more types of cancer than any other class of chemotherapy agents. They are used to treat a wide range of cancers, including leukemias, lymphomas, and breast, uterine, ovarian, and lung cancers. They have many adverse side effects which limit their usefulness, including heart damage (cardiotoxicity) and vomiting. Nanoparticle formulations of doxorubicin are widely used to mitigate side effects, increase delivery efficiency, and to target and image cancer cells [380].

Artemisinin is an anticancer drug abstracted from traditional plants that have been used for thousands of years as sources of medicine. Artemisinin has strong antitumor activity against melanoma, breast, ovarian, prostate, central nervous system, and renal cancer cell lines, but presents bioavailability problems because of hydrophobicity, low solubility, and instability.

These problems have been overcome by using polyelectrolyte capsules made with layer-by-layer self-assembly. The polyelectrolyte vesicles have several advantages over simpler encapsulation methods: (1) film thickness and capsule size can be controlled to within a few nanometers, allowing tuning of the release rate and enabling production of capsules small enough for injection (<1 μm); (2) hydrophilicity of particles can be improved with polyelectrolyte coatings; (3) aggregation and clumping are avoided because the coated capsules have like electrostatic surface charges, and thus repel each other; (4) capsules can be functionalized for imaging and targeting; and (5) organic solvents and other toxic materials are not needed for production [381].

Taxol is another anticancer drug derived from natural products, which we have discussed earlier [104–106]. Taxol, paclitaxel, levobetaxolol, and other variants are widely formulated in nanoparticles and nanocapsules to increase solubility, reduce toxicity and side effects, and lower required dosages, using layer-by-layer assemblies and other techniques [382].

Curcumin, a yellow polyphenol extracted from the rhizome of the turmeric (*Curcuma longa*), has potent anticancer properties, but clinical application has been limited due to poor aqueous solubility. In a collaborative research effort between Johns Hopkins, Baltimore, Maryland and the University of Delhi, Delhi, India, a nanoencapsulated formulation of curcumin, nanocurcumin, has been made using the micellar aggregates of cross-linked and random copolymers of N-isopropylacrylamide (NIPAAM), with N-vinyl-2-pyrrolidone (VP) and poly(ethyleneglycol)monoacrylate (PEG-A). By enabling aqueous dispersion, nanocurcumin provides an opportunity to use curcumin in preclinical tests on vivo models of cancer and other diseases [383].

Another example of a natural product–derived drug that can be enhanced by nanoparticle delivery is the promising compound ß-lapachone, an o-naphthoquinone found in the bark of the South American lapacho tree. ß-lapachone is known to induce cytotoxic effects in a wide variety of malignant human cell types including colon, lung, prostate, breast, pancreatic, ovarian, and bone cancers, as well as some blood cancers and retinoblastoma [384].

Dr. David Boothman and his colleagues at the University of Texas Southwestern Medical Center, Dallas, Texas found that ß-lapachone interacts with an enzyme called NQO1 (NAD(P)H:quinone oxidoreductase), which is present at high levels in certain types of solid cancer tumors. In tumors, the compound is metabolized by NQO1 and produces cell death but does not initiate apoptosis in noncancerous tissues, since they normally do not express this enzyme. In the tumor cells, ß-lapachone induces a novel apoptotic pathway dependent on NQO1, which reduces ß-lapachone to an unstable hydroquinone that rapidly undergoes a two-step oxidation back to the parent compound, perpetuating a self-sustaining redox cycle. A deficiency or inhibition of NQO1, such as is the case in normal cells, protects them from the effects of ß-lapachone—but when ß-lapachone interacts with NQO1 in the tumor cell, the cell kills itself [385].

Thus, ß-lapachone has great potential for the treatment of specific cancers with elevated NQO1 levels. (e.g., breast, non-small-cell lung, pancreatic, colon, and prostate cancers). Dr. Boothman's team is developing ß-lapachone mono(arylimino) prodrug derivatives, specifically a derivative converted in a tumor-specific manner (i.e., in the acidic local environment of the tumor tissue), in order to reduce normal tissue toxicity while eliciting tumor-selective cell killing by NQO1 bioactivation [386].

In order to ensure delivery of ß-lapachone and its derivatives to the local environment of the tumor without losing or diluting them in the body, one could simply inject them into the tumor. But experiments showed that the drug is carried away by the blood circulation relatively rapidly, before it has time to fully react with a large number of tumor cells. Dr. Boothman and his group are developing a variety of nanoparticle formulations to target and release the anticancer drug in an effective manner. The group is also exploring the use of multifunctional nanoparticles for targeting, imaging, and delivering anticancer therapies [387].

5.5.13 Focus on Nanoparticle Therapies for Types of Cancers

With cancer, just as with other types of diseases, nanotechnology and nanoparticle drug delivery is impacting a wide range of therapies for different types of disease in different organ systems of the body. It is of interest to have a quick overview oriented by type of disease to get an appreciation of where and how nanoparticles are producing results and being pursued for research in cancer medicine.

We mentioned earlier that targeting of nanoparticles is especially effective where disease is affecting a special type of tissue that has distinguishing hormonal or metabolic characteristics. Because hormone-producing tissues have a more active and complex metabolism they tend to be more prone to the disruptions that lead to cancer. This is also true for epithelial tissue with the added risks of exposure to external carcinogenic influences. So nanoparticle therapies are found to be in very active development for gonadal and epithelial cancers, although they are being explored for many other types of carcinoma as well.

5.5.13.1 *Pancreatic Cancer*

Cancer of the pancreas is one of the most difficult cancers to treat. Nanoparticles are being formulated in efforts to find an effective therapy for this type of cancer. Approaches using peptide conjugates [388] and using multivalent nanoparticles with small molecule drugs are being evaluated [389].

5.5.13.2 *Ovarian and Gynecological Cancers*

Breast, ovarian, and cervical cancers represent the most life-threatening gynecological malignant disorders endangering women throughout the world.

One of the problems in ovarian cancer, as with many others, is development of drug resistance to anticancer agents by carcinoma cells with repeated courses of chemotherapy. Biodegradable polymeric nanoparticles are being used for coadministration of two strong anticancer drugs, paclitaxel and ceramide, in a targeted delivery system to overcome drug resistance in ovarian cancers [390].

At the same time, earlier and more accurate diagnosis is being aided by new and specific contrast agents. Detection of cancer in the early stages before metastatic spread gives much better treatment options and more positive outcomes. Traditional contrast agents are not very effective in detecting primary metastatic tumors and cells due to a lack of specificity and sensitivity. Nanomedicine-based contrast agents are being developed with improved solubility, cell-specific targeting, toxicities, and immunological responses. These nanomedicine-based agents include multifunctional inorganic and polymeric nanohybrids, which can combine molecular imaging with direct and targeted application of therapy [391].

5.5.13.3 Breast Cancer

Knowledge of the genetic disposition that leads to vulnerability to certain types of breast cancers has enabled the design of nanoparticles targeted to cell receptors that are overexpressed in the cancer cells. Using this approach, for example, the Her-2/neu receptor in breast cancer cells can be targeted with functionalized iron oxide nanoparticles, which can enhance imaging of the tumors and which also can be used for hyperthermal therapy to destroy tumor cells [392].

5.5.13.4 Prostate Cancer

Prostate cancer is an increasingly common type of cancer, partly due to demographic factors. This type of cancer can be targeted using unique cell markers, with various types of nanoparticles, including drug carriers such as nanoparticle–aptamer bioconjugates, and magnetic nanoparticles for hyperthermia. Nanoparticles are also being used to detect clinically occult lymph-node metastases, a major danger with prostate and other cancers [393–397].

5.5.13.5 Lung Cancer

Paclitaxel has demonstrated effectiveness in shrinking many types of lung tumors, but some of the earlier emulsion formulations of paclitaxel caused allergic reactions. This was found to be associated with a surfactant used to make the nanoparticles (Cremophor). A Cremophor-free particle formulation of paclitaxel (Abraxane) is now available, with promising results. The nanoparticles are composed of paclitaxel bonded with albumin to minimize any source of allergic reaction [398].

5.5.13.6 Nanoparticle Targeting of Folic Acid Receptors
for a Variety of Cancers

Folic acid receptors exhibit limited expression on healthy cells but are often present in large numbers on cancer cells. Folic acid receptors are overexpressed on epithelial cancers and cancers of the ovary, mammary gland, colon, lung, prostate, nose, throat, and brain. Attaching folic acid on various nanoparticles in combination with anticancer drugs and other therapies has been found an effective means of targeting these types of cancer. For example, folic acid has been attached to gold nanoparticles using noncovalent interaction via different PEG backbones to target cancer cells for drug delivery and photothermal therapy [399].

5.5.13.7 Epithelial Cancers Targeted by Hyperthermia
and Photothermal Therapy

Eighty-five percent of all cancers in the United States are epithelial cancers, including oral and throat cancers, gastrointestinal cancer, pulmonary cancer and skin cancer. Hyperthermia and photothermal therapies are somewhat easier to apply for epithelial cancers than for cancers inside solid organs, because of accessibility (on the skin or via endoscopic access), and because of lower risk to surrounding healthy tissue where the tumor presents on the surface of an epithelial layer. For these reasons, phototherapy and hyperthermia are being increasingly used for treatment of the various types of epithelial cancers. A recent investigation was conducted to determine the minimum temperature required to selectively destroy cancer cells using photothermal energy with immunotargeted gold nanoparticles [400].

For epithelial and other cancers, multifunctional nanoparticles with immune- or receptor-mediated targeting, imaging capability, and the ability to delivery thermal or radiation therapy and multiple drugs are being developed to increase the odds of successfully eliminating cancer cells with multiple modes of attack.

5.6 Theranostics

Increasingly sophisticated ways of fabricating nanoparticles are leading to new concepts in drug delivery, imaging, and therapeutics. Nanotechnology integrated with biotechnology is blurring the distinctions between diagnosis, therapy, and management of disease.

The term "theranostics" grew out of the molecular genomics pharmaceutical arena [401,402], and is increasingly being applied in the nanomedicine context to the combination of diagnostic and therapeutic capabilities in multifunctional nanodevices for diagnosis, treatment, and management of health and disease [403–405]. The term combines the ideas of "therapy," including thermal, radiotherapies, microsurgery, and tissue engineering as well as drugs, with "diagnostics" in the sense of capability for imaging, genetic, and immunological biomarker matching to identify and target diseases.

Theranostics also applies to a broader and deeper approach to healthcare than merely combining multiple functions in a single nanoparticle or nanodevice. It encompasses the idea of "personalized medicine" in which molecular medicines are targeted precisely based on the genetic and phenotypic biomarkers of the patient and disease [406–410].

An integrated personalized medicine is based on three capabilities: (1) ability to determine the genomic and proteomic coding and status of the patient; (2) ability to identify and monitor biomarkers for signaling and metabolic processes in healthy and diseased cells; and (3) ability to deliver therapies precisely and selectively to targets. Nanotechnology contributes crucially to the implementation of all three of these capabilities.

We look at some examples of the type of genome profiling and custom proteomic targeting that are fundamental to the theranostics and personalized medicine paradigms, but first it is helpful to review the technological capabilities of the nanotechnology which provides much of the basis for diagnostic sensing and therapeutic actions that can make personalized medicine a reality.

5.6.1 Multifunctional Nanoparticles for Imaging and Therapy

From origins as simple conjugates and capsules, nanomedicines have been developed to incorporate multiple functions—imaging, targeting, drug delivery, photo- and magnetic therapy activity—on a single formulation, so they have grown from being mere nanoparticles to the point that they may be described as nanodevices.

Multifunctional nanoparticles and nanomedicines began with imaging and targeting on particles such as gold nanodots [37] or polymers [411], and combining targeting with drug delivery [412,413], and then advanced to combining imaging, targeting, drug delivery, photothermal action, and other functionality on the same nanostructure [414–416]. In the examples of the previous sections, there were multifunctional nanoparticles with targeting based on specific biomarkers in cells, combined with selective drug release triggered by pH, light, enzyme activity, or other biomolecular interactions with specific targets within the selected cells.

Multifunctional particles for imaging can expand macroscale diagnostics to probe for information about biological systems at the molecular and cellular levels. For example, nanoparticles have been designed to incorporate multiple imaging modalities including MRI, positron emission tomography (PET), and CT, and fluorescence tags on the same particle platforms. Starting with a simple magnetic nanoparticle for MRI enhancement as a core, other functional moieties are overlaid, including fluorescence tags, radionuclides, and other biomolecules for multimodal imaging, gene delivery, and cellular trafficking. With this design approach, a fluorescent dye-doped silica core surrounded by magnetic nanoparticles is used to image the distribution of neuroblastoma cancer cells via MRI along with subcellular information via fluorescence imaging [417]. Magnetic nanoparticles coupled to radionuclides for MRI–PET dual-modal probes can accurately detect cancer metastasis in lymph nodes. In vivo MRI/PET images using these nanoparticles can identify metastasis nodes as small as 3 mm diameter along with precise anatomical information.

5.6.2 Nanocapsules and Bioreactors with Active Elements

The most elaborate and sophisticated of the nanocarriers can rightly be called "nanoreactors," "nanosize bioreactors" [418], "nano cargo ships for drug delivery" [419], and similar names describing their complex and "smart" dynamic functionality [420]. (However, in the spirit of "sonic hedgehog" genes and other playful names, some have called their nanocarriers "nanoworms" [421], "knedels" [422], "nanodumplings," (Figure 5.12) [423] or "doughnut deliveries" [186], etc.)

5.6.3 Chemically Activated Release

For example, the nanoreactor drug carriers designed at the University of Basel, Basel, Switzerland are drug loaded nanocontainers that release their

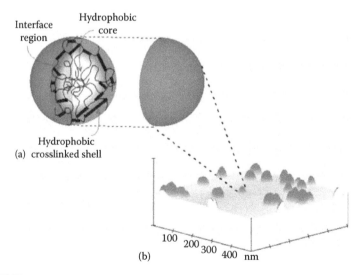

FIGURE 5.12
Nanodumpling: (a) Internal structure and (b) size distribution determined by AFM. (From Senior, K., *Mol. Med. Today*, 4, 321, 1998. With permission.)

payloads in response to specific physiological signals, such as a biochemical marker or enzyme characteristic of tumor cells [424]. And nanoworms, designed by a team at the University of California at San Diego, not only self-assemble into worm-like chain particles, but they also use biomimetic homing to find tumors. The nanoworms are an instructive example of how nanoparticles can be programmed to carry out quite sophisticated macromolecular engineering—they not only attach to targeted biomarkers, but once attached, they send signals to amplify their own accumulation at the target site. By amplifying their own homing on the target, they resemble platelets, mimicking the mechanism by which blood clots are formed [425].

Other examples of device nanoengineering are microporous silica particle designs with pores capped with chitosan hydrogel or other materials that can open and close in response to pH changes or enzymes, thereby releasing drugs such as insulin or chemotherapy agents [249,426–428].

Another example is a nanoparticle architecture with controlled functionalization of internal and external sites in nanoscale cage-like structures, with the ability to selectively uptake and release guest molecules. The cages are synthetic analogues of viral capsids. The uptake and release of large and small molecules in the polymer cage is controlled by tailored placement of functional groups at well-defined positions within the nanostructural framework. The chemistry of the cage framework is altered by covalent attachment of selected lipids and acrylic acid residues to enhance uptake of hydrophobic guest molecules into the cage. By attaching lipids with selected polar functional groups, the polarity of the encapsulated lipid domains within the cage could be controlled. This particular work is being carried out at Washington University in Saint Louis [422,429]. This and similar work being done elsewhere represent the leading edge of nanoparticle engineering, involving synthetic polymer biochemistry and molecular biology applied to construction of extremely sophisticated macromolecular nanostructures with subtle functionality.

5.6.4 Photonic Release

Multifunctional nanoparticles are also designed to deliver targeted therapies using magnetism, radiation, and light along with other functions. Magnetic or electromagnetic energy may be used to guide particles or as an initiating mechanism for activation of imaging and drug delivery functions.

One example is the use of light-triggered release of drugs. We saw examples of photo- and thermal therapy in the earlier review of nanoparticles, in Section 5.3 of this chapter. In addition to direct use of light or heat action for therapy, light irradiation can be used in more subtle ways, with drug release triggered by photochemical reactions after a nanocarrier has reached its target. Here, the light does not act directly on the cell—it acts on the nanoparticle to release the active agent.

One design mechanism for photonically triggered release is called photochemical internalization. It improves the efficiency for release of therapeutic molecules into the cell, by photochemically opening capsules such as liposomes once they have entered into the cytoplasm. Nanocapsules, which can easily enter cells, may not always be efficient at releasing their cargo, but if the capsules contain a photosensitive component with bonds that are opened by specific wavelengths of light, then irradiation with the selected wavelength can be applied after incubation and ingestion of the capsules. This method has been used to efficiently deliver drugs such as ribosome-inactivating proteins, enzymes, and green fluorescent protein marker from endosomes and lysosomes into the cytosol [430]. A related method uses photosensitive bonding agents to conjugate drugs to nanoparticles such as solid particles or polymers. The drug is released by photochemical breaking of the bonds after the particles have been absorbed into or attached to their targeted cells [431]. In methods that rely on photochemical release, the photosensitizer and its activating wavelength must be chosen for efficient transmittal into the tissues involved and for minimal photochemical damage to healthy cells.

Another type of photoactivation uses light-activated motion in molecules to open gates or induce motion in nanoparticles. The California NanoSystems Institute at the University of California at Los Angeles, Los Angeles, California has been especially productive in exploring the possibilities of this approach, and have dubbed their creations "nanoimpellers." Photoactivated moving parts based on the photoisomerization of large planar molecules such as azobenzene derivatives are used with mesoporous silica nanoparticles to regulate drug delivery from pores in the silica. The azobenzene derivatives, with substituents ranging from hydrogen atoms to dendrimers, transition from trans to cis isomers when interacting with the electromagnetic oscillation of a light beam. The change in conformation and size between the trans and cis isomers can be used to regulate the transport of molecules through pores to electrodes. A light-induced back-and-forth wagging motion has been demonstrated to act as a molecular impeller that regulates the release of molecules from the pores of silica nanoparticles under "remote control" upon photoexcitation [432–434]. This type of particle has been used experimentally to take up drugs and deliver them into cancer cells [435].

Photostimulation to manipulate the vibration, rotation, and folding of large molecules requires less energy input than that needed for photochemical breaking of bonds, and is therefore somewhat less invasive. Bond dissociation energies fall in the ultraviolet (UV) light range, but rotational, vibrational, and conformation spectra are in the infrared (IR) to microwave region. The available wavelengths for applying UV photoactivation must be chosen to avoid damage to cellular molecules such as DNA. The use of IR avoids this problem, but a large number of possible infrared spectral absorption and emission modes are shared by many common cellular constituents, leaving only a few IR windows available for use in nanoparticle manipulation. This increases the difficulty of designing IR-driven photoactivation for practical use, but does not make it impossible. Another design consideration is making the activation resilient to random IR noise and thermal effects, both of which could interact with the low-energy transitions from cis to trans configurations and other molecular conformational states. This is a potential source of interference with control of the particle activation, which makes the design of molecular gates a sophisticated process.

5.6.5 Nanosensor Particle Systems for In Vivo Diagnostics

The second leg of an integrated nanomedicine is in vivo molecular scale diagnostics, which include not only imaging, but information on physiology and body chemistry at the molecular and genetic level. This goal requires the capability of tracking individual molecules—single molecule microscopy and spectroscopy. Then, it will be feasible to know the dynamic state of the body and its systems at the cellular level, to monitor how well it is maintaining its rhythms and homeostasis, in order to be able to apply therapy intelligently and effectively. Nanotechnology and nanoscale probes are playing an important part as single molecule probes are becoming a central activity in biomedical nanotechnology and molecular sensing [436–438]. Optical detection of a single molecule is difficult; spatial resolution limitations must be overcome, and the signal must be extracted from the background arising from billions of other molecules. One way to extract the signal is to attach a marker label to the molecule of interest. The ideal label must fulfill the contradictory requirements of generating a detectable signal with minimal perturbation of the observed biological system.

Nanoprobes, along with fluorescent molecular tags and green fluorescent protein, make it possible to apply recent advances in single molecule microscopy to living biological tissues and cells. There continue to be many advances in microscopy and nanotechnology which make manipulation of subcellular structures and single molecules possible, including advances in microscopy and cell manipulation by optical tweezers and electrophoresis [439–441], which are used in conjunction with the ability to image on the molecular scale.

Nanoparticles and nanoscale devices can be used to make extremely powerful sensors for physiological and biochemical information. The physical properties of particles, fibers, thin films, and surfaces at the nanoscale are influenced by their environment while being free from the overwhelming influence of bulk material of their own composition, unlike matter on the macroscale. The optical, mechanical, and electromagnetic properties of structured and functionalized nanosurfaces are very sensitive to the influence of a small amount of neighboring or absorbed matter, and of small amounts of energy (heat, force, or light).

Why focus on nanoparticle sensor systems as a key enabling technology for an integrated personalized medicine? Nanoparticles and nanoprobes can play an important role in elucidating the physical and molecular basis for health and disease, because they are small enough to enter and sample local sites within cells and intimate cellular environments. Where conventional instrumentation can give only an averaged measurement of many molecules, nanoscale sensors offer one way to obtain precise readings relevant to the molecular mechanisms of cellular architecture. Nanoprobes can localize spectroscopy and electrochemical measurements to the scale of molecular biology, and can enhance and increase the resolution of MRI and nuclear imaging. And discrete particulate or fiber nanoprobes can be targeted and inserted or even released into living cell environments to report on physical status and events in context. Thus, nanoprobes can enable or complement other powerful approaches to single molecule microscopy, with techniques such as environmental electron microscopy, laser microdissection, nanoprobe mass spectroscopy, and atomic force or tunneling microscopy. Many challenges remain in obtaining the goal, for example, of the sub-thousand dollar genetic profile, but progress is expanding and even exploding on many fronts.

In the earlier sections, we discussed the use of nanoparticles such as quantum dots for enhancement of conventional diagnostic images to show anatomical features and identify tumor cells [31–45,410]. Fluorescent quantum dot bioconjugates are useful not only for diagnostic imaging and photothermal therapy, but also for sensing and probing cellular processes. All of the advantages of nanodots for conventional radiology image enhancement are equally applicable for molecular scale sensing: signal strength, absence of photobleaching, stability under in vivo conditions, emission wavelength tunable with small variations in particle size, and simultaneous excitation of multiple wavelengths [40,61,442,443]. Although larger than fluorescent molecules, quantum dots are useful because they are still small enough to enter cells with minimal disruption, and can be attached to target proteins and structures with minimal alteration of the target's movement and less impact on its chemical properties.

Nanodot particles have been widely applied as imaging probes in immunoassays, and as noted earlier, to detect signaling pathway components and cellular processes (apoptosis and degranulation) in inflammatory and cancer cells [40,444,445]. Nanoparticles with a wide range of resonance frequencies from UV through visible and IR have been synthesized for use as imaging agents to study cell signaling pathways, using various core and shell materials including gold, carbon nanotubes and fullerenes, nanodiamonds, CdSe–ZnS semiconductors, ceramics, and dye-doped silica nanoparticles. They have been used extensively for imaging of immune cells, tumor cells, and other cells to study the details of normal and disease processes, by labeling of organelles and other internal cell structures. Surface modifications are used to target different structures within the cells. The information gained in research today may become useful tomorrow for diagnostic testing, or may help understanding of the mechanism of actions of drugs and other therapies.

A novel technique using small quantum dots (~10 nm) has been developed that represents a significant advance in the ability to image single molecules within cells: it is based on using photothermal interference contrast, rather than using nanodot fluorescence directly [446]. This method relies on the strong optical absorption of a nanodot at its plasma resonance, giving rise to a photothermal-induced change in temperature around the particle when it is illuminated by an energizing laser beam. This temperature change leads to a variation of the local index of refraction that can be optically detected when combining high-frequency modulation and polarization interference contrast by using a second laser beam.

The researchers at the University of Bordeaux, Bordeaux, France who developed the photothermal interference contrast technique were able to demonstrate 3D imaging of receptor proteins stained with individual 10 nm gold particles in the plasma membrane of cells. The ability to resolve single proteins could open the way to new experiments on complex biological systems, gaining access to molecular heterogeneity, dynamical fluctuations, diffusion patterns, conformational changes, and other important features of cellular mechanisms.

Besides nanodots, other types of multifunctional nanoparticles that are useful as enhanced therapy vehicles are equally useful for diagnostic probes. Magnetic nanoparticles for MRI contrast enhancement can selectively target and highlight aspects of cellular metabolism with the addition of other functional moieties such as targeting ligands, fluorescence tags, and radionuclides. Each component of such multimodal probes complements the other modalities for in vitro and in vivo biological measurements. Systems using multicomponent nanoparticles modified with biomolecules can monitor gene expression and other markers in cell therapeutics studies. The migration and fate of stem cells can be monitored with MRI using hybrid stem cell-magnetic nanoparticles. Hybrid probes of magnetic nanoparticles with adenovirus and green fluorescent protein can detect cells targeted for gene therapy and can monitor gene delivery using combined MRI and optical imaging [417].

Molecular-level detection with nanosensors can also be useful when carried by probes that are inserted into cells or that monitor blood and other body fluids. These types of nanosensors for monitoring enzymes and proteins have been developed based on porous silicon [447], carbon nanotubes [448] and carbon fiber nanowires and cantilevers, and use a variety of nanoscale effects. Such probes can be based on optics, electrochemistry, impedance, surface acoustic resonance, and other effects that can be very sensitive and selective at the nanoscale. They can be readily integrated into microelectronics and microfluidic devices [7–10]. We discuss them in detail in Chapter 9 on medical monitoring and genetic profiling.

5.6.6 Nanotechnology for Genetic Screening and Therapy

The third leg of an integrated nanomedicine is genomic and proteomic assessment and therapy. The underlying program of the body's metabolism and structure is coded in the genome and expressed at the first level in the

RNA and the proteome. Although the phenotype is significantly influenced by meta- and epigenetic factors, the genome contains important information to guide diagnosis and treatment. Nanotechnology is producing many powerful genomic and proteomic technologies that make it feasible to examine heterogeneity, genetic instability, and the mutational state of cancer compared with normal cells. And nanotechnology is providing new ways to modify the genome to correct mutations by gene therapy. The eventual goal is to be able to design and deliver highly effective individual therapies based on the genetic profile of the disease, as determined in the individual patient [410].

Nanoparticles are used in the detection of genetic patterns and in delivery of genes into cells [449,450]. These capabilities in genetic marker identification and gene therapy are analogous to the use of nanoparticles in diagnostic imaging and drug therapy, and are based on similar principles and properties. Nanoparticles can be targeted to locate short genetic sequences by attachment of DNA tags that are the complement of a target sequence, along with a reporter ligand that can give a fluorescent signal to indicate where the particle has located a matching segment. Thus, nanoparticles can be used for diagnostic screening for known genetic markers.

A number of nanotechnology strategies have been developed and evaluated as alternatives to viral delivery of genetic material, to avoid the known risks of mutations and oncogenes with viral gene modifications. Nonviral gene delivery systems, such as DNA incorporated in lipids, polycation complexes, or nanoparticles, are safer and easier to produce and use than viral vectors— but these systems are much less efficient in delivering DNA and initiating gene expression than the viruses. The viral vectors are much more capable of overcoming the many barriers for gene delivery into a cell. Therefore, a number of strategies are being tried to overcome the barriers [451–453].

One approach for DNA delivery uses magnetic nanoparticles. DNA is incorporated into the magnetic particles and a strong magnetic field is applied near the target cells. The magnetic field increases particle internalization and gene expression. The exact mechanism by which the magnetic field increases gene uptake has not been completely elucidated, but it is known to increase transfection efficiency by several hundred times. Studies have indicated that the magnetic forces lead to an accelerated sedimentation of magnetofectins on the cell surface but do not directly affect the endocytic uptake mechanism [454–456].

Some safe and nontoxic polymer nanoparticles have been developed to activate selected cell signaling pathways and harness cell trafficking machinery for transport of DNA into the cell nucleus. A nonionic block copolymer of poly(ethylene oxide) and poly(propylene oxide), Pluronic, was found to be capable of activating a transcription factor in cells and enhancing gene expression without inducing a cytotoxic effect [457]. DNA is bound by transcription factors which transport it across the cytoplasm–nucleus barrier by means of nuclear membrane transport machinery. It was found that Pluronic enhanced cellular uptake and nuclear transport of DNA delivered into cells with DNA in polycation complexes. Thus, by combining Pluronic with existing nonviral vectors, the efficiency of gene delivery can be safely increased.

The most promising alternative nonviral strategy effectively bypasses gene therapy by using epigenetics. Cells can be effectively reprogrammed using epigenetic factors without classical gene therapy. Instead of modifying the genome, epigenetic factors alter the expression of genes at later stages of transcription. Gene expression is regulated by many factors, including influence by proteins produced by other genes, and other regulating molecules. One recent line of research uses nanoassembled programming macromolecules consisting of cell-penetrating peptides (or transduction peptides), assembled with protein epigenetic factors, which can regulate genetic expression if delivered into the right cell compartments where transcription and gene expression take place. Transduction peptides, modeled on peptides produced by some viruses to penetrate and deliver material into cells, have been developed into delivery tools for small molecule drugs since their discovery in the 1980s [458,459]. The demonstrated ability to reprogram cells using semiochemical or epigenetic factors is relatively recent. These factors include molecules such as peptides, microRNA, and other substances that interact with the gene expression and transcription process. Nanotechnologies have enabled the actions of these compounds to be traced, captured, isolated, and further studied to understand how they can be used for therapeutic benefit. The goal is to regenerate diseased or damaged tissues by reprogramming cells, which would be a truly revolutionary development. How gene therapy, epigenetics, and other cell therapies are used in conjunction with nanotechnologies to support cell environments will be a subject in Chapter 7 on tissue regeneration and integrated nanotherapies.

5.7 Conclusion: Nanomedicines Have a Broad Impact Throughout Medicine

Nanoparticle formulations are having a significant impact in diagnosis and treatment for infectious, degenerative, inflammatory, and other conditions in many areas of medicine, of which we have given only a small sample here. The interested reader may find many other examples throughout medicine in reviews and articles cited in the references at the end of this chapter [460,461]. We have limited our discussion in this chapter only to nanoparticles, but there is a continuum between molecular drugs, nanoparticles, scaffolds, and nano- and micro-devices. In this chapter, we have focused on nanoparticles for diagnosis and drug delivery; in Chapters 6 and 7 we move up the continuum somewhat to discuss the application of nanotechnology in devices, guides, scaffolds, and support materials for surgery, tissue regeneration and artificial organ development.

References

1. Naomi Halas, *Working with Nanoshells,* Interview on PBS *Nova,* http://www.pbs.org/wgbh/nova/sciencenow/3209/03-nanoshells.html (2005).
2. N. A. Peppas, J. Z. Hilt, and J. B. Thomas (eds.), *Nanotechnology in Therapeutics,* Horizon Bioscience, Wymondham, U.K., 2007.
3. K. Nakamoto, M. Tsuboi, and G. D. Strahan, *Drug–DNA Interactions,* John Wiley & Sons, Inc., Hoboken, NJ, 2008.
4. P. Suetens, *Fundamentals of Medical Imaging,* 2nd edn., Cambridge University Press, Cambridge, U.K., 2009.
5. R. R. H. Coombs and D. W. Robinson (eds.), *Nanotechnology in Medicine and the Biosciences,* Informa Healthcare, London, U.K., 1996.
6. T. Vo-Dinh (ed.), *Nanotechnology in Biology and Medicine*: *Methods, Devices and Applications,* CRC Press, Boca Raton, FL, 2007.
7. J. Moore and G. Zouridakis (eds.), *Biomedical Technology and Devices Handbook,* CRC Press, Boca Raton, FL, 2004.
8. R. S. Greco, F. B. Prinz, and R. L. Smith (eds.), *Nanoscale Technology in Biological Systems,* CRC Press, Boca Raton, FL, 2004.
9. N. H. Malsch (ed.), *Biomedical Nanotechnology,* CRC Press, Boca Raton, FL, 2005.
10. G. L. Hornyak, J. J. Moore, H. F. Tibbals, and J. Dutta, *Fundamentals of Nanotechnology,* CRC Press, Boca Raton, FL, 2008.
11. C. T. Badea, S. Samei, K. Ghaghada, R. Saunders, H. Yuan, Y. Qi, L. W. Hedlund, and S. Mukundan, Utility of a prototype liposomal contrast agent for x-ray imaging of breast cancer: A proof of concept using micro-CT in small animals, in J. Hsieh and E. Samei (eds.), *Proceedings of the SPIE on Medical Imaging 2008*: *Physics of Medical Imaging,* Vol. 6913, San Diego, CA, 2008, pp. 691303-1–691303-9.
12. J. U. Leike, A. Sachse, and K. Rupp, Characterization of continuously extruded iopromide-carrying liposomes for computed tomography blood-pool imaging, *Investigational Radiology,* 36, 303–308 (2001).
13. A. T. Yordanov, A. L. Lodder, E. K. Woller, M. J. Cloninger, N. Patronas, D. Milenic, and M. W. Brechbiel, Novel iodinated dendritic nanoparticles for computed tomography (CT) imaging, *Nano Letters,* 2, 595–599 (2002).
14. Ulrich Speck, Contrast agents: X-ray contrast agents and molecular imaging— A contradiction?, in W. Semmler and M. Schwaiger (eds.), *Molecular Imaging I. Handbook of Experimental Pharmacology 185/I,* Springer-Verlag, Berlin/Heidelberg, Germany, 2008, pp. 167–175.
15. A. M. Schwartzberg, T. Y. Olson, C. E. Talley, and J. Z. Zhang, Synthesis, characterization, and tunable optical properties of hollow gold nanospheres, *Journal of Physical Chemistry B,* 110, 19935–19944 (2006).
16. W. Dong, H. Dong, Z. Wang, P. Zhan, Z. Yu, X. Zhao, Y. Zhu, and N. Ming, Ordered array of gold nanoshells interconnected with gold nanotubes fabricated by double templating, *Advanced Materials,* 18, 755–759 (2006).
17. Y. Hao, C. Huang, J. Jiang, M. Lu, L. Sun, E. I. Meletis, J. Nyagilo, D. P. Dave, M. Xiao, and X. Sun, Hollow gold nanoparticles as theranostic agent, *Second International Conference from Nanoparticles and Nanomaterials to Nanodevices and Nanosystems, and Aegean Nanoscience and Nanotechnology Workshop (Second IC4N2009),* Rhodes, Greece, June 28–July 3, 2009, p. 65, Abstracts.

18. C. Loo, A. Lin, L. Hirsch, M.-H. Lee, E. Chang, J. West, N. Halas, and R. Drezek, Gold nanoshell bioconjugates for molecular imaging in living cells, *Optics Letters*, 30, 1012–1014 (2005).
19. M. L. Brongersma, Nanoshells: Gifts in a gold wrapper, *Nature Materials*, 2, 296–297 (2003).
20. J. Pérez-Juste, I. Pastoriza-Santos, L. M. Liz-Marzán, and P. Mulvaney, Gold nanorods: Synthesis, characterization and applications, *Coordination Chemistry Reviews*, 249, 1870–1819 (2005).
21. A. Gole, J. W. Stone, W. R. Gemmill, H.-C. zur Loye, and C. J. Murphy, Iron oxide coated gold nanorods: Synthesis, characterization, and magnetic manipulation, *Langmuir*, 24, 6232–6237 (2008).
22. F. K. Kálmán, M. Woods, P. Caravan, P. Jurek, M. Spiller, G. Tircsó, R. Király, E. Brücher, and A. D. Sherry, Potentiometric and relaxometric properties of a gadolinium-based MRI contrast agent for sensing tissue pH, *Inorganic Chemistry*, 46, 5260–5270 (2007).
23. J. W. M. Bulte and D. L. Kraitchman, Iron oxide MR contrast agents for molecular and cellular imaging, *NMR in Biomedicine*, 17, 484–499 (2004).
24. R. M. Petoral Jr., F. Söderlind, A. Klasson, A. Suska, M. A. Fortin, P.-O. Käll, M. Engström, and K. Uvdal, Synthesis and characterization of Tb3+ doped Gd_2O_3 nanocrystals: A bifunctional material with combined fluorescent labeling and MRI contrast agent properties, *Journal of Physical Chemistry C*, 113, 6913–6920 (2009).
25. A. Klasson, M. Ahrén, E. Hellqvist, F. Söderlind, A. Rosén, P.-O. Käll, K. Uvdal, and M. Engström, Positive MRI contrast enhancement in THP-1 cells with Gd_2O_3 nanoparticles, *Contrast Media & Molecular Imaging*, 3, 106–111 (2008).
26. F. Söderlind, M.-A Fortin, R. M. Petoral Jr., A. Klasson, T. Veres, M. Engström, K. Uvdal, and P.-O. Käll, Colloidal synthesis and characterization of ultrasmall perovskite $GdFeO_3$ nanocrystals, *Nanotechnology*, 19, 085608 (2008).
27. M. S. Girguis, P. W. Baron, A. C. Cottrell, I. Kjellin, and G. A. Kirk, Gadodiamide-associated nephrogenic systemic fibrosis: why radiologists should be concerned, *AJR: American Journal of Roentgenology*, 188, 586–592 (2007).
28. M.-A. Fortin, R. M. Petoral Jr., F. Söderlind, A. Klasson, M. Engström, T. Veres, P.-O. Käll, and K. Uvdal, PEG-covered ultra-small Gd_2O_3 nanoparticles for positive contrast at 1.5 T MR clinical scanning, *Nanotechnology*, 18, 1–9, 2007.
29. S. Eroglu, B. Gimi, L. Leoni, B. Roman, G. Friedman, T. Desai, and R. L. Magin, NMR imaging of biocapsules for monitoring the performance of cell and tissue implants, in *Proceedings of the Second Annual International IEEE-EMB Special Topic Conference on Microtechnology in Medicine and Biology*, Madison, WI, 2002, pp. 193–198.
30. E. Immel, G. Lorenz, M. Friebe, and A. Melzer, Inductively Coupled MR Visualization of the Stent Lumen, *Proceedings of the 18th International Conference: Society for Medical Innovation & Technology (SMIT 2006)*, May 11–14, 2006, Pacific Grove, CA, 2006, http://www.biophan.com/dmdocuments/Immel.pdf (2009).
31. C. Z. Hotz and M. Bruchez (eds.), *Quantum Dots: Applications in Biology*, Springer Verlag, Berlin, Germany, 2007.
32. M. N. Rhyner, A. M. Smith, X. Gao, H. Mao, L. Yang, and S. Nie, Quantum dots and multifunctional nanoparticles: New contrast agents for tumor imaging, *Nanomedicine*, 1, 209–217 (2006).

33. C. Loo, A. Lin, L. Hirsch, M.-H. Lee, J. Barton, N. Halas, J. West, and R. Drezek, Nanoshell-enabled photonics-based imaging and therapy of cancer, *Technology in Cancer Research and Treatment*, 3, 33–40 (2004).

34. C. Loo, A. Lowery, N. Halas, J. West, and R. Drezek, Immunotargeted nanoshells for integrated cancer imaging and therapy, *Nano Letters*, 5, 709–711 (2005).

35. P. Sharma, S. Brown, G. Walter, S. Santra, and B. Moudgil, Nanoparticles for bioimaging, *Advances in Colloid and Interface Science*, 123, 471–485 (2006).

36. J. W. M. Bulte and M. M. J. Modo (eds.), *Nanoparticles in Biomedical Imaging, Emerging Technologies and Applications Series: Fundamental Biomedical Technologies*, Vol. 3, Springer Verlag, Berlin, Germany, 2008.

37. W. C. W. Chan, D. J. Maxwell, X. Gao, R. E. Bailey, M. Han, and S. Nie, Luminescent quantum dots for multiplexed biological detection and imaging, *Current Opinion in Biotechnology*, 13, 40–46 (2002).

38. J. S. Aaron, N. Nitin, K. Travis, S. Kumar, T. G. Collier, S. Y. Park, M. J. Yacaman et al., Plasmon resonance coupling of metal nanoparticles for molecular imaging of carcinogenesis in vivo, *Journal of Biomedical Optics*, 12, 034007 (2007).

39. C. J. Murphy, T. K. Sau, A. M. Gole, C. J. Orendorff, J. Gao, L. Gou, S. E. Hunyadi, and T. Li, Anisotropic metal nanoparticles: Synthesis, assembly, and optical applications, *Journal of Physical Chemistry B*, 109, 13857–13870 (2005).

40. B. A. Hernandez-Sanchez, T. J. Boyle, T. N. Lambert, S. D. Daniel-Taylor, J. M. Oliver, B. S. Wilson, D. S. Lidke, and N. L. Andrews, Synthesizing biofunctionalized nanoparticles to image cell signaling pathways, *IEEE Transactions on Nanobioscience*, 5, 222–230 (2006).

41. W. J. Mulder, A. W. Griffioen, G. J. Strijkers, D. P. Cormode, K. Nicolay, and Z. A. Fayad, Magnetic and fluorescent nanoparticles for multimodality imaging, *Nanomedicine*, 2, 307–324 (2007).

42. K.-T. Yong, J. Qian, I. Roy, H. H. Lee, E. J. Bergey, K. M. Tramposch, S. He, M. T. Swihart, A. Maitra, and P. N. Prasad, Quantum rod bioconjugates as targeted probes for confocal and two-photon fluorescence imaging of cancer cells, *Nano Letters*, 7, 761–765 (2007).

43. X. Qu, J. Wang, Z. Zhang, N. Koop, R. Rahmanzadeh, and G. J. Hüttmann, Imaging of cancer cells by multiphoton microscopy using gold nanoparticles and fluorescent dyes, *Journal of Biomedical Optics*, 13, 031217 (2008).

44. J. Oh, M. D. Feldman, J. Kim, H. W. Kang, P. Sanghi, and T. E. Milner, Magnetomotive detection of tissue-based macrophages by differential phase optical coherence tomography, *Lasers in Surgery and Medicine*, 39, 266–272 (2007).

45. J. Oh, M. D. Feldman, J. Kim, P. Sanghi, D. Do, J. J. Mancuso, N. Kemp, M. Cilingiroglu, and T. E. Milner, Detection of macrophages in atherosclerotic tissue using magnetic nanoparticles and differential phase optical coherence tomography, *Journal of Biomedical Optics*, 13, 054006 (2008).

46. J. Liu, A. L. Levine, J. S. Mattoon, M. Yamaguchi, R. J. Lee, X. Pan, and T. J. Rosol, Nanoparticles as image enhancing agents for ultrasonography, *Physics in Medicine and Biology*, 51, 2179–2189 (2006).

47. L. Wang, *Photoacoustic Imaging and Spectroscopy*, CRC Press, Boca Raton, FL, 2009.

48. Y. V. Zhulina, A novel algorithm of surface eliminating in undersurface optoacoustic imaging, *EURASIP Journal on Applied Signal Processing*, 2004, 2684–2695 (2004).

49. J. J. Niederhauser, Real-time biomedical optoacoustic imaging, Dissertation, Technische Wissenschaften, Eidgenössische Technische Hochschule ETH Zürich, Nr. 15572, Zurich, Switzerland, 2004, http://e-collection.ethbib.ethz.ch/view/eth:27339 (2009).

50. T. Khamapirad, P. M. Henrichs, K. Mehta, T. G. Miller, A. T. Yee, and A. A. Oraevsky, Diagnostic imaging of breast cancer with LOIS: Clinical feasibility, *SPIE Photonics Plus Ultrasound: Imaging and Sensing*, 5697, 35–44 (2005).

51. A. Stein, P. Otto, M. McCorvey, T. Khamapirad, M. Leonard, and A. Oraevsky, Optoacoustic imaging system for diagnostic imaging of breast cancer, in *Poster Presented at San Antonio Breast Symposium*, San Antonio, TX, December 10–14, 2008, http://www.senomedical.com/downloads/SanAntonio_BreastSymposium_Poster.pdf (2009).

52. J. A. Copland, M. Eghtedari, V. L. Popov, N. Kotov, N. Mamedova, M. Motamedi, and A. A. Oraevsky, Bioconjugated gold nanoparticles as a molecular based contrast agent: Implications for imaging of deep tumors using optoacoustic tomography, *Molecular Imaging and Biology*, 6, 341–349 (2004).

53. M. Eghtedari, A. Oraevsky, J. A. Copland, N. A. Kotov, A. Conjusteau, and M. Motamedi, High sensitivity of in vivo detection of gold nanorods using a laser optoacoustic imaging system, *Nano Letters*, 7, 1914–1918 (2007).

54. R. G. Rayavarapu, W. Petersen, C. Ungureanu, J. N. Post, T. G. van Leeuwen, and S. Manohar, Synthesis and bioconjugation of gold nanoparticles as potential molecular probes for light-based imaging techniques, *Journal of Biomedical Imaging*, 2007, 5 (2007).

55. D. E. J. G. J. Dolmans, D. Fukumura, and R. K. Jain, Photodynamic therapy for cancer. *Nature Reviews Cancer*, 3, 380–387 (2003).

56. A. C. S. Samia, X. Chen, and C. Burda, Semiconductor quantum dots for photodynamic therapy, *Journal of the American Chemical Society*, 125, 15736–15737 (2003).

57. D. Pissuwan, S. M. Valenzuela, and M. B. Cortie, Prospects for gold nanorod particles in diagnostic and therapeutic applications, *Biotechnology and Genetic Engineering Reviews*, 25, 93–112 (2008).

58. E. Sassaroli, K. C. P. Li, and B. E. O'Neill, Numerical investigation of heating of a gold nanoparticle and the surrounding microenvironment by nanosecond laser pulses for nanomedicine applications, *Physics in Medicine and Biology*, 54, 5541–5560 (2009).

59. J. L. West and N. J. Halas, Engineered nanomaterials for biophotonics applications: Improving sensing, imaging, and therapeutics, *Annual Review of Biomedical Engineering*, 5, 285–292 (2003).

60. A. M. Gobin, M. H. Lee, N. D. Halas, W. D. James, R. A. Drezek, and J. L. West, Near-infrared resonant nanoshells for combined optical imaging and photothermal cancer therapy, *Nano Letters*, 7, 1929–1934 (2007).

61. D. Gao, R. R. Agayan, H. Xu, M. A. Philbert, and R. Kopelman, Nanoparticles for two-photon photodynamic therapy in living cells, *Nano Letters*, 6, 2383–2386 (2006).

62. Y. Namiki, T. Namiki, M. Date, K. Yanagihara, M. Yashiro, and H. Takahashi, Enhanced photodynamic anti-tumor effect on gastric cancer by a novel photosensitive stealth liposome. *Pharmacolical Research*, 50, 65–76 (2004).

63. W. Chen and J. Zhang, Using nanoparticles to enable simultaneous radiation and photodynamic therapies for cancer treatment, *Journal of Nanoscience and Nanotechnology*, 6, 1159–1166 (2006).

64. I. Safarik and M. Safarik, Use of magnetic techniques for the isolation of cells, *Journal of Chromatography B*, 722, 33–53 (1999).

65. M. Lewin, N. Carlesso, C.-H. Tung, X.-W. Tang, D. Cory, D. T. Scadden, and R. Weissleder, Tat peptide-derivatized magnetic nanoparticles allow in vivo tracking and recovery of progenitor cells, *Nature Biotechnology*, 18, 410–414 (2000).

66. Z. M. Saiyed, S. D. Telang, and C. N. Ramchand, Application of magnetic techniques in the field of drug discovery and biomedicine, *BioMagnetic Research and Technology*, 1, 1–2 (2003).

67. B. Molnar, F. Sipos, O. Galamb, and Z. Tulassay, Molecular detection of circulating cancer cells: Role in diagnosis, prognosis and follow-up of colon cancer patients, *Digestive Diseases*, 21, 320–325 (2003).

68. Q. A. Pankhurst, J. Connolly, S. K. Jones, and J. Dobson, Applications of magnetic nanoparticles in biomedicine, *Journal of Physics D: Applied Physics*, 36, R167–R181 (2003).

69. D. Wang, J. He, N. Rosenzweig, and Z. Rosenzweig, Fe2O3 beads-CdSe/ZnS quantum dots core-shell nanocomposite particles for cell separation, *Nano Letters*, 4, 409–413 (2004).

70. A. S. Lübbe, C. Alexiou, and C. Bergemann, Clinical applications of magnetic drug targeting, *Journal of Surgical Research*, 95, 200–206 (2001).

71. U. Häfeli, W. Schütt, J. Teller, and M. Zborowski (eds.), *Scientific and Clinical Applications of Magnetic Carriers*, Springer Verlag, Berlin, Germany, 1997.

72. T. Neuberger, B. Schopf, H. Hofmann, M. Hoffmann, and B. von Rechenberg, Superparamagnetic nanoparticles for biomedical applications: Possibilities and limitations of a new drug delivery system, *Journal of Magnetism and Magnetic Materials*, 293, 483–496 (2005).

73. M. Shinkai and A. Ito, Functional magnetic particles for medical application, *Advances in Biochemical Engineering/Biotechnology*, 91, 191–220 (2004).

74. B.-I. Haukanes and C. Kvam, Application of magnetic beads in bioassays, *BioTechnology*, 11, 60–63 (1993).

75. V. H. L. Lee, Nanotechnology: Challenging the limit of creativity in targeted drug delivery *Advanced Drug Delivery Reviews*, 56, 1527–1528 (2004).

76. S. Vinogradov, The second annual symposium on nanomedicine and drug delivery: Exploring recent developments and assessing major advances, August 19–20, 2004, Polytechnic University, Brooklyn, NY, *Expert Opinion on Drug Delivery*, 1, 181–184 (2004).

77. G. A. Hughes, Nanostructure-mediated drug delivery, *Nanomedicine: Nanotechnology, Biology, and Medicine*, 1, 22–30 (2005).

78. C. Shaffer, Nanomedicine transforms drug delivery, *Drug Discovery Today*, 10, 1581–1582 (2006).

79. R. Mozafari (ed.), *Nanocarrier Technologies: Frontiers of Nanotherapy*, Springer Verlag, Berlin, Germany, 2006.

80. C. G. Thanos and D. F. Emerich, The pinpoint promise of nanoparticle-based drug delivery and molecular diagnosis, *Biomolecular Engineering*, 23, 171–184 (2006).

81. K. D. Nelson, A. A. Romero-Sanchez, G. M. Smith, N. Alikacem, D. Radulescu, P. Waggoner, and Z. Hu, Drug releasing biodegradable fiber implant, U.S. Patent 6,596,296, 2003.

82. R. Lam, M. Chen, E. Pierstorff, H. Huang, E. Osawa, and D. Ho, Nanodiamond-embedded microfilm devices for localized chemotherapeutic elution, *ACS Nano*, 2, 2095–2102 (2008).

83. H. F. Edelhauser, J. H. Boatright, J. M. Nickerson, and the Third ARVO/Pfizer Research Institute Working Group, Drug delivery to posterior intraocular tissues: Third annual ARVO/Pfizer Ophthalmics Research Institute conference, *Investigative Ophthalmology and Visual Science*, 49, 4712–4720 (2008).

84. W. E. Bawarski, E. Chidlowsky, D. J. Bharali, and S. A. Mousa, Emerging nanopharmaceuticals, *Nanomedicine: Nanotechnology, Biology and Medicine*, 4, 273–282 (2008).

85. Z. Ye and R. I. Mahato, Role of nanomedicines in cell-based therapeutics, *Nanomedicine*, 3, 5–8 (2008).

86. K. Ulbrich and V. Subr, Polymeric anticancer drugs with pH-controlled activation, *Advanced Drug Delivery Reviews*, 56, 1023–1050 (2004).

87. M. C. Garnett and P. Kallinteri, Nanomedicines and nanotoxicology: Some physiological principles, *Occupational Medicine*, 56, 307–311 (2006).

88. D. F. Emerich and C. G. Thanos, Targeted nanoparticle-based drug delivery and diagnosis, *Journal of Drug Targeting*, 15, 163–183 (2007).

89. E. Igarashi, Factors affecting toxicity and efficacy of polymeric nanomedicines, *Toxicology and Applied Pharmacology*, 229, 121–134 (2008).

90. S. D. Caruthers, S. A. Wickline, and G. M. Lanza, Nanotechnological applications in medicine, *Current Opinion in Biotechnology*, 18, 26–30 (2007).

91. S. Vijayaraghavalu, D. Raghavan, and V. Labhasetwar, Nanoparticles for delivery of chemotherapeutic agents to tumors, *Current Opinion in Investigational Drugs*, 8, 477–484 (2007).

92. G. L. Hornyak, H. F. Tibbals, J. Dutta, and J. J. Moore, Introduction to medical nanotechnology, in *Introduction to Nanoscience and* Nanotechnology, Chapter 27, CRC Press, Boca Raton, FL, 2009.

93. J. Kreuter, Nanoparticles—A historical perspective, *International Journal of Pharmaceutics*, 331, 1–10 (2007).

94. R. Langer, New methods of drug delivery, *Science*, 249, 1527–1533 (1990).

95. T. M. Fahmy, P. M. Fong, A. Goyal, and W. M. Saltzman, Targeted for drug delivery, *Materials Today*, 8, 18–26 (2005).

96. G. L. Hornyak, J. J. Moore, H. F. Tibbals, and J. Dutta, Targeting with magic bullets, Section 12.1.2, in *Fundamentals of Nanotechnology*, CRC Press, Boca Raton, FL, 2009.

97. J. R. Heath and M. E. Davis, Nanotechnology and cancer, *Annual Review of Medicine*, 59, 251–265 (2008).

98. P. Geher, C. Mühlfeld, B. Rother-Rutishauser, and F. Blank (eds.), *Particle-Lung Interactions*, 2nd edn., Informa Healthcare, Inc., New York, 2010.

99. G. Oberdörster, V. Stone, and K. Donaldson, Toxicology of nanoparticles: A historical perspective, *Nanotoxicology*, 1, 2–25 (2007).

100. K. R. Vega-Villa, J. K. Takemoto, J. A. Yáñez, C. M. Remsberg, M. L. Forrest, and N. M. Davies, Clinical toxicities of nanocarrier systems, *Advanced Drug Delivery Reviews*, 60, 929–938 (2008).

101. T. Morris, M. Stables, and D. W. Gilroy, New perspectives on aspirin and the endogenous control of acute inflammatory resolution, *Scientific World Journal*, 6, 1048–1065 (2006).

102. M. Paul-Clark, T. V. Cao, N. Moradi-Bidhendi, D. Cooper, and D. W. Gilroy, 15-epi-lipoxin A4-mediated induction of nitric oxide explains how aspirin inhibits acute inflammation, *Journal of Experimental Medicine*, 200, 69–78 (2004).

103. M. K. Al-Shawi and H. Omote, The remarkable transport mechanism of P-glycoprotein: A multidrug transporter, *Journal of Bioenergetics and Biomembranes*, 37, 489–496 (2005).

104. P. M. Jones and A. M. George, The ABC transporter structure and mechanism: Perspectives on recent research, *Cellular and Molecular Life Sciences*, 61, 682–699 (2004).

105. A. Ponte-Sucre (ed.), *ABC Transporters in Microorganisms*, Caister Academic Press, Norfolk, U.K., 2009.

106. N. Kumar, Taxol-induced polymerization of purified tubulin, *The Journal of Biological Chemistry*, 256, 10435–10441 (1981).

107. S. B. Horwitz, Mechanism of action of taxol, *Trends in Pharmacological Sciences*, 13, 134–136 (1992).

108. J. Goodman and V. Walsh, *The Story of Taxol: Nature and Politics in the Pursuit of an Anti-Cancer Drug*, Cambridge University Press, Cambridge, U.K., 2001.

109. N. A. Peppas and L. Brannon-Peppas, Drug Delivery Biomaterials, in *Encyclopedia of Materials: Science and Technology*, Elsevier, Amsterdam, the Netherlands, pp. 2351–2355, 2008.

110. M. L. Hans and A. M. Lowman, Biodegradable nanoparticles for drug delivery and targeting, *Current Opinion in Solid State and Materials Science*, 6, 319–327 (2002).

111. W. Dong, T. Zhang, A. Cogbill, J. Kasbohm, C. Padilla, R. Njabon, M. Udoetuk, and Z. R. Tian, New nanobiomaterials for potential applications in therapeutic, diagnostic, and regenerative nanomedicines, *Nanomedicine: Nanotechnology, Biology and Medicine*, 2, 274–275 (2006).

112. R. Langer and N. A. Peppas, Advances in biomaterials, drug delivery, and bionanotechnology, *AIChE Journal*, 49, 2990–3006 (2003).

113. N. A. Peppas, Intelligent therapeutics: Biomimetic systems and nanotechnology in drug delivery, *Advanced Drug Delivery Reviews*, 56, 1529–1531 (2004).

114. D. Thassu, M. Deleers, and Y. Pathak (eds.), *Nanoparticulate Drug Delivery Systems*, Informa Healthcare, New York, 2007.

115. M. M. de Villiers, P. Aramwit, and G. S. Kwon (eds.), *Nanotechnology in Drug Delivery*, Springer, New York, 2008.

116. S. Wu-Pong, and Y. Rojanasakul (eds.), *Biopharmaceutical Drug Design and Development*, Humana Press, Totowa, NJ, 2008.

117. A. H. Farajia, and P. Wipf, Nanoparticles in cellular drug delivery, *Bioorganic & Medicinal Chemistry*, 17, 2950–2962 (2009).

118. J.-U. A. H. Junghanns and R. H Müller, Nanocrystal technology, drug delivery and clinical applications, *International Journal of Nanomedicine*, 3, 295–310 (2008).

119. K. Garber, Rapamycin's resurrection: A new way to target the cancer cell cycle, *Journal of the National Cancer Institute*, 93, 1517–1519 (2001).

120. J. Camardo, Tribute to Suren Sehgal, *Transplantation Proceedings*, 35, S2–S4 (2003).

121. S. Das, R. Banerjee and J. Bellare, Aspirin loaded albumin nanoparticles by coacervation: Implications in drug delivery, *Trends in Biomaterials and Artificial Organs*, 18, 203–212 (2005).

122. N. A. Peppas, Gels for drug delivery, in *Encyclopedia of Materials: Science and Technology*, Pergamon Press, Oxford, U.K., 2008, pp. 3492–3495.

123. B. J. Boyd, Past and future evolution in colloidal drug delivery systems, *Expert Opinion on Drug Delivery*, 5, 69–85 (2008).

124. A. Elaissari (ed.), *Colloidal Biomolecules, Biomaterials, and Biomedical Applications*, CRC Press, Boca Raton, FL, 2003.

125. R. H. Muller, S. Benita, and B. Bohm (eds.), *Emulsions and Nanosuspensions for the Formulation of Poorly Soluble Drugs*, Medpharm Scientific Publishers, Stuttgart, Germany, 1998.
126. M. Malmsten, *Surfactants and Polymers in Drug Delivery*, Marcel Dekker, New York, 2002.
127. H. Chen, X. Chang, D. Du, J. Li, H. Xu, and X. Yang, Microemulsion-based hydrogel formulation of ibuprofen for topical delivery, *International Journal of Pharmaceutics*, 315, 52–58 (2006).
128. H. Chen, D. Mou, D. Du, X. Chang, D. Zhu, J. Liu, H. Xu, and X. Yang, Hydrogel thickened microemulsion for topical administration of drug molecule at an extremely low concentration, *International Journal of Pharmaceutics*, 341, 78–84 (2007).
129. R. Lam and D. Ho, Nanodiamonds as vehicles for systemic and localized drug delivery, *Expert Opinion on Drug Delivery*, 6, 883–895 (2009).
130. J. Zeng, X. Xu, X. Chen, Q. Liang, X. Bian, L. Yang, and X. Jing, Biodegradable electrospun fibers for drug delivery, *Journal of Controlled Release*, 92, 227–231 (2003).
131. M. M. Hussain and S. S. Ramkumar, Physicochemical characteristics of drug-laden nanofibers for controlled drug delivery, in *AICHE Annual Meeting, 2006*, San Francisco, CA, November 12, 2006, p. 323.
132. J. Venugopal, M. P. Prabhakaran, S. Low, A. T. Choon, Y. Z. Zhang, G. Deepika, and S. Ramakrishna, Nanotechnology for nanomedicine and delivery of drugs, *Current Pharmaceutical Design*, 14, 2184–200 (2008).
133. J. B. Melanko, M. E. Pearce, and A. K. Salem, Nanotubes, nanorods, nanofibers, and fullerenes for nanoscale drug delivery, in M. M. de Villiers, P. Aramwit, and G. S. Kwon (eds.), in *Nanotechnology in Drug Delivery*, Chap. 4, Springer, New York, 2008, pp. 105–127.
134. D. Losic and S. Simovic, Self-ordered nanopore and nanotube platforms for drug delivery applications, *Expert Opinion on Drug Delivery*, 6, 1363–1381 (2009).
135. J. H. Fendler (ed.), *Nanoparticles and Nanostructured Films*, Wiley-VCH, Weinheim, Germany, 1998.
136. Y. F. Mei, X. L. Wu, X. F. Shao, G. G. Siu, and X. M. Bao, Formation of an array of isolated alumina nanotubes, *Europhysics Letters*, 62, 595–599 (2003).
137. A. K. Patri, J. F. Kukowska-Latallo, and J. R. Baker Jr., Targeted drug delivery with dendrimers: Comparison of the release kinetics of covalently conjugated drug and non-covalent drug inclusion complex, *Advanced Drug Delivery Reviews*, 57, 2203–2214 (2005).
138. H. L. Crampton and E. E. Simanek, Dendrimers as drug delivery vehicles: Non-covalent interactions of bioactive compounds with dendrimers, *Polymer International*, 56, 489–496 (2007).
139. J. Das, J. M. J. Fréchet, and A. K. Chakraborty, Self-assembly of dendronized polymers, *Journal of Physical Chemistry B*, 113, 13768–13775 (2009).
140. R. Esfand and D. A. Tomali, Poly(amidoamine) (PAMAM) dendrimers: From biomimicry to drug delivery and biomedical applications, *Drug Discovery Today*, 6, 427–436 (2001).
141. E. Chiellini, J. Sunamoto, C. Migliaresi, and R. M. Ottenbrite (eds.), *Biomedical Polymers and Polymer Therapeutics*, Springer Verlag, Berlin, Germany, 2001.
142. P. J. Tarcha, *Polymers for Controlled Drug Delivery*, CRC Press, Boca Raton, FL, 1990.

143. M. V. Chaubal, Synthetic polymer-based ion exchange resins: Excipients and actives, *Drug Delivery Technology*, 3, 6–8 (2003), http://www.drugdeliverytech.com/ (2009).

144. K. S. Soppimath, T. M. Aminabhavi, A. R. Kulkarni, and W. E. Rudzinski, Biodegradable polymeric nanoparticles as drug delivery devices, *Journal of Controlled Release*, 70, 1–20 (2001).

145. M. Thanou and R. Duncan, Polymer-protein and polymer-drug conjugates in cancer therapy, *Current Opinion in Investigational Drugs*, 4, 701–709 (2003).

146. R. Duncan, M. J. Vicent, F. Greco, and R. I. Nicholson, Polymer-drug conjugates: Towards a novel approach for the treatment of endrocine-related cancer, *Endocrine-Related Cancer*, 12, S189–S199 (2005).

147. J. R. Robinson and V. H. L. Lee (eds.), *Controlled Drug Delivery: Fundamentals and Applications*, 2nd edn., Informa Healthcare, New York, 1987.

148. R. Duncan, Polymer conjugates as anticancer nanomedicines, *Nature Reviews: Cancer*, 6, 688–701 (2006).

149. V. Cuchelkar, P. Kopecková, and J. Kopecek, Synthesis and biological evaluation of disulfide-linked HPMA copolymer-mesochlorin e6 conjugates, *Macromolecular Bioscience*, 8, 375–383 (2008).

150. B. P. Koppolu, M. Rahimi, S. P. Nattama, A. Wadajkar, and K. Nguyen, Development of multiple-layer polymeric particles for targeted and controlled drug delivery, *Nanomedicine: Nanotechnology, Biology and Medicine*, 6, 355–361 (2009).

151. M. J. Vicent and R. Duncan, Polymer conjugates: Nanosized medicines for treating cancer, *Trends in Biotechnology*, 24, 39–47 (2006).

152. H. Maeda, SMANCS and polymer-conjugated macromolecular drugs: Advantages in cancer chemotherapy, *Advanced Drug Delivery Reviews*, 46, 169–185 (2001).

153. V. M. Lenaerts and R. Gurny, *Bioadhesive Drug Delivery Systems*, CRC Press, Boca Raton, FL, 1990.

154. C. de Duve, T. de Barsy, B. Poole, A. Trouet, P. Tulkens, and F. Van Hoof, Lysosomotropic agents, *Biochemical Pharmacology*, 23, 2495–2531 (1974).

155. H. Ringsdorf, Structure and properties of pharmacologically active polymers, *Journal of Polymer Science: Polymer Symposia*, 51, 135–153 (1975).

156. R. Duncan, Designing polymer conjugates as lysosomotropic nanomedicines, *Biochemical Society Transactions*, 35, 56–60 (2007).

157. K. Cho, X. Wang, S. Nie, Z. G. Chen, and D. M. Shin, Therapeutic nanoparticles for drug delivery in cancer, *Clinical Cancer Research*, 14, 1310–1316 (2008).

158. P. Roxburgh and T. R. J. Evans, Systemic therapy of hepatocellular carcinoma: Are we making progress?, *Advances in Therapy*, 25, 1089–1104 (2008).

159. C. Li and S. Wallace, Polymer-drug conjugates: Recent development in clinical oncology, *Advanced Drug Delivery Reviews*, 60, 886–898 (2008).

160. H. Wang, S. Wang, H. Su, K.-J. Chen, A.-L. Armijo, W.-Y. Lin, Y. Wang, J. Sun, K. Kamei, J. Czernin, C. G. Radu, and H.-R. Tseng, A supramolecular approach for preparation of size-controlled nanoparticles, *Angewandte Chemie International Edition*, 48, 4344–4348 (2009).

161. A. Das, Y. Zhou, A. A. Ivanov, R. L. Carter, T. K. Harden, and K. A. Jacobson, Enhanced potency of nucleotide–dendrimer conjugates as agonists of the P2Y$_{14}$ receptor: Multivalent effect in G protein-coupled receptor recognition, *Bioconjugate Chemistry*, 20, 1650–1659 (2009).

162. P. Singh, U. Gupta, A. Asthana, and N. K. Jain, Folate and folate–PEG–PAMAM dendrimers: Synthesis, characterization, and targeted anticancer drug delivery potential in tumor bearing mice, *Bioconjugate Chemistry*, 19, 2239–2252 (2008).

163. K. Kono, M. Liu, and J. M. J. Fréchet, Design of dendritic macromolecules containing folate or methotrexate residues, *Bioconjugate Chemistry*, 10, 1115–1121 (1999).

164. E. K. Woller and M. J. Cloninger, The lectin-binding properties of six generations of mannose-functionalized dendrimers, *Organic Letters*, 4, 7–10 (2002).

165. B. Le Droumaguet and K. Velonia, Click Chemistry: A powerful tool to create polymer-based macromolecular chimeras, *Macromolecular Rapid Communications*, 29, 1073–1089 (2008).

166. K. Gupta, V. P. Singh, R. K. Kurupati, A. Mann, M. Ganguli, Y. K. Gupta, Y. Singh, K. Saleem, S. Pasha, and S. Maiti, Nanoparticles of cationic chimeric peptide and sodium polyacrylate exhibit striking antinociception activity at lower dose, *Journal of Controlled Release*, 134, 47–54 (2009).

167. V. J. Venditto, C. A. S. Regino, and M. W. Brechbiel, PAMAM dendrimer based macromolecules as improved contrast agents, *Molecular Pharmaceutics*, 2, 302–311 (2005).

168. S. Shukla, G. Wu, M. Chatterjee, W. Yang, M. Sekido, L. A. Diop, R. Müller et al., Synthesis and biological evaluation of folate receptor-targeted boronated PAMAM dendrimers as potential agents for neutron capture therapy, *Bioconjugate Chemistry*, 14, 158–167 (2003).

169. M. Massignani, C. LoPresti, A. Blanazs, J. Madsen, S. P. Armes, A. L. Lewis, and G. Battaglia, Controlling cellular uptake by surface chemistry, size, and surface topology at the nanoscale, *Small*, 5, 2424–2432 (2009).

170. D. Needham, Lipid membranes: Biological inspiration for micro and nano encapsulation technologies, especially drug delivery, *Materials Research Society Symposium—Proceedings*, 774, 173–202 (2003).

171. C. P. Reis, R. J. Neufeld, A. J. Ribeiro, and F. Veiga, Nanoencapsulation I. Methods for preparation of drug-loaded polymeric nanoparticles, *Nanomedicine: Nanotechnology, Biology and Medicine*, 2, 8–21 (2006).

172. C. P. Reis, R. J. Neufeld, A. J. Ribeiro, and F. Veiga, Nanoencapsulation II. Biomedical applications and current status of peptide and protein nanoparticulate delivery systems, *Nanomedicine: Nanotechnology, Biology and Medicine*, 2, 53–65 (2006).

173. V. Torchilin, Micellar nanocarriers: Pharmaceutical perspectives, *Pharmaceutical Research*, 24, 1–16 (2007).

174. N. T. Huynh, C. Passirani, P. Saulnier, and J. P. Benoit, Lipid nanocapsules: A new platform for nanomedicine, *International Journal of Pharmaceutics*, 379, 201–209 (2009).

175. B. Mishra, B. B. Patel, and S. Tiwari, Colloidal nanocarriers: A review on formulation technology, types and applications toward targeted drug delivery, *Nanomedicine: Nanotechnology, Biology and Medicine*, 6, 9–24 (2009), doi:10.1016/j.nano.2009.04.008.

176. S. Khurana, P. Utreja, A. K. Tiwary, N. K. Jain, and S. Jain, Nanostructured lipid carriers and their application in drug delivery, *International Journal of Biomedical Engineering and Technology*, 2, 152–171 (2009).

177. V. P. Torchilin, Targeted polymeric micelles for delivery of poorly soluble drugs, *Cellular and Molecular Life Sciences*, 61, 2549–2559 (2004).

178. Z. Ge and S. Liu, Supramolecular self-assembly of nonlinear amphiphilic and double hydrophilic block copolymers in aqueous solutions, *Macromolecular Rapid Communications*, 30, 1523–1532 (2009).

179. A. J. Hell, D. J. A. Crommelin, W. E. Hennink, and E. Mastrobattista, Stabilization of peptide vesicles by introducing inter-peptide disulfide bonds, *Pharmaceutical Research*, 26, 2186–2193 (2009).

180. Y. Bae and K. Kataoka, Intelligent polymeric micelles from functional poly(ethylene glycol)-poly(amino acid) block copolymers, *Advanced Drug Delivery Reviews*, 61, 768–784 (2009).

181. M. Yokoyama, Drug targeting with nano-sized carrier systems, *Journal of Artificial Organs*, 8, 77–84 (2005).

182. Y. Noguchi, J. Wu, R. Duncan, J. Strohalm, K. Ulbrich, T. Akaike, and H. Maeda, Early phase tumor accumulation of macromolecules: A great difference in clearance rate between tumor and normal tissues, *Cancer Science*, 89, 307–314 (2005).

183. U.S. National Institutes of Health, National Cancer Institute, Drug dictionary website: http://www.cancer.gov/drugdictionary/?CdrID=434427 (2009).

184. Y. Tsukioka, Y. Matsumura, T. Hamaguchi, H. Koike, F. Moriyasu, and T. Kakizoe, Pharmaceutical and biomedical differences between micellar doxorubicin (NK911) and liposomal doxorubicin (Doxil), *Japanese Journal of Cancer Research*, 93, 1145–1153 (2002).

185. S. Danson, D. Ferry, V. Alakhov, J. Margison, D. Kerr, D. Jowle, M. Brampton, G. Halbert, and M. Ranson, Phase I dose escalation and pharmacokinetic study of pluronic polymer-bound doxorubicin (SP1049C) in patients with advanced cancer, *British Journal of Cancer*, 90, 2085–2091 (2004).

186. S. de Bono and B. de Bono, Doughnut delivery, *Trends in Biochemical Sciences*, 26, 14 (2001).

187. S. C. Basu and M. Basu (eds.), *Liposome Methods and Protocols*, Humana Press, Totowa, NJ, 2002.

188. A. Agarwal, Y. Lvov, R. Sawant, and V. Torchilin, Stable nanocolloids of poorly soluble drugs with high drug content prepared using the combination of sonication and layer-by-layer technology, *Journal of Controlled Release*, 128, 255–260 (2008).

189. J. Leng, S. U. Egelhaaf, and M. E. Cates, Kinetics of the micelle-to-vesicle transition: Aqueous lecithin-bile salt mixtures, *Biophysics Journal*, 85, 1624–1646 (2003).

190. G. Gregoriadis (ed.), *Liposome Technology, Volume I: Liposome Preparation and Related Techniques*, 3rd edn., CRC Press, Boca Raton, FL, 2006.

191. L. A. Meure, R. Knott, N. R. Foster, and F. Dehghani, The depressurization of an expanded solution into aqueous media for the bulk production of liposomes, *Langmuir*, 25, 326–337 (2009).

192. M. R. Mozafari and S. M. Mortazavi, *Nanoliposomes: From Fundamentals to Recent Developments*, Trafford Publishing, Oxford, U.K., 2005.

193. J. C. Colas, W. L. Shi, V. S. N.M. Rao, A. Omri, M. R. Mozafari, and H. Singh, Microscopical investigations of nisin-loaded nanoliposomes prepared by Mozafari method and their bacterial targeting, *Micron*, 38, 841–847 (2007).

194. A. A. Gabizon, Stealth liposomes and tumor targeting: One step further in the quest for the magic bullet, *Clinical Cancer Research*, 7, 223–225 (2001).

195. P. K. Jayanna, V. P. Torchilin, and V. A. Petrenko, Liposomes targeted by fusion phage proteins, *Nanomedicine: Nanotechnology, Biology and Medicine*, 5, 83–89 (2009).

196. A. Samad, Y. Sultana, and M. Aqil, Liposomal drug delivery systems: An update review, *Current Drug Delivery*, 4, 297–305 (2007).
197. D. Peer, A. Florentin, and R. Margalit, Hyaluronan is a key component in cryoprotection and formulation of targeted unilamellar liposomes, *Biochimica et Biophysica Acta*, 1612, 76–82 (2003).
198. D. Peer and R. Margalit, Tumor-targeted hyaluronan nanoliposomes increase the antitumor activity of liposomal doxorubicin in syngeneic and human xenograft mouse tumor models, *Neoplasia*, 6, 343–353 (2004).
199. S.-M. Lee, H. Chen, C. M. Dettmer, T. V. O'Halloran, and S.-B. T. Nguyen, Polymer-caged liposomes: A pH-responsive delivery system with high stability, *Journal of the American Chemical Society*, 129, 15096–15097 (2007).
200. C. P. O'Neil, T. Suzuki, D. Demurtas, A. Finka, and J. A. Hubbell, A novel method for the encapsulation of biomolecules into polymersomes via direct hydration, *Langmuir*, 25, 9025–9029 (2009).
201. D. E. Discher and F. Ahmed, Polymersomes, *Annual Review of Biomedical Engineering*, 8, 323–341 (2006).
202. D. H. Levine, P. P. Ghoroghchian, J. Freudenberg, G. Zhang, M. J. Therien, M. I. Greene, D. A. Hammer, and R. Murali, Polymersomes: A new multi-functional tool for cancer diagnosis and therapy, *Methods*, 46, 25–32 (2008).
203. D. A. Christian, S. Cai, D. M. Bowen, Y. Kim, J. D. Pajerowski, and D. E. Discher, Polymersome carriers: From self-assembly to siRNA and protein therapeutics, *European Journal of Pharmaceutics and Biopharmaceutics*, 71, 463–474 (2009).
204. E. Boisselier and D. Astruc, Gold nanoparticles in nanomedicine: Preparations, imaging, diagnostics, therapies and toxicity, *Chemical Society Reviews*, 38, 1759–1782 (2009).
205. H. M. E. Azzazy, M. M. H. Mansour, and S. C. Kazmierczak, From diagnostics to therapy: Prospects of quantum dots, *Clinical Biochemistry*, 40, 917–927 (2007).
206. V. N. Mochalin and Y. Gogotsi, Wet chemistry route to hydrophobic blue fluorescent nanodiamond, *Journal of the American Chemical Society*, 131, 4594–4595 (2009).
207. S. A. Wissinga, O. Kayserb, and R. H. Müller, Solid lipid nanoparticles for parenteral drug delivery, *Advanced Drug Delivery Reviews*, 56, 1257–1272 (2004).
208. N. Anton, P. Saulnier, C. Gaillard, E. Porcher, S. Vrignaud, and J. P. Benoit, Aqueous-core lipid nanocapsules for encapsulating fragile hydrophilic and/or lipophilic molecules, *Langmuir*, 25, 11413–11419 (2009).
209. T. A. Desai, S. Sharma, R. J. Walczak, A. Boiarski, M. Cohen, J. Shapiro, T. West et al., Nanoporous implants for controlled drug delivery, in *BioMEMS and Biomedical Nanotechnology: Therapeutic Micro/Nanotechnology*, Vol. 3, Springer, New York, 2007, pp 263–286.
210. J. Guan, H. He, B. Yu, and L. J. Lee, Polymeric nanoparticles and nanopore membranes for controlled drug and gene delivery, in K. E. Gonsalves, C. R. Halberstadt, C. T. Laurencin and L. S. Nair (eds.), *Biomedical Nanostructures*, John Wiley & Sons, Inc., Hoboken, NJ, 2008.
211. K. Raemdonck, J. Demeester, and S. De Smedt, Advanced nanogel engineering for drug delivery, *Soft Matter*, 5, 707–715 (2009).
212. J. K. Oh, D. I. Lee, and J. M. Park, Biopolymer-based microgels/nanogels for drug delivery applications, *Progress in Polymer Science*, 34, 1261–1282 (2009).
213. B. R. Saunders, N. Laajam, E. Daly, S. Teow, X. Hu, and R. Stepto, Microgels: From responsive polymer colloids to biomaterials, *Advances in Colloid and Interface Science*, 147–148, 251–262 (2009).

214. J. K. Oh, C. Tang, H. Gao, N. V. Tsarevsky, and K. Matyjaszewski, Inverse miniemulsion ATRP: A new method for synthesis and functionalization of well-defined water-soluble/cross-linked polymeric particles, *Journal of the American Chemical Society*, 128, 5578–5584 (2006).

215. J. K. Oh, D. J. Siegwart, H. Lee, G. Sherwood, L. Peteanu, J. O. Hollinger, K. Kataoka, and K. Matyjaszewski, Biodegradable nanogels prepared by atom transfer radical polymerization as potential drug delivery carriers: Synthesis, biodegradation, in vitro release, and bioconjugation, *Journal of the American Chemical Society*, 129, 5939–5945 (2007).

216. A. V. Kabanov and S. V. Vinogradov, Nanogels as pharmaceutical carriers: Finite networks of infinite capabilities, *Angewandte Chemie International Edition*, 48, 5418–5429 (2009).

217. S. Salmon and S. M. Hudson, Crystal morphology, biosynthesis, and physical assembly of cellulose, chitin, and chitosan, *Polymer Reviews*, 37, 199–276 (1997).

218. G. L. Hornyak, J. Dutta, H. F. Tibbals, and A. Rao, *Introduction to Nanoscience*, CRC Press, Boca Raton, FL, 2008.

219. S. A. Agnihotri, N. N. Mallikarjuna, and T. M. Aminabhavi, Recent advances on chitosan-based micro- and nanoparticles in drug delivery, *Journal of Controlled Release*, 100, 5–28 (2004).

220. Y. Zheng, Y. Wu, W. Yang, C. Wang, S. Fu, and X. Shen, Preparation, characterization, and drug release in vitro of chitosan-glycyrrhetic acid nanoparticles, *Journal of Pharmaceutical Sciences*, 95, 181–191 (2005).

221. Q. Gan and T. Wang, Chitosan nanoparticle as protein delivery carrier—Systematic examination of fabrication conditions for efficient loading and release, *Colloids and Surfaces B: Biointerfaces*, 59, 24–34 (2007).

222. E. M. M. Del Valle, Cyclodextrins and their uses: A review, *Process Biochemistry*, 39, 1033–1046 (2004).

223. R. Challa, A. Ahuja, J. Ali, and R. K. Khar, Cyclodextrins in drug delivery: An updated review, *AAPS PharmSciTech*, 6, E329–E357 (2005).

224. H. Dodziuk (ed.), *Cyclodextrins and Their Complexes; Chemistry, Analytical Methods, Applications*, Wiley-VCH, Weinheim, Germany, 2006.

225. A. F. Soares, R. de Albuquerque-Carvalho, and F. Veiga, Oral administration of peptides and proteins: Nanoparticles and cyclodextrins as biocompatible delivery systems, *Nanomedicine*, 2, 183–202 (2007).

226. A. Rasheed, A. Kumar, and C. K. Sravanthi, Cyclodextrins as drug carrier molecule: A review, *Scientia Pharmaceutica*, 76, 567–598 (2008).

227. F. Theeuwes, Elementary osmotic pump, *Journal of Pharmaceutical Science*, 64, 1987–1991 (1975).

228. H. T. Hammel, and W. M. Schlegel, Osmosis and solute–solvent drag: Fluid transport and fluid exchange in animals and plants, *Cell Biochemistry and Biophysics*, 42, 277–345 (2005).

229. Y. Gan, W. Pan, M. Wei and R. Zhang, Cyclodextrin complex osmotic tablet for glipizide delivery, *Drug Development and Industrial Pharmacy*, 28, 1015–1021 (2002).

230. A. Mehramizi, M. E. Asgari, M. Pourfarzib, K. Bayati, F. A. Dorkoosh, and M. Rafiee-Tehrani, Influence of β-cyclodextrin complexation on lovastatin release from osmotic pump tablets (OPT), *Daru Pharmacy Journal*, 15, 71–78 (2007).

231. L. Liu and X. Wang, Solubility-modulated monolithic osmotic pump tablet for atenolol delivery, *European Journal of Pharmaceutics and Biopharmaceutics*, 68, 298–302 (2008).

232. M. C. Gohel, R. K. Parikh, and N. Y. Shah, Osmotic drug delivery: An update, *Pharmainfo.net Latest Reviews*, 7(2) (2009), published on-line at website: http://www. pharmainfo.net/reviews/osmotic-drug-delivery-update (2009).

233. F. Bellia, D. La Mendola, C. Pedone, E. Rizzarelli, M. Saviano, and G. Vecchio, Selectively functionalized cyclodextrins and their metal complexes, *Chemical Society Reviews*, 38, 2756–2781 (2009).

234. B. G. De Geest, B. G. Sukhorukov, and H. Möhwald, The pros and cons of polyelectrolyte capsules in drug delivery, *Expert Opinion on Drug Delivery*, 6, 613–624 (2009).

235. T. Douglas and M. Young, Making friends with old foes, *Science*, 312, 873–875 (2006).

236. F. Ahmed, P. J. Photos, and D. E. Discher, Polymersomes as viral capsid mimics, *Drug Development Research*, 67, 4–14 (2006).

237. Y. Ren, S.-M. Wong, and L.-Y. Lim, In vitro-reassembled plant virus-like particles for loading of polyacids, *Journal of General Virology*, 87, 2749–2754 (2006).

238. E. R. Ballister, A. H. Lai, R. N. Zuckermann, Y. Cheng, and J. D. Mougous, Nanotubes from biomimetically bioengineered viruses for drug delivery: In vitro self-assembly of tailorable nanotubes from a simple protein building block, *Proceedings of the National Academy of Sciences*, 105, 3733–3738 (2008).

239. V. Huter, M. P. Szostak, J. Gampfer, S. Prethaler, G. Wanner, F. Gabor, and W. Lubitz, Bacterial ghosts as drug carrier and targeting vehicles, *Journal of Controlled Release*, 61, 51–63 (1999).

240. S. Paukner, G. Kohl, and W. Lubitz, Bacterial ghosts as novel advanced drug delivery systems: Antiproliferative activity of loaded doxombicin in human Caco-2 cells, *Journal of Controlled Release*, 94, 63–74 (2004).

241. D. Akin, J. Sturgis, K. Ragheb, D. Sherman, K. Burkholder, J. P. Robinson, A. K. Bhunia, S. Mohammed, and R. Bashir, Bacteria-mediated delivery of nanoparticles and cargo into cells, *Nature Nanotechnology*, 2, 441–449 (2006).

242. B. Rapp, Manipulating diatoms, *Materials Today*, 7, 13 (2004).

243. M. R. Choi, K. J. Stanton-Maxey, J. K. Stanley, C. S. Levin, R. Bardhan, D. Akin, S. Badve et al., A cellular Trojan Horse for delivery of therapeutic nanoparticles into tumors, *Nano Letters*, 7, 3759–3765 (2007).

244. MagForce Nanotechnologies AG, www.magforce.de/ (2009).

245. D. Gong, V. Yadavalli, M. Paulose, M. Pishko, and C. A. Grimes, Controlled molecular release using nanoporous alumina capsules, *Biomedical Microdevices*, 5, 75–80 (2003).

246. P. M. Sinha and M. Ferrari, Sacrificial Oxide Layer for Drug Delivery, in A. P. Lee and L. J. Lee (eds.), *BioMEMS and Biomedical Nanotechnology: Biological and Biomedical Nanotechnology*, Vol. 1, Chap. 5, Springer-Verlag, New York, 2005.

247. V. S.-Y. Lin, Nanomedicine: Veni, vidi, vici and then… vanished, *Nature Materials*, 8, 252–253 (2009).

248. J.-H. Park, L. Gu, G. von Maltzahn, E. Ruoslahti, S. N. Bhatia, and M. J. Sailor, Biodegradable luminescent porous silicon nanoparticles for in vivo applications, *Nature Materials*, 8, 331–336 (2009).

249. S. Angelos, Y.-W. Yang, K. Patel, J. F. Stoddart, and J. I. Zink, pH-responsive supramolecular nanovalves based on cucurbit[6]uril pseudorotaxanes, *Angewandte Chemie*, 47, 2222–2226 (2008).

250. G. A. Urban, Nanotechnologie in der Medizin, *Praxis*, 41, 1591–1593 (2005).

251. P. Couvreur and C. Vauthier, Nanotechnology: Intelligent design to treat complex disease, *Pharmaceutical Research*, 23, 1417–1450 (2006).

252. J. L. Gilmore, X. Yi, L. Quan, and A. V. Kabanov, Novel nanomaterials for clinical neuroscience, *Journal of Neuroimmune Pharmacology*, 3, 83–94 (2008).
253. R. Sykes, 'Towards the magic bullet.' Hamao Umezawa memorial award lecture, *International Journal of Antimicrobial Agents*, 14, 1–12 (2000).
254. R. B. Sykes, The magic bullet in the new millennium—Cause for optimism, *Journal of Infection and Chemotherapy*, 8, 121–124 (2002).
255. H. Tomioka and K. Namba, Development of antituberculous drugs: Current status and future prospects, *Kekkaku*, 81, 753–774 (2006).
256. M. Okada and K. Kobayashi, Recent progress in mycobacteriology, *Kekkaku*, 82, 783–799 (2007).
257. M. Ma, Y. Cheng, Z. Xu, P. Xu, H. Qu, Y. Fang, T. Xu, and L. Wen, Evaluation of polyamidoamine (PAMAM) dendrimers as drug carriers of anti-bacterial drugs using sulfamethoxazole (SMZ) as a model drug, *European Journal of Medicinal Chemistry*, 42, 93–98 (2007).
258. T. Thomas and G. Foster, Nanomedicines in the treatment of chronic hepatitis C—Focus on pegylated interferon alpha-2a, *International Journal of Nanomedicine*, 2, 19–24 (2007).
259. J.-J. Yu, B. Nolting, Y. H. Tan, L. Xue, J. Grvay-Hague, and G. Lu, Polyvalent interactions of HIV-gp120 protein and nanostructures of carbohydrate ligands, *NanoBioTechnology*, 1, 1551–1286 (2005).
260. D. J. Owen, Dendrimers: New opportunities to treat and prevent human diseases, *Nanomedicine: Nanotechnology, Biology and Medicine*, 3, 338 (2007).
261. L. J. Peek, C. R. Middaugh, and C. Berkland, Nanotechnology in vaccine delivery, *Advanced Drug Delivery Reviews*, 60, 915–928 (2008).
262. Z. Cui and R. J. Mumper, Topical immunization using nanoengineered genetic vaccines, *Journal of Controlled Release*, 81, 173–184 (2002).
263. R. H. G. Baxter, C.-I. Chang, Y. Chelliah, S. Blandin, E. A. Levashina, and J. Deisenhofer, Structural basis for conserved complement factor-like function in the antimalarial protein TEP1, *Proceedings of the National Academy of Sciences*, 104, 11615–11620 (2007).
264. G. L. Hornyak, H. F. Tibbals, J. Dutta, and J. J. Moore, *Fundamentals of Nanoscience and Nanotechnology: Adaptive Protein Grippers as Anti-Parasite Weaponry*, Section 26.2.6, pp. 1361–1364, CRC Press, Boca Raton, FL, 2009.
265. L. Dinesen and S. Travis, Targeting nanomedicines in the treatment of Crohn's disease: Focus on certolizumab pegol (CDP870), *International Journal of Nanomedicine*, 2, 39–47 (2007).
266. T. Barnes and R. Moots, Targeting nanomedicines in the treatment of rheumatoid arthritis: Focus on certolizumab pegol, *International Journal of Nanomedicine*, 2, 3–7 (2007).
267. H. Onyüksel, F. Séjourné, H. Suzuki, and I. Rubinstein, Human VIP-alpha: A long-acting, biocompatible and biodegradable peptide nanomedicine for essential hypertension, *Peptides*, 27, 2271–2275 (2006).
268. N. Popovic and P. Brundin, Therapeutic potential of controlled drug delivery systems in neurodegenerative diseases, *International Journal of Pharmaceutics*, 314, 120–126 (2006).
269. N. Singh, C. A. Cohen, and B. A. Rzigalinski, Treatment of neurodegenerative disorders with radical nanomedicine, *Annals of the New York Academy of Sciences*, 1122, 219–230 (2008).

270. S. A. Wickline and G. Lanza, Nanotechnology for molecular imaging and targeted therapy, *Circulation*, 107, 1092–1095 (2003).

271. F. A. Jaffer, P. Libby, and R. Weissleder, Molecular and cellular imaging of atherosclerosis: Emerging applications, *Journal of the American College of Cardiology*, 47, 1328–1338 (2006).

272. X. Yang, Nano- and microparticle-based imaging of cardiovascular interventions: Overview, *Radiology*, 243, 340–347 (2007).

273. M. D. Kuo, J. M. Waugh, C. J. Elkins, and D. S. Wang, Translating nanotechnology to vascular disease, in R. S. Greco, F. B. Prinz and R. L. Smith (eds.), *Nanoscale Technology in Biological Systems*, Chap. 17, CRC Press, Boca Raton, FL, 2004, pp. 386–416.

274. S. A. Wickline, A. M. Neubauer, P. Winter, S. Caruthers, and G. Lanza, Applications of nanotechnology to atherosclerosis, thrombosis, and vascular biology, *Atherosclerosis, Thrombosis, and Vascular Biology*, 26, 435–441 (2006).

275. G. M. Lanza, P. M. Winter, S. D. Caruthers, M. S. Hughes, T. Cyrus, J. N. Marsh, A. M. Neubauer, K. C. Partlow, and S. A. Wickline, Nanomedicine opportunities for cardiovascular disease with perfluorocarbon nanoparticles, *Nanomedicine*, 1, 321–329 (2006).

276. G. Lanza, P. Winter, T. Cyrus, S. Caruthers, J. Marsh, M. Hughes, and S. Wickline, Nanomedicine opportunities in cardiology, *Annals of the New York Academy of Sciences*, 1080, 451–465 (2006).

277. W. J. M. Mulder and Z. A. Fayad, Nanomedicine captures cardiovascular disease, *Arteriosclerosis, Thrombosis, and Vascular Biology*, 28, 801–802 (2008).

278. R. T. Sataloff and C. Wei, Nanomedicine: Important new concepts for otolaryngology, *Ear, Nose & Throat Journal*, 86, 528–531 (2007), on website at: http://www.thefreelibrary.com/Nanomedicine:+important+new+concepts+for+otolaryngology.-a0169824141 (2009).

279. G. L. Hornyak, Nanotechnology in otolaryngology, *Otolaryngologic Clinics of North America*, 38, 273–293 (2005).

280. A. Zimmer and J. Kreuter, Microspheres and nanoparticles used in ocular delivery systems, *Advanced Drug Delivery Reviews*, 16, 61–73 (1995).

281. Th. F. Vandamme, Microemulsions as ocular drug delivery systems: Recent developments and future challenges, *Progress in Retinal and Eye Research*, 21, 15–34 (2002).

282. D. Ghate and H. F. Edelhauser, Ocular drug delivery, *Expert Opinion on Drug Delivery*, 3, 275–287 (2006).

283. J. Vandervoort and A. Ludwig, Ocular drug delivery: Nanomedicine applications, *Nanomedicine*, 2, 11–21 (2007).

284. Y. Ogura, Drug delivery to the posterior segments of the eye, *Advanced Drug Delivery Reviews*, 52, 1–3 (2001).

285. T. K. De and A. S. Hoffman, An ophthalmic formulation of a beta-adrenoceptor antagonist, levobetaxolol, using poly(acrylic acid) nanoparticles as carrier: Loading and release studies, *Journal of Bioactive and Compatible Polymers*, 16, 20–31 (2001).

286. R. S. Navath, Y. E. Kurtoglu, B. Wang, S. Kannan, R. Romero, and R. M. Kannan, Dendrimer-drug conjugates for tailored intracellular drug release based on glutathione levels, *Bioconjugate Chemistry*, 19, 2446–2455 (2008).

287. R. D. Simoni, R. L. Hill, and M. Vaughan, The discovery of insulin: The work of Frederick Banting and Charles Best, *Journal of Biological Chemistry*, 277, 26 (2002).

288. G. L. Hornyak, H. F. Tibbals, J. Dutta, and J. J. Moore, Section 27.1.5. Nanoparticles and nanoencapsulation for insulin delivery, pp. 1423–1426, in [S. Vijayaraghavalu, D. Raghavan, and V. Labhasetwar, Nanoparticles for delivery of chemotherapeutic agents to tumors, *Current Opinion in Investigational Drugs*, 8, 477–484 (2007)] (2009).

289. R. S. Spangler, Insulin administration via liposomes, *Diabetes Care*, 13, 911–922 (1990).

290. S. Furtado, D. Abramson, L. Simhkay, D. Wobbekind, and E. Mathiowitz, Subcutaneous delivery of insulin loaded poly(fumaric-co-sebacic anhydride) microspheres to type 1 diabetic rats, *European Journal of Pharmaceutics and Biopharmaceutics*, 63, 229–236 (2006).

291. E. Allémann, J.-C. Leroux and R. Gurny, Polymeric nano- and microparticles for the oral delivery of peptides and peptidomimetics, *Advanced Drug Delivery Reviews*, 43, 171–189 (1998).

292. B. Sarmentoa, A. Ribeirob, F. Veiga, and D. Ferreira, Development and characterization of new insulin containing polysaccharide nanoparticles, *Colloids and Surfaces B: Biointerfaces*, 53, 193–202 (2006).

293. M. Aboubakar, F. Puisieux, P. Couvreur, M. Deyme, and C. Vauthier, Study of the mechanism of insulin encapsulation in poly(isobutylcyanoacrylate) nanocapsules obtained by interfacial polymerization, *Journal of Biomedical Materials Research*, 47, 568–576 (1999).

294. S. Watnasirichaikul, N. M. Davies, T. Rades, and I. G. Tucker, Preparation of biodegradable insulin nanocapsules from biocompatible microemulsions, *Pharmaceutical Research*, 17, 684–689 (2000).

295. G. P. Carino, J. S. Jacob, and E. Mathiowitz, Nanosphere based oral insulin delivery, *Journal of Controlled Release*, 65, 261–269 (2000).

296. J. S. Jacob, Y. S. Jong, D. T. Abramson, E. Mathiowitz, C. A. Santos, M. J. Bassett, and S. Furtardo, Nanoparticulate therapeutic biologically active agents, U.S. Patent 20,050,181,059, Spherics, Inc., Mansfield, MA, 2004.

297. E. Merisko-Liversidge, S. L. McGurk, and G. G. Liversidge, Insulin Nanoparticles: A novel formulation approach for poorly water soluble Zn-insulin, *Pharmaceutical Research*, 21, 1545–1553 (2004).

298. N. K. Kavitha Raj and C. P. Sharma, Oral insulin—A perspective, *Journal of Biomaterials Applications*, 17, 183–196 (2003).

299. Z. T. Bloomgarden, Insulin treatment and type 1 diabetes topics, *Diabetes Care*, 29, 936–944 (2006).

300. S. L. Tao and T. A. Desai, Microfabrication of multilayer, asymmetric, polymeric devices for drug delivery, *Advanced Materials*, 17, 1625 (2005).

301. R. A. Shimkunas, E. Robinson, R. Lam, S. Lu, X. Xu, X.-Q. Zhang, H. Huang, E. Osawa, and D. Ho, Nanodiamond–insulin complexes as pH-dependent protein delivery vehicles, *Biomaterials*, 30, 5720–5728 (2009).

302. N. J. Kavimandan, E. Losi, and N. A. Peppas, Novel delivery system based on complexation hydrogels as delivery vehicles for insulin-transferrin conjugates, *Biomaterials*, 27, 3846–3854 (2006).

303. B. Kim and N. A. Peppas, In vitro release behavior and stability of insulin in complexation hydrogels as oral drug delivery carriers, *International Journal of Pharmaceutics*, 266, 29–37 (2003).

304. T. M. Kumar, W. Paul, C. P. Sharma, and M. A. Kuriachan, Bioadhesive, pH responsive micromatrix for oral delivery of insulin, *Trends in Biomaterials and Artificial Organs*, 18, 199–202 (2005).

305. L. Serra, J. Doménech, and N. A. Peppas, Engineering design and molecular dynamics of mucoadhesive drug delivery systems as targeting agents, *European Journal of Pharmaceutics and Biopharmaceutics*, 71, 519–528 (2009).
306. E. Renard, G. Costalat, and J. Bringer, From external to implantable insulin pump, can we close the loop? *Diabetes & Metabolism*, 28, S19–S25 (2002).
307. J. D. Zahn, Y.-C. Hsieh, and M. Yang, Components of an integrated microfluidic device for continuous glucose monitoring with responsive insulin delivery, *Diabetes Technology & Therapeutics*, 7, 536–545 (2005).
308. J. Z. Hilt and N. A. Peppas, Microfabricated drug delivery devices, *International Journal of Pharmaceutics*, 306, 15–23 (2005).
309. Debiotech S. A., Insulin pump breakthrough: The nanopump, http://www.debiotech.com/ (2009).
310. STMicroelectronics and Debiotech announce first prototypes of disposable insulin nanopump, June 23, 2008, http://www.st.com/stonline/stappl/cms/press/news/year2008/t2301.htm (2008).
311. Insulet Corporation, http://www.myomnipod.com/ (2009).
312. E. Dassau, C. C. Palerm, H. Zisser, B. A. Buckingham, L. Jovanovic, and F. J. Doyle III, In silico evaluation platform for artificial pancreatic β-cell development—A dynamic simulator for dlosed-loop control with hardware-in-the-loop, *Diabetes Technology & Therapeutics*, 11, 187–194 (2009).
313. J. C. Pickup, Z.-L. Zhi, F. Khan, T. Saxl, and D. J. S. Birch, Nanomedicine and its potential in diabetes research and practice, *Diabetes/Metabolism Research and Reviews*, 24, 604–610 (2008).
314. M. Koch, F. F.-F. Schmid, V. Zoete, and M. Meuwly, Insulin: A model system for nanomedicine? *Nanomedicine*, 1, 373–378 (2006).
315. A. R. DeGroot and R. J. Neufeld, Encapsulation of urease in alginate beads and protection from a-chymotrypsin with chitosan membranes. *Enzyme and Microbial Technology*, 29: 321–327 (2001).
316. E. J. A. Pope, K. Braun, and C. M. Peterson, Bioartificial organs I: Silica gel encapsulated pancreatic islets for the treatment of diabetes mellitus, *Journal of Sol-Gel Science and Technology*, 8, 635–639 (1997).
317. T. A. Desai, W. H. Chu, J. K. Tu, G. M. Beattie, A. Hayek, and M. Ferrari, Mircofabricated immunoisolating biocapsules, *Biotechnology and Bioengineering*, 57, 118–120 (1998).
318. T. A. Desai, W. H. Chu, G. Rasi, P. Sinibaldi-Vallebona, E. Guarino, and M. Ferrari, Microfabricated biocapsules provide short-term immunoisolation of insulinoma xenografts, *Biomedical Microdevices*, 1, 131–138 (1999).
319. F. J. Martin and C. Grove, Microfabricated drug delivery systems: Concepts to improve clinical benefit, *Biomedical Microdevices*, 3, 97–108 (2001).
320. K. E. La Flamme, G. Mor, D. Gong, T. La Tempa, V. A. Fusaro, C. A. Grimes, and T. A. Desai, Nanoporous alumina capsules for cellular macroencapsulation: Transport and biocompatibility, *Diabetes Technology & Therapeutics*, 7, 684–694 (2005).
321. K. E. La Flamme, K. C. Popat, L. Leoni, E. Markiewicz, T. J. La Tempa, B. B. Roman, C. A. Grimes, and T. A. Desai, Biocompatibility of nanoporous alumina membranes for immunoisolation, *Biomaterials*, 28, 2638–2645 (2007).
322. F. Lim and A. M. Sun, Microencapsulated islets as bioartificial endocrine pancreas, *Science*, 210, 908–910 (1980).
323. H. Uludag, P. De Vos, and P. A. Tresco, Technology of mammalian cell encapsulation *Advanced Drug Delivery Reviews*, 42, 29–64 (2000).

324. W. T. Godbey and A. Atala, In vitro systems for tissue engineering, *Annals of the New York Academy of Sciences*, 961, 10–26 (2002).
325. C. Smith, R. Kirk, T. West, M. Bratzel, M. Cohen, F. Martin, A. Boiarski, and A. A. Rampersaud, Diffusion characteristics of microfabricated silicon nanopore membranes as immunoisolation membranes for use in cellular therapeutics, *Diabetes Technology & Therapeutics*, 7, 151–162 (2005).
326. A. I. Silva, A. N. de Matos, I. G. Brons, and M. Mateus, An overview on the development of a bio-artificial pancreas as a treatment of insulin-dependent diabetes mellitus, *Medicinal Research Reviews*, 26, 181–222 (2005).
327. G. Erdodi, J. Kang, B. Yalcin, M. Cakmak, K. S. Rosenthal, S. Grundfest-Broniatowski, and J. P. Kennedy, A novel macroencapsulating immunoisolatory device: The preparation and properties of nanomat-reinforced amphiphilic conetworks deposited on perforated metal scaffold, *Journal Biomedical Microdevices*, 11, 297–312 (2009).
328. B. Gimi, T. Leong, Z. Gu, M. Yang, D. Artemov, Z. M. Bhujwalla, and D. H. Gracias, Self-assembled three dimensional radio frequency (RF) shielded containers for cell encapsulation, *Biomedical Microdevices*, 7, 341–345 (2005).
329. P. de Vos, A. F. Hamel, and K. Tatarkiewicz, Considerations for successful transplantation of encapsulated pancreatic islets, *Diabetologia*, 45, 159–173 (2002).
330. P. de Vos and P. Marchetti, Encapsulation of pancreatic islets for transplantation in diabetes: The untouchable islets, *Trends in Molecular Medicine*, 8, 363–366 (2002).
331. A. S. Narang and R. I. Mahato, Biological and biomaterial approaches for improved islet transplantation, *Pharmacological Reviews*, 58, 194–243 (2006).
332. S. Schneider, P. J. Feilen, F. Brunnenmeier, T. Minnemann, H. Zimmermann, U. Zimmermann, and M. M. Weber, Long-term graft function of adult rat and human islets encapsulated in novel alginate-based microcapsules after transplantation in immunocompetent diabetic mice, *Diabetes*, 54, 687–693 (2005).
333. D. Dufrane, R.-M. Goebbels, A. Saliez, Y. Guiot, and P. Gianello, Six-month survival of microencapsulated pig islets and alginate biocompatibility in primates: Proof of concept, *Transplantation*, 81, 1345–1353 (2006).
334. H. Zimmermann, S. G. Shirley, and U. Zimmermann, Alginate-based encapsulation of cells: Past, present, and future, *Current Diabetes Reports*, 7, 314–320 (2007).
335. A. Murua, A. Portero, G. Orive, R. M. Hernández, M. de Castro, and J. L. Pedraz, Cell microencapsulation technology: Towards clinical application, *Journal of Controlled Release*, 132, 76–83 (2008).
336. J. T. Wilson and E. L. Chaikof, Challenges and emerging technologies in the immunoisolation of cells and tissues, *Advanced Drug Delivery Reviews*, 60, 124–145 (2008).
337. J. O.-H. Shama, Y. Zhang, W. H. Finlay, W. H. Roa, and R. Löbenberg, Formulation and characterization of spray-dried powders containing nanoparticles for aerosol delivery to the lung, *International Journal of Pharmaceutics*, 269, 457–467 (2004).
338. Y. Y. Huang and C. H. Wang, Pulmonary delivery of insulin by liposomal carriers, *Journal of Controlled Release* 113, 9–14 (2006).
339. G. T. McMahon and R. A. Arky, Inhaled insulin for diabetes mellitus, *New England Journal of Medicine*, 356, 497–502 (2007).
340. J. C. Sung, B. L. Pulliam, and D. A. Edwards, Nanoparticles for drug delivery to the lungs, *Trends in Biotechnology*, 25, 563–570 (2007).

341. W. Yang, J. I. Peters, and R. O. Williams III, Inhaled nanoparticles—A current review, *International Journal of Pharmaceutics*, 356, 239–247 (2008).

342. A. Mistry, S. Stolnik, and L. Illum, Nanoparticles for direct nose-to-brain delivery of drugs, *International Journal of Pharmaceutics*, 379, 146–157 (2009).

343. L. Illum, Nasal drug delivery—Possibilities, problems and solutions, *Journal of Controlled Release*, 87, 187–198 (2003).

344. D. Filmore, Breaching the blood–brain barrier, *Modern Drug Discovery*, 5, 22–27 (2002).

345. M. J. Alonso, Nanomedicines for overcoming biological barriers, *Biomédecine & Pharmacothérapie*, 58, 168–172 (2004).

346. J. Kreuter, Drug transport(ers) and the diseased brain: Application of nanoparticles for the delivery of drugs to the brain, *International Congress Series*, 1277, 85–94 (2005).

347. N. D. Doolittle, L. E. Abrey, W. A. Bleyer, S. Brem, T. P. Davis, P. Dore-Duffy, L. R. Drewes et al., New frontiers in translational research in neuro-oncology and the blood–brain barrier: Report of the tenth annual blood–brain barrier disruption consortium meeting, *Clinical Cancer Research*, 11, 421–428 (2005).

348. L. L. Muldoon, P. G. Tratnyek, P. M. Jacobs, N. D. Doolittle, G. A. Christoforidis, J. A. Frank, M. Lindau et al., Imaging and nanomedicine for diagnosis and therapy in the central nervous system: Report of the eleventh annual blood–brain barrier disruption consortium meeting, *American Journal of Neuroradiology*, 27, 715–721 (2006).

349. K. K. Jain, Nanobiotechnology-based drug delivery to the central nervous system, *Neuro-Degenerative Diseases*, 4, 287–291 (2007).

350. G. A. Silva, Nanotechnology approaches for drug and small molecule delivery across the blood brain barrier, *Surgical Neurology*, 67, 113–116 (2007).

351. C. Roney, P. Kulkarni, V. Arora, P. Antich, F. Bonte, A. Wu, N. N. Mallikarjuana et al., Targeted nanoparticles for drug delivery through the blood–brain barrier for Alzheimer's disease, *Journal of Controlled Release*, 108, 193–214 (2005).

352. G. Xu, K.-T. Yong, I. Roy, S. D. Mahajan, H. Ding, S. A. Schwartz, and P. N. Prasad, Bioconjugated quantum rods as targeted probes for efficient transmigration across an in vitro blood?brain barrier, *Bioconjugate Chemistry*, 19, 1179–1185 (2008).

353. J. M. Koziara, P. R. Lockman, D. D. Allen, and R. J. Mumper, Paclitaxel nanoparticles for the potential treatment of brain tumors, *Journal of Controlled Release*, 99, 259–269 (2004).

354. O. C. Farokhzad and R. Langer, Nanomedicine: Developing smarter therapeutic and diagnostic modalities, *Advanced Drug Delivery Reviews*, 58, 1456–1459 (2006).

355. S. Logothetidis, Nanotechnology in medicine: The medicine of tomorrow and nanomedicine, *Hippokratia*, 10, 7–21 (2006).

356. D. M. Brown (ed.), *Drug Delivery Systems in Cancer Therapy*, Humana Press, Totowa, NJ, 2004.

357. D. Peer, J. Karp, S. Hong, O. Farokhzad, R. Margalit, and R. Langer, Nanocarriers as an emerging platform for cancer therapy, *Nature Nanotechnology*, 2, 751–760 (2007).

358. K. Y. Kim, Nanotechnology platforms and physiological challenges for cancer therapeutics, *Nanotechnology, Biology and Medicine*, 3, 103–110 (2007).

359. K. K. Jain, Recent advances in nanooncology, *Technology in Cancer Research & Treatment*, 7, 1–13 (2008).

360. R. K. Zee-Cheng and C. C. Cheng, Delivery of anticancer drugs, *Methods and Findings in Experimental and Clinical Pharmacology*, 11, 439–529 (1989).

361. C. K. Kim and S. J. Lim, Recent progress in drug delivery systems for anticancer agents, *Archives of Pharmacal Research*, 25, 229–239 (2002).

362. E. S. Kawasaki and A. Player, Nanotechnology, nanomedicine, and the development of new, effective therapies for cancer, *Nanomedicine: Nanotechnology, Biology and Medicine*, 1, 101–109 (2005).

363. M. M. Amiji, *Nanotechnology for Cancer Therapy*, CRC Press, Boca Raton, FL, 2006.

364. M. Conti, V. Tazzari, C. Baccini, G. Pertici, L. P. Serino, and U. De Giorgi, Anticancer drug delivery with nanoparticles, *In vivo*, 20, 697–701 (2006).

365. S. Nie, Y. Xing, G. J. Kim, and J. W. Simons, Nanotechnology applications in cancer *Annual Review of Biomedical Engineering*, 9, 257–288 (2007).

366. J. Larocque, D. Bharali, and S. Mousa, Cancer detection and treatment: The role of nanomedicines, *Molecular Biotechnology*, 42, 358–366 (2009).

367. A. I. Freeman and E. Mayhew, Targeted drug delivery, *Cancer*, 58(Suppl 2), 573–583 (1986).

368. K. K. Jain, Targeted drug delivery for cancer, *Technology in Cancer Research & Treatment*, 4, 311–454 (2005).

369. J. R. Baker, A. Quintana, L. Piehler, M. Banazak-Holl, D. Tomalia, and E. Raczka, The synthesis and testing of anti-cancer therapeutic nanodevices, *Biomedical Microdevices*, 3, 61–69 (2001).

370. M. Shi, J. Lu, and M. S. Shoichet, Organic nanoscale drug carriers coupled with ligands for targeted drug delivery in cancer, *Journal of Materials Chemistry*, 19, 5485–5498 (2009).

371. D. Sutton, N. Nasongkla, E. Blanco, and J. Gao, Functionalized micellar systems for cancer targeted drug delivery, *Pharmaceutical Research*, 24, 1029–1046 (2007).

372. E. Blanco, C. W. Kessinger, B. D. Sumer, J. Gao, Multifunctional micellar nanomedicine for cancer therapy, *Experimental Biology and Medicine*, 234, 123–131 (2009).

373. R. Krishna and L. D. Mayer, The use of liposomal anticancer agents to determine the roles of drug pharmacodistribution and P-glycoprotein (PGP) blockade in overcoming multidrug resistance (MDR), *Anticancer Research*, 19, 2885–2891 (1999).

374. C. Mamot, D. C. Drummond, K. Hong, D. B. Kirpotin, J. W. Park, Liposome-based approaches to overcome anticancer drug resistance, *Drug Resistance Updates*, 6, 271–279 (2003).

375. E. Ristorcelli, E. Beraud, P. Verrando, C. Villard, D. Lafitte, V. Sbarra, D. Lombardo, and A. Verine, Human tumor nanoparticles induce apoptosis of pancreatic cancer cells, *The FASEB Journal*, 22, 3358–3369 (2008).

376. F. Ahmed, R. I. Pakunlu, A. Brannan, F. Bates, T. Minko, and D. E. Discher, Biodegradable polymersomes loaded with both paclitaxel and doxorubicin permeate and shrink tumors, inducing apoptosis in proportion to accumulated drug, *Journal of Controlled Release*, 116, 150–158 (2006).

377. L. H. Reddy, J.-M. Renoir, V. Marsaud, S. Lepetre-Mouelhi, D. Desmaele, and P. Couvreur, Anticancer efficacy of squalenoyl gemcitabine nanomedicine on 60 human-tumor cell panel and on experimental tumor, *Molecular Pharmaceutics*, 6, 1526–1535 (2009).

378. J. Wang, D. Mongayt, and V. P. Torchilin, Polymeric micelles for delivery of poorly soluble drugs: Preparation and anticancer activity in vitro of paclitaxel incorporated into mixed micelles based on poly(ethylene glycol)-lipid conjugate and positively charged lipids, *Journal of Drug Targeting*, 13, 73–80 (2005).

379. K. Margulis-Goshen, and S. Magdassi, Formation of simvastatin nanoparticles from microemulsion, *Nanomedicine: Nanotechnology, Biology and Medicine*, 5, 274–281 (2009).

380. J.-H. Park, G. von Maltzahn, E. Ruoslahti, S. N. Bhatia, and M. J. Sailor, Micellar hybrid nanoparticles for simultaneous magnetofluorescent imaging and drug delivery, *Angewandte Chemie International Edition*, 47, 7284–7288 (2008).

381. Y. Chen, X. Lin, H. Park, and R. Greever, Study of artemisinin nanocapsules as anticancer drug delivery systems, *Nanomedicine: Nanotechnology, Biology and Medicine*, 5, 316–322 (2009).

382. G. K. Gupta, V. Jain, and P. R. Mishra, Paclitaxel delivery by micro/nano encapsulation using layer-by-layer assembly, *Nature Proceedings*, <http://dx.doi.org/10.1038/npre.2009.2812.1> (2009).

383. S. Bisht, G. Feldmann, S. Soni, R. Ravi, C. Karikar, A. Maitra, and A. Maitra, Polymeric nanoparticle-encapsulated curcumin ("nanocurcumin"): A novel strategy for human cancer therapy, *Journal of Nanobiotechnology*, 5, 3 (2007) online at website: http://www.jnanobiotechnology.com/content/5/1/3 (2009).

384. P. Merritt and L. A. Snyder, Pharmacology of ß-lapachone and lapachol, Cyberbotanica, URL: http://biotech.icmb.utexas.edu/botany/beta.html, BioTech Resources, Austin, TX (2008).

385. D. A. Boothman and A. B. Pardee, Inhibition of radiation-induced neoplastic transformation by ß-lapachone, *Proceedings of the National Academy of Sciences*, 86, 4963–4967 (1989).

386. K. E. Reinicke, E. A. Bey, M. S. Bentle, J. J. Pink, S. T. Ingalls, C. L. Hoppel, R. I. Misico et al., Development of ß-lapachone prodrugs for therapy against human cancer cells with elevated NAD(P)H: Quinone oxidoreductase 1 levels, *Clinical Cancer Research*, 11, 3055–3064 (2005).

387. D. Sutton, S. Wang, N. Nasongkla, J. Gao, and E. E. Dormidontova, Doxorubicin and ß-lapachone release and interaction with micellar core materials: Experiment and modeling, *Experimental Biology and Medicine*, 232, 1090–1099 (2007).

388. X. Montet, R. Weissleder, L. Josephson, Imaging pancreatic cancer with a peptide-nanoparticle conjugate targeted to normal pancreas, *Bioconjugate Chemistry*, 17, 905–911 (2006).

389. R. Weissleder, K. Kelly, E. Y. Sun, T. Shtatland, and L. Josephson, Cell-specific targeting of nanoparticles by multivalent attachment of small molecules, *Nature Biotechnology*, 23, 1418–1423 (2005).

390. H. Devalapally, Z. Duan, M. V. Seiden, and M. M. Amiji, Paclitaxel and ceramide co-administration in biodegradable polymeric nanoparticulate delivery system to overcome drug resistance in ovarian cancer, *International Journal of Cancer*, 121, 1830–1838 (2007).

391. V. V. Mody, M. I. Nounou, and M. Bikram, Novel nanomedicine-based MRI contrast agents for gynecological malignancies, *Advanced Drug Delivery Reviews*, 61, 795–807 (2009).

392. D. Artemov, N. Mori, B. Okollie, and Z. M. Bhujwalla, MR molecular imaging of the Her-2/neu receptor in breast cancer cells using targeted iron oxide nanoparticles, *Magnetic Resonance in Medicine*, 49, 403–408 (2003).

393. O. C. Farokhzad, S. Jon, A. Khademhosseini, T.-N. T. Tran, D. A. LaVan, and R. Langer, Nanoparticle-aptamer bioconjugates—A new approach for targeting prostate cancer cells, *Cancer Research*, 64, 7668–7672, (2004).

394. M. Johannsen, U. Gneveckow, L. Eckelt, A. Feussner, N. Waldöfner, R. Scholz, S. Deger, P. Wust, S. A. Loening, and A. Jordan, Clinical hyperthermia of prostate cancer using magnetic nanoparticles: Presentation of a new interstitial technique, *International Journal of Hyperthermia*, 21, 637–647 (2005).

395. M. Johannsen, B. Thiesen, U. Gneveckow, K. Taymoorian, N. Waldöfner, R. Scholz, S. Deger, K. Jung, S. A. Loening, and A. Jordan, Thermotherapy using magnetic nanoparticles combined with external radiation in an orthotopic rat model of prostate cancer, *The Prostate*, 66, 97–104 (2005).

396. M. Johannsen, U. Gneveckow, B. Thiesen, K. Taymoorian, C. H. Cho, N. Waldöfner, R. Scholz, A. Jordan, S. A. Loening, and P. Wust, Thermotherapy of prostate cancer using magnetic nanoparticles: Feasibility, imaging, and three-dimensional temperature distribution, *European Urology*, 52, 1653–1662 (2007).

397. M. G. Harisinghani, J. Barentsz, P. F. Hahn, W. M. Deserno, S. Tabatabaei, C. H. van de Kaa, J. de la Rosette, and R. Weissleder, Noninvasive detection of clinically occult lymph-node metastases in prostate cancer, *New England Journal of Medicine*, 348, 2491–2499 (2003).

398. M. R. Green, G. M. Manikhas, S. Orlov, B. Afanasyev, A. M. Makhson, P. Bhar, and M. J. Hawkins, Abraxane®, a novel Cremophor®-free, albumin-bound particle form of paclitaxel for the treatment of advanced non-small-cell lung cancer, *Annals of Oncology*, 17, 1263–1268 (2006).

399. R. Bhattacharya, C. Patra, A. Earl, S. Wang, A. Katarya, L. Lu, J. Kizhakkedathu, M. Yaszemski, P. Greipp, and D. Mukhopadhyay, Attaching folic acid on gold nanoparticles using noncovalent interaction via different polyethylene glycol backbones and targeting of cancer cells, *Nanomedicine: Nanotechnology, Biology and Medicine*, 3, 224–238 (2007).

400. X. Huang, P. K. Jain, I. H. El-Sayed, and M. A. El-Sayed, Determination of the minimum temperature required for selective photothermal destruction of cancer cells with the use of immunotargeted gold nanoparticles, *Photochemistry and Photobiology*, 82, 412–417 (2006).

401. F. J. Picard and M. G. Bergeron, Rapid molecular theranostics in infectious diseases, *Drug Discovery Today*, 7, 1092–1101 (2002).

402. S. Warner, Diagnostics + therapy = theranostics, *The Scientist*, 18, 38 (2004).

403. J. W. Hooper, The genetic map to theranostics, *MLO: Medical Laboratory Observer*, 38, 22–25 (2006).

404. B. Sumer and J. Gao, Theranostic nanomedicine for cancer, *Nanomedicine*, 3, 138–140 (2008).

405. J. R. Heath, M. E. Davis, and L. Hood, Nanomedicine targets cancer, *Scientific American*, 300, 44–51 (2009).

406. C. Plank, Nanomedicine: Silence the target, *Nature nanotechnology*, 4, 544–545 (2009).

407. K. K. Jain, Role of nanobiotechnology in developing personalized medicine for cancer, *Technology in Cancer Research & Treatment*, 4, 645–650 (2006).

408. H. M. Warenius, L. Seabra, L. Kyritsi, R. White, and R. Dormer, Theranostic proteomic profiling of cyclins, cyclin dependent kinases and Ras in human cancer cell lines is dependent on p53 mutational status, *International Journal of Oncology*, 32, 895–907 (2008).

409. K. K. Jain, *Textbook of Personalized Medicine*, Springer Verlag, Berlin, Germany, 2009.

410. H. M. Warenius, Technological challenges of theranostics in oncology, *Expert Opinion on Medical Diagnostics*, 3, 381–393 (2009).

411. C. Khemtong, C. W. Kessinger, and J. Gao, Polymeric nanomedicine for cancer MR imaging and drug delivery, *Chemical Communalizations*, 2009, 3497–3510 (2009).

412. O. M. Koo, I. Rubinstein, and H. Onyuksel, Role of nanotechnology in targeted drug delivery and imaging: A concise review, *Nanomedicine: Nanotechnology, Biology and Medicine*, 1, 193–212 (2005).

413. Z.-R. Lu, F. Ye, and A. Vaidya, Polymer platforms for drug delivery and biomedical imaging, *Journal Controlled Release*, 122, 269–277 (2007).

414. V. P. Torchilin, Multifunctional nanocarriers, *Advanced Drug Delivery Reviews*, 58, 1532–1555 (2006).

415. V. P. Torchilin (ed.), *Multifunctional Pharmaceutical Nanocarriers*, Springer-Verlag, Berlin, Germany, 2008.

416. J. Gao, H. Gu, and B. Xu, Multifunctional magnetic nanoparticles: Design, synthesis, and biomedical applications, *Accounts of Chemical Research*, 42, 1097–1107 (2009).

417. J. Cheon and J. H. Lee, Synergistically integrated nanoparticles as multimodal probes for nanobiotechnology, *Accounts of Chemical Research*, 41, 1630–1640 (2008).

418. P. Broz, S. Driamov, J. Ziegler, N. Ben-Haim, S. Marsch, W. Meier, and P. Hunziker, Toward intelligent nanosize bioreactors: A pH-switchable, channel-equipped, functional polymer nanocontainer, *Nano Letters*, 6, 2349–2353 (2006).

419. S. O. Meade, M. S. Yoon, K. H. Ahn, and M. J. Sailor, Porous silicon photonic crystals as encoded microcarriers, *Advanced Materials*, 16, 1811–1814 (2004).

420. M. J. Sailor and J. R. Link, Smart dust: Nanostructured devices in a grain of sand, *Chemical Communications*, 2005, 1375–1383 (2005).

421. J.-H. Park, G. von Maltzahn, L. Zhang, A. M. Derfus, D. Simberg, T. J. Harris, S. N. Bhatia, E. Ruoslahti, and M. J. Sailor, Systematic surface engineering of magnetic nanoworms for in vivo tumor targeting, *Small*, 5, 694–700 (2009).

422. K. Senior, Nanodumpling with drug delivery potential, *Molecular Medicine Today*, 4, 321 (1998).

423. A. M. Nyströma and K. L. Wooley, Thiol-functionalized shell crosslinked knedel-like (SCK) nanoparticles: A versatile entry for their conjugation with biomacromolecules, *Tetrahedron*, 64, 8543–8552 (2008).

424. A. Ranquin, W. Versées, W. Meier, J. Steyaert, and P. Van Gelder, Therapeutic nanoreactors: Combining chemistry and biology in a novel triblock copolymer drug delivery system, *Nano Letters*, 5, 2220–2224 (2005).

425. D. Simberg, T. Duza, J. H. Park, M. Essler, J. Pilch, L. Zhang, A. M. Derfus et al., Biomimetic amplification of nanoparticle homing to tumors, *Proceedings of the National Academy of Sciences*, 104, 932–936 (2007).

426. J. Wu and J. M. Sailor, Chitosan hydrogel-capped porous SiO_2 as a pH-responsive nano-valve for triggered release of insulin, *Advanced Functional Materials*, 19, 733–741 (2009).

427. K. Patel, S. Angelos, W. R. Dichtel, A. Coskun, Y. Yang, J. I. Zink, and J. F. Stoddart, Enzyme-responsive snap-top covered silica nanocontainers, *Journal of the American Chemical Society*, 130, 2382–2383 (2008).

428. M. Liong, J. Lu, M. Kovochich, T. Xia, S. G. Ruehm, A. E. Nel, F. Tamanoi, and J. I. Zink, Multifunctional inorganic nanoparticles for imaging, targeting, and drug delivery, *ACS Nano*, 2, 889–896 (2008).

429. J. L. Turner, Z. Chen, and K. L. Wooley, Regiochemical functionalization of a nanoscale cage-like structure: Robust core-shell nanostructures crafted as vessels for selective uptake and release of small and large guests, *Journal of Controlled Release*, 109, 189–202 (2005).

430. K. Berg, P. K. Selbo, L. Prasmickaite, T. E. Tjelle, K. Sandvig, J. Moan, G. Gaudernack et al., Photochemical internalization: A novel technology for delivery of macro-molecules into cytosol, *Cancer Research*, 59, 1180–1183 (1999).

431. M. K. K. Oo, H. Wang, and H. Du, Photosensitiser conjugated gold nanoparticles, *Pharma Focus Asia*, 8, 31–34, 2008, http://www.pharmafocusasia.com/research_development/gold_nanoparticles_targeted_delivery.html

432. J. Lu, E. Choi, F. Tamanoi, and J. I. Zink, Light-activated nanoimpeller-controlled drug release in cancer cells, *Small*, 4, 421–426 (2008).

433. Y. Klichko, M. Liong, E. Choi, S. Angelos, A. E. Nel, J. F. Stoddart, F. Tamanoi, and J. I. Zink, Mesostructured silica for optical functionality, nanomachines, and drug delivery, *Journal of the American Ceramic Society*, 92, S2–S10 (2009).

434. S. Angelos, M. Liong, E. Choi, and J. I. Zink, Mesoporous silicate materials as substrates for molecular machines and drug delivery, *Chemical Engineering Journal*, 137, 4–13 (2008).

435. J. Lu, M. Liong, S. Sherman, T. Xia, M. Kovochich, A. E. Nel, J. I. Zink, and F. Tamanoi, Mesoporous silica nanoparticles for cancer therapy: Energy-dependent cellular uptake and delivery of paclitaxel to cancer cells, *Nano-biotechnology*, 3, 89–95 (2008).

436. W. E. Moerner, A dozen years of single-molecule spectroscopy in physics and chemistry and biophysics, *Journal of Physical Chemistry B*, 106, 910–927 (2002).

437. N. G. Walter, J. C. Meiners, E. Meyhofer, R. R. Neubig, N. C. Perkins, D. G. Steel, R. K. Sunahara, and J. A. Swanson, At the single molecule frontier: Integration in biology and nanotechnology, *Biopolymers*, 85, 106–114 (2007).

438. N. G. Walter, Future of biomedical sciences: Single molecule microscopy, *Biopolymers*, 85, 103–105 (2007).

439. S. Ram, E. S. Ward, and R. J. Ober, Beyond Rayleigh's criterion: A resolution measure with application to single-molecule microscopy, *Proceedings of the National Academy of Sciences*, 103, 4457–4462 (2006).

440. A. E. Cohen and W. E. Moerner, Suppressing Brownian motion of individual biomolecules in solution, *Proceedings of the National Academy of Sciences*, 103, 4362–4365 (2006).

441. S. C. Kuo, Using optics to measure biological forces and mechanics, *Traffic*, 2, 757–763 (2001).

442. X. Gao, L. Yang, J. A. Petros, F. F. Marshall, J. W. Simons, and S. Nie, In vivo molec-ular and cellular imaging with quantum dots, *Current Opinion in Biotechnology*, 16, 63–72 (2005).

443. H. Matoussia, Use of quantum dot-bioconjugates for sensing and probing cellu-lar processes, *Nanomedicine: Nanotechnology, Biology and Medicine*, 2, 282 (2006).

444. A. Hoshino, N. Manabe, K. Fujioka, K. Suzuki, M. Yasuhara, and K. Yamamoto, Use of fluorescent quantum dot bioconjugates for cellular imaging of immune cells, cell organelle labeling, and nanomedicine: Surface modification regulates biological function, including cytotoxicity, *Journal of Artificial Organs*, 10, 149–157 (2007).

445. A. M. Smith, H. Duan, A. M. Mohs, and S. Nie, Bioconjugated quantum dots for in vivo molecular and cellular imaging, *Advanced Drug Delivery Reviews*, 60, 1226–1240 (2008).

446. L. Cognet, C. Tardin, D. Boyer, D. Choquet, P. Tamarat, and B. Lounis, Single metallic nanoparticle imaging for protein detection in cells, *Proceedings of the National Academy of Sciences*, 100, 11350–11355 (2003).

447. M. M. Orosco, C. Pacholski, and M. J. Sailor, Real-time monitoring of enzyme activity in a mesoporous silicon double layer, *Nature Nanotechnology*, 4, 255–258 (2009).

448. M. J. Schulz, Y. Yun, A. Bange, W. R. Heineman, H. B. Halsall, V. N. Shanov, Z. Dong et al., An impedance biosensor based on carbon nanotubes, *Nanomedicine: Nanotechnology, Biology and Medicine*, 2, 280 (2006).

449. D. V. Schaffer and D. A. Lauffenburger, Targeted synthetic gene delivery vectors, *Current Opinion in Molecular Therapeutics*, 2, 155–161 (2000).

450. M. M. Amiji, *Polymeric Gene Delivery: Principles and Applications*, CRC Press, Boca Raton, FL (2004).

451. S. Jin and K. Ye, Nanoparticle-mediated drug delivery and gene therapy, *Biotechnology Progress*, 23, 32–41 (2007).

452. E. N. Gal-Yam, Y. Saito, G. Egger, and P. A. Jones, Cancer epigenetics: Modifications, screening, and therapy, *Annual Review of Medicine*, 59, 267–280 (2008).

453. R. Garzon, G. A. Calin, and C. M. Croce, MicroRNAs in cancer, *Annual Review of Medicine*, 60, 167–179 (2009).

454. F. Krötz, C. de Wit, H.-Y. Sohn, S. Zahler, T. Gloe, U. Pohl, and C. Plank, Magnetofection: A highly efficient tool for antisense oligonucleotide delivery in vitro and in vivo, *Molecular Therapy*, 7, 700–710 (2003).

455. Y. Namiki, T. Namiki, H. Yoshida, Y. Ishii, A. Tsubota, S. Koido, K. Nariai et al., A novel magnetic crystal–lipid nanostructure for magnetically guided in vivo gene delivery, *Nature Nanotechnology*, 4, 598–606 (2009).

456. S. Huth, J. Lausier, S. W. Gersting, C. Rudolph, C. Plank, U. Welsch, and J. Rosenecker, Insights into the mechanism of magnetofection using PEI-based magnetofectins for gene transfer, *The Journal of Gene Medicine*, 6, 923–936 (2004).

457. Z. Yang, G. Sahay, S. Sriadibhatla, and A. V. Kabanov, Amphiphilic block copolymers enhance cellular uptake and nuclear entry of polyplex-delivered DNA, *Bioconjugate Chemistry*, 19, 1987–1994 (2008).

458. Ü. Langel (ed.), *Handbook of Cell Penetrating Peptides*, 2nd edn., CRC Press, Boca Raton, FL, 2007.

459. P. Koch, Z. Kokaia, O. Lindvall, and O. Brüstle, Emerging concepts in neural stem cell research: Autologous repair and cell-based disease modeling, *The Lancet Neurology*, 8, 819–829 (2009).

460. R. I. Mahato (ed.), *Biomaterials for Delivery and Targeting of Proteins and Nucleic Acids*, CRC Press, Boca Raton, FL, 2004.

461. A. Lewis (ed.), *Drug Device Combination Products: Delivery Technologies and Applications*, CRC Press, Boca Raton, FL, 2010.

462. G. Orive, E. Anitua, J. L. Pedraz, and D. F. Emerich, Biomaterials for promoting brain protection, repair and regeneration, *Nature Reviews Neuroscience*, 10, 682–692 (2009).

6

Intervention: Nanotechnology in Reconstructive Intervention and Surgery

> While some may dream of nanorobots circulating in the blood, the immediate applications in medicine will occur at the interfaces among ...nanotechnology, micro-electronics, microelectromechanical systems (MEMS) and microopticalelectro-mechanical systems (MOEMS). ... The bounty will not be realized until those trained in these new paradigms begin to ... address basic medical and scientific questions.
>
> **D.A. LaVan and R. Langer, MIT, NSF Symposium 2001**

6.1 Introduction

We started our discussion of medical nanotechnology in Chapter 5 with nanoparticles and nanomedicines for imaging and drug delivery. In this chapter, we look at medical applications of nanotechnology beyond nanomedicine particles. First, we explore in the direction of greater spatial extension of nanomaterials, to fibers, tubes, networks, films, and 3D scaffolds. Then, as we add increasing complexity to these linear, planar, and solid structures, we can fabricate drug-releasing films and scaffolds, nanodevices, MEMS, smart materials, robotics, and artificial tissues and organs.

In this chapter, we will explore the area of medical nanotechnology that includes those materials, devices, and methodologies whose fabrication and/or action depends in significant ways on nanotechnology. Our purpose in reviewing these medical technologies is to identify the opportunities and challenges for application of the results of nanotechnology to medicine.

6.2 Nanoengineered Materials in Surgical and Restorative Applications

Nanoparticles have a great many medical applications, as we have seen in Chapter 5, for imaging, drug delivery, and tissue engineering. Extension of nanoengineering to the formation of fibers, sheets, and volume-filling materials such as gels, networks, and scaffolds can create many useful constructions and devices for tissue repair and restoration. These materials and devices may range in size up to macroscales, but their properties and fabrication depend on nanoscale features; hence they are referred to as nanomaterials [1–5].

A range of new nanomaterials are useful in surgical and wound healing applications. The science and technology of nanomaterials is continuous with the established body of knowledge on biomaterials engineering; it merely extends that knowledge to take advantage of newly learned properties on the nanoscale [6–14].

Biomaterials are used for the restoration of connective and epithelial tissues, muscle, bone [15–19], and for tissue engineering in restoration of organs such as liver and pancreas [20–22]. Special materials and techniques make up the biomaterials armatorium for repair of skin, connective tissues, and internal organs such as the bladder, blood vessels, and the eye [23–27]. Substances such as polymers, ceramics, glasses, and natural materials can be used as the base materials, with many fabrication techniques [28–33]. For some applications, such as joint replacements, durability and inertness are important; for others such as soft-tissue regeneration, biodegradability is required. A key factor is controlling the interface between the tissue and the implant to provide the optimal environment [34–39]. Nanotechnology gives new tools and techniques for producing a wider range of materials options to meet these needs.

Nanotechnology is employed to design and synthesize novel materials with unique properties of porosity, biodegradability, lightweight, strength, toughness, and biocompatibility for tissue replacement and repair. Nanoengineered materials have proven very useful for making passive implants as tissue replacements for bone and cartilage, because their load-bearing properties, resistance to wear and crack propagation, and surface properties for interfacing to tissue can be controlled to produce high performance based on their nanostructure.

Nanotechnology has contributed to the design of highly versatile surgical glues, connective fibers, webs, and scaffolds for wound healing and surgical interventions in many types of tissue. The nanoscale surface topography of macroscale objects can be engineered to control the degree to which materials are hydrophobic or hydrophilic, adhesive or lubricating, antifouling, anticlotting, promoting of cell growth, supporting of laminar flow in narrow channels, and other properties. Nanofabrication of organic and polymer materials can be used to create materials, which release growth-stimulating substances, antibiotics, and other cell-protecting and cell-promoting molecules by novel mechanisms.

Nanomaterials are especially useful in supportive and bioactive implants, to which cells can attach to form strong connections, or grow into the implant to replace it with new tissue, especially if the material is biodegradable. The most basic type of bioactivity starts with surface properties that are friendly to cell attachment and growth. Surfaces can be nanoengineered to mimic the environment needed by the cells that will replace the damaged or missing tissue, so that growth of new tissue is supported and stimulated. Nanofabrication facilitates the design of materials with external surfaces that are cell-friendly, while maintaining strength and resiliency of the overall structure.

6.3 Bridging the Gap between Drugs and Surgery with Endoscopic MEMS

In Chapter 1, we recalled Feynman's description of the fundamental dilemma facing the task of nanomedicine—it is difficult "because we are too big." The gap between the chemical scale and the microbiological scale is vast, as pointed out in numerous sources in Chapter 5. This gap is being bridged by nanoscience and medical nanotechnology. For medicine at the molecular scale, nanoscience is helping to create and deliver drugs that are more selective and targeted than traditional chemical therapeutics. And from the macroscale downward, nanotechnology is producing materials and devices that extend the ability for precise surgery and tissue engineering, and even for manipulation of subcellular structures and processes.

By bridging the gap between the molecular and anatomical scales, nanotechnology is blurring the distinction between drugs and surgical intervention, as well as between diagnosis and therapy. Extension of the concept of drugs into nanomedicines and nanoparticles is making them more targeted and specific in their therapeutic actions, including precise manipulation of the nanoscale cellular environment—procedures that can be thought of in terms of nanosurgery. Diagnosis and therapy are being merged by combination of sensors, targeting, and image enhancement with therapeutic actions such as drug release, photothermal, or magnetic therapy in a single nanoparticle design.

Another important way in which nanotechnology is affecting surgery is by implementing more powerful miniaturization of electronics, sensors, and electromechanical actuators, which can be used in minimally invasive endoscopic and robotics-assisted surgery systems. These include microelectromechanical systems (MEMS) used to make advanced electromechanical robotics and image-guided controls (mechatronics). Although this is the least direct mode by which nanotechnology contributes to surgery, it is among the first ways in which nanotechnology has made a significant impact. As we review medical technologies, we see that technology is being adopted first where it is most needed to augment existing capabilities for care and healing.

6.3.1 Endoscopy, Endoscopic Surgery, and Natural Orifice Translumenal Endoscopy (NOTES)

Endoscopy is the use of imaging probes for enhanced observation inside a patient's body [40–43]. Endoscopy is used in examination of the gastrointestinal tract [44–46], in urology [47,48], in gynecology [49,50], in otolaryngology [51], and in orthopedics [52]. Endoscopy is also used for examination of the spinal column, but there are still some barriers to widespread clinical use [53–59]. The term endoscopy is sometimes used to include both diagnostic and surgical procedures; modern endoscopic instruments integrate the two functionalities.

Laparoscopic surgery is performed by making small incisions and inserting and manipulating surgical instruments through the openings, without the necessity of cutting an incision large enough for the surgeon's hands or exposing the organs (laparotomy) [60–62]. Endoscopic surgery combines endoscopy with laparoscopic surgery [63]. Historically, laparoscopic surgery originated with fishing for bullets or shrapnel without the aid of imaging or endoscopy. Laparoscopic surgery can be performed today by using x-ray or MRI to guide the surgeon in real time, or by stereotaxy, using images obtained in advance, combined with stereotaxic fixtures to maintain accurate positioning and guidance of the surgical probes.

NOTES is a new approach to endoscopic surgery in which natural orifices are used as entry points for incisions, thus avoiding damage to the skin and/or wall of the abdomen or thorax, and eliminating external surgical scars. NOTES can be performed through internal incisions in the stomach, bladder, vagina, navel, as well as transnasal endoscopic surgery [64,65].

Percutaneous refers to any medical procedure by which access to inner organs or other tissue is obtained via needle puncture of the skin. Laparoscopic surgery is generally performed with the aid of a trocar, a sleeve or tube resembling a large needle which holds the incision open and protects the surrounding tissue from damage due to instrument exchanges and motion. There is some overlap between the use of the terms percutaneous and laparoscopic, and between needles and trocars (for example, the term percutaneous endoscopic gastrostomy, PEG [66]). In recent practice, percutaneous usually refers to access to blood vessels and the spinal column, and laparoscopic refers to access to larger body compartments.

Modern laparoscopic surgical techniques employ sophisticated designs for trocars or surgical sleeves, some with multiple ports or lumens for holding tools, illumination, and endoscopes. Multiple lumen sleeves can reduce the number of incisions required to perform a laparoscopic operation [67].

6.3.1.1 Endoscopic Diagnostic and Surgical Techniques

Advances in miniaturized and flexible imaging have transformed endoscopy from the early dependence on rigid examining tubes that could extend a short distance into the body. Today endoscopes are flexible, small, and can contain multiple ports and tools for imaging with cold light illumination and perform biopsies and surgical procedures. Instruments require less sedation and can reach further and into smaller anatomies [68,69].

The field of minimally invasive surgery has grown because of advances in microelectronics. Each new generation of digital cameras and illumination systems make it possible to probe ever smaller compartments and vessels of the body. New minimally invasive endoscopic surgical and diagnostic techniques can now be used for procedures that formerly required open surgery, reducing traumatic impact and recovery times. These advances depend only indirectly on the nanotechnology that went into development of their instrumentation: they are still macroscopic procedures. In Chapter 7 we look at the interface between nanotechnology and cellular structure and development in detail as applied to tissue regeneration. For now, we survey surgical and related areas impacted by biomedical nanotechnologies.

6.3.1.2 Endoscopic Instrumentation

Over the past two decades, digital cameras based on charged-coupled devices (CCDs) have been advancing in density of sensors while shrinking in power and size requirements. Beginning in the 1990s, advances in microelectronics drove the replacement of fiber optic bundle endoscopes by instruments with CCD video camera chips. Even though fiber bundles with diameters of 4 mm or less can be made with thousands of fibers, technical issues limiting high resolution use include packing density, core-to-core coupling, and fragility of fibers [70,71]. The resolution that can be achieved with fiber optic bundles is in practice much less than the number of fibers. But advances in fiber technology have been useful for improved illumination and phototherapy, coupled with improvements in light emitting diode (LED) devices. These advances, along with improved signal processing and wireless microelectronics, are making it possible to shrink the size and extend the reach of endoscopic diagnostic and surgical instruments [72–75].

The current state of the art in CCD endoscopic instruments includes features such as more than 5 million pixels of image resolution, with high color definition and brightness optimized by digital signal processing, voice activation and device control, and wireless communication with auxiliary displays [76].

Flexible endoscopes with diameters of 5–6 mm are replacing common 9.5 mm scopes for gastrointestinal endoscopy, and pediatric and prototype endoscopes with diameters of 3–4 mm are available [43]. Fiber endoscopes with outer diameters as small as 0.5–1.4 mm have been made for experimental laboratory investigation in spinal examination [53]. Endoscopes with diameters of less than 1 mm have been produced for dental and craniofacial applications [77–79]. Sterilization and exposure to radiation can create problems for endoscopes. Shorter endoscopes can be used with disposable sheaths to minimize sterilization problems [80,81].

Endoscopes are manufactured with lengths up to 110 cm for gastrointestinal use, allowing examination and procedures in the nasopharynx, oropharynx, hypopharynx, esophagus, stomach, and duodenum. Working ports enable biopsy specimens of the mucosal surface to be obtained and surgical procedures to be performed. Smaller diameter endoscopes reduce the need for sedation during diagnostic examination, thus reducing morbidity, time lost from work, and resource demands on personnel and facilities [82,83]. Smaller endoscopes have also permitted upper gastrointestinal endoscopy to become a routine procedure in pediatrics [84,85].

Miniaturized remotely operated tools for endoscopic procedures have been developed for sewing stitches, stapling, band ligation, anastomosis, knot tying, endoscopic mucosal resection, thread cutting, full thickness resection, and gastroplasty for obesity [86]. Cauterization and coagulation by electrosurgery with lasers and gas discharges are well adapted for endoscopic surgery [87].

Advanced endoscopic instruments are manufactured by a number of companies, including Karl Storz Medical, Stryker Instruments, Olympus, Pentax, Sony, Fujimon, Covidien/Autosuture, Fiegert Endotech, ACMI, among others. The instruments designed for different specialized uses are referred to as gastroendoscopes, colonoscopes, and arthoscopes.

6.3.1.3 MEMS (Microelectromechanical Systems) for Endoscopic Imaging and Sensing Modalities

In addition to conventional video imaging, endoscopy can be used with other imaging modalities such as ultrasound, infrared, and multispectral 3D holography. All of these modalities have been made possible and improved in capability and usefulness due to advances in nanotechnology-based MEMS for sensors, transducers, and electronics.

MEMS technologies have extended the functionality of endoscopy beyond visual imaging to infrared and other modalities. For example, in neurosurgery, MEMS for side-viewing IR reflectometry have been developed to aid the registration of probe locations against MRI imagery when performing operations such as destruction of loci in the brain for treatment of Parkinson's disease and epilepsy. Infrared scanning MEMS have been fabricated as prototypes for OCT (optical coherence tomography) tips on endoscopes, which can be used to image layers beneath the surface of the gastrointestinal tract, blood vessels, and other tissues. As nanotechnology delivers smaller and more powerful devices, more types of imaging modalities, sensors, and surgical functions can be made available to endoscopic surgery. Smaller probes will be able to reach into bile ducts, the liver, kidneys, smaller blood vessels, craniofacial recesses, and the vesicles of the brain, by minimally invasive routes that do not involve opening the abdomen or skull.

Endoscopic ultrasound is one of the best established and most widely used endoscopic procedures. Ultrasound sources are normally applied to the exterior of the body, but when the ultrasound probe is small enough to be inserted into, for example, a blood vessel, much more detailed information about the condition of the tissue can be obtained [88–90]. Endoscopic ultrasonography has been found especially useful in imaging of the interior of soft tissue, where x-ray methods can only give shadow images. For this reason, it is the imaging method of choice in detecting, staging, and follow-up for cancers of the pancreas and esophagus [91,92]. Nanoscale devices can vibrate extremely rapidly, and use lasers to energize materials, generating frequencies in the gigahertz range, high enough to produce optoacoustical effects [93–97]. High-frequency ultrasound can be used therapeutically, producing free radicals which can enhance the effect of drugs and produce chemical effects to destroy cancer cells [98,99].

Interest in infrared endoscopy arises because infrared radiation can penetrate tissue and give information about blood oxygenation, temperature, and other physiological and anatomical properties. (This is the basis of pulse oximetry, which uses the absorption of red and infrared light by hemoglobin to measure blood oxygen.) This information can be useful in diagnosing conditions and locating lesions that are beneath the surface of the epithelial layer of, for example, the gastrointestinal tract. Another potential advantage of working in the infrared spectrum is that the tissue emits infrared heat radiation continuously, so passive thermometry imaging should be possible, like that used in night vision systems, eliminating the need for illuminating the field of observation. A third useful aspect of infrared endoscopy is that intense infrared laser light can be used as a microscopic laser scapel. External passive thermal imaging of the skin is used to locate tumors and infections, but thus far no clinical system for infrared endoscopy imaging is available. Several experimental infrared endoscopy systems have been developed, however [100]. One of the challenges for imaging with an infrared system is that the longer wavelengths of infrared are subject to absorption, scattering, and reradiation, limiting the available resolution compared with visible light. Another challenge is producing fiber-optic cable that can transmit infrared without loss or distortion, for use with low levels of ambient light in passive mode. This is another area in which nanotechnology is producing advances, through new methods of fabricating fibers [4].

Active infrared scanning can be used in optical coherence tomography (OCT) to produce images of the subsurface tissues a few cells deep. Nanotechnology can be used to fabricate electrothermal micromirrors for OCT small enough to be attached to the tip of fiber optics for endoscopic use [101].

Even without imaging, infrared spectral measurement with endoscopic instruments can be useful. A system has been developed to measure the absorption and reflectance of infrared wavelengths emitted from a probe used in brain surgery [102–105]. Different parts of the brain, such as white matter, grey matter, and blood vessels have distinguishable patterns of interaction with infrared light, so a simple probe to measure light intensity can be useful for navigating along a straight path planned using MRI or tomography imaging of the brain.

The infrared data is used to verify the location of the probe in the brain by comparing the intensity with that expected based on the previously obtained brain image, ensuring a more accurate localization of the surgical procedure.

This technology has been used in laparoscopic brain surgeries in which a small number of neurons are destroyed in order to eliminate the active source of disorders such as Parkinson's tremors and epileptic seizures.

Three-dimensional holographic endoscopic imaging has the potential to give the surgeon a virtual reality immersion in the anatomy of the patient, including the microanatomical detail. This could improve diagnosis and treatment of conditions where the normal anatomy is complex, or where injury or tumor has led to complex surgical challenges. Nanotechnology has enabled fabrication of MEMS holography light systems small enough for endoscopy [106]. MEMS holography systems can also be used to image and measure individual cells for pathology and diagnostic purposes [107].

6.3.2 Access by Catheters: Nanotechnology Impacts

A catheter is any small tube that is inserted into the body for medical purposes, such as to provide a route for drainage from a blocked cavity. Catheters are used in trauma and urological procedures, where prevention of infection is a primary concern. Antimicrobial silver nanoparticle coatings have recently been developed to prevent introduction of infection in catheters. The silver nanoparticles are produced by a proprietary process and do not require a binder, since the nanoparticles adhere to the catheter material by means of surface forces [108].

Catheters can also be used for diagnostic and treatment procedures as probes and carriers for very small surgical and imaging instruments. The Swan–Ganz catheter is inserted into the pulmonary artery to monitor critical heart functions, for example. Instruments and procedures have been developed for insertion of catheters into blood vessels and the heart, where they can deliver imaging enhancement agents, drugs, or electrical stimulation. Vascular catheters can also be tipped with ablative tools, balloons, or stents to clear blocked vessels. Miniaturization of transducers has made possible catheters equipped to deliver laser, radiofrequency, or ultrasonic ablative energy to remove plaques, clots, or other obstructions [109–112].

Percutaneous procedures are widely used in cardiac catheterization, where they can be monitored by x-ray imaging in real time for angiography (imaging of the blood vessels). Coronary angioplasty, in which arteries are cleared of obstructions, and insertion of stents to keep arteries from re-closing (restenosis) are two of the most common medical procedures performed in the United States. By using the minimially invasive catheterization procedures, access to the heart and its blood vessels and chambers can be attained without surgery.

Although digital imaging for guiding and analyzing cardiac angiography was available from the 1970s, it was not widely accepted for use until advances in image quality and processing speed met the clinical needs by the mid-1990s [113]. Before that time, digital technologies could not come close to the performance of analog x-ray film in order to capture, display, and store images of the beating heart with sufficient speed, artifact-free detail, and resolution for observation and diagnosis of fine arterial details [114]. Real-time guidance of the angiography procedure was available on video monitors, but the cardiologist had to wait for developed film to see crucial details, resulting in delays and sometimes requiring a second session.

Availability of clinical quality digital images of the moving heart brought great advantages in efficiency of obtaining, analyzing, and reviewing cardiac angiography. This is another area in which nanotechnology-based advances in electronics, computers, and sensors has made an indirect but significant impact on medicine [115,116].

In the meantime, computational and sensor scanning advances have enabled high-resolution magnetic resonance and x-ray computer tomography images of the heart by noninvasive procedures, reducing the need even for minimally invasive cardiac catheterization for angiography [117,118]. Such is the pace of advances in the performance of digital technology that what seemed an enormous challenge can become routine with the passage of just a few years.

Cardiac catheters can be inserted percutaneously into any of several major arteries (usually entering at the leg or arm) and pushed with sheaths and guidewires to reach the heart. Catheters are manufactured in diameters from 0.4 mm to more that 2 mm and are inserted into blood vessels through a special hypodermic needle or access port. Using multiple wires and mechanical linkages to exert differential tension, the tips of catheters can be controlled from the far end to bend, rotate, and thus be steered through curved passages in the vasculature. The manipulation and guidance of a catheter in this manner is a surgical skill that must be learned with practice. The fabrication and manufacture of catheters and steering linkages capable of being threaded smoothly through small diameter guide sheaths over a distance on the order of 1 m requires materials with special properties, another area where nanotechnology fabrication is contributing.

Endoscopes used in gastrointestinal and other procedures contain ports through which catheters can be threaded for access to tissues in the viewing field. The catheters can be tipped with transducers or surgical tools for biopsies or other procedures. Gallstones or the gallbladder can be removed endoscopically by this technique.

6.3.3 Techniques for Cerebrospinal Navigation and Endoscopy

Endoscopic surgery has been used experimentally and clinically for a number of interventions in the spinal column [53–58,119–122]. In addition, procedures have been developed for insertion of small-diameter catheters and endoscopes into the cerebrospinal column at the base of the spine, and for traversal up the spinal column into the base of the brain and the cerebral ventricles [123–126]. This technique is also being used experimentally to gain access to the interior of the skull and brain to perform endoscopic surgical procedures in the brain, pituitary, etc. If this technique, called percutaneous intraspinal navigation (PIN), can be developed into a proven safe surgical route, it would eliminate the need in many cases for open skull surgery or drilling through the skull to perform brain surgery or cerebral shunts for treatment of hydrocephalus. It would provide a much less traumatic access route than is currently available for diagnostic and surgical access to the interior of the skull for many other types of procedures.

6.4 Robotics in Surgery: The Technology

Endoscopy combined with advanced controls has made it feasible to perform surgeries with robotic aids [127–131]. Robotic surgery is not based on nanoscale robots circulating in the body, but on augmenting the capabilities of the surgeon with advanced nanotechnology-based sensors, imaging, navigation, and actuators. The advances being made in robotic-assisted surgery, telerobotic surgery, and autonomous robotic surgery would not be possible without the huge gains made in solid-state electronics and sensor technology, which are tied to advances in nanotechnology. Surgical robotics in its present state of the art is not itself nanotechnology, but it is made possible by underlying nano-technologies that go into the development of its control, actuation, sensing, and communication capabilities, which continue to expand at a rapid pace.

As important as sensors and actuators are the spatial navigation systems and user interfaces, based on integration of advanced computer processors, software, graphics displays, and interactive devices which enable the surgeon to accurately visualize, plan, and direct the movement of surgical tools in the body. In some areas, such as precise machining of receptacle spaces in bone for implants, robotic surgery has been found useful in autonomous modes of operation, once guided to position by the surgeon.

There are some advances being made in surgical robotics based on unte-thered automated surgical tools positioned and actuated by wireless radio-frequency or magnetic controls, but first we look at systems with laparoscopic and endoscopic tools, connected and integrated into a control interface so as to perform like an enhanced extension of the surgeon's eyes and hands.

Examples of robotic surgery systems include, among others, the following:

1. The da Vinci, a widely used robotic surgical system, produced by Intuitive Surgical Incorporated with three or four arms for laparo-scopic surgery [132,133].
2. The ZEUS system, integrated with the AESOP voice-controlled endo-scopic camera and the HERMES platform for manipulating multiple instruments under voice control (Its developer, Computer Motion,

merged with Intuitive in 2003, and the ZEUS is superseded by the da Vinci system) [134–136].

3. The NeuroArm system developed at the University of Calgary (Advances include usability in MRI environments) [137].

4. The Laprotek system produced by endoVia Medical, Inc. of Norwood, Massachusetts [138].

5. The TraumaPOD, an advanced medical telerobot developed for military medicine sponsored by the United States Defense Department [139].

6. The PathFinder (Prosurgics, United Kingdom), a robotic arm with six degrees of freedom designed to assist stereotaxic surgery [140].

7. The Stereotaxis, Inc. Niobe electrophysiology magnetic guidance catheter system, integrated with the Webster Biosense and the Siemens AXIOM Artis navigation systems (which, unlike the previous examples, guides catheter tips rather than laparoscopic instruments) [141–143].

8. Catheter Robotics for remote guidance of conventional catheters (tested at the University of chicago and used for atrial surgery at Leicester University and Glenfield Hospital Leicester, U.K.) [144].

9. The Hansen Sensei system, which enables surgeons to guide special catheter tips (Artisan Extend catheters) mechanically from an ergonomic console, out of the x-ray imaging field, with navigation visualization [145].

10. The VikY system, a small and easily deployable robotic holder for endoscopic surgery developed at CHU de Grenoble [146].

11. The ARTEMIS system developed by the Eberhard Karls University, Tübingen [147].

12. The TransPort endoscopic platform with ShapeLock locking over-tube, with grasping tools for endoscopic surgery, developed by USGI Medical, San Capistrano, California [148].

In addition to the above systems, a number of other systems have been developed for robotic surgery, both by companies and research institutions [148–153].

The advantages of robotic-assisted and robotic surgery include

1. Minimally invasive surgery with smaller and fewer incisions, resulting in less pain and scarring and faster recovery (For example, a typical cardiac bypass procedure can be performed with three incisions of about 1 cm each with robotics, compared with a 30 cm incision that requires distension of the rib cage for a conventional procedure.).

2. Extremely precise and accurate movements, free of tremor, flinch, fatigue, or lapse, and the ability to deal with microscopic and/or convoluted

anatomies that are difficult to reach, visualize, and manipulate with the unaided human eye and hand.

3. Robotic systems can provide the surgeon operating positions that are ergonomically superior to those required by traditional laparoscopy or open surgery. The surgeon's fingers can be connected, in a virtual manner, directly to the tips of the surgical instruments' jaws, instead of manipulating them with handles on the opposite sides of hinges or shanks. This direct virtual connection provides for maximum control and dexterity with seven full degrees of freedom in motion. This is a significant advantage, especially in minimally invasive laparoscopic surgery, where the hands would otherwise have to manipulate instruments from outside of the body. Software interfaces are developed to make tip movement intuitive and true to the surgeon's intentions, and ensure that the surgeon's orientation is never lost.

4. Ability to track and compensate for patient's body and organ movement.

5. Shorter procedure times, with less blood loss (and less radiation exposure in the case of fluoroscopy guided procedures).

6. Improved work flow and utilization of operating room and staff resources.

7. Ability to perform simulated operations with visualizations for training and procedure planning.

8. Ability in special circumstances to perform operations remotely (telerobotic surgery), extending surgical experience and skill to remote or dangerous locations (telepresence).

Areas that are actively being pursued for further improvements and development include

1. Advanced 3D visualization and navigation.

2. Improved automated instrument collision avoidance.

3. Improved tracking and adaptation of tissue and organ movement.

4. Improvements in user interfaces, including haptics and live endoscopic imaging at the instrument working areas.

5. Greater variety of imaging and surgical tools on the robotic arms, including MEMS for in-depth tissue imaging and procedures.

6. Ability for microelectronic imaging and actuator components to work in radiation and magnetic fields with longer device lifetimes and less interference, for enhanced real-time imaging and visualization with minimal radiation exposure.

7. Generally greater precision, accuracy, reliability, speed, and safety of procedures. The use of robotics in a human environment, with

intimate contact and harmful, even fatal consequences of failure presents the greatest possible challenge to engineers and designers. Nanotechnology and the advances in electronics and sensors which are constantly progressing are making it possible and economical to implement redundancy and deep design and control strategies to help minimize flaws and adverse outcomes.

8. Lowering costs, including costs of setup and training time.

9. Development of ability to work within the MRI imaging field environment [154,155]. Two challenges are confined space and high magnetic fields within the imaging [156]. Researchers at Johns Hopkins have developed an MRI-compatible robotics system (ACUBOT) using pneumatic actuators for MRI compatibility [157]. Researchers at Kyushu University in Japan have also developed an MRI-guided laparoscopic and robotic surgery system with an MRI-compatible endoscope [158].

6.4.1 The Human Interface

Robotic mechatronics increases precision and speed, but at the cost of imposing physical separation between surgeon and patient. Reconnecting visuomotor sensory feedback is essential for safe and effective use of surgical robotics, and for improved performance and acceptance by surgeons [159]. Achieving improved human interfaces for optimal surgical performance and safety demands the best technologies in ergonomics, haptics, and imaging systems.

6.4.2 Ergonomics

A basic but important advantage of robotics in surgery is the increased potential for ergonomic modes in performing the challenging work of surgery. Surgeons are able to sit at an ergonomic console rather than stand for long operations. Not only can delicate movements be performed precisely by the robotics, but their initiation and control can be executed with optimal hand positions and arm support. Optimal performance of demanding tasks can be maintained and improved with the aid of ergonomically designed actuator controls, unconstrained by the necessity of reaching into the patient's anatomy [160–162].

6.4.3 Haptics

Adding haptic feedback is one of the challenging priorities for development in surgical robotics. At present, most commercially available robotic surgical systems lack this capability. To fill this gap, a number of projects have added force sensors to existing surgical robots to provide sensory force feedback [163,164]. Other developments are studying needs and benefits to determine desirable approaches to robotic surgical haptics and build systems that include sensory force feedback in the design [165,166].

6.4.4 Immersive Imaging Systems and Augmented Environments

One of the critical elements of surgical robotics is the imaging environment. Much work has been done to supplement the mechanical aspects of surgical robots with platforms for augmented human interaction for the surgeon. Computer displays give the ability to view the surgical field from many angles without the restrictions of confined spaces and limited field of view. These systems give the user the sense of immersion in the work environment with freedom to explore and assess at selected magnifications and illuminations [167].

Computer-aided imaging systems provide image fusion and overlay, position tracking, and metrology capability to improve the precision and accuracy of minimally invasive surgery. Other important capabilities provided by the user interface are 3D feedback of spatial position of surgical targets, and predictive ability to guide laparoscopic dissection along the ideal surgical plane, with built-in safety checks and balances. An example is the European EndoCAS (Endoscopic Computer Aided Surgery) project [168].

The most sophisticated and advanced techniques in human factors engineering are being applied to bridge the separation between surgeon and patient. For example, in the Royal Society Wolfson Medical Image Computing Laboratory at Imperial College London, a system is been developed based on a novel gaze contingent framework with real-time haptic feedback to transform visual sensory information into physical constraints that interact with motor sensory channels. Motor tracking of deforming tissue can be made more effective and accurate through the use of gaze-contingent motor channeling. The method also uses dynamic tracking of 3D eye gaze to prescribe and update safety boundaries during robotic-assisted surgery without requiring prior knowledge of the soft-tissue morphology. This technique has been validated on simulated and robotic-assisted phantom procedures to demonstrate its valuable clinical potential [169].

Continuing system developments of this type to enhance soft-tissue navigation are needed for progression of surgical robotic systems from experimental use into standard clinical practice. At present, widely available abdominal navigation systems are still considered too imperfect for daily surgical routine in many cases [170]. To meet these needs for improved predictive surgical navigation, developers are calling on the latest techniques in augmented reality from areas such as aircraft piloting simulators and computer gaming [171].

6.4.5 Virtual Reality Simulators for Training and Planning

Another augmentation possible with surgical robotics is the ability to simulate operations for training and planning [172–175]. Skills can be learned, sharpened, and evaluated with accurate and objective feedback. New strategies and approaches can be tried out in simulation before going to animal, cadaver, or human trials [176,177]. Sophisticated and realistic simulators enable the study and evaluation of cognitive ergonomic factors such as task workload, sensory overload, and distraction without going into the operating room [178–180]. Simulators can record details of movements and timing to comparatively evaluate ergonomic and technical effects. All of these capabilities would be much more difficult or impossible without the power of computer simulation with visuomotor feedback.

6.4.6 Telerobotics and Telesurgery

Telerobotics is the ability to manipulate the robot from a distance. Much surgical robotics can be described as telerobotic in the sense that surgery is performed from a control console rather than directly over the patient. This capability can be extended to remote distances with advanced high-speed communications for real-time control, imaging, and feedback. The concept of remote telerobotics is being developed and evaluated for extension of skilled medical and surgical care, training, and mentoring across distances to places where resources are not available or to dangerous locations such as conflict zones or disaster areas [181–186].

6.4.7 Critiques of Surgical Robotics and Technical Barriers to Be Overcome

Robotic surgery has been adopted relatively rapidly for such a revolutionary medical technology, but it is by no means universal. A number of medical, technical, and economic barriers to its use still exist despite continuing rapid development and improvements. Any new medical technology will not become adopted as standard practice until its benefits, safety, and efficacy have been well established—this is something that must be kept in mind for all nanotechnology-related technologies applied to medicine. Medical professional bodies and regulatory agencies are monitoring and setting guidelines to ensure that robotic surgery systems provide real benefits and are safe and efficacious. Where there is enthusiasm for new technologies, it must be moderated by cautious evaluation.

Feedback from practitioners is invaluable in the development of any new medical technology to guide improvements and new developments. The feedback thus far from many published evaluations of individual systems and surgical robotics in general is still mixed. The first question for any new technology is whether it is really an advance—do the risks outweigh any benefits? The second is whether it is justifiable economically— do the benefits outweigh the risks and costs? Numerous evaluations agree on the benefits of the currently available surgical robotic systems as having improved ergonomics, elimination of tremor, 3D vision, more degrees of freedom with lesser fulcrum effect, and greater accuracy and speed for many if not all operation procedures. Any remaining concerns can only be addressed by long-term feasibility and efficacy studies. The time and cost of such evaluations is complicated by the many different procedures, specialties, and agencies involved [152–153,186–188].

Cost is a recurring negative factor in most environments: initial investment as well as training and operating expenses, although actual published number in studies show only slightly higher costs for most procedures and lower costs for some, as will be seen by reviewing evaluations for specific types of operations.

Initial costs for complete robotic surgical instrumentation can run near $1 million, prohibitive for many hospital systems. The long-term trend of lower costs for computers and electronics will tend to lower this investment, but it may be offset by increasing features and capabilities in controls, haptics, and software. Potential future upgrades and compatibility with existing tools and equipment and with systems from other manufacturers is a concern, which may need to be addressed by development of standards. At present, lack of certain special tools compatible with the robotic arms can require human assistants to perform parts of the surgery.

Costs of integration of the present generation of robotic systems includes more than the price tag for the instrumentation. Some of the machines are large, and space for movement of the robotic arms must be allowed in already crowded operating rooms. This is a problem that will be addressed by further miniaturization of robotic arms made possible by improved actuators, and in any case it will gradually be accommodated by newly designed and constructed operating rooms if robotics gains general adoption. But it is an initial barrier to adoption that is significant.

The need for changes to operating procedures and training are also cited as barriers. These are acknowledged as transitory. But in today's environment, improvements in costs are needed for more rapid widespread adoption.

Technical barriers are most readily overcome. Critiques of early versions of robotic systems included that they lacked haptic feedback, had too few arms, and the instrument diameters were too large. Other problems included external collisions in the robotic devices and visual disparity in multiple planes. All of these technical issues are being dealt with in new versions and releases of the systems [187,188].

A potentially more fundamental problem is the challenge of dealing with unexpected bleeding, leading to the possible necessity of conversion of the operation to a more invasive surgery in mid-procedure. This can be a problem in any laparoscopic procedure, but recognition of the problem and conversion for a robotic procedure can be more involved and take more time, increasing risk to the patient.

Advances based on nanotechnology, like any technological progressions, have a way of breaking through and leapfrogging obstacles. Before describing some new technologies that may supersede current concepts of surgical robotics, we should briefly review where the technology is currently being used in medical practice, with some of its advantages and challenges.

Feedback and evaluation of experience with medical technology tends to be very focused on specific procedures and practices, so we include reviews for a number of surgical specialties.

6.5 Robotics in Surgical Practice

Robotics are being used and/or evaluated in almost every type of internal surgery. Their use has been pioneered in fields where laparoscopic surgery has been widely used, such as urological, gastrointestinal, and esophageal surgeries and they have been evaluated and used in many other procedures [189,190], from adrenalectomy to varicocelectomy. Robotic surgery is impacting clinical practice in general surgery [191,192], and specialist training for perioperative robotics nursing is being proposed [193]. Robotics for catheter manipulation has also been very widely adopted in cardiology, as well as laparoscopic robotics for some heart and thoracic surgeries. We start with the most widely used procedures and review highlights of robotic surgery evaluations and experience.

This overview of medical application areas is meant to illustrate how newly available technologies, which are the fruits of nanoscience advances, are being applied in a pragmatic, needs-driven way to different medical specialties with different challenges. Some medical areas such as ocular and vascular surgeries need the tremor-free micro-precision of miniaturized robotics; others such as bone surgery need the combination available in robotics of high strength with high precision. For many parts of the body, access for delicate and precise procedures without invasive open surgery is provided by small and dextrous laparoscopic robotic instrumentation. In these and other cases, the need is not only to extend the hands of the surgeon, but also the eyes and visualization; in these areas high-fidelity endoscopy probes offer guidance. With complex soft tissues such as the liver, navigation, and virtual reality based on accurate models of the internal structures of the organ are critical augmentations. The body and its disorders are varied and complex, presenting many grand challenges to medicine. The role of technology is to augment the ability to respond to those challenges.

6.5.1 Surgical Robotics in Cardiology and Cardiothoracic Surgery

Surgical robotics, especially magnetic telerobotic control of catheter tips, has made a significant impact on cardiothoracic surgery and catheterization procedures for cardiovascular surgery [194–196]. Remote image-guided magnetic catheter guidance systems have been used for mapping and ablative surgery to treat atrial fibrillation [196] and tachycardia conditions [197–200]. Robotic-assisted catheter surgery has been used extensively for mitral valve repair [201–203]. Robotic catheter guidance has been employed in minimally invasive surgery for coronary artery stenoses [204] and to facilitate navigation in septal ablation for hypertrophic obstructive cardiomyopathy [205], a condition in which the heart muscle thickens, associated with sudden cardiac death syndrome.

A particularly interesting development is the use of robotic magnetic navigation with echocardiology to guide catheter ablation of atrial fibrillation, without the use of x-ray fluoroscopy [206]. Guidance of a catheter without the aid of magnetic navigation requires the fine definition and high-resolution images provided by x-rays; the demonstration that this procedure can be done with magnetic navigation using only sonography imaging could lead to similar surgeries with no exposures to ionizing radiation and lower costs.

Cardiac catheterization procedures approach the interior of the heart through major blood vessels. Other minimally invasive approaches have been developed using endoscopic robotics for closed chest access to the outer vessels of the heart, for coronary artery bypass operations [207–211]. These procedures have been performed with closed chest perfusion of the arrested heart, as well as on the beating heart [212–214]. Closed chest surgery is much less traumatic than open chest procedures which involve extensive rib spreading, so recovery is more rapid and less painful. A compromise between straight percutaneous laparoscopic access and open chest surgery with rib spreading has been developed, involving a small thoracic incision (thoracotomy) without rib spreading [215]. With the aid of surgical robotics, the small incision can be used to harvest internal mammary arteries and graft them onto the heart for some bypass procedures. In general, recovery and long-term outcomes have been found to be good for all types of robotically aided heart bypass surgeries [207–211,216,217].

6.5.2 Tracking the Beating Heart

Robotic tracking and compensation for the movement of a beating heart can be considered a grand challenge for robotics, one which has been largely met in recent years, even though there will always be room for improvement. This has been due to increasingly sophisticated mathematical and adaptive control strategies for robotic tracking and movement [218–220]. The implementation of these advanced algorithms in real time is dependent on nanotechnology-based advances in faster computing and control electronics, sensors, and actuators. As these capabilities continue to develop, there is a rich trove of control theory available for application to track the movement of the heart, the eye, and other body systems for surgery and other therapies and diagnostics [221–226].

It is a matter of differing opinions among experts whether it is better to arrest the heart, thus lowering oxygen demand while perfusing the heart muscle to maintain circulation, or to perform surgery on the beating heart. In either case, the availability of less traumatic route to perform more significant surgical procedures on the heart will increase availability and access to surgeries that can counter the impact of coronary disease on quality of life, by lowering risks and costs.

6.5.3 Electrophysiology

In addition to heart surgery, robotic navigation is beginning to be adopted for guiding catheters in electrophysiology procedures, which are used to measure or stimulate the cardiac rhythms, as well as for spinal and vascular procedures [227].

6.5.4 Neurology and Neurosurgery

Robotics was adopted early for neurosurgery to aid in guiding stereotaxic procedures for brain surgery and other neurosurgical areas. Use of laparoscopic robotic arms has been more limited in neurosurgery compared to stereotaxic navigation aids, due to the precision required and the complexity and vital functions of the embedded and surrounding anatomy in the surgical field [228,229].

In brain surgery in particular, care must be taken to avoid collateral damage. Unnecessary exposure of brain area must be avoided if possible; localization must be precise and accurate. Stereotaxic frames used for fixation in brain surgery typically have an accuracy within 2 mm. Frame-based targeting methods can lead to greater inaccuracy in patients with movement disorders [230]. For neurosurgical robotics an accuracy of 2 mm or better is needed, comparable to what is achievable with fixation frames, and within the range of resolution of CT and MR images on which navigation is based, and for targeting specific brain structures.

6.5.5 Head and Neck Surgery and Otorhinolaryngology

Skull base surgery and transnasal approaches are relevant to both neurosurgery and otolaryngology. The endonasal route has been adopted as a useful approach for transsphenoidal surgery targeting the pituitary. An image-guided robotics system for skull base access has been developed at the University of Erlangen-Nuremberg and tested experimentally with a reproducible navigation accuracy of 1.53 mm, based on redundant navigational controls. The system was designed for use in skull base surgery using telemanipulation as well as automated image-guided procedures. Tests in which sphenoidotomies were successfully performed were conducted on cadaveric heads [231].

The use of robotic surgery improves the precision of procedures, offering surgeons a more comfortable working position, particularly for longer procedures, without the need for an assistant to hold the camera. The AESOP robotic surgery system was found to be a good system as a microscope positioning and navigation system for skull base surgery targeting the sella (on the sphenoid bone at the base of the skull) [232]. The learning curve for the system was short, and the positioning was stable and accurate. A useful feature in this case was the ability to save up to three operating positions, enabling the system to return to a previous location with a single voice command. Elimination of tremor reduced collisions, and having a stable microscope holder allowed the surgeon to use both hands for the actual procedure. Another advantage noted was that the system had a small footprint, taking up little space in the operating room. Tests on cadaver heads were done in which a single neurosurgeon was able to maneuver the endoscope, visualize key anatomical features in the sphenoid, and resect skull base lesions after the approach was made by an otolaryngologist, without needing an assistant to position the microscope.

The AESOP system has also been found useful for endoscopic laryngosurgery. Various standard rigid endolaryngeal telescopes can be attached to the robotic arm for video-assisted surgery. The system was found to be particularly useful for patients with difficult laryngeal exposure [233].

In other otolaryngology applications, the da Vinci robotic surgery system has been evaluated and reported with good results on a new surgical technique for transoral radical tonsillectomy [234], and for upper aerodigestive tract neoplasms [235].

Robotic surgery is beginning to be evaluated and used in ear surgery [236]. Experimental robots have been built and evaluated for milling cavities for implants, and robotic systems to aid cochlear implant surgery have been developed and used [237,238].

6.5.6 Ophthalmology

In ophthalmic surgery, the surgeon has direct visualization of the structures of most ocular sites through the cornea; therefore one of the main advantages of laparoscopic robotic surgery—endoscopic imaging—is not applicable to most eye surgeries. Ophthalmic surgery requires precise and accurate manipulation of microsurgical instrumentation—an area in which robotics excels. Robotic surgical instrumentation can be valuable in eye surgery by removing tremor, providing remote access to subspeciality training and mentoring, and in surgical training and planning through simulation. At present, precision of commercially available robots is on the order of 1 mm. For many ophthalmologic surgeries, accuracy on the order of microns will be required. Thus there is room for technological advances based on improved nanotechnologies [239–241].

6.5.7 Oral and Maxillofacial Surgery

In surgery of the face and upper jaw, robotics is being used for planning in orthognathic surgeries to correct deformations of the face and jaw [242,243]. Robotic metrology systems can rapidly and accurately determine biometrics and aid in evaluation of orthognathic changes through surgery modeling in the planning stages. Active robotics is also being used experimentally for more invasive types of maxillofacial surgery [244].

An area closely related to surgery in maxillofacial medicine is oral rehabilitation. Researchers in Japan have designed and built a robot to provide massage to the facial tissues in therapy for conditions such as temperomandibular joint disorder (at the junction of the jaw and skull) and dry mouth (due to lowered activity of saliva glands). The computer controlled robot can automatically generate massage trajectories and delivers massage to the masseter and temporal muscles and to the parotid gland and duct. It has 2 six degree-of-freedom arms with virtual compliance control. Experimental evaluation has been reported [245].

Computer-assisted systems for planning and performing dental implants have also been developed [246].

6.5.8 Orthodontics

Orthodontics, like facial orthognathics, requires precise and careful measurements and planning to be successful. With the aid of computer-aided measurement, fixtures and braces can be custom generated to fit the patient's measurements, and to exert therapeutic forces according to a pre-evaluated plan that can be simulated based on computer-aided force calculations and automated design and fabrication. Several companies now offer computer-aided systems for lingual orthodontics, including computer-aided 3D measurement and simulation of the patient's dental anatomy, forming a digital model which can be examined, manipulated, and used to automatically manufacture fixtures [247–253]. This is an application of computer-aided metrology, design, and fabrication, which translates directly from industrial to medical use, with corresponding improvements in accuracy and productivity.

6.5.9 Craniofacial Surgery

High levels of precision, skill, and experience are necessary in order to perform maxillofacial interventions successfully. Craniofacial surgery can require complex bone cut trajectories, which require distinct and precise orientations of cutting and milling instruments. Exact bone cuts are needed in reconstructive procedures for bone repositioning in the human skull [254].

Robotic systems can aid the surgeon by generation of preoperative plans using 3D computer models of the patient's skull. Precise location and repositioning capabilities are required of the robotic system for craniofacial surgery. To implement complex multiphase surgical plans, robotic surgery systems must have the flexibility to allow for changes in the patient's position during interoperative phases, integrated with computer models and imaging for referencing and registration of the position and orientation of the patient.

Thus, design and implementation of robotic systems for craniofacial surgery is a complex task that must be approached by integrating the system into the surgical workflow [255–257].

As in all surgeries, the prime concern has to be safety for the human patients and caregivers. With surgery on the face, special care must be given to accuracy and avoidance of undesired and unnecessary interventions, because of the special role that the human face has in personal identity and social communication.

6.5.10 Plastic and Reconstructive Surgery

Reconstructive surgery in particular can involve complex tasks that must be done with the aid of surgical microscopes, such as reconnection of very small nerves and blood vessels (microvascular anastomosis). Researchers at Johns Hopkins have reported experimental use of surgical robotics for performing microvascular anastomoses in animal models, as an alternative to manual instruments under surgical microscopes [258].

Use of surgical robotics is also becoming adopted for microsurgical procedures in plastic surgery, primarily to avoid tremor and irregular hand motion in delicate tasks where minimization of scarring is important, and also for reducing procedure times, training, planning, and remote telementoring [259,260].

6.5.11 Orthopedic Surgery

Robotics in orthopedic surgery is used for accurate cutting, drilling, and milling of cavities to receive implants [261]. Orthopedic surgery requires accurate registration using fiducial markers (metal pins) or points on the surface of the bone. Since the bone can be treated as a fixed object, computer control of robotic surgery is simplified. The surgeon has to connect the robot to the bone and expose the bone for access and secure fixation of the robot to the bone, requiring careful soft-tissue management [262,263]. Computer-assisted and robotic surgery aids these tasks to produce greater spatial accuracy and more reliable and reproducible outcomes. The ability of robots to combine high precision with strong forces is especially appropriate for surgery involving large structural bone tissues. Computer-assisted orthopedic surgery can assist non-robotic surgery for guidance and planning; however, robot-assisted orthopedic surgery can achieve levels of accuracy, precision, and safety not capable with computer assistance alone [264].

Orthopedic surgery was an early area for development of robotics, starting with the ROBODOC collaborative project begun in 1986 between IBM's Thomas J. Watson Research Center and researchers at the University of California, Davis. The ROBODOC robotic surgery system has been in use in Europe since 1994, and in 2008 it received U.S. FDA 510K clearance for total hip arthroplasty procedures [265,266].

Another commercially available system developed for orthopedic robotic surgery is the Acrobot, which has been successfully used in total knee replacement surgery [267,268]. Other systems that have been used for knee replacement surgery include the CASPAR system developed and used in Europe [269,270].

One of the most valuable aspects of computer and robotic-assisted systems for orthopedics is the ability to map and plan the operation with 3D visualization [271–274]. These systems have also been used for navigation in placement of implants for the spine, in rotator cuff surgery (shoulder arthroscopy) and repair of ligaments in the knee (anterior cruciate ligament) [272–274].

6.5.12 Gastrointestinal

In gastrointestinal surgery practice, robotic-assisted laparoscopic surgery has been generally reported as safe and efficacious. Specific advantages compared with conventional laparoscopic operations are not marked, but advantages that are recognized are surgical simulations and augmented-reality surgery to aid in deep tissue visualization and navigation [275]. Evaluations and clinical experiences that have been reported include gastric bypass [276,277], surgical repair of "upside down stomach," a condition in which hiatal and paraesophageal hernias may displace the stomach in the thoracic cavity [278,279], and surgical treatment for gastroesophageal reflux disease and/or obesity [279–282].

For the comparatively less complicated gastric bypass [283], an evaluation found that use of a commercial robotic surgical system was a superior alternative to the standard laparoscopic procedure, and had a faster learning curve, although total costs were about 15% higher [276].

Antireflux surgery usually involves fundoplication, in which a portion of the stomach is pulled up and attached around the base of the esophagus to support a weakened lower esophageal spinchter [279–282]. A number of evaluations have reported that robotic-assisted fundoplication is comparable to the standard laparoscopic procedure in terms of feasibility and outcome, but operating times are longer and costs are higher. Some surgeons found the robotic procedure superior despite longer operating times, but the disadvantages that were generally cited were the time needed for training and the need for exact trocar positioning to accommodate robotic arms. The main disadvantage, cited as preventing robotic surgery becoming the standard for these types of operation, was high cost.

6.5.13 Hernia

A pilot study has been conducted for robotic-assisted laparoscopic mesh repair of incisional hernias with exclusive intracorporeal suturing in 11 human patients with no conversions to open surgery and no mortality [284]. In this one reported study of using robot-assisted mesh fixation, the technique was shown to be feasible, with absence of chronic postoperative pain. Further randomized studies would be required to assess the benefits.

6.5.14 Gallbladder: Cholecystectomy

In 2001, cholecystectomy—surgical removal of the gallbladder—was chosen to successfully demonstrate and evaluate the first transoceanic telesurgery. The operation was successfully performed across the Atlantic on a pig [285]. Since then, a number of other robotic surgical innovations have been first evaluated with cholecystectomy, a procedure that is usually performed by general surgeons as an outpatient procedure, using conventional laparoscopic instrumentation. The traditional approach commonly requires the use of four separate small incisions, but trails are being conducted to evaluate NOTES and single-incision cholecystectomy [286].

In evaluations reported from Korea, Europe, and North America, robotic-assisted gallbladder surgery has been found to be reliable and safe, but not justifiable in terms of operating room resources [287–290]. In Canada, the chief value was considered to be for training and allowing inexperienced surgeons to gain confidence in performing robotic procedures. A meta study in 2009 reviewed a large database to compare the safety of robot assist versus human assistants in laparoscopic cholecystectomy and to assess whether the robot can substitute for the human assistant, concluding that although robot-assisted laparoscopic cholecystectomy appears safe, there are no significant advantages over human-assisted laparoscopic cholecystectomy [291].

6.5.15 Liver Surgery

Laparoscopic surgery on the liver has remained an experimental procedure until the first decade of the 2000s, with techniques for dealing with bleeding still being developed for this highly vascularized organ [292]. Recent progress with improved methods of vascular clamping, navigation, and reconstruction has been rapid [293–302], and the first experiences with robotic laparoscopic surgery of the liver have started to be reported [303–305].

Relatively few cases have been published on robotic-assisted liver surgery, but the results are promising. In the first case in Latin America, a 72 year-old male with cryptogenic liver cirrhosis and hepatocellular carcinoma had a 2.2 cm tumor with decreased liver size and signs of portal hypertension. Robotic surgery via five trocars was used to transect the liver, remove the tumor, and apply interrupted stitches for hemostasis of raw surface areas. Operative time was 120 min, blood loss was minimal, and the patient did not receive transfusion. The recovery was uneventful and the patient was discharged on the third postoperative day without ascites (abdominal fluid). Robotic-assisted laparoscopic approaches such as this may enable liver resection in patients with cirrhosis and evidence of liver failure that would be likely to contraindicate open surgery, which would involve transection of major abdominal collaterals [306]. Experience and controlled trials with many more cases will be necessary to confirm whether such remarkable results can be generally achieved. In the meantime, other cases are being reported in North America, Asia, and Europe [307].

As laparoscopic procedures in liver surgery move into practice, more robotic-assisted and imaging guided methods are being developed. A point that is frequently made in regard to robotic-aided laparoscopic surgery is that successful application requires skill and experience in conventional and laparoscopic surgery; this is especially true for the liver and other complex soft-tissue organs. Such skills can be enhanced and augmented by mapping and guidance technologies whose development requires cross-disciplinary collaboration between medical science, control science, micromechanics, human factors, and information technologies. Computer-driven presentation of 3D virtual environments in advanced displays has been enabled by microdevices such as light projector microchips incorporating nanotechnology cantilevers and fast-switching optoelectronic filters [308–313]. For example, a detailed anatomic map can be projected onto the patient's abdomen or onto a phantom alongside the operating table, or a 3D image showing internal structure based on prior imaging can be viewed in a stereoscopic imaging system to guide surgery around critical vessels and to the tumors.

The liver is a large complex and richly vascular organ, with soft and deformable tissues, leading to navigation challenges for conventional as well as robotic laparoscopic surgery. Here is a place where it is critical to augment visualization and mapping capabilities before attempting physical entry and surgery. Much creative and sophisticated effort goes into applying the most advanced imaging, computational mapping, and visualization to provide the surgeon with 3D virtual reality navigation aids for planning and guiding surgery on the liver. This is a case where mapping of each individual patient is necessary, as well as tracking changes and deformations caused by surgical intrusions. These technologies are extending the reach of surgeons to smaller and smaller tumors [314].

Ultrasound is a good imaging modality for soft tissue, and a system providing 3D navigation based on optoelectric ultrasound has been developed and used in liver resection by a team of medical researchers in Berlin. The system is designed to support vessel-oriented surgery with visualization for vasculature and tumor margins for removal of liver metastases, facilitating preservation of liver parenchyma and improving oncological outcome. The system uses high precision 3D models constructed from preoperative data. It has been used successfully on 32 of 33 patients [315].

A guidance system for radiofrequency ablation of liver tumors based on CT sonography with magnetic navigation control of the instrument probe has been developed and used in Japan [316].

The technologies developed for navigation and robotic-assisted surgery in the liver are being used for pancreatic surgery, where vascularization and need to preserve specialized tissues is at a premium. An initial published case for robotic-assisted pancreatic resection reported minimal blood loss and patient discharge 4 days after a subtotal pancreatectomy to remove an intraductal pancreatic neoplasm located in the neck of the pancreas, causing atrophy of the body and tail and an acute pancreatitis episode [317]. Long-term follow-up and many controlled studies will be necessary to determine more general results.

One cause of liver cancer is metastasis of primary colon cancer, requiring surgery on both organs. A pilot study of robotic-assisted surgery for primary colon cancer and synchronous liver metastases suggests that laparoscopic one-stage colon and liver resection is feasible and safe. Robotic assistance was used to facilitate liver resection, increasing the number of patients who could benefit from a one-stage minimally invasive operation [318].

6.5.16 Colorectal Surgery

In 2004, the results of a study were reported which compared laparoscopically assisted and open colectomy for colon cancer, concluding no significant differences in outcomes or complications, but with significantly shorter hospital stays for laparoscopically treated patients [319]. Since then, laparoscopic colorectal resection has become widely adopted, and techniques for robotic colorectal surgery have been developed and evaluated, including total mesorectal excision for rectal cancer using four robotic arms [320–325]. Short-term results of a pilot randomized trial with 36 patients were reported in 2008 concluding that tumor-specific mesorectal excision was performed safely and effectively using the robotic system and the perioperative outcomes were acceptable. Hospital stays were shorter for the robotic group (6.9 ± 1.3 days in the robotic group and 8.7 ± 1.3 days for conventional laparoscopy) [326].

6.5.17 Urology

Robot-assisted surgery has gained immense popularity in urology, a field in which laparoscopic surgery has already been well established, especially for surgery on the prostate. The Da Vinci system and other laparoscopic robots are well suited for many urologic procedures where laparoscopic access is gained through a minimal number of incisions in the abdomen. Robotic-assisted laparoscopic surgery has been used in nearly all urological areas, including prostate, renal, bladder (cystectomy), and urogynecology. In urology, the advantages of robotic surgery are similar to those in other internal medicine areas: safety, more homogeneous outcomes with less variability of surgery, shorter recovery times, and new tools and procedures giving greater access to more types of surgery. For the surgeon, there is the advantage of shorter learning curve, reduced fatigue, and the opportunity to perform complex procedures that would be difficult using conventional laparoscopy. Robotic systems provide better precision and ergonomics than conventional laparoscopy. Training and remote mentoring possibilities are made feasible by robotic surgical systems in many areas [327–330].

The goal of lower overall costs is another potential advantage that has not always been realized; economic concerns remain the major drawbacks of medical robotic systems, as the clinical benefits must be weighed against higher investment and operating costs. Other disadvantages are lack of haptics and limitations of 3D vision capabilities. Newer systems are advancing with haptics, improved instruments, and better image guidance and navigation systems, and systems are expected to continue to advance rapidly in these areas [331,332]. With advances in the capabilities and benefits available with robotic surgery systems, robotics training programs are being integrated into surgical training, including nursing and technical specialists to support the operating environment [333].

6.5.18 Renal Surgery

Robot-assisted techniques have been described for almost all renal-related procedures, but use of robotics for kidney surgery has been slower than for the prostate. This has been due partly to costs and partly to the perception that robotics does not offer significant benefits over open surgery or laparoscopic surgery for most kidney procedures [334,335]. But with advancement in minimally invasive techniques, laparoscopic and robotic surgeries are performed with the advantage of decreased morbidity while maintaining the same oncologic principles as those of open surgery.

Robotic procedures and techniques that have been described for renal surgery include radical and partial nephrectomy, pyeloplasty, radical nephroureterectomy, and others [336–340]. Initial feasibility studies and some evaluations have been published on robot-assisted laparoscopic nephrectomy for diseased kidneys. Many early cases of robot-assisted laparoscopic nephrectomy were carried out in live donors for renal transplantation. Experience with robot-assisted laparoscopic pyeloplasty is more mature. Robot-assisted laparoscopic partial nephrectomy is continuing to evolve. Robot assistance seems to have a role in reconstructive renal procedures such as pyeloplasty and partial nephrectomy, due mainly to the precise suturing ability [335].

6.5.19 Nephrectomy

In treatment for tumors or disease of the kidney, it is a goal to preserve functional portions of the kidney if possible. If some of the nephrons that perform its filtration work are intact, the patient may retain at least partial kidney function. Partial nephrectomy has become the standard of treatment for renal tumors less than 4 cm in size, and more recently this technique has been applied to larger tumors as well. Laparoscopic and robotic-assisted techniques are increasingly being used for complex nephron-sparing surgeries for kidney tumors, including complex renal tumors, such as hilar and endophytic lesions [341]. Some feasibility studies are indicating that robot-assisted partial nephrectomy is feasible, with immediate oncologic results and peri-operative outcomes comparable with more mature laparoscopic methods. Short hospital stays and short learning curves are also reported [341–343]. Even with the advantages of robotics, however, laparoscopic partial nephrec-tomy is still an advanced procedure with potential for complications, requir-ing considerable experience with reconstructive laparoscopy [344]. Further studies will be required to determine if reduction in procedure complexity warrants the expense of robotic technology.

The development of single port and NOTES techniques for nephrectomies and other renal procedures has demonstrated advantages such as elimina-tion of the need for laparoscopic triangulation for intracorporeal suturing, decreased recovery times, reduced pain and scarring, and less morbidity. Robotic-assisted laparoscopic surgery has been used to perform radical pros-tatectomy, dismembered pyeloplasty, radical nephrectomy, vesicourethral anastomosis, and pelvi-ureteric anastomosis through single ports, including transumbilical ports [345,346]. Robotic NOTES for renal surgery is currently in the experimental stage [347].

6.5.20 Adrenalectomy

Techniques have been developed for use of robotics-assisted removal of the adrenal gland [348]. Robotic surgery has been found to be a safe and effective alternative to conventional laparoscopic procedures for adrenalectomy [349]. Techniques and multi-patient studies have reported shorter hospital stays; costs were not significantly higher than for conventional laparoscopy, and were lower than for open surgery [350].

6.5.21 Prostatectomy

Robotic-assisted prostatectomy is one of the most widely used applications for laparoscopic robotic-assisted surgery. The basic techniques are well established [351,352], and more advanced techniques have been developed, for example, for preservation of function by nerve grafts [353]. Experience gained with large numbers of cases at some centers has contributed to lower complication rates and shorter operation times than for unassisted laparos-copy. Widespread experience has led to dissemination of surgical technique and management of complications, and the morbidity of robotic-assisted radical prostatectomy is comparable to conventional laparoscopic proce-dures, and both compare favorably to open surgery [354].

6.5.22 Reproductive Medicine

Robotic surgery has been widely adopted in reproductive surgery with improvement of outcomes at leading medical centers. It has been applied in tubal ligation and reversals, vasectomy and vasovasostomy (reversal surgery), varicocelectomy, myomectomy (uterine fibroid removal), radical hysterectomy, and specialized hysterectomies for cervical and uterine cancers [355–357].

6.5.22.1 Varicocelectomy

Varicocelectomy is the most common operation performed for male infertility. The standard is open microsurgery. Microsurgical varicocele repairs need reliable identification and preservation of the testicular arteries and lymphatic channels and reliable identification of all internal spermatic veins and gubernacular veins. Minimally invasive aproscopic and robotic-assisted methods are being developed with the goal of eliminating tremor, reducing recovery time and lowering costs [358].

6.5.22.2 Vasovasostomy

Vasovasostomy is surgery to reverse blockage or ligation of the vas deferens (usually as a result of a previous vasectomy procedure). Robotic-assisted vasovasostomy microsurgery is an experimental procedure developed on animal models, which has recently been used on human patients [359–361]. The challenges and prospective benefits are similar to those for varicocelectomy.

6.5.22.3 Gynecology

Nearly all gynecologic procedures can now be performed routinely by laparoscopy. Relatively simple procedures such as tubal ligation, treatment of ectopic pregnancy, lysis of mild adhesions, and cautery of endometriosis are performed by most gynecologists. Until recently, open surgery was still typically used for many more complicated conditions such as hysterectomy, myomectomy, incontinence, and prolapse procedures, distal tuboplasty and microsurgical tubal anastomosis, ovarian cystectomy, extensive adhesiolysis, and advanced endometriosis. But with support from significant experience and peer-reviewed publications, laparoscopy is replacing laparotomy in gynecologic surgery for an increasing number of surgeries [362–365].

The development of robotic surgical systems is aimed as overcoming the shortcomings of conventional laparoscopy: robotic technology is an enhancement along the continuum of laparoscopic technological advances. Robotic surgery systems were designed to address some of the difficulties associated with the performance of laparoscopic operations. Benefits include 3D imaging, improved instrument articulation and dexterity, downscaling of movements, decrease of fatigue and tension tremor, and comfort for the surgeon, assistant, and surgical nursing staff. Disadvantages include costs and time to assemble and disassemble the instruments. Before robotic technologies are accepted wholeheartedly, their true merit and objective benefits to patients must be established by well-designed studies with long-term clinical outcomes, including complications, cost, pain, return to normal activity, and quality of life [366–368].

The use of robotics in gynecologic surgery is increasing, but is still not widely adopted in clinical practice. Procedures such as hysterectomy are still performed predominantly via laparotomy. Robotic technology is gaining preference in some centers over conventional laparoscopic instrumentation for the surgical treatment of gynecologic malignancies and for procedures such as benign hysterectomy, myomectomy, and surgery for invasive pelvic endometriosis. Reported robotic-assisted laparoscopic surgeries in gynecology also include tubal reanastomoses, radical hysterectomy, lymph node dissection, and sacrocolpopexies. Recent publications include case series and comparative studies demonstrating the feasibility of this particular type of surgery. Although individual studies vary, robot-assisted gynecologic surgery is generally reported as having similar clinical outcomes, decreased blood loss, and shorter hospital stay compared with conventional laparoscopic procedures [369–371].

Robotic techniques have been developed and evaluated as specialized alternative treatments with laparoscopic pyeloplasty for symptomatic ureteropelvic junction obstruction [372], where laparscopy using conventional instrumentation is complex because of rigid instruments and difficulty in providing strong layered closures for incisions.

In gynecologic oncology, robotic surgery for endometrial cancer has been reported for a year-long series of more than 100 patients, with lower blood loss and shorter hospital stays compared with open endometrial staging, resulting in overall efficiencies and expansion of practice. Lymph node yields and complications were comparable [373]. Another series study of 65 patients reported no change in surgical volume compared to the year before adoption of robotic surgery for management of endometrial cancer, but did report significant improvement in several perioperative outcomes when compared to laparotomy and laparoscopy. Complication rates and blood loss were significantly lower with robotic surgery than with laparotomy, and operating time was significantly less than for laparoscopy. Total number of perioperative inpatient days decreased from 331 to 150 in 1 year following the transition to predominantly robotic surgery [374].

Recent studies with steadily improving robotic technology have demonstrated the feasibility and safety of applying robotics to a broad range of gynecologic procedures. Although robotic procedures seem to confer the same benefits as laparoscopic surgery without additional complications, it is unclear whether robotic surgery in general imparts significant benefits versus costs when compared with conventional laparoscopic techniques. Benefits driving application of robotics include shorter recovery times and less scarring. Barriers cited for wider adoption include costs, training, and credentialing. Simulation is being developed to provide efficiencies in training and evaluation on new robotic technology, allowing simulated placement of uterine manipulator, robot docking and positioning, port placement, instrument changes, and console operation [375]. Additional rigorous scientific studies and long-term data will be needed to determine the most appropriate applications of robotics in gynecology and obstetrics [376,377].

6.5.22.4 Obstetrics

The chief benefit derived from application of robotics in obstetrics is the provision of realistic simulation for training and methods evaluation [375,378]. Simulation tools developed for obstetrics include instrumented forceps and a childbirth simulator [379,380]. The simulator and forceps have been used in training and evaluation of skill transfer and techniques [381].

6.5.22.5 Pediatrics

Since pediatric surgery can involve smaller anatomy than adult procedures, robotics can offer advantages in complex procedures that involve areas that are difficult to access and in procedures in which dissection of delicate anatomic structures is required. This has been confirmed in early assessment studies of a number of robotically assisted, laparoscopic and thoracic procedures performed by surgeons experienced in the technique. Robotic surgery was found to be feasible and safe for a number of routine pediatric procedures, and advantages were seen in complex procedures involving challenges for access to small and delicate structures. But the initial study did not demonstrate superior clinical outcomes for robotic surgeries compared to conventional laparoscopic and open surgery [382].

Successful experience reported in other studies has led to expanded use of robotic surgery in pediatric urology, for procedures that include pyeloplasty, ureteral reimplantation, abdominal testis surgery, and partial or total nephrectomy. These procedures are only performed at select centers offering robotic expertise combined with expert experience in pure laparoscopy, which is still essential in the event of a mechanical malfunction. Complex reconstructive pediatric surgeries such as appendicovesicostomy, antegrade continent enema creation, and augmentation cystoplasty are being developed using robotics, but are still in their infancy, as reported by Pasquale Casale of Children's Hospital of Philadelphia [383].

Indications for surgery in cases of varicoceles in adolescence can be controversial, but the use of color Doppler ultrasound has provided an objective tool in the assessment of such patients based on the determination of varicocele size, venous flow patterns, testicular volume, and resistance index, leading to more precise targeting of surgery and improved outcomes [384]. Improved diagnostic capabilities, plus technical modifications to robotic technique, have been developed to enable robotic-assisted single-port surgery for pediatric varicocoelectomy [385].

Robotic surgery techniques have been developed for treatment of congenital urologic defects and other areas of pediatric urology, where it provides increased magnification and dexterity for in situ minimally invasive surgery. Robotic-assisted laparoscopic surgery has been used in pyeloplasty for ureteropelvic junction obstruction. Robotic-assisted pyeloplasty in children has been demonstrated to be feasible and to have satisfactory results. The short-term data suggest that outcomes are similar to those of open pyeloplasty in children [386,387].

Surgery for hepatobiliary anomalies is complex and difficult with standard laparoscopic instruments. Robotic surgery has been found to be well suited to intracorporeal hepatic surgery in children, especially with the aid of 3D imaging. Surgery for a number of complex liver defects in children has been reported and found safe and effective [388].

6.5.23 Image-Guided Robotics in Radiation Oncology

Robotic control of movement in concert with 3D image–based navigation can be used to guide sources and beams for radiation. Robotic computerized controls are used in radiation oncology for radiosurgery to deliver precisely shaped beams of ionizing radiation into the skull, spine, or other parts of the body that are difficult to reach by direct physical access [389–391]. Radiosurgery is also used for treatment of tumors that are not addressable by conventional surgery, for example, for inoperable lung cancer [392]. Radiosurgery is also used in conjunction with surgical resection where all of the tumor cannot be removed [393,394].

The ability to generate and focus extremely thin diameter beams of ionizing radiation has only recently been made possible by advanced electronics, engineering, and materials science. Several systems offer different capabilities and types of therapy. Other limitations that have been overcome to make precise robotic radiosurgery possible are reduction in the size and weight of accelerators needed to produce the radiation, and more powerful and precise magnetics and electronics for beam focusing.

The CyberKnife system, Gamma Knife, BrainLAB, and Varian Trilogy all offer different versions of this capability. They differ from previous generations of radiation therapy instrumentation in their ability to focus and control extremely fine and powerful convergent beams, precisely targeted into tissue. With superior beam control, more radiation can be directed into a tumor or lesion with less damage to other tissue. This capability is especially powerful in the Gamma Knife, because it uses powerful intensity short-wavelength gamma radiation.

Another capability that has become available through advances in mechatronics is robotic control for precise access and placement of localized sources of radiation therapy in the body (brachytherapy) in the form of small capsules or pins containing radioactive emitters. This allows implantation of these powerful sources of ionizing radiation directly into tumors where they bombard the cancer cells at close range from the inside, without a radiation beam having to traverse the body to reach the tumor [395].

6.5.24 Summary of Surgical Robotics in Medical Practice

Reviewing where surgical robotics is being used in current and translational medicine gives an idea of the current transformations that are taking place in surgery, based on new technologies that are arising out of the ability to make robotics and mechatronics smaller and more capable. These capabilities are coming from advancements that enable electronic sensors and actuators to be fabricated with nanoscale geometries, resulting in new devices that are faster, denser, and more energy efficient for building computers, displays, sensors, actuators, and communications links to give robotics and navigation tools with ever-accelerating power.

We have noted how these robotic and navigation capabilities are being applied pragmatically and specifically to each branch of surgery, with customized capabilities to meet medical needs; there is not a general capability for medical robotics. Each special part of the body and each disease has its unique combination of requirements.

It appears that the truly revolutionary impact of robotics in surgery so far is not in autonomous nanobots but in tools to augment and enhance the capabilities of the surgeon, extending the capabilities for perceiving, visualizing, and navigating complex structures from the macro down to the microscopic scale, and providing the ability to effectively and safely manipulate organs and tissues. In some cases, robotics provides strength, speed, precision, and accuracy for large tasks; in others, microscopic precision and intricate navigation and manipulation for microscopic procedures. In all cases, the robotics are serving to execute the work desired and conceptualized by the surgeon, overcoming the manual and visual limitations of our unaided senses and hands.

6.6 Recent Advances and Emerging Technologies in Surgical and Endoscopic Navigation

We have been looking in a rather narrow focus at surgical robotics, following the path of implementation and application of the laparoscopic robotic model, with occasional asides to consider guidance of catheters, radiosurgery, and related topics. Before leaving the discussion of the current impact of robotics, mechatronics, and augmented visualization technologies, we should also look at some emerging directions these technologies are taking. These include using robotics and 3D imaging to guide miniaturized and flexible robotics for catheter and endoscope control, robotics for NOTES, untethered robotic and sensor devices that can navigate in the body, and integration of surgical robotics with imaging and fabrication capabilities. In this section, we explore some very new nanotechnology-enabled instrumentation that is just entering experimental medical use. We also cover some conceptual and proposed medical devices based on MEMS and other nanotechnologies.

6.6.1 Miniaturized and Distributed Control for Laparoscopic Robotics

Advances in MEMS and other nanotechnology-driven electronics, sensors, and actuators are allowing miniaturization of the laparoscopic robot architecture. As motors become smaller and electronic communication and control become faster with higher throughput, sensors, actuators, and motor drives can be made smaller and distributed over the robotic arms to provide greater flexibility, dexterity, and responsiveness. Some recent surgical robotics designs already represent steps toward a more distributed control and actuator design, with slave instrument motor drive packs mounted on the existing bed rails of the operating table, taking up much less space than the normal robotic arms [396,397].

The ultimate extension of this capability and concept will lead to multiple jointed robotic arms like tentacles with actuators distributed over the arm, capable of snake or wormlike ability to execute multiple turns and curves to follow complex anatomical pathways, while capable of performing surgical operations at the end or along the arm. Implementation of such designs useful for surgery awaits further miniaturization of actuators and management of distributed control and communications. Inexpensive mote processors that are small, require minimal power, and are capable of communicating with many other motes are already being produced and used in distributed communications networks and automation systems. Surgical robotics devices will benefit from mote-based control used in biomimetic designs that emulate movement mechanisms found in animals, plants, and cells.

6.6.2 Robotics for NOTES and LESS

New technologies for control and visualization are propelling NOTES [398,399] and laproendoscopic single site surgery (LESS) [400,401] from the evaluation and development status into clinical usefulness. A look at how implementation is progressing is informative in relation to the many other new medical procedures that are and will shortly be arriving due to nanotechnology-driven advances. NOTES, like any new medical technology which involves major changes in procedure, is being treated with caution until the benefits are proven. Leaders of the American Society of Gastrointestinal Endoscopy (ASGE) and the Society of American Gastrointestinal and Endoscopic Surgeons (SAGES) met in 2005 to identify the challenges to NOTES adoption as a clinical procedure, and set up a monitoring organization to establish guidelines and standards (with the acronym NOSCAR for Natural Orifice Surgery Consortium for Assessment and Research [402]). In the meantime, results of experiments and trails continue to be reported, evaluations are given, and new techniques are being refined, making NOTES a moving target [403–409].

Most commercially available surgical robotics systems were designed before the development of NOTES. As a result, the most widely used laparoscopic surgical robotics systems rely on from three to five or more endoscopic ports to perform minimally invasive surgeries. More recently, developers are designing robotic surgery to accommodate the needs of NOTES and other single-port surgical procedures [410–413].

To work with a single port, designers can take several approaches. A single incision port can be used to accommodate a trocar with multiple channels or lumen [67,396,409,412]. Additional robotic actuators can be designed to increase the articulation and flexibility of the instruments within the body, eliminating external collisions, and the need to work around a single-port fulcrum. For some functions, small-diameter flexible instruments, endoscopes, or catheters can be employed [414]. Directional and functional control of internal robotic arm movements can be through wireless communication linkages, reducing the number of wires for control signal connections. This allows for completely flexible endoscopic probes introduced through a single small port [415]. This is a logical extension of the basic idea of the fiber endoscope [416]. Early versions of the externally guided flexible endoscope concept date back to the 1990s [417–423].

Finally, the surgical probes can be completely wireless for many functions, freeing some instrument modules from connections via the port—the ultimate in flexibility. Physical congestion and collisions caused by the need to control multiple instruments through a single multi-lumen port are eliminated, leaving the port for essential connected functions such as irrigation, aspiration, introduction of tools, and retrieval of tissue and instruments. The concept of a wireless ingestible sensor for physiology measurements dates back to the 1950s [424–426]. Wireless endoscopic systems were first introduced as gastrointestinal diagnostic imaging devices, and have more recently been developed for endoscopic surgical functions [427–433].

Design and application of wireless robotic surgical instruments for use within the body present their own technical challenges. Only recently have advances in microelectronics for wireless communication reached the levels of size, signal strength, and minimal power requirements to enable feasibility of a unit small enough to be introduced through a trocar and operate within an abdominal cavity with any useful surgical functions. Wireless communication frequencies must penetrate the tissues with wavelengths and power intensities that are not significantly absorbed and do not cause heating or physiological damage. Untethered wireless robotic instruments must be fixable in order to maintain stable positions and exert leverage for surgical tasks. Fixation and navigation techniques must be developed that do not damage tissue.

Examples of many types of flexible endoscopic instruments have been proposed, designed, built, and tested experimentally. Conceptual design proposals for untethered freely navigating medical microrobots, such as once found only in science fiction, have become more realistic and feasible with maturation of underlying technology.

6.6.3 Flexible Robotics: Robotic Activated Endoscopes and Catheters

A number of robotic systems with flexible steerable endoscopic arms have been designed and several are commercially available [6,7,10,434]. Although most of the commercial devices were designed primarily for electrophysiology or gastrointestinal procedures, a number of medical researchers have pursued the adaptation of these robotic endoscopic devices to other more general applications in NOTES and LESS surgeries [434–437].

Novel approaches to robotic NOTES surgery can be taken by combining and adapting instrumentation developed for other endoscopic procedures. Flexible endoscopic tubes as small as 2.5 mm are designed for ureteroscopes, and have been used in diagnosis, management, and treatment for uteral and renal stones and tumors, using lasers, electrofulguration, and electrohydraulic lithotripsy [438,439]. In 2008, Desai and coworkers used a custom-modified fiber-optic ureteroscope placed through the small working lumen of a steerable robotic catheter, in order to successfully fragment calculi in porcine models [440].

These flexible endoscopy approaches have generated much interest in the possibilities for performing simple procedures with NOTES surgeries by adapting currently available tools.

Other researchers have evaluated the adaptation to NOTES of flexible six degree-of-freedom, long-shafted instruments with haptic feedback that run alongside a standard gastroscope or colonoscope. In preliminary validation studies on animal models, it was found that such instruments were difficult to introduce into the gastrointestinal tract and manipulation forces were insufficient for procedures. Further design work for a second generation system is being done based on results of these studies [441].

Other approaches also use flexible robotic manipulators that can be attached to an endoscope. Several such designs have been proposed and simulated; some prototypes have been built and tested in animal models [442–445], including ergonomic designs for NOTES control consoles to aid intuitive and safe control [446]. These devices tend to look like the business end of a praying mantis attached to the tip of the endoscope, with two or more effectors with multiple degrees of freedom on either side of a central head housing the camera (or lens port for the fiber optic column), illumination, and lumens for tools, suction, and irrigation. Control and actuation is through mechanical or electronic cabling running through or parallel to the flexible endoscopic arm, which may have various degrees of freedom for forming and holding curved configurations.

6.6.4 In Vivo Robotics: Wireless Robotic Navigation
for Diagnosis and Surgery

Two lines of development have taken place in parallel for wireless endoluminal or intracorporeal devices: one is the invention and increasing sophistication of ingestible capsules for diagnostic sensing and imaging in the gastrointestinal tract; the other is the design of increasingly capable wireless robotic devices to aid surgery. Both are referred to by the term in vivo robotics. As more and more functional capabilities are added, both lines of development are tending to merge toward multipurpose endoscopic theranostic robotic devices—larger versions of the multifunctional theranostic nanoparticles we looked at in Section 5.6 of Chapter 5.

6.6.4.1 Capsule Endoscopy

Wireless endoscopy capsules are self-contained ingestable cameras that can transmit images from within the gastrointestinal tract [447–450]. This type of endoscopy device was made possible as microelectronics advanced to reduce size and power requirements for all kinds of circuits, including imaging and communications devices. Beginning in the 1950s, experiments were made with wireless transmission of temperature, pressure, and pH from sensors in the body [424–426,451]. Small radiofrequency transmitters developed for covert communications were adapted in the 1980s by Paul Swain and Tim Mills at University College London to transmit pH measurements from a wireless capsule in the gastrointestinal tract [452].

With the availability of small CCD video cameras in the early 1990s, it became possible to transmit images wirelessly as radiofrequency signals from a camera module to a receiver. This concept was adopted by Gavriel J. Iddan in Israel for sending images from within the body with a freely traveling endoscopic camera communicating with a monitor outside of the body [453,454]. In practice, this ability required extreme miniaturization of camera, encoding circuitry, power source, and radiofrequency transmitter, and solving optical problems such as how to keep a lens clean in a freely traveling camera capsule. A key factor was the development of complementary metal oxide semiconductor (CMOS) technology at this time, which reduced the size and power requirements of imaging and computing circuits compared with previous CCD technologies. Also important were improvements in batteries and computing performance to implement power-saving strategies [453].

6.6.4.1.1 The PillCam

In 1997, Swain joined a new company, Given Imaging, being formed by Iddan and a team in Israel to develop the first endoscopic capsule camera, or PillCam, a video camera with radiofrequency transmitter and antenna that fit into a capsule 11 mm in diameter and 26 mm in length, about the size of a large vitamin pill, and weighing 3.7 g. The early versions of the capsule had a color video camera with a viewing angle of 140°, a wireless radiofrequency transmitter and antenna, four LED lights, and enough battery power to take 57,000 color images at a rate of 2 frames/s during an 8 h journey through the digestive tract. Preparation for the procedure was much simpler than for a conventional endoscopy. Data was collected by a small battery-powered recorder worn around the waist, attached to an array of sensors positioned on the body [454].

By this time, endoscopes were being used to examine the gastrointestinal tract from colon upward, and from the esophagus and stomach downward, but most of the small intestine was inaccessible by endoscopy because of distance and torturous geometry. Even for more accessible portions of the digestive tract anatomy, examination by endoscope was uncomfortable and time consuming for patient and caregiver. So a means of obtaining images of the interior of the body by simply ingesting a pill, even a large one, was welcomed. The system was shown to be useful in obtaining diagnostic images of small intestinal bleeding, early signs of Crohn's disease, and other pathologies and abnormalities of the small bowel [455–458].

Later versions of Given Imaging's PillCam increased efficiency and coverage by adding a second camera and light source, taking images in opposite directions from both ends of the capsule. It incorporated improvements to sense when the pill was in motion and adapt the image capture rate, thus reducing redundancy of images, optimizing battery and storage usage, and making the diagnostic use of the image data easier. Software was improved to allow automatic classification of images by recognizing signs of bleeding. A system for providing localization coordinates was added to reduce the difficulty of precisely locating pathologies. Versions were produced with delays, which activated the camera to cover different parts of the digestive tract: the PillCam ESO for the esophagus, the PillCam SB for the small intestine, and most recently, the PillCam Colon, which was given the European CE mark in 2009 [459].

The PillCam created a great deal of enthusiasm and excitement because it was a revolutionary demonstration of the power of miniaturized electronics, as well as for its medical diagnostic advances. For many, it seemed to be the first step toward realizing the visions of miniature medical robots. In designing the PillCam, the developers acknowledged using nanotechnology from firms such as MEMSCAP for key components of the system.

In the community of medical researchers and practitioners, it was carefully evaluated in clinical trials and meta-analyses, and found to be effective, safe, and generally superior for many diagnostic purposes to other methods in the small bowel, such as barium enhanced x-ray imaging. Cost remained an issue, especially with lagging acceptance by insurers. And while the PillCam has definitely proven useful for small bowel diagnosis, it has been slower to gain acceptance for the colon and esophagus, where conventional endoscopy can compete with an established record of practice [460].

Improvements continue to be made in capsule endoscopy systems, including external magnetic steering mechanisms [461–463]. For example, the NORIKA system developed in Japan has a mechanism for controlling rotation, for more efficient capture of images [464]. In addition, improvements are being made in software for analysis and management of the high volume of image data obtained [465].

6.6.4.1.2 *Capsules for pH and Impedance Monitoring*

In the meantime, instrumented wireless capsules have been applied by Medtronic (Minneapolis, Minnesota) to measurement of pH for diagnosis and monitoring of gastroesophageal reflux disease (GERD), which can lead to ulceration and cancer of the esophagus. The Bravo system is a diagnostic wireless capsule with pH sensing, which is temporarily attached to the wall of the esophagus by a surgical stapling mechanism. The Bravo capsule remains in place for 48 h or more, and allows the patient to eat and speak normally – unlike the alternative conventional monitors, which must be connected to a monitor via a transnasal cable. In December of 2008, Given Imaging acquired the Bravo product line from Medtronic, complementing the PillCam products' diagnostic capabilities [466].

The ability to monitor for symptoms of GERD with wireless capsules was a great advance, which enabled continuous monitoring to understand the course and management of the disease with much less discomfort to the patient. Clinical studies suggest that impedance is of at least equal importance to pH in diagnosis and monitoring of GERD [467]. To meet the need to monitor GERD more completely, new capsules are being developed that measure impedance as well as pH [468].

6.6.4.2 **Wireless Robotic Modules for Endoscopic Surgery**

In parallel with the advances in wireless capsules for endoscopic sensing and imaging, researchers have been developing mobile wireless robotics to aid in endoscopic surgery. This development includes robotic modules with magnetic guidance and fixation as well as more elaborate robots with inchworm-like self-propulsion. Wireless cameras and instruments can eliminate the need to manipulate endoscopic instruments via connections through incisions. Any wireless device that can be passed through a single incision and deployed wirelessly reduces the instrumental congestion at the incision, making the surgery easier and safer, and reducing the size and number of incisions needed. Application of this concept started with the simplest functions, such as fixed illumination or anchoring points for leverage, where the device could be inserted, left in place during the surgery, and removed afterward [469–471].

Extension of this concept to active robotic wireless devices has been made feasible by shrinking size and power requirements, concomitant with increased performance in electronics, wireless communications, and robotic controls. A number of wireless robotic modules have been developed, all of which operate under remote control by magnetic or radiofrequency links. Autonomous medical robots are still speculative, but accomplishment of surgical functions by remote wireless control is quite challenging and impressive enough, and calls on the latest in miniaturized technology [472–474].

Miniature wireless in vivo surgical robots have been used experimentally for NOTES surgery, where they appear to overcome many of the limitations of working laparoscopically through a single incision trocar port [475–477]. Current advanced experimental designs for in vivo surgical robotics feature both mobile and fixed base devices that fit entirely inside the abdominal cavity. Modular wireless platforms can accommodate a variety of instruments including biopsy graspers, staplers and clamps, video cameras, and physiological sensors. These tools have been integrated with a common wireless platform and tested in vivo in a porcine model [478].

6.6.4.2.1 Modular Reconfigurable Multiunit Endoluminal Robotic Surgical Systems

The simplest design for wireless in vivo surgical robots would consist of a single unit with multiple functionalities, such as imaging, active locomotion, and surgical intervention. But a single surgical robot operating within the body would be limited in leverage and degrees of freedom for its functional components. Sets of modular endoluminal surgical robots have the possibility to be employed cooperatively from optimal positions and angles for surgical tasks [479].

Multidisciplinary research groups are addressing the opportunities and challenges in designs for sets of interworking multiunit in vivo surgical robots. Coordination of multiple units by remote wireless control is similar in principle to the task of coordinating multiple surgical tools with physical connections; in some ways, the task faced for wireless coordination should be simpler, because collisions and interferences of robotic arms and endoscopic columns extending to the outside of the body are eliminated. But coordination of independently moving tools introduces its own complexities—it is like going from coordinating rail traffic to air traffic control. Plus, it is not enough merely to avoid interference; the tools must be orchestrated smoothly on a single focused task. Each module must be able to communicate wirelessly with a directing surgical team, and in some cases interact with some or all of its neighbors—increasing the complexity of the design. Even if the robotic surgical unit has some autonomous functions, the need for communication with an external management cannot be eliminated for a useful medical system.

This design problem is currently the object of a number of theoretical and experimental studies.

Some of these studies have designed self-assembling robotic building blocks that can be introduced as units into the body where they are fabricated into larger surgical tools. In the ARES (assembling reconfigurable endoluminal surgical) system, the individual building blocks are designed to be ingestible for work in the gastrointestinal tract, and thus are of similar size to an endoscope capsule (11 mm in diameter and 26 mm in length) [480].

Some early prototypes have been designed and fabricated, with modular units containing battery power and robotic motors. The prototypes have been used to evaluate bending and rotational motion capabilities in the assemblies [481].

6.6.4.2.2 Modes of Locomotion and Propulsion for In Vivo Robotic Modules

Another challenging design problem is how surgical robots can move through the body with controlled navigation and without causing unintended penetration or injury to tissues and organs. This is a problem faced in different ways by robotic arms, endoscopes, catheters, individual robotic modules, or self-assembling endoluminal robots. It is summed up nicely in the title of an excellent recent review: How should microrobots swim? [482]

Researchers have been exploring ways to give greater control over mobility for wireless robotics to aid in endoscopic imaging and surgery. This development started with robotic modules with magnetically guided or inchworm-like self-propulsion in the digestive tract—as contrasted with the freely floating ingestible capsule, which depends on peristalsis to move it through the gut.

A large number of proposed mechanisms for propulsion of in vivo robotics have been studied, simulated and in some cases built experimentally, both for self-propelled modules and for units driven and directed by external forces such as magnetic fields. Typical modes of robotic locomotion evaluated for in vivo microrobots include legged capsules, propellers, fins, eel-like undulation, and biomimetic flagella [445,483–485]. An unusual proposed method for endoscopic capsule propulsion used static and magnetic field forces in an MR imaging system [486]. Detailed computer simulations of motion have also been developed and evaluated for biologically inspired continuum robots [487].

6.6.4.2.3 Magnetic Technologies for NOTES

One approach to wireless control for NOTES and LESS uses external magnets to manipulate endoscopic devices to perform surgical tasks. The devices may be completely untethered, and control is via magnetic forces through the abdominal wall, so a dedicated surgical port is not required, reducing the number of incisions needed. The magnetically positioned and controlled devices can be an illumination source, a fixed "third hand" to retract and hold tissue, or devices with actuators such as staplers, sensors, or complex and multifunctional tools. Cameras, illumination devices, irrigation and suction tubes, lasers, and electrocauterization devices can have lightweight flexible cabling if needed to serve their functions, but do not need to be pushed into position by endoscopic shanks or tubing. Advanced versions of cameras can send images by wireless radiofrequency links through the body, and illumination and other power requirements can be supplied by batteries, reducing the connections required [473,488].

The advantages of magnetic anchoring and manipulation of endoscopic surgical instruments include (1) minimizing incisions: multiple instruments can be introduced and retrieved through a single incision (reducing blood loss, trauma to tissue, and recovery time); (2) additional instruments and anchoring points for leverage can be provided without additional incisions (a "third hand" for triangulation, without compromising operating space); (3) improved operating space (in conventional laparoscopic surgery, the working envelope is limited to an inverted cone with limited degrees of freedom by the fulcrum motion centered through each incision port); (4) reduction of instrument collisions: attached handles or pushable cables are not required, reducing internal and external collision and congestion (reducing operation time, reducing complexity of procedures); and (5) imaging and instrument fidelity can be maintained equal to that for conventional laparoscopy [488–491].

This type of system depends only indirectly on nanotechnology, but it is clear that future developments in this direction will rely more and more on nanotechnology, which is making possible the implementation of higher performance batteries, light sources, and computer controls for the untethered surgical modules, as well as more powerful and flexible magnets, using correlated magnetics [492]. The current magnetically controlled wireless endoscopic surgical instruments represent a step toward more flexible semiautonomous robotic surgical tools.

An experimental magnetic anchoring and guidance system (MAGS) for NOTES and LESS was developed jointly at the University of Texas Southwestern Medical Center and the University of Texas at Arlington [488–490]. MAGS uses strong handheld magnets on the outside of the abdomen to anchor and move devices with magnetically tagged instruments that are inserted into the abdomen through a single incision port. These deployable intracorporeal instruments included illumination sources, cameras, retractors, and cautery dissectors. Continued development has been aimed at improving the number and performance of instruments and potentially eliminating the need for any laparoscopic assistance in the single port operations. The MAGS system deploys multiple instruments through a single 15 mm trocar. A number of experimental surgeries using MAGS on porcine models were carried out and evaluated [493,494]. Recently a laparoscopic nephrectomy and appendectomy were performed successfully in two human patients [495].

Another magnetic anchoring and guidance system for single port surgery has been developed at the Clinic of the Trinity-Mitre in Buenos Aires, Argentina, where it was successfully used on a human patient [496]. The chief motivation for development of this system was to avoid bile duct injury during laparoscopic surgery, a recognized problem [497,498]. The system consists of a series of clip assemblies connected to a linear array of spherical magnetic elements connected by washers threaded on a cable, terminated by a magnetic anchoring element, with tools for holding the clip assembly in place and manipulating it [499,500]. The magnetic grasper assembly is designed to give the same security of grip as with a conventional laparoscopic forceps, while avoiding biliary injury caused by manipulation of the forceps.

6.6.4.2.4 Autonomous Guidance of Surgical Robots by Ultrasound

Ultrasound may be an alternative to endoscopy for guiding minimally invasive surgery externally from a remote control console, either by cable or wireless [501,502]. In a novel development, an autonomous robotic surgery system has been designed with guidance by ultrasound. The system has been demonstrated in feasibility tests to be able to guide robot arms to touch two needle tips together with high accuracy in a water tank [503]. It has also been able to locate a ferromagnetic needle fragment (simulating shrapnel) and guide a robotic surgery probe to the fragment [504].

6.6.4.2.5 *Robotic Laser Microsurgery*

Laser microsurgery is a well-established technique in neuroscience [505,506], cell biology [507,508], and medical applications such as ophthalmology and treatment of cancers of the mouth and throat, where access to surgical targets is unobstructed [509–511]. Endoscopic laser surgery is also well established, and instrumentation for laser ablation and cutting are available for use through the working ports of endoscopes [512–514]. Recent advances in materials engineering and fiber optics have extended the range of wavelengths available for laser endoscopic surgery, making it more practical for precise neurosurgery [515]. Advanced pulsed lasers can be used to form laser nanoscissors for nanosurgery on cytoskeletons and other subcellular structures within individual living cells [516–518].

Femtosecond pulsed lasers have now been developed with capabilities of forming microplasmas with highly localized ionization and energy transfer. These lasers can be used to create cold plasmas which open new possibilities for medical applications, such as surface sterilization and laser surgery with minimal damage to living tissue [519–522]. Combined fluorescence microscopy and femtosecond laser microsurgery form a powerful "seek and treat" tool for microsurgery [523].

Advanced pulsed lasers are capable of very precise tissue cutting with minimal damage to adjacent tissues [524,525]. These capabilities, coupled with the lack of mechanical complexity and advances in miniaturization and power consumption, have led to consideration of laser surgery for use with in vivo surgical robotics [526,527].

A significant obstacle to feasibility of robotic laser surgery is the need for stability and extreme accuracy of positioning in order to avoid injury and take advantage of the high precision possible with micro-focused surgical lasers. Recent advances in ultrashort pulsed lasers make it possible to achieve selective cutting effects inside tissue while leaving adjacent layers intact [522–525]. Advances in dynamic stabilization of microrobots are also being made, based on nano-cantilever controls and motors [528,529]. The convergence of these technologies is making possible realistic design proposals for microcapsule in vivo robotic instruments with surgical capabilities.

6.6.4.2.6 *Thermal and Chemically Actuated Microrobotics for Surgery*

Another approach to wireless robotic surgery uses materials that change the shape or volume with temperature and/or interaction with chemicals. Shape memory alloys have been explored for some surgical applications, such as stapling [530]. Shape memory polymers, which have a more biocompatible range of activation temperatures than metal alloys, have been investigated for cytological and other biology applications [531]. Tetherless thermobiochemical microgrippers capable of picking up microscopic beads and cells embedded in tissue have been developed and evaluated as a step toward the development of autonomous surgical microtools. The microgrippers can be fabricated en masse by lithography, with stressed bimetallic thin film actuation. They could be the basis for future microtools for biopsy sampling or other microsurgical tasks [532].

Thermochemically driven nanoelectromechanical systems based on relative motion of carbon nanotubes have also been proposed as actuators for medical nanorobots [533]. Various forms of artificial muscle have also been explored in theoretical designs for medical robotics, for example, biomimetic designs based on spider silks [534].

Protein biomolecular nanoengines have also been proposed as the basis for surgical or theranostic robots. But once we enter the small world of protein engines, we are at the level of cell membranes and cellular biology, and thus have left medical surgery and entered the realms of macromolecular therapeutics and immunology. For example, thioester protein nanogrippers that attach to malaria parasites are being explored for the design of antimalarial drugs [535], and natural and synthetic optical switches are being investigated for the control of gated ion channels in cell membranes [536,537].

We will discuss the nanomedical aspects of protein interactions at the cellular level in Chapter 7 on nanotechnology in regenerative medicine. We will look at artificial muscle applications in Chapter 8, dealing with functional nanomaterials for tissue engineering and prosthetics.

6.6.5 Integration of Robotics with Biological Materials Engineering

Another direction in which surgical robotics is advancing is in the integration of imaging, metrology, and surgery with fabrication and manufacturing of implants. This integration is already taking place for dental orthodontics, as we saw earlier. It is beginning to be developed for dental and other implants as well. Computer-based measurement, processing, and control of manufacturing machinery, such as rapid prototyping 3D printers and computer-controlled materials working and molding machinery enable rapid and economical custom fabrication of implants. This technology is being developed initially in the field of dental and bone implants. A system has been described for integrated fabrication of frontotemporal bone implants based on real-time imaging and automated fabrication of exact shapes for custom skull implants [538].

Implants may be made from metals, or from plastics or ceramics. Conceptually, machinery could be made to fabricate biodegradable tissue scaffolding to desired sizes and shapes. Mesh, sleeves, or stents could be generated and dispensed during the surgical procedure as needed, guided by imagery and commands from the surgeon. The concept of systems for integrated imaging, fabrication, and surgical application, using automated imaging, assembly and robotics, could be extended in principle to the generation of nanoengineered materials or even to assembly of tissue replacement scaffolding containing live cells. This brings us back from our foray into robotics, returning full circle to biomaterials.

6.7 Summary of Translational Development of Nanoengineered Regenerative Tissue Therapy

Robotic systems are gaining acceptance in their appropriate role of extending the capabilities of surgeons and healthcare teams. Future development in surgical robots promises greater application of robotic devices to increasingly more difficult procedures and hard-to-access anatomical sites, with significant improvement in patient outcomes. These systems will continue to improve in capability and reliability as nanotechnology produces increasingly more powerful controls, sensors, and actuators [539].

But robots will never work alone in the operating theatre like industrial manufacturing robots. Although mechatronic systems do not fatigue, and can react faster and vibrate less than humans, a surgical team can keep the overview and react in situations that may well go beyond the capabilities of technical systems. Therefore, robot systems will be designed to work in tight cooperation with human surgeons and be integrated into medical practice. Science fiction robots that could replace physicians and surgeons entirely are far from being a reality. Medicine will continue to demand physician competence, outcomes measurement, medical error reduction, and cost containment. Any new surgical technology must support these goals to improve patient care [540,541].

Wireless devices are suggesting images of medical nanobots—but it must be kept in mind that effective medical devices are going to be on the macro to micro scale. When our devices shrink to the size of cells—a few hundred micrometers—they come into interaction with the body's cellular machinery. At even smaller sizes—the nanoscale—unique surface and chemical forces come into play alongside familiar mechanical and electronic forces, and we enter the world of nanoparticles—a step further into the divide between chemistry and surgery, as we saw previously in Chapter 5. But at the level of the cell, there are many unique forms of interaction governed by nanoscale geometries and forces, and we will look at them in Chapter 7, on nanotechnology for tissue scaffolds, cellular growth guidance, and cellular nanoengineering.

References

1. F. Gelain, Novel opportunities and challenges offered by nanobiomaterials in tissue engineering, *International Journal of Nanomedicine*, 3, 415–424 (2008).
2. K. Gonsalves, C. Halberstadt, C. T. Laurencin, and L. Nair (eds.), *Biomedical Nanostructures*, John Wiley & Sons, New York, 2007.
3. K. K. Jain, *The Handbook of Nanomedicine*, Humana Press, New York, 2008.
4. G. L. Hornyak, H. F. Tibbals, J. Dutta, and J. J. Moore, *Introduction to Nanoscience and Nanotechnology*, CRC Press, Boca Raton, FL, 2009.
5. V. Torchilin and M. Amiji, *Handbook of Materials for Nanomedicine*, Pan Stanford Publishing, Singapore/Malaysia, 2009.
6. S. Ramakrishna, M. Ramalingam, T. S. S. Kumar, and W. O. Soboyejo, *Biomaterials: A Nano Approach*, CRC Press, Boca Raton, FL, 2010.
7. S. V. Bhat, *Biomaterials*, Kluwer Academic Publishers, Dordrecht, the Netherlands, 2002.
8. J. B. Park and J. D. Bronzino (eds.), *Biomaterials: Principles and Applications*, CRC Press, Boca Raton, FL, 2002.
9. T. S. Hin, *Engineering Materials for Biomedical Applications*, World Scientific Publishing, Singapore, 2004.
10. B. D. Ratner, A. S. Hoffman, F. J. Schoen, and J. E. Lemons, *Biomaterials Science: An Introduction to Materials in Medicine*, 2nd edn., Elsevier Academic Press, London, U.K., 2004.
11. G. E. Wnek and G. L. Bowlin (eds.), *Encyclopedia of Biomaterials and Biomedical Engineering*, 2nd edn., 4 Vols., Informa Healthcare, London, U.K., 2008.
12. S. A. Guelcher and J. O. Hollinger (eds.), *An Introduction to Biomaterials*, CRC Press, Boca Raton, FL, 2005.
13. J. Y. Wong and J. D. Bronzino, *Biomaterials*, CRC Press, Boca Raton, FL, 2007.
14. J. S. Temenoff and G. Mikos, *Biomaterials: The Intersection of Biology and Materials Science*, Prentice-Hall, Upper Saddle Lake, NJ, 2008.
15. J. Vincent, *Structural Biomaterials*, Revised edn., Princeton University Press, Princeton, NJ, 1990.
16. D. L. Wise, D. J. Trantolo, K.-U. Lewandrowski, J. D. Gresser, M. V. Cattaneo, and M. J. Yaszemski (eds.), *Biomaterials Engineering and Devices: Human Applications. Volume 2: Orthopedic, Dental, and Bone Graft Applications*, Humana Press, Totowa, NJ, 2000.
17. S. W. Shalaby and U. Salz (eds.), *Polymers for Dental and Orthopedic Applications*, CRC Press, Boca Raton, FL, 2006.
18. R. V. Curtis and T. F. Watson (eds.), *Dental Biomaterials: Imaging, Testing and Modeling*, CRC Press, Boca Raton, FL, 2008.
19. J. A. Planell, S. M. Best, D. Lacroix, and A. Merolli (eds.), *Bone Repair Biomaterials*, CRC Press, Boca Raton, FL, 2009.
20. D. Shi (ed.), *Biomaterials and Tissue Engineering*, Springer Verlag, Berlin, Germany, 2004.
21. J. D. Bronzino (ed.), *Tissue Engineering and Artificial Organs*, 3rd edn., CRC Press, Boca Raton, FL, 2006.
22. L. L. Hench and J. R. Jones (eds.), *Biomaterials, Artificial Organs and Tissue Engineering*, CRC Press, Boca Raton, FL, 2005.

23. D. Orgill and C. Blanco, *Biomaterials for Treating Skin Loss*, CRC Press, Boca Raton, FL, 2009.
24. J. Denstedt and A. Atala (eds.), *Biomaterials and Tissue Engineering in Urology*, CRC Press, Boca Raton, FL, 2009.
25. C. Archer and J. Ralphs (eds.), *Regenerative Medicine and Biomaterials for the Repair of Connective Tissues*, CRC Press, Boca Raton, FL, 2010.
26. T. Gourlay and R. Black (eds.), *Biomaterials and Devices for the Circulatory Systems*, CRC Press, Boca Raton, FL, 2010.
27. T. V. Chirila (ed.), *Biomaterials and Regenerative Medicine in Ophthalmology*, CRC Press, Boca Raton, FL, 2010.
28. S. Dumitriu (ed.), *Polymeric Biomaterials*, Revised and Expanded, CRC Press, Boca Raton, FL, 2001.
29. M. I. Shtilman, *Polymeric Biomaterials*: *Polymer Implants*, Part I, Brill Academic Publishers, Leiden, the Netherlands, 2003.
30. S. W. Shalaby and K. J. L. Burg, *Absorbable and Biodegradable Polymers*, CRC Press, Boca Raton, FL, 2003.
31. P. K. Chu and X. Liu (eds.), *Biomaterials Fabrication and Processing Handbook*, CRC Press, Boca Raton, FL, 2008.
32. S. C. Anand, J. F. Kennedy, M. Miraftab, and S. Rajendran (eds.), *Medical Textiles and Biomaterials for Healthcare*, CRC Press, Boca Raton, FL, 2005.
33. M. Razeghi, *The MOCVD Challenge*, 2nd edn., CRC Press, Boca Raton, FL, 2010.
34. J. E. Ellingsen and S. P. Lyngstadaas, *Bio-Implant Interface*: *Improving Biomaterials and Tissue Reactions*, CRC Press, Boca Raton, FL, 2003.
35. P. Vadgama, *Surfaces and Interfaces for Biomaterials*, CRC Press, Boca Raton, FL, 2005.
36. P. Chen (ed.), *Molecular Interfacial Phenomena of Polymers and Biopolymers*, CRC Press, Boca Raton, FL, 2005.
37. K. C. Dee, D. A. Puleo, and R. Bizios, *An Introduction to Tissue-Biomaterial Interactions*, 2nd edn., John Wiley & Sons, New York, 2008.
38. D. A. Puleo and R. Bizios, *Biological Interactions on Materials Surfaces*: *Understanding and Controlling Protein, Cell, and Tissue Responses*, Springer Verlag, Berlin, Germany, 2009.
39. L. Di Silvio (ed.), *Cellular Response to Biomaterials*, CRC Press, Boca Raton, FL, 2009.
40. J. Cohen, *Comprehensive Atlas of High Resolution Endoscopy and Narrow Band Imaging*, Wiley Interscience, Malden, MA, 2008.
41. M. A. Reuter, H. J. Reuter, and R. M. Engel, *History of Endoscopy*, Vols. 1–4, Karl Storz, GmbH & Co. KG, Tuttlingen, Germany, 1998.
42. M. A. Reuter, H. J. Reuter, and R. M. Engel, *History of Endoscopy*, Vols. 5–7, Karl Storz, GmbH & Co. KG, Tuttlingen, Germany, 2003.
43. J. R Saltzman, The future of endoscopic technology, *Digestive Disease Week 2004*, http://www.medscape.com/viewarticle/478425 (2009).
44. K. F. R. Schiller, R. Cockel, R. H. Hunt, and B. F. Warren (eds.), *Atlas of Gastrointestinal Endoscopy and Related Pathology*, 2nd edn., Blackwell Science, Malden, MA, 2002.
45. P. B. Cotton and C. B. Williams, *Practical Gastrointestinal Endoscopy*: *The Fundamentals*, Blackwell Science, Malden, MA, 2003.
46. H. Tajiri, H. Niwa, M. Nakajima, and K. Yasuda, *New Challenges in Gastrointestinal Endoscopy*, Springer, New York, 2009.

47. R. A. Natalin and J. Landman, Where next for the endoscope? History of endoscopic urology, *Nature Reviews Urology*, 6, 622–628, (2009).
48. J. G. Gow and H. H. Hopkins, *Handbook of Urological Endoscopy*, Elsevier Health Sciences, New York, 1978.
49. P. L. Dwyer, *Atlas of Urogynecological Endoscopy*, Informa Healthcare, London, U.K., 2007.
50. S. Gordts, H. C. Verhoeven, R. Camp, I. Brosens, and P. Puttemans, *Atlas of Transvaginal Endoscopy*, Karl Storz, GmbH & Co. KG, Tuttlingen, Germany, 2007.
51. S. D. Salman, *An Atlas of Diagnostic Nasal Endoscopy*, The Parthenon Publishing Group, New York, 2004.
52. G. Laytai, S. J. Snyder, G. R. Applegate, G. Aitzetmüller, and C. Gerber, *Shoulder Arthroscopy*, Karl Storz, GmbH & Co. KG, Tuttlingen, Germany, 2006.
53. S. Uchiyama, K. Hasegawa, T. Homma, H. E. Takahashi, and K. Shimoji, Ultrafine flexible spinal endoscope (myeloscope) and discovery of an unreported subarachnoid lesion, *Spine*, 23, 2358–2362 (1998).
54. T. Eguchi, N. Tamaki, and H. Kurata, Endoscopy of spinal cord and posterior fossa by a lumbar percutaneous approach: Endoscopic anatomy in cadavers, *Minimally Invasive Neurosurgery*, 42, 74–78 (1999).
55. T. Eguchi, N. Tamaki, and H. Kurata, Endoscopy of the spinal cord: Cadaveric study and clinical experience, *Minimally Invasive Neurosurgery*, 42, 146–151 (1999).
56. T. Fujimoto, B. P. Giles, R. E. Replogle, H. Fujimoto, S. L. Miller, and P. D. Purdy, Visualization of sacral nerve roots via percutaneous intraspinal navigation (PIN), *American Journal of Neuroradiology*, 26, 2420–2424 (2005).
57. A. Fast and D. Goldsher, *Navigating the Adult Spine: Bridging Clinical Practice and Neuroradiology*, Demos Medical Publishing, LLC, New York, 2007.
58. P. A. Hardy, K. Ellisa, and S. Workman, Spinal endoscopy, a treatment looking for a disease? *Regional Anesthesia and Pain Medicine*, 32. S57 (2007).
59. G. Schütze, *Epiduroscopy: Spinal Endoscopy*, Springer Medizin Verlag, Heidelberg, Germany, 2008.
60. K. A. Zucker, *Surgical Laproscopy*, 2nd edn., Lippincott Williams & Wilkins, Philadelphia, PA, 2000.
61. J. Cueto-Garcia, M. Jacobs, and M. Gagner, *Laproscopic Surgery*, McGraw-Hill Professional, New York, 2003.
62. D. B. Jones, J. S. Wu, and N. J. Soper (eds.), *Laproscopic Surgery: Principles and Procedures*, 2nd edn., Revised and Expanded, Marcel Dekker, New York, 2004.
63. N. J. Soper, L. L. Swanström, and W. S. Eubanks, *Mastery of Endoscopic and Laparoscopic Surgery*, 3rd edn., Lippincott Williams & Wilkins, Philadelphia, PA, 2008.
64. S. A. Giday, P. Magno, and A. N. Kalloo, NOTES: The future, *Gastrointestinal Endoscopy Clinics of North America*, 18, 387–395 (2008).
65. I. Halim and A. Tavakkolizadeh, NOTES: The next surgical revolution? *International Journal of Surgery*, 6, 273–276 (2008).
66. J. L. Ponsky and M. W. Gauderer, Percutaneous endoscopic gastrostomy: A nonoperative technique for feeding gastrostomy, *Gastrointestinal Endoscopy*, 27, 9–11 (1981).
67. J. E. Varela, Single-site laparoscopic sleeve gastrectomy: Preclinical use of a novel multi-access port device, *Surgical Innovation*, 16, 207–210 (2009).
68. C. Y. Kim, R. W. O'Rourke, E. Y. Chang, and B. A. Jobe, Unsedated small-caliber upper endoscopy: An emerging diagnostic and therapeutic technology, *Surgical Innovation*, 13, 31–39 (2006).

69. Y. Tatsumi, A. Harada, T. Matsumoto, T. Tani, and H. Nishida, Current status and evaluation of transnasal esophagogastroduodenoscopy, *Digestive Endoscopy*, 21, 141–146 (2009).
70. J. B. Pawley (ed.), *Handbook of Biological Confocal Microscopy*, 3rd edn., Springer Academic Press, New York, 2006.
71. X. Chen, K. L. Reichenbach, and C. Xu, Experimental and theoretical analysis of core-to-core coupling on fiber bundle imaging, *Optics Express*, 16, 21598–21607 (2008).
72. J. Moore and G. Zouridakis, *Biomedical Technology and Devices Handbook*, CRC Press, Boca Raton, FL, 2003.
73. J. D. Bronzino (ed.), *Medical Devices and Systems*, 3rd edn., CRC Press, Boca Raton, FL, 2006.
74. Microscopix Limited, Endoscope design and assembly, web site at: http://www.ebme.co.uk/arts/scopes/index.htm (2009).
75. J. Baillie, The endoscope, *Gastrointestinal Endoscopy*, 65, 886–893 (2007).
76. M. J. Bruno, Magnification endoscopy, high resolution endoscopy, and chromoscopy; towards a better optical diagnosis, *Gut*, 52, iv7–iv11 (2003).
77. R. V. Stambaugh, G. C. Myers, J. Watenabe, C. Lass, and K. A. Stambaugh, Clinical response to scaling and root planning aided by the dental endoscope, *Journal of Dental Research*, 79, 2762 (2000).
78. R. V. Stambaugh, G. Myers, W. Ebling, B. Beckman, and K. A. Stambaugh, Endoscope visualization of the subgingival dental sulcus and tooth root surface, *Journal of Periodontology*, 73, 374–382 (2002).
79. R. V. Stambaugh, The dental endoscope creates the opportunity for successful periodontal therapy and offers the dental hygienist a tool to aid in definitive scaling and root planning, *Dimensions of Dental Hygiene*, 1, 12–16 (2003).
80. M. D. Noar, Full screen digital image CCD chip transnasal esophagoscopy with disposable endosheath (TNE/DE) is equal to standard video endoscopy as initial screening tool in chronic GERD patients, *Gastrointestinal Endoscopy*, 67, AB129–AB130 (2008).
81. M. D. Noar, Full screen digital image CCD chip transnasal esophagoscopy with disposable endosheath (TNE/DE) is superior to ESO Pillcam (ESO) as screening tool for esophageal pathology, *Gastrointestinal Endoscopy*, 67, AB123 (2008).
82. A. Catanzaro, A. Faulx, G. A. Isenberg, R. C. K. Wong, G. Cooper, M. V. Sivak Jr., and A. Chak, Prospective evaluation of 4-mm diameter endoscopes for esophagoscopy in sedated and unsedated patients, *Gastrointestinal Endoscopy*, 57, 300–304 (2003).
83. N. Yamamoto, K. Hashimoto, C. Hayashi, Y. Ohda, N. Hida, K. Hori, T. Sakagami, H. Ishikawa, T. Matsumoto, and H. Miwa, Does slim endoscope improve the tolerance of patients or do we still need conscious sedation?—A randomized double-blind placebo-controlled study, *Gastrointestinal Endoscopy*, 65, AB322 (2007).
84. G. Gershman and M. E. Ament, Pediatric upper gastrointestinal endoscopy: State of the art, *Acta Paediatrica Taiwanica*, 40, 369–392 (1999).
85. J. E. Pollina, J. A. E. Ibarz, N. G. Martínez-Pardo, M. R. de Temiño Bravo, and R. E. Villacampa, Pediatric endoscopy: State of the art, *Cirugía Pediátrica*, 20, 29–32 (2007).
86. F. F. Willingham and W. R. Brugge, Taking NOTES: Translumenal flexible endoscopy and endoscopic surgery: State-of-the-art procedures, *Current Opinion in Gastroenterology*, 23, 550–555 (2007).

87. J. Raiser and M. Zenker, Argon plasma coagulation for open surgical and endoscopic applications: State of the art, *Journal of Physics D: Applied Physics*, 39, 3520–3523 (2006).

88. M. S. Bhutani and J. C. Deutsch, *Digital Human Anatomy and Endoscopic Ultrasonography*, B. C. Decker, Hamilton, Canada, 2005.

89. C. F. Dietrich (ed.), *Endoscopic Ultrasound: An Introductory Manual and Atlas*, Georg Thieme Verlag, Stuttgart, Germany, 2006.

90. F. Gress and T. Savides (eds.), *Endoscopic Ultrasonography*, Wiley-Blackwell, Chichester, U.K., 2009.

91. J. DeWitt, B. Devereaux, M. Chriswell, K. McGreevy, T. Howard, T. F. Imperiale, D. Ciaccia et al., Comparison of endoscopic ultrasonography and multidetector computed tomography for detecting and staging pancreatic cancer, *Annals of Internal Medicine*, 141, 753–763 (2004).

92. C. J. Lightdale and K. G. Kulkarni, Role of endoscopic ultrasonography in the staging and follow-up of esophageal cancer, *Journal of Clinical Oncology*, 23, 4483–4489 (2005).

93. S. A. Wilson, R. P. J. Jourdain, Q. Zhang, R. A. Dorey, C. R. Bowen, M. Willander, Q. U. Wahab et al., New materials for micro-scale sensors and actuators: An engineering review, *Materials Science and Engineering: R: Reports*, 56, 1–129 (2007).

94. G. de Graaf, L. Mol, L. A. Rocha, E. Cretu, and R. F. Wolffenbuttel, Pre-distorted sinewave-driven parallel-plate electrostatic actuator for harmonic displacement, *Journal of Micromechanics and Microengineering*, 15, S103–S108 (2005).

95. Y. Hou, J.-S. Kim, S.-W. Huang, S. Ashkenazi, L. J. Guo, and M. O'Donnell, Characterization of a broadband all-optical ultrasound transducer—From optical and acoustical properties to imaging, *IEEE Transactions on Ultrasonics, Ferroelectrics, and Frequency Control*, 55, 1867–1877 (2008).

96. T. Pedersen, E. V. Thornsen, T. Zawada, K. Hansen, and R. Lou-Moeller, New technique for fabrication of high frequency piezoelectric micromachined ultrasound transducers, in *Proceedings of the 2008 IEEE International Ultrasonics Symposium*, Beijing, China, 2008, pp. 2115–2118.

97. T. Siu, R. N. Rohling, and M. Chiao, Power density requirement of a 4 MHz micro-ultrasonic transducer for sonodynamic therapy, *Biomedical Microdevices*, 10, 89–97 (2008).

98. S. Vaezy, M. Andrew, P. Kaczkowski, and L. Crum, Image-guided acoustic therapy, *Annual Review of Biomedical Engineering*, 3, 375–390 (2001).

99. I. Rosenthal, J. Z. Sostaric, and P. Riesz, Sonodynamic therapy—A review of the synergistic effects of drugs and ultrasound, *Ultrasonics Sonochemistry*, 11, 349–363 (2004).

100. L. Kociszewski, Passive endoscopes: Idea and state of the art, *Proceedings of the SPIE*, 5566, 127–131 (2004).

101. L. Wu and H. Xie, An electrothermal micromirror with dual reflective surfaces for circumferential scanning endoscopic imaging, *Journal of Micro/Nanolithography, MEMS, and MOEMS*, 8, 013030 (2009).

102. M. Johns, C. A. Giller, and H. Liu, In-vivo optical reflectance measurement of human brain tissue with calculation of absorption and scattering coefficients, in T. Vo-Dinh, W. S. Grundfest, D. A. Benaron, S. T. Charles, R. D. Bucholz, and M. W. Vannier (eds.), *SPIE Proceedings on Biomedical Diagnostic, Guidance, and Surgical-Assist Systems*, Vol. 3595, San Jose, CA, 1999, pp. 70–78.

103. M. Johns, C. A. Giller, and H. Liu, Calculation of hemoglobin saturation from in vivo human brain tissues using a modified diffusion theory model, in T. Vo-Dinh, W. S. Grundfest, and D. A. Benaron (eds.), *SPIE Proceedings on Biomedical Diagnostic, Guidance, and Surgical-Assist Systems III*, Vol. 4254, San Jose, CA, 2001, pp. 194–203.

104. C. A. Giller, L. Hanli, P. Gurnani, S. Victor, U. Yazdani, and D. C. German, Validation of a near-infrared probe for detection of thin intracranial white matter structures, *Journal of Neurosurgery*, 98, 1299–1306 (2003).

105. A. N. Bahadur, C. A. Giller, D. Kashyap, and H. Liu, Determination of optical probe interrogation field of near-infrared reflectance: Phantom and Monte Carlo study, *Applied Optics*, 46, 5552–5561 (2007).

106. E. Kolenovic, W. Osten, R. Klattenhoff, S. Lai, C. von Kopylow, and W. Jüptner, Miniaturized digital holography sensor for distal three-dimensional endoscopy, *Applied Optics*, 42, 5167–5172 (2003).

107. B. Rappaz, F. Charrière, T. Colomb, C. Depeursinge, P. J. Magistretti, and P. Marquet, Simultaneous cell morphometry and refractive index measurement with dual-wavelength digital holographic microscopy and dye-enhanced dispersion of perfusion medium, *Optics Letters*, 33, 744–746 (2008).

108. AcryMed, Beaverton, OR, web site at: http://www.acrymed.com/medical.html (2009).

109. R. Butler, M. Gunning, and J. Nolan, *Essential Cardiac Catheterization*, Oxford University Press, Oxford, U.K., 2007.

110. D. S. Baim (ed.), *Grossman's Cardiac Catheterization, Angiography, and Intervention*, 7th edn., Lippincott Williams & Wikins, Philadelphia, PA, 2006.

111. C. E. Mullins, *Cardiac Catheterization in Congenital Heart Disease: Pediatric and Adult*, Blackwell Science, Malden, MA, 2005.

112. M. J. Stern, *The Interventional Cardiac Catheterization Handbook?*, 2nd edn., Mosby/Elsevier, Philadelphia, PA, 2004.

113. G. B. J. Mancini, Digital coronary angiography: Advantages and limitations, in J. H. Reiber and P. W. Serruys (eds.), *Quantitative Coronary Arteriography*, Springer, New York, 1991, pp. 23–42.

114. L. A. J. Verhoeven, Digital cardiac imaging, *Medicamundi*, 32, 111–116 (1987).

115. G. G. Gensini, *Coronary Angiography*, Futura Publishing, Mount Kisco, NY, 1996.

116. W. C. Sheldon, Trends in cardiac catheterization laboratories in the United States, *Catheterization and Cardiovascular Interventions*, 53, 46–47 (2001).

117. O. M. Weber, A. J. Martin, and C. B. Higgins, Whole-heart steady-state free precession coronary artery magnetic resonance angiography, *Magnetic Resonance in Medicine*, 50, 1223–1228 (2003).

118. G. L. Raff, M. J. Gallagher, W. W. O'Neill, and J. A. Goldstein, Diagnostic accuracy of noninvasive coronary angiography using 64-slice spiral computed tomography, *Journal of the American College of Cardiology*, 46, 552–557 (2005).

119. J. M. Mathis (ed.), *Image-Guided Spine Interventions*, Springer, New York, (2003).

120. D. Kim, R. Fessler, and J. Regan (eds.), *Endoscopic Spine Surgery and Instrumentation*, Thieme Medical Publishers, New York, 2004.

121. H. M. Mayer (ed.), *Minimally Invasive Spine Surgery: A Surgical Manual*, 2nd edn., Springer Verlag, Berlin, Germany, 2005.

122. D. Samartzis, F. H. Shen, M. J. Perez-Cruet, and D. G. Anderson, Minimally invasive spine surgery: A historical perspective, *Orthopedic Clinics of North America*, 38, 305–326 (2007).

123. P. D. Purdy, R. E. Replogle, G. L. Pride Jr., C. Adams, S. Miller, and D. Samson, Percutaneous intraspinal navigation: Feasibility study of a new and minimally invasive approach to the spinal cord and brain in cadavers, *American Journal of Neuroradiology*, 24, 361–365 (2003).

124. P. D. Purdy, T. Fujimoto, R. E. Replogle, B. P. Giles, H. Fujimoto, and S. L. Miller, Percutaneous intraspinal navigation for access to the subarachnoid space: Use of another natural conduit for neurosurgical procedures, *Neurosurgical Focus*, 19, E11 (2005).

125. P. Purdy, Lumbosacral fiberscope, *Journal of Neurosurgery*, 110, 374–374 (2009).

126. K. Shimoji, M. Ogura, S. Gamou, S. Yunokawa, H. Sakamoto, S. Fukuda, and S. Morita, A new approach for observing cerebral cisterns and ventricles via a percutaneous lumbosacral route by using fine, flexible fiberscopes, *Journal of Neurosurgery*, 110, 376–381 (2009).

127. R. D. Howe and Y. Matsuoka, Robotics for surgery, *Annual Review of Biomedical Engineering*, 1, 211–240 (1999).

128. B. Davies, A review of robotics in surgery, *Proceedings of the Institution of Mechanical Engineers—Part H Journal of Engineering in Medicine*, 214, 129–140 (2000).

129. R. A. Faust (ed.), *Robotics in Surgery: History, Current and Future Applications*, Nova Science Publishers, New York, 2006.

130. F. Gharagozloo and F. Najam, *Robotic Surgery*, McGraw-Hill Professional, New York, 2008.

131. V. Bozovic (ed.), *Medical Robotics*, Tech Education & Publishing, Vienna, Austria, 2008.

132. Intuitive Surgical, The development of robotic-assisted surgery, web site at: http://www.intuitivesurgical.com/products/robotic/index.aspx (Retrieved 26 March 2009).

133. G. H. Ballantyne and F. Moll, The da Vinci telerobotic surgical system: The virtual operative field and telepresence surgery, *Surgical Clinics of North America*, 83, 1293–1304 (2003).

134. S. W. Unger, H. M. Unger, and R. T. Bass, AESOP robotic arm, *Surgical Endoscopy*, 8, 1131 (1994).

135. L. K. Jacobs, V. Shayani, and J. M. Sackier, Determination of learning curve of AESOP robot, *Surgical Endoscopy*, 11, 54–55 (1997).

136. B. M. Kraft, C. Jager, K. Kraft, B. J. Leibl, and R. Bittner, The AESOP robot system in laparoscopic surgery: Increased risk or advantage for surgeon and patient? *Surgical Endoscopy*, 18, 1216–1223 (2004).

137. The University of Calgary, NeuroArm web site at: http://www.neuroarm.org/project.php (2009).

138. R. J. Franzino, The Laprotek surgical system and the next generation of robotics, *Surgical Clinics of North America*, 83, 1317–1320 (2003).

139. P. Garcia, J. Rosen, C. Kapoor, M. Noakes, G. Elbert, M. Treat, T. Ganous et al., Trauma pod: A semi-automated telerobotic surgical system, *International Journal of Medical Robotics and Computer Assisted Surgery*, 5, 136–146 (2009).

140. M. S Eljamel, Validation of a neurosurgical robot using a phantom, *International Journal of Medical Robotics*, 3, 372–377 (2007).

141. M. N. Faddis, W. Blume, J. Finney, A. Hall, J. Rauch, J. Sell, K. T. Bae, M. Talcott, and B. Lindsay, Novel, magnetically guided catheter for endocardial mapping and radiofrequency catheter ablation, *Circulation*, 106, 2980–2985 (2002).

142. M. N. Faddis and B. D. Lindsay, Magnetic catheter manipulation, *Coronary Artery Disease*, 14, 25–27 (2003).

143. M. N. Faddis, J. Chen, J. Osborn, M. Talcott, M. E. Cain and B. D. Lindsay, Magnetic guidance system for cardiac electrophysiology, *Journal of the American College of Cardiology*, 42, 1952–1958 (2003).

144. B. Knight, G. M. Ayers, and T. J. Cohen, Robotic positioning of standard electrophysiology catheters: A novel approach to catheter robotics, *Journal of Invasive Cardiology*, 20, 250–253 (2008), See also Catheter Robotics, Inc., Budd, NJ, http://catheterrobotics.com/ (2010).

145. Y. Okumura, S. Johnson and D. Packer, An analysis of catheter tip/tissue contact force-induced distortion of three-dimensional electroanatomical mapping created using the Sensei robotic catheter system, *Heart Rhythm*, 4, S318 (2007), See also Hansen Medical, Mountain View, CA, web site at: http://www.hansen-medical.com/company/default.aspx (2009).

146. J. A. Long, P. Cinquin, J. Troccaz, S. Voros, P. Berkelman, J. L. Descotes, C. Letoublon, and J. J. Rambeaud, Development of miniaturized light endoscope-holder robot for laparoscopic surgery, *Journal of Endourology*, 21, 911–914 (2007).

147. M. O. Schurr, G. F. Buess, B. Neisius, and U. Voges, Robotics and telemanipulation technologies for endoscopic surgery: A review of the ARTEMIS project: Advanced robotic telemanipulator for minimally invasive surgery, *Surgical Endoscopy*, 14, 375–381 (2000).

148. K. M. Reavis and W. S. Melvin, Advanced endoscopic technologies, *Surgical Endoscopy*, 22, 1533–1546 (2008).

149. Scribd, Surgical Robotics—Groups & Work in Progress, web site at: http://www.scribd.com/doc/8053351/Surgical-Robotics-Groups-Work-in-Progress (2009).

150. D. R. Ewing, A. Pigazzi, Y. Wang, and G. H. Ballantyne, Robots in the operating room—The history, *Surgical Innovation*, 11, 63–71 (2004).

151. A. R. Lanfranco, A. E. Castellanos, J. P. Desai, and W. C. Meyers, Robotic surgery—A current perspective, *Annals of Surgery*, 239, 14–21 (2004).

152. K. C. Curley, An overview of the current state and uses of surgical robots, *Operative Techniques in General Surgery*, 7, 155–164 (2005).

153. H. W. R. Schreuder and R. H. M. Verheijen, Robotic surgery, *BJOG: An International Journal of Obstetrics and Gynaecology*, 116, 198–213 (2008).

154. E. Hempel, H. Fischer, L. Gumb, T. Höhn, H. Krause, U. Voges, H. Breitwieser et al., An MRI-compatible surgical robot for precise radiological interventions, *Computer Aided Surgery*, 8, 180–191 (2003).

155. S. Zangos, C. Herzog, K. Eichler, R. Hammersting, A. Lukoschek, S. Guthmann, B. Gutmann, U. J. Schoepf, P. Costello, and T. J. Vogl, MR-compatible assistance system for function in a high-field system: Device and feasibility of transgluteal biopsies of the prostate gland, *European Radiology*, 17, 1118–1124 (2007).

156. H. Elhawary, Z. T. H. Tse, A. Hamed, M. Rea, B. L. Davies, and M. U. Lamperth, The case for MR-compatible robotics: A review of the state of the art, *International Journal of Medical Robotics and Computer Assisted Surgery*, 4, 105–113 (2008).

157. D. Stoianovici, D. Song, D. Petrisor, D. Ursu, D. Mazilu, M. Mutener, M. Schar, and A. Patriciu, 'MRI Stealth' robot for prostate interventions, *Minimally Invasive Therapy & Allied Technologies*, 16, 241–248 (2007).

158. M. Hashizume, MRI-guided laparoscopic, and robotic surgery for malignancies, *International Journal of Clinical Oncology*, 12, 94–98 (2007).

159. D. Manzey, S. Röttger, J. E. Bahner-Heyne, D. Schulze-Kissing, A. Dietz, J. Meixensberger, and G. Strauss, Image-guided navigation: The surgeon's perspective on performance consequences, and human factors issues, *International Journal of Medical Robotics and Computer Assisted Surgery*, 5, 297–308 (2009).

160. G. Hubens, H. Coveliers, L. Balliu, M. Ruppert, and W. Vaneerdeweg, A performance study comparing manual and robotically assisted laparoscopic surgery using the da Vinci system, *Surgical Endoscopy*, 17, 1595–1599 (2003).

161. K. Moorthy, Y. Munz, A. Dosis, J. Hernandez, S. Martin, F. Bello, T. Rockall, and A. Darzi, Dexterity enhancement with robotic surgery, *Surgical Endoscopy*, 18, 790–795 (2004).

162. L. Golenberg, A. Cao, R. D. Ellis, M. Klein, G. Auner, and A. K. Pandya, Hand position effects on precision and speed in telerobotic surgery, *International Journal of Medical Robotics and Computer Assisted Surgery*, 3, 217–223 (2007).

163. M. Tavakoli, R. V. Patel, and M. Moallem, Haptic interaction in robot-assisted endoscopic surgery: A sensorized end-effector, *International Journal of Medical Robotics*, 1, 53–63 (2005).

164. S. Shimachi, S. Hirunyanitiwatna, Y. Fujiwara, A. Hashimoto, and Y. Hakozaki, Adapter for contact force sensing of the da Vinci® robot, *International Journal of Medical Robotics and Computer Assisted Surgery*, 4, 121–130 (2008).

165. E. P. Westebring-van der Putten, R. H. Goossens, J. J. Jakimowicz, and J. Dankelman, Haptics in minimally invasive surgery—A review, *Minimally Invasive Therapy & Allied Technologies*, 17, 3–16 (2008).

166. O. A. van der Meijden and M. P. Schijven, The value of haptic feedback in conventional and robot-assisted minimal invasive surgery and virtual reality training: A current review, *Surgical Endoscopy*, 23, 1180–1190 (2009).

167. T. M. Buzug (ed.), *Medical Robotics, Navigation, and Visualization (MRNV 2004)*, Book of abstracts, Verlag Kreartive Konzepte, Remagen, Germany, 2004.

168. G. Megali, V. Ferrari, C. Freschi, B. Morabito, F. Cavallo, G. Turini, E. Troia et al. EndoCAS navigator platform: A common platform for computer and robotic assistance in minimally invasive surgery, *International Journal of Medical Robotics and Computer Assisted Surgery*, 4, 242–251 (2008).

169. G. P. Mylonas, K. W. Kwok, A. Darzi, and G. Z. Yang, Gaze-contingent motor channelling and haptic constraints for minimally invasive robotic surgery, *Medical Image Computing and Computer Assisted Intervention*, 11, 676–683 (2008).

170. D. Teber, M. Baumhauer, E. O. Guven, and J. Rassweiler, Robotic and imaging in urological surgery, *Current Opinion in Urology*, 19, 108–113 (2009).

171. O. Ukimura and I. S. Gill, Image-fusion, augmented reality, and predictive surgical navigation, *Urological Clinics of North America*, 36, 115–123 (2009).

172. J. R. Korndorffer Jr., D. J. Hayes, J. B. Dunne, R. Sierra, C. L. Touchard, R. J. Markert, and D. J. Scott, Development and transferability of a cost-effective laparoscopic camera navigation simulator, *Surgical Endoscopy*, 19, 161–167 (2005).

173. J. R. Korndorffer Jr., J. B. Dunne, R. Sierra, D. Stefanidis, C. L. Touchard, and D. J. Scott, Simulator training for laparoscopic suturing using performance goals translates to the OR, *Journal of the American College of Surgeons*, 201, 23–29 (2005).

174. L. M. Sutherland, P. F. Middleton, A. Anthony, J. Hamdorf, P. Cregan, D. Scott, and G. J. Maddern, Surgical simulation—A systematic review, *Annals of Surgery*, 243, 291–300 (2006).

175. J. M. Albani and D. I. Lee, Virtual reality-assisted robotic surgery simulation, *Journal of Endourology*, 21, 285–287 (2007).

176. R. A. Bareeq, S. Jayaraman, B. Kiaii, C. Schlachta, J. D. Denstedt, and S. E. Pautler, The role of surgical simulation and the learning curve in robot-assisted surgery, *Journal of Robotic Surgery*, 2, 11–15 (2008).

177. D. W. Lin, J. R. Romanelli, J. N. Kuhn, R. E. Thompson, R. W. Bush, and N. E. Seymour, Computer-based laparoscopic and robotic surgical simulators: Performance characteristics and perceptions of new users, *Surgical Endoscopy*, 23, 209–214 (2009).

178. D. Stefanidis, R. Haluck, T. Pham, J. B. Dunne, T. Reinke, S. Markley, J. R. Korndorffer Jr., P. Arellano, D. B. Jones, and D. J. Scott, Construct and face validity and task workload for laparoscopic camera navigation: Virtual reality versus videotrainer systems at the SAGES Learning Center, *Surgical Endoscopy*, 21, 1158–1164 (2007).

179. S. N. Buzink, S. M. B. I. Botden, J. Heemskerk, R. H. M. Goossens, H. de Ridder, and J. J. Jakimowicz, Camera navigation and tissue manipulation; are these laparoscopic skills related? *Surgical Endoscopy*, 23, 750–757 (2009).

180. J. R. Pluyter, S. N. Buzink, A.-F. Rutkowski, and J. J. Jakimowicz, Do absorption and realistic distraction influence performance of component task surgical procedure? *Surgical Endoscopy*, 24, 902–907 (2009).

181. G. H. Ballantyne, Robotic surgery, telerobotic surgery, telepresence, and telementoring, *Surgical Endoscopy*, 16, 1389–1402 (2002).

182. S. Kumar and J. Marescaux, *Telesurgery*, Springer Verlag, Berlin, Germany, 2008.

183. M. C. Cavusoglu, W. Williams, F. Tendick, and S. S. Sastry, Robotics for telesurgery: Second generation Berkeley/UCSF laparoscopic telesurgical workstation and looking towards the future applications, in *Proceedings of the 39th Allerton Conference on Communication, Control and Computing*, October 3–5, 2001, Monticello, IL, 2001.

184. M. J. H. Lum, D. C. W. Friedman, G. Sankaranarayanan, H. King, K. Fodero, R. Leuschke, B. Hannaford, J. Rosen, and M. N. Sinanan, The RAVEN: Design and validation of a telesurgery system, *International Journal of Robotics Research*, 28, 1183–1197 (2009).

185. C. Nguan, B. Miller, R. Patel, P. P. W. Luke, and C. M. Schlachta, Pre-clinical remote telesurgery trial of a da Vinci telesurgery prototype, *International Journal of Medical Robotics and Computer Assisted Surgery*, 4, 304–309 (2009).

186. J. A. Van Koughnett, S. Jayaraman, R. Eagleson, D. Quan, A. van Wynsberghe, and C. M. Schlachta, Are there advantages to robotic-assisted surgery over laparoscopy from the surgeon's perspective? *Journal of Robotic Surgery*, 3, 79–82 (2009).

187. J. N. Afthinos, M. J. Latif, F. Y. Bhora, C. P. Connery, J. J. McGinty, A. Burra, M. Attiyeh, G. J. Todd, and S. J. Belsley, What technical barriers exist for realtime fluoroscopic and video image overlay in robotic surgery? *International Journal of Medical Robotics and Computer Assisted Surgery*, 4, 368–372 (2008).

188. F. Corcione, C. Esposito, D. Cuccurullo, A. Settembre, N. Miranda, F. Amato, F. Pirozzi, and P. Caiazzo, Advantages and limits of robot-assisted laparoscopic surgery: Preliminary experience, *Surgical Endoscopy*, 19, 117–119 (2005).

189. M. A. Talamini, S. Chapman, S. Horgan, and W. S. Melvin, A prospective analysis of 211 robotic-assisted surgical procedures, *Surgical Endoscopy*, 17, 1521–1524 (2003).

190. G. B. Cadierre and J. Himpens, Feasibility of robotic laparoscopic surgery: 146 cases, *World Journal of Surgery*, 25, 1467–1477 (2001).

191. J. W. Hazey and W. S. Melvin, Robot-assisted general surgery, *Seminars in Laparoscopic Surgery*, 11, 107–112 (2004).

192. P. C. Giulianotti, A. Coratti, M. Angelini, F. Sbrana, S. Cecconi, T. Balestracci, and G. Caravaglios, Robotics in general surgery: Personal experience in a large community hospital. *Archives of Surgery*, 138, 777–784 (2003).
193. P. Francis, The evolution of robotics in surgery and implementing a perioperative robotics nurse specialist role, *AORN Journal*, 83, 629–650 (2006).
194. D. G. Pennington, The impact of new technology on cardiothoracic surgical practice, *Annals of Thoracic Surgery*, 81, 10–18 (2006).
195. S. Ernst, The future of atrial fibrillation ablation, *Heart*, 95, 158–163 (2009).
196. J. D. Burkhardt and A. Natale, New technologies in atrial fibrillation ablation, *Circulation*, 120, 1533–1541 (2009).
197. S. Ernst, F. Ouyang, C. Linder, K. Hertting, F. Stahl, J. Chun, H. Hachiya, D. Bänsch, M. Antz, and K.-H. Kuck, Initial experience with remote catheter ablation using a novel magnetic navigation system, *Circulation*, 109, 1472–1475 (2004).
198. C. Pappone, G. Vicedomini, F. Manguso, F. Gugliotta, P. Mazzone, S. Gulletta, N. Sora et al., Robotic magnetic navigation for atrial fibrillation ablation, *Journal of the American College of Cardiology*, 47, 1390–1400 (2006).
199. R. Kerzner, J. M. Sánchez, J. L. Osborn, J. Chen, M. N. Faddis, M. J. Gleva, B. D. Lindsay, and T. W. Smith, Radiofrequency ablation of atrioventricular nodal reentrant tachycardia using a novel magnetic guidance system compared with a conventional approach, *Heart Rhythm*, 3, 261–267 (2006).
200. A. Aryana, A. d'Avila, E. K. Heist, T. Mela, J. P. Singh, J. N. Ruskin, and V. Y. Reddy, Remote magnetic navigation to guide endocardial and epicardial catheter mapping of scar-related ventricular tachycardia, *Circulation*, 115, 1191–1200 (2007).
201. W. R. Chitwood Jr., E. Rodriguez, M. W. A. Chu, A. Hassan, T. B. Ferguson, P. W. Vos, and L. W. Nifong, Robotic mitral valve repairs in 300 patients: A single-center experience, *Journal of Thoracic and Cardiovascular Surgery*, 136, 436–441 (2008).
202. W. R. Chitwood Jr. and E. Rodriguez, Minimally invasive and robotic mitral valve surgery, *Cardiac Surgery in the Adult*, 3, 1079–1100 (2008).
203. T. Mihaljevic, A. M. Gillinov, C. Jarrett, L. Seto, R. Savage, and P. DeVilliers, Endoscopic robotically-assisted mitral valve repair, *Multimedia Manual of Cardiothoracic Surgery*, 2009(0914), 3608 (September 14, 2009).
204. K. Tsuchida, H. M. García-García, W. J. van der Giessen, E. P. McFadden, M. van der Ent, G. Sianos, H. Meulenbrug, A. T. L. Ong, and P. W. Serruys, Guidewire navigation in coronary artery stenoses using a novel magnetic navigation system: First clinical experience, *Catheterization and Cardiovascular Interventions*, 67, 356–363 (2006).
205. R. G. Bach, C. Leach, S. A. Milov, and B. D. Lindsay, Use of magnetic navigation to facilitate transcatheter alcohol septal ablation for hypertrophic obstructive cardiomyopathy, *Journal of Invasive Cardiology*, 18, E176–E178 (June 03, 2006), Published online at: http://www.invasivecardiology.com/article/5741 (2006).
206. J. D. Ferguson, A. Helms, J. M. Mangrum, S. Mahapatra, P. Mason, K. Bilchick, G. McDaniel, D. Wiggins, and J. P. DiMarco, Catheter ablation of atrial fibrillation without fluoroscopy using intracardiac echocardiography and electroanatomic mapping, *Circulation: Arrhythmia and Electrophysiology*, 2, 611–619 (2009).
207. L. W. Tang, G. D'Ancona, J. Bergsland, A. Kawaguchi, and H. L. Karamanoukian, Robotically assisted video-enhanced-endoscopic coronary artery bypass graft surgery, *Angiology*, 52, 99–102 (2001).

208. S. Dogan, T. Aybek, E. Andreßen, C. Byhahn, S. Mierdl, K. Westphal, G. Matheis, A. Moritz, and G. Wimmer-Greinecker, Totally endoscopic coronary artery bypass grafting on cardiopulmonary bypass with robotically enhanced tele-manipulation: Report of forty-five cases, *Journal of Thoracic and Cardiovascular Surgery*, 123, 1125–1131 (2002).

209. D. de Cannière, G. Wimmer-Greinecker, R. Cichon, V. Gulielmos, F. Van Praet, U. Seshadri-Kreaden, and V. Falk, Feasibility, safety, and efficacy of totally endoscopic coronary artery bypass grafting: Multicenter European experience, *Journal of Thoracic and Cardiovascular Surgery*, 134, 710–716 (2007).

210. Y. K. Mishra, H. Wasir, M. Rajneesh, K. K. Sharma, Y. Mehta, and N. Trehan, Robotically enhanced coronary artery bypass surgery, *Journal of Robotic Surgery*, 1, 221–226 (2007).

211. B. Caynak, E. Sagbas, B. Onan, I. S. Onan, I. Sanisoglu, and B. Akpinar, Robotically enhanced coronary artery bypass grafting: The feasibility and clinical outcome of 196 procedures, *International Journal of Medical Robotics and Computer Assisted Surgery*, 5, 170–177 (2009).

212. R. P. Casula, T. Athanasiou, A. Cherian, R. Bacon, R. Foale, and A. Darzi, Totally endoscopic robotically enhanced coronary artery bypass on the beating heart, *Journal of the Royal Society of Medicine*, 96, 400–401 (2003).

213. M. V. Bashkirov and E. Bennett-Guerrero, Pro: Robotically-assisted CABG is the optimal treatment for coronary artery disease, *Journal of Cardiothoracic and Vascular Anesthesia*, 17, 546–548 (2003).

214. W. Wisser, T. Fleck, D. Hutschala, and E. Wolner, The 3rd hand—A simple but useful tool for beating heart total endoscopic coronary bypass graft-ing (BH-TECAB), *Interactive CardioVascular and Thoracic Surgery*, 5, 519–520 (2006).

215. N. Nesher, I. Bakir, F. Casselman, I. Degrieck, R. De Geest, F. Wellens, W. Willert, Y. Vermeulen, H. Vandrmen, and F. Van Praet, Robotically enhanced minimally invasive direct coronary artery bypass surgery: A winning strategy? *Journal of Cardiovascular Surgery*, 48, 333–338 (2007).

216. A. P. Kypson, Recent trends in minimally invasive cardiac surgery, *Cardiology*, 107, 147–158 (2007).

217. N. Bonaros, T. Schachner, D. Wiedemann, A. Oehlinger, E. Ruetzler, G. Feuchtner, C. Kolbitsch et al., Quality of life improvement after robotically assisted coro-nary artery bypass grafting, *Cardiology*, 114, 59–66 (2009).

218. C. W. Kennedy, T. Hu, J. P. Desai, A. S. Wechsler, and J. Y. Kresh, A novel approach to robotic cardiac surgery using haptics and vision, *Cardiovascular Engineering*, 2, 15–22 (2002).

219. J. Marescaux and L. Soler, Image-guided robotic surgery, *Surgical Innovation*, 11, 113–122 (2004).

220. T. Ortmaier, M. Groger, D. H. Boehm, V. Falk, and G. Hirzinger, Motion estima-tion in beating heart surgery, *IEEE Transactions on Biomedical Engineering*, 52, 1729–1740 (2005).

221. O. Bebek and M. C. Cavusoglu, Intelligent control algorithms for robotic-assisted beating heart surgery, *IEEE Transactions on Robotics*, 23, 468–480 (2007).

222. R. Richa, Philippe Poignet, and Chao Liu, Three-dimensional motion track-ing for beating heart surgery using a thin-plate spline deformable model, *International Journal of Robotics Research*, 29, 218–230 (2010).

223. M. W. Spong and M. Vidyasagar, *Robot Dynamics and Control*, Wiley, New York, 1989.

224. F. L. Lewis, S. Jagannathan, and A. Yesildirek, *Neural Network Control of Robot Manipulators and Nonlinear Systems*, Taylor & Francis, London, 1999.

225. G. A. D. Lopes and D. E. Koditschek, Visual servoing for nonholonomically constrained three degree of freedom kinematic systems, *International Journal of Robotics Research*, 26, 715–736 (2007).

226. H. F. Ho, Y. K. Wong, and A. B. Rad, Robust fuzzy tracking control for robotic manipulators, *Simulation Modelling Practice and Theory*, 15, 801–816 (2007).

227. B. Schmidt, K. R. J. Chun, R. R. Tilz, B. Koektuerk, F. Ouyang, and K.-H. Kuck, Remote navigation systems in electrophysiology, *Europace*, 10 (suppl_3), iii57–iii61 (2008).

228. N. Nathoo, T. Pesek, and G. H. Barnett, Robotics and neurosurgery, *Surgical Clinics of North America*, 83, 1–8 (2003).

229. L. Zamorano, Q. Li, S. Jain, and G. Kaur, Robotics in neurosurgery: State of the art and future technological challenges, *International Journal of Medical Robotics*, 1, 7–22 (2004).

230. M. S. Eljame, Robotic neurological surgery applications: Accuracy and consistency or pure fantasy? *Stereotactic and Functional Neurosurgery*, 87, 88–93 (2009).

231. K. Bumm, J. Wurm, J. Rachinger, T. Dannenmann, C. Bohr, R. Fahlbusch, H. Iro, and C. Nimsky, An automated robotic approach with redundant navigation for minimal invasive extended transsphenoidal skull base surgery, *Minimally Invasive Neurosurgery*, 48, 159–164 (2005).

232. C.-A. O. Nathan, V. Chakradeo, K. Malhotra, H. D'Agostino, and R. Patwardhan, The voice-controlled robotic assist scope holder AESOP for the endoscopic approach to the sella, *Skull Base*, 16, 123–131 (2006).

233. M. Alessandrini, A. De Padova, B. Napolitano, A. Camillo, and E. Bruno, The AESOP robot system for video-assisted rigid endoscopic laryngosurgery, *European Archives of Oto-Rhino-Laryngology*, 265, 1121–1123 (2008).

234. G. S. Weinstein, B. W. O'Malley Jr., W. Snyder, E. Sherman, and H. Quon, Transoral robotic surgery—Radical tonsillectomy, *Archives of Otolaryngology—Head and Neck Surgery*, 133, 1220–1226 (2007).

235. B. A. Boudreaux, E. L. Rosenthal, J. S. Magnuson, J. R. Newman, R. A. Desmond, L. Clemons, and W. R. Carroll, Robot-assisted surgery for upper aerodigestive tract neoplasms, *Archives of Otolaryngology—Head and Neck Surgery*, 135, 397–401 (2009).

236. A. Parmar, D. G. Grant, and P. Loizou, Robotic surgery in ear nose and throat, *European Archives of Oto-Rhino-Laryngology*, 267, 625–633 (2010).

237. P. A. Federspil, U. W. Geisthoff, D. Henrich, and P. K. Plinkert, Development of the first force-controlled robot for otoneurosurgery, *The Laryngoscope*, 113, 465–471 (2003).

238. J. Zhang. K. Xu, N. Simaan, and S. Manolidis, A pilot study of robot-assisted cochlear implant surgery using steerable electrode arrays, *Medical Image Computing and Computer-Assisted Intervention*, 9, 33–40 (2006).

239. A. Tsirbas, C. Mango, and E. Dutson, Robotic ocular surgery, *British Journal of Ophthalmology*, 91, 18–21 (2007).

240. R. Douglas, Robotic surgery in ophthalmology: Reality or fantasy? *British Journal of Ophthalmology*, 91, 1 (2007).

241. V. Swetha, E. Jeganathan, and S. Shah, Robotic technology in ophthalmic surgery. *Current Opinion in Ophthalmology*, 21, 75–80 (2010).

242. T. Theodossy and M. A. Bamber, Model surgery with a passive robot arm for orthognathic surgery planning, *Journal of Oral and Maxillofacial Surgery*, 61, 1310–1317 (2003).

243. A. Metaxas, Advances in the diagnosis of facial asymmetries, *International Journal of Computer Assisted Radiology and Surgery*, 3, 205–211 (2008).

244. A. Hein and T. C. Lueth, Robot control in maxillofacial surgery, in *Experimental Robotics VI*, Lecture Notes in Control and Information Sciences, Vol. 250, Springer Verlag, Berlin, Germany, 2000, pp. 173–182.

245. H. Ishii, H. Koga, Y. Obokawa, J. Solis, A. Takanishi, and A. Katsumata, Development and experimental evaluation of oral rehabilitation robot that provides maxillofacial massage to patients with oral disorders, *International Journal of Robotics Research*, 28, 1228–1239 (2009).

246. A. Azari and S. Nikzad, Computer-assisted implantology: Historical background and potential outcomes—A review, *International Journal of Medical Robotics and Computer Assisted Surgery*, 4, 95–104 (2008).

247. D. Wiechmann, V. Rummel, A. Thalheim, J.-S. Simon, and L. Wiechmann, Customized brackets and archwires for lingual orthodontic treatment, *American Journal of Orthodontics and Dentofacial Orthopedics*, 124, 593–599 (2003).

248. E. Kuo and R. J. Miller, Automated custom-manufacturing technology in orthodontics, *American Journal of Orthodontics and Dentofacial Orthopedics*, 123, 578–581 (2003).

249. M. Y. Hajeer, D. T. Millett, A. F Ayoub, and J. P. Siebert, Applications of 3D imaging in orthodontics: Part II, *Journal of Orthodontics*, 31, 154–162 (2004).

250. A. J. Miller, K. Maki, and D. C. Hatcher, New diagnostic tools in orthodontics, *American Journal of Orthodontics and Dentofacial Orthopedics*, 126, 395–396 (2004).

251. M. Magali, C. Fauquet, C. Galletti, C. Palot, D. Wiechmann, and J. Mah, Digital design and manufacturing of the Lingualcare bracket system, *Journal of Clinical Orthodontics*, 39, 375–382 (2005).

252. H. S. McCrostie, Lingual orthodontics: The future, *Seminars in Orthodontics*, 12, 211–214 (2006).

253. J. M. Palomo, C.-Y. Yang, and M. G. Hans, Clinical application of three-dimensional craniofacial imaging in orthodontics, *Journal of Medical Science*, 25, 269–278 (2005), online at: http://jms.ndmctsgh.edu.tw/2506269.pdf (2009).

254. D. Engel, J. Raczkowsky, and H. Worn, A safe robot system for craniofacial surgery, in *Proceedings of the 2001 ICRA IEEE International Conference on Robotics and Automation*, Vol. 2, May 21–26, 2001, Seoul, Korea, 2001, pp. 2020–2024.

255. D. Engel, W. Korb, J. Raczkowsky, S. Hassfeld, and H. Woern, Location decision for a robot milling complex trajectories in craniofacial surgery, *International Congress Series*, 1256, 760–765 (2003).

256. A. Pernozzoli, C. Burghart, J. Brief, S. Hassfeld, J. Raczkowsky, J. Mühling, U. Rembold, and H. Wörn, A real-time CORBA based system architecture for robot assisted craniofacial surgery, *Studies in Health Technology and Informatics*, 70, 253–255 (2000).

257. H. Wörna and J. Mühling, Computer- and robot-based operation theatre of the future in cranio-facial surgery, *International Congress Series*, 1230, 753–759 (2001).

258. R. D. Katz, J. A. Taylor, G. D. Rosson, P. R. Brown, and N. K. Singh, Robotics in plastic and reconstructive surgery: Use of a telemanipulator slave robot to perform microvascular anastomoses, *Journal of Reconstructive Microsurgery*, 22, 053–058 (2006).

259. T. Grunwald, T. Krummel, and R. Sherman, Advanced technologies in plastic surgery: How new innovations can improve our training and practice, *Plastic and Reconstructive Surgery*, 114, 1556–1567 (2004).

260. S. Saraf, Role of robot assisted microsurgery in plastic surgery, *Indian Journal of Plastic Surgery*, 39, 57–61 (2006).

261. W. L. Bargar, Robots in orthopaedic surgery: Past, present, and future, *Clinical Orthopedics and Related Research*, 463, 31–36 (2007).

262. R. H. Taylor, L. Joskowicz, B. Williamson, A. Guéziec, A. Kalvin, P. Kazanzides, R. Van Vorhis et al., Computer-integrated revision total hip replacement surgery: Concept and preliminary results, *Medical Image Analysis*, 3, 301–319 (1999).

263. A. Bauer, Robot-assisted total hip replacement in primary and revision cases, *Operative Techniques in Orthopaedics*, 10, 9–13 (2000).

264. A. Adili, Robot-assisted orthopedic surgery, *Seminars in Laparosc Surgery*, 11, 89–98 (2004).

265. C. M. Bach, P. Winter, M. Nogler, G. Göbel, C. Wimmer, and M. Ogon, No functional impairment after Robodoc total hip arthroplasty: Gait analysis in 25 patients, *Acta Orthopaedica Scandinavica*, 73, 386–391 (2002).

266. F. Rodriguez y Baena and B. Davies, Robotic surgery: From autonomous systems to intelligent tools, *Robotica*, 28, 163–170 (2010), online at http://dx.doi.org/10.1017/S0263574709990427

267. M. Jakopec, S. J. Harris, F. Rodriguez y Baena, P. Gomes, J. Cobb, and B. L. Davies, The first clinical application of a hands-on robotic knee surgery system, *Computer Aided Surgery*, 6, 329–339 (2001).

268. J. Cobb, J. Henckel, P. Gomes, S. Harris, M. Jakopec, F. Rodriguez, A. Barrett, and B. Davies, Hands-on robotic unicompartmental knee replacement, a prospective, randomised, controlled study of the ACROBOT system, *Journal of Bone and Joint Surgery*, 88-B, 188–197 (2006).

269. W. Siebert, S. Mai, R. Kober, and P. F. Heeckt, Technique and first clinical results of robot-assisted total knee replacement, *The Knee*, 9, 173–180 (2002).

270. W. Siebert, S. Mai, and P. F. Heeckt, Robotics in total knee arthroplasty, in G. R. Scuderi and A. J. Tria (eds.), *Minimally Invasive Surgery in Orthopedics*, Section VI, Chap. 80, Springer Science and Business Media, New York, 2010, pp. 675–681.

271. M. J. Seel, M. A. Hafez, K. Eckman, B. Jaramaz, D. Davidson, and A. M. DiGioia III, Three-dimensional planning and virtual radiographs in revision total hip arthroplasty for instability, *Clinical Orthopaedics and Related Research*, 442, 35–38 (2006).

272. A. L. Carl, and M. Matsumoto, Computer-assisted guidance systems for spinal instrumentation, *Current Opinion in Orthopedics*, 10, 154–161 (1999).

273. Y. Ito, Y. Nakao, T. Manaka, Y. Naka, I. Matsumoto, and K. Takaoka, Advantages of a navigation system to create portals for shoulder arthroscopy: A preliminary investigation *Current Orthopaedic Practice*, 19, 677–681, (2008).

274. A. D. Pearle and M. Citak, Navigation for anterior cruciate ligament surgery, *Current Orthopaedic Practice*, 21, 11–16 (2010).

275. G. H. Ballantyne, Telerobotic gastrointestinal surgery: Phase 2—Safety and efficacy. *Surgical Endoscopy*, 21, 1054–1062 (2007).

276. C. J. Mohr, G. S. Nadzam, R. S. Alami, B. R. Sanchez, and M. J. Curet, totally robotic laparoscopic Roux-en-Y gastric bypass: Results from 75 patients, *Obesity Surgery*, 16, 690–696 (2006).
277. M. J. Curet, H. Solomon, G. Lui, and J. M. Morton, Comparison of hospital charges between robotic, laparoscopic stapled, and laparoscopic handsewn Roux-en-Y gastric bypass, *Journal of Robotic Surgery*, 3, 75–78 (2009).
278. C. Braumann, C. Menenakos, J. C. Rueckert, J. M. Mueller, and C. A. Jacobi, Computer-assisted laparoscopic repair of "upside-down" stomach with the Da Vinci system, *Surgical Laparoscopy Endoscopy & Percutaneous Techniques*, 15, 285–289 (2005).
279. J. Hartmann, C. A. Jacobi, C. Menenakos, M. Ismail, and C. Braumann, Surgical treatment of gastroesophageal reflux disease and upside-down stomach using the Da Vinci® robotic system, A prospective study, *Journal of Gastrointestinal Surgery*, 12, 504–509 (2007).
280. D. Stefanidis, J. R. Korndorffer, and D. J. Scott, Robotic laparoscopic fundoplication, *Current Treatment Options in Gastroenterology*, 8, 71–83 (2005).
281. M. Morino, L. Pellegrino, C. Giaccone, C. Garrone, and F. Rebecchi, Randomized clinical trial of robot-assisted versus laparoscopic Nissen fundoplication, *British Journal of Surgery*, 93, 553–558 (2006).
282. J. Hartmann, C. Menenakos, J. Ordemann, M. Nocon, W. Raue, and C. Braumann, Long-term results of quality of life after standard laparoscopic vs. robot-assisted laparoscopic fundoplications for gastro-oesophageal reflux disease, A comparative clinical trial, *International Journal of Medical Robotics and Computer Assisted Surgery*, 5, 32–37 (2009).
283. J. E. Varela, M. W. Hinojosa, and N. T. Nguyen, Laparoscopic fundoplication compared with laparoscopic gastric bypass in morbidly obese patients with gastroesophageal reflux disease, *Surgery for Obesity and Related Diseases*, 5, 139–143 (2009).
284. C. Tayar, M. Karoui, D. Cherqui, and P. L. Fagniez, Robot-assisted laparoscopic mesh repair of incisional hernias with exclusive intracorporeal suturing: A pilot study, *Surgical Endoscopy*, 21, 1786–1789 (2007).
285. J. Marescaux, J. Leroy, M. Gagner, F. Rubino, D. Mutter, M. Vix, S. E. Butner, and M. K. Smith, Transatlantic robot-assisted telesurgery, *Nature*, 413, 379–380 (2001).
286. J. E. Everhart, Cancer of the gallbladder, National Institute of Diabetes and Digestive and Kidney Diseases (NIDDK), http://www2.niddk.nih.gov/NR/rdonlyres/E9E791A3-AC4E-4B91-9664-63E513B22758/0/BurdenDD_ch11_Jan2009.pdf (2009).
287. V. B. Kim, W. H. Chapman, R. J. Albrecht, B. M. Bailey, J. A. Young, L. W. Nifong, and W. R. Chitwood Jr., Early experience with telemanipulative robot-assisted laparoscopic cholecystectomy using da Vinci, *Surgical Laparoscopy, Endoscopy & Percutaneous Techniques*, 12, 33–40 (2002).
288. T. J. Vidovszky, W. Smith, J. Ghosh, and M. R. Ali, Robotic cholecystectomy: Learning curve, advantages, and limitations, *Journal of Surgical Research*, 136, 172–178 (2006).
289. C. M. Kang, H. S. Chi, W. J. Hyeung, K. S. Kim, J. S. Choi, W. J. Lee, and B. R. Kim, The first Korean experience of telemanipulative robot-assisted laparoscopic cholecystectomy using the da Vinci system, *Yonsei Medical Journal*, 48, 540–545 (2007).

290. S. Jayaraman, W. Davies, and C. M. Schlachta, Getting started with robotics in general surgery with cholecystectomy: The Canadian experience, *Canadian Journal of Surgery*, 52, 374–378 (2009).
291. K. S. Gurusamy, K. Samraj, G. Fusai, and B. R. Davidson, Robot assistant for laparoscopic cholecystectomy, *Cochrane Database of Systematic Reviews*, (1), CD006578, (2009), doi: 10.1002/14651858.CD006578.pub2.
292. J. F. Buell, M. J. Thomas, T. C. Doty, K. S. Gersin, T. D. Merchen, M. Gupta, S. M. Rudich, and E. S. Woodle, An initial experience and evolution of laparoscopic hepatic resectional surgery, *Surgery*, 136, 804–811 (2004).
293. D. Cherqui and J. Belghiti, La chirurgie hépatique. Quels progrès? Quel avenir? *Gastroentérologie Clinique et Biologique*, 33, 896–902 (2009).
294. M. Pai, G. Navarra, A. Ayav, C. Sommerville, S. K. Khorsandi, O. Damrah, and J. R. Jiao, Habib Laparoscopic Habib 4X: A bipolar radiofrequency device for bloodless laparoscopic liver resection, *HPB (Oxford)*, 10, 261–264 (2008).
295. H. M. Abu, T. Underwood, M. G. Taylor, K. Hamdan, H. Elberm, and N. W. Pearce, Bleeding and hemostasis in laparoscopic liver surgery, *Surgical Endoscopy*, 24, 572–577 (2010).
296. P. O. Szavaya, T. Luithle, S. W. Warmann, H. Geerlings, B. M. Ure, and J. Fuchs, Impact of pedicle clamping in pediatric liver resection, *Surgical Oncology*, 17, 17–22 (2008).
297. A. Besirevic, S. Schlichting, V. Martens, P. Hildebrand, U. J. Roblick, L. Mirow, C. G. Bürk, A. Schweikard, H.-P. Bruch, and M. Kleemann, Design and development of sterilisable adapters for navigated visceral (liver) surgery and first practical experiences, *International Journal of Computer Assisted Radiology and Surgery*, 2, S273–S275 (2007).
298. S. Weber, M. Markert, S. Nowatschin, and T. C. Lueth, Concepts for application of a navigated ultrasound aspirator (CUSA) in soft tissue surgery, *International Journal of Computer Assisted Radiology and Surgery*, 2, S275–S277 (2007).
299. M. Feuerstein, T. Mussack, S. M. Heining, and N. Navab, Intraoperative laparoscope augmentation for port placement and resection planning in minimally invasive liver resection, *IEEE Transactions on Medical Imaging*, 27, 355–369 (2008).
300. K. T. Nguyen, T. C. Gamblin, and D. A. Geller, World review of laparoscopic liver resection—2804 patients, *Annals of Surgery*, 250, 831–841 (2009).
301. I. Dagher, N. O'Rourke, D. A. Geller, D. Cherqui, G. Belli, T. C. Gamblin, P. Lainas et al., Laparoscopic major hepatectomy: An evolution in standard of care, *Annals of Surgery*, 250, 856–860 (2009).
302. M. R. Marvin and J. F. Buell, Laparoscopic liver surgery, *Advances in Surgery*, 43, 159–173 (2009).
303. S. Luncă, G. Bouras, and A. C. Stănescu, Gastrointestinal robot-assisted surgery: A current perspective, *Romanian Journal of Gastroenterology*, 14, 385–391 (2005).
304. S. Vasile, O. Sgarbur, V. Tomulescu, and I. Popescu, The robotic-assisted left lateral hepatic segmentectomy: The next step, *Chirurgia*, 103, 401–405 (2008).
305. S. B. Choi, J. S. Park, J. K. Kim, W. J. Hyung, K. S. Kim, D. S. Yoon, W. J. Lee, and B. R. Kim, Early experiences of robotic-assisted laparoscopic liver resection, *Yonsei Medical Journal*, 49, 632–638 (2008).
306. M. A. Machado, F. F. Makdissi, R. C. Surjan, and R. Z. Abdalla, First robotic-assisted laparoscopic liver resection in Latin America (Ressecção hepática robótica. Relato de experiência pioneira na América Latina), *Arquivos de Gastroenterológica*, 46, 78–80 (2009).

307. G. Testa, W. Malago, and E. Benedetti, Liver transplantation—the donor—surgical procedures, adult donor to adult recipient, in R. W. G. Gruessner and E. Benedetti (eds.), *Living Donor Organ Transplantation*, McGraw-Hill, New York, 2007, pp. 477–481.

308. D. Selle, B. Preim, A. Schenk, and H. O. Peitgen, Analysis of vasculature for liver surgical planning, *IEEE Transactions on Medical Imaging*, 21, 1344–1357 (2002).

309. M. Markert, S. Weber, and T. C. Lueth, Manual registration of ultrasound with CT/planning data for hepatic surgery, *Studies in Health Technology and Informatics*, 125, 319–321 (2007).

310. N. Navab, J. Traub, T. Sielhorst, M. Feuerstein, and C. Bichlmeier, Action- and workflow-driven augmented reality for computer-aided medical procedures, *IEEE Computer Graphics and Applications*, 27, 10–14 (2007).

311. B. Dagon, C. Baur, and V. Bettschart, A framework for intraoperative update of 3D deformable models in liver surgery, in *Proceedings of the 30th IEEE Conference of Engineering in Medicine and Biology Society*, Vol. 30, August 20–24, 2008, Vancouver, Canada, 2008, pp. 3235–3238.

312. C. Hansen, J. Wieferich, F. Ritter, C. Rieder, and H.-O. Peitgen, Illustrative visualization of 3D planning models for augmented reality in liver surgery, *International Journal of Computer Assisted Radiology and Surgery*, 5, 133–141 (2010).

313. E. Samset, D. Schmalstieg, J. Vander Sloten, A. Freudenthal, J. Declerck, S. Casciaro, Ø. Rideng, and B. Gersak, Augmented reality in surgical procedures, in *SPIE Proceedings on Medical Imaging*, 6806, 1–12 (2008), doi:10.1117/12.784155.

314. K. J. Oldhafer, G. A. Stavrou, G. Prause, H.-O. Peitgen, T. C. Lueth and S. Weber, How to operate a liver tumor you cannot see, *Langenbeck's Archives of Surgery*, 394, 489–494 (2009).

315. S. Beller, M. Hünerbein, T. Lange, S. Eulenstein, B. Gebauer, and P. M. Schlag, Image-guided surgery of liver metastases by three-dimensional ultrasound-based optoelectronic navigation, *British Journal of Surgery*, 94, 866–875 (2007).

316. Y. Minami, H. Chung, M. Kudo, S. Kitai, S. Takahashi, T. Inoue, K. Ueshima, and H. Shiozaki, Radiofrequency ablation of hepatocellular carcinoma: Value of virtual CT sonography with magnetic navigation, *American Journal of Roentgenology*, 190, W335–W341 (2008).

317. M. A. Machado, F. F. Makdissi, R. C. Surjan, and R. Z. Abdalla, Robotic resection of intraductal neoplasm of the pancreas, *Journal of Laparoendoscopic and Advanced Surgical Techniques*, 19, 771–775 (2009).

318. A. Patriti, G. Ceccarelli, A. Bartoli, A. Spaziani, L. M. Lapalorcia, and L. Casciola, Laparoscopic and robot-assisted one-stage resection of colorectal cancer with synchronous liver metastases: A pilot study, *Journal of Hepato-Biliary-Pancreatic Surgery*, 16, 450–457 (2009).

319. Clinical Outcomes of Surgical Therapy Study Group, A comparison of laparoscopically assisted and open colectomy for colon cancer, *New England Journal of Medicine*, 350, 2050–2059 (2004).

320. S. H. Baik, C. M. Kang, W. J. Lee, N. K. Kim, S. K. Sohn, H. S. Chi, and C. H. Cho, Robotic total mesorectal excision for the treatment of rectal cancer, *Journal of Robotic Surgery*, 1, 99–102 (2007).

321. A. L. Rawlings, J. H. Woodland, R. K. Vegunta, and D. L. Crawford, Robotic versus laparoscopic colectomy, *Surgical Endoscopy*, 21, 1701–1708 (2007).

322. M. H. Whiteford and L. L. Swanstrom, Emerging technologies including robotics and natural orifice transluminal endoscopic surgery (NOTES) colorectal surgery, *Journal of Surgical Oncology*, 96, 678–683 (2007).

323. G. Spinoglio, M. Summa, F. Priora, R. Quarati, and S. Testa, Robotic colorectal surgery: First 50 cases experience, *Diseases of the Colon and Rectum*, 51, 1627–1632 (2008).

324. S. H. Baik, Robotic colorectal surgery, *Yonsei Medical Journal*, 49, 891–896 (2008).

325. S. H. Baik, W. J. Lee, K. H. Rha, N. K. Kim, S. K. Sohn, H. S. Chi, C. H. Cho et al., Robotic total mesorectal excision for rectal cancer using four robotic arms, *Surgical Endoscopy*, 22, 792–797 (2008).

326. S. H. Baik, Y. T. Ko, C. M. Kang, W. J. Lee, N. K. Kim, S. K. Sohn, H. S. Chi, and C. H. Cho, Robotic tumor-specific mesorectal excison of rectal cancer: Short-term outcome of a pilot randomized trial, *Surgical Endoscopy*, 22, 1601–1608 (2008).

327. A. Renda and G. Vallancien, Principles and advantages of robotics in urologic surgery, *Current Urology Reports*, 4, 114–118 (2003).

328. M. M. Nguyen and S. Das, The evolution of robotic urologic surgery, *Urologic Clinics of North America*, 31, 653–658 (2004).

329. H. L. Kim and P. Schulam, The PAKY, HERMES, AESOP, ZEUS, and Da Vinci robotic systems, *Urologic Clinics of North America*, 31, 659–669 (2004).

330. S. Kaul and M. Menon, Robotics in laparoscopic urology, *Minimally Invasive Therapy & Allied Technologies*, 14, 62–70 (2005).

331. V. R. Patel (ed.), *Robotic Urologic Surgery*, Springer Verlag, London, U.K., 2007.

332. P. Mozera, J. Troccazb, and D. Stoianovicia, Urologic robots and future directions, *Current Opinion in Urology*, 19, 114–119 (2009).

333. A. Amodeo, Q. A. Linares, J. V. Joseph, E. Belgrano, and H. R. Patel, Robotic laparoscopic surgery: Cost and training, *Minerva Urologica e Nefrologica*, 61, 121–128 (2009).

334. J. Warren, V. da Silva, Y. Caumartin, and P. P. W. Luke, Robotic renal surgery: The future or a passing curiosity? *Canadian Urological Association Journal*, 3, 231–240 (2009).

335. K. Sairam, O. Elhage, D. Murphy, B. Challacombe, N. Hegarty, and P. Dasgupta, Robotic renal surgery, *Minerva Urologica e Nefrologica*, 60, 185–196 (2008).

336. C. K. Phillips, S. S. Taneja, M. D. Stifelman, Robot-assisted laparoscopic partial nephrectomy: The NYU technique, *Journal of Endourology*, 19, 441–445 (2005).

337. K. Rose, S. Khan, H. Godbole, J. Olsburgh, and P. Dasgupta, Robotic assisted retroperitoneoscopic nephroureterectomy—First experience and the hybrid port technique, *International Journal of Clinical Practice*, 60, 12–14 (2005).

338. S. Kaul, R. Laungani, R. Sarle, H. Stricker, J. Peabody, R. Littleton, and M. Menon, Da Vinci-assisted robotic partial nephrectomy: Technique and results at a mean of 15 months of follow-up, *European Urology*, 51, 186–192 (2007).

339. C. G. Rogers, A. Singh, A. M. Blatt, W. M. Linehan, and P. A. Pinto, Robotic partial nephrectomy for complex renal tumors: Surgical technique, *European Urology*, 53, 514–523 (2008).

340. M. N. Patel, S. A. Kaul, R. Laungani, D. Eun, M. Bhandari, M. Menon, and C. G. Rogers, Retroperitoneal robotic renal surgery: Technique and early results, *Journal of Robotic Surgery*, 3, 1–5, (2009).

341. M. Carini, A. Minervini, and S. Serni, Nephron-sparing surgery: Current developments and controversies, *European Urology*, 51, 12–14 (2007).

342. C. G. Rogers, M. Menon, E. S. Weise, M. T. Gettman, I. Frank, D. L. Shephard, H. M. Abrahams, J. M. Green, D. J. Savatta, and S. B. Bhayani, Robotic partial nephrectomy: A multi-institutional analysis, *Journal of Robotic Surgery*, 2, 141–143 (2008).

343. L. A. Deane, H. J. Lee, G. N. Box, O. Melamud, D. S. Yee, J. B. A. Abraham, D. S. Finley et al., Robotic versus standard laparoscopic partial/wedge nephrectomy: A comparison of intraoperative and perioperative results from a single institution, *Journal of Endourology*, 22, 947–952 (2008).

344. I. S. Gill, K. Kamoi, M. Aron, and M. M. Desai, 800 laparoscopic partial nephrectomies: A single surgeon series, *Journal of Urology*, 183, 34–42 (2010).

345. J. H. Kaouk and R. K. Goel, Single-port laparoscopic and robotic partial nephrectomy, *European Urology*, 55, 1163–1169 (2009).

346. J. H. Kaouk, R. K. Goel, G. P. Haber, S. Crouzet, and R. J. Stein, Robotic single-port transumbilical surgery in humans: Initial report, *British Journal of Urology International*, 103, 366–369 (2009).

347. G. P. Haber, S. Crouzet, K. Kamoi, A. Berger, M. Aron, R. Goel, D. Canes, M. Desai, J. S. Gill, and J. H. Kaouk, Robotic NOTES (Natural Orifice Translumenal Endoscopic Surgery) in reconstructive urology: Initial laboratory experience, *Urology*, 71, 996–1000 (2008).

348. A. D'Annibale, V. Fiscon, P. Trevisan, M. Pozzobon, V. Gianfreda, G. Sovernigo, E. Morpurgo, C. Orsini, and D. Del Monte, The da Vinci Robot in right adrenalectomy: Considerations on technique, *Surgical Laparoscopy, Endoscopy & Percutaneous Techniques*, 14, 38–41 (2004).

349. S. S. Zafar and R. Abaza, Robot-assisted laparoscopic adrenalectomy for adrenocortical carcinoma: Initial report and review of the literature, *Journal of Endourology*, 22, 985–990 (2008).

350. J. M. Winter, M. A. Talamini, C. L. Stanfield, D. C. Chang, J. D. Hundt, A. P. Dackiw, K. A. Campbell, and R. D. Schulick, Thirty robotic adrenalectomies, *Surgical Endoscopy*, 20, 119–124 (2006).

351. C.-C. Abbou, A. Hoznek, L. Salomon, L. E. Olsson, A. Lobontiu, F. Saint, A. Cicco, P. Antiphon, and D. Chopin, Laproscopic radial prostatectomy with a remote controlled robot, *Journal of Urology*, 165, 1964–1966 (2001).

352. A. Tewari, J. Peabody, R. Sarle, G. Balakrishnan, A. Hemal, A. Shrivastava, and M. Menon, Technique of da vinci robot-assisted anatomic radical prostatectomy, *Urology*, 60, 569–572 (2002).

353. J. H. Kaouk, M. M. Desai, S. C. Abreu, F. Papay, and I. S. Gill, Robotic assisted laparoscopic sural nerve grafting during radical prostatectomy: Initial experience, *The Journal of Urology*, 170, 909–912 (2003).

354. J. C. Hu, R. A. Nelson, T. G. Wilson, M. H. Kawachi, S. A. Ramin, C. Lau, and L. E. Crocitto, Perioperative complications of laparoscopic and robotic assisted laparoscopic radical prostatectomy, *The Journal of Urology*, 175, 541–546 (2006).

355. T. Falcone and J. M. Goldberg, Robotic surgery, *Clinical Obstetrics and Gynecology*, 46, 37–43 (2003).

356. T. Falcone, Future directions and development in reproductive surgery, *International Congress Series*, 1266, 107–110 (2004).

357. S. P. Dharia and T. Falcone, Robotics in reproductive medicine, *Fertility and Sterility*, 84, 1–11 (2005).

358. T. Shu, S. Taghechian, and R. Wang, Initial experience with robot-assisted varicocelectomy, *Asian Journal of Andrology*, 10, 146–148 (2008).

359. J. Schiff, P. S. Li, and M. Goldstein, Robotic microsurgical vasovasostomy and vasoepididymostomy: A prospective randomized study in a rat model, *Journal of Urology*, 171, 1720–1725 (2004).

360. C. Fleming, Robot-assisted vasovasostomy, *Urologic Clinics of North America*, 31, 769–772 (2004).

361. G. De Naeyer, P. Van Migem, P. Schatteman, P. Carpentier, E. Fonteyne, and A. Mottrie, Robotic assistance in urological microsurgery: Initial report of a successful in-vivo robot-assisted vasovasostomy, *Journal of Robotic Surgery*, 1, 161–162 (2007).

362. T. Falcone and J. M. Goldberg, Robotics in gynecology, *Surgical Clinics of North America*, 83, 1483–1489 (2003).

363. C. Nezhat, N. S. Saberi, B. Shahmohamady, and F. Nezhat, Robotic-assisted laparoscopy in gynecological surgery, *Journal of the Society of Laparoendoscopic Surgeons*, 10, 317–320 (2006).

364. C. E. Bedient, J. F. Magrina B. N. Noble, and R. M. Kho, Comparison of robotic and laparoscopic myomectomy, *American Journal of Obstetrics and Gynecology*, 201, 566.e1–566.e5 (2009).

365. A. R. Cooper, M. A. Powell, P. T. Jimenez, M. D. Johnson, A. Rabinov, and A. S. Graseck, Comparison of robotic and laparoscopic myomectomy by Bedient et al., *American Journal of Obstetrics and Gynecology*, 201, 625–627 (2009).

366. J. F. Magrina, Robotic surgery in gynecology, *European Journal of Gynaecology and Oncology*, 28, 77–82 (2007).

367. A. P. Advincula and A. Song, The role of robotic surgery in gynecology, *Current Opinion in Obstetrics and Gynecology*, 19, 331–336 (2007).

368. Y. T. Kim, S. W. Kim, and Y. W. Jung, Robotic surgery in gynecologic field, *Yonsei Medical Journal*, 49, 886–890 (2008).

369. A. G. Visco and A. P. Advincula, Robotic gynecologic surgery, *Obstetrics and Gynecology*, 112, 1369–1384 (2008).

370. R. W. Holloway, S. D. Patel, and S. Ahmad, Robotic surgery in gynecology, *Scandinavian Journal of Surgery*, 98, 96–109 (2009).

371. C. Nezhat, O. Lavie, M. Lemyre, E. Unal, C. H. Nezhat, and F. Nezhat, Robot-assisted laparoscopic surgery in gynecology: Scientific dream or reality? *Fertility and Sterility*, 91, 2620–2622 (2009).

372. W. Bentas, M. Wolfram, R. Bräutigam, M. Probst, W.-D. Beecken, D. Jonas, and J. Binder, Da Vinci robot assisted Anderson-Hynes dismembered pyeloplasty: Technique and 1 year follow-up, *World Journal of Urology*, 21, 133–138 (2003).

373. D. S. Veljovich, P. J. Paley, C. W. Drescher, E. N. Everett, C. Shah, and W. A. Peters III, Robotic surgery in gynecologic oncology: Program initiation and outcomes after the first year with comparison with laparotomy for endometrial cancer staging, *American Journal of Obstetrics and Gynecology*, 198, 679.e1–679.e10 (2008).

374. A. V. Hoekstra, A. Jairam-Thodla, A. Rademaker, D. K. Singh, B. M. Buttin, J. R. Lurain, J. C. Schink, and M. P. Lowe, The impact of robotics on practice management of endometrial cancer: Transitioning from traditional surgery, *International Journal of Medical Robotics and Computer Assisted Surgery*, 5, 392–397 (2009).

375. S. T. Lipskind, A. V. Hoekstra, J. M. Morgan, M. P. Milad, and M. P. Lowe, Robotics in obstetrics and gynecology: Training residents in new surgical technology, *Fertility and Sterility*, 92, S124–S125 (2009).

376. A. P. Advincula and K. Wang, Evolving role and current state of robotics in minimally invasive gynecologic surgery, *Journal of Minimally Invasive Gynecology*, 16, 291–301 (2009).

377. C. C. G. Chen and T. Falcone, Robotic surgery: Past, present and future, *Clinical Obstetrics and Gynecology*, 52, 335–343 (2009).

378. R. Gardner and D. B. Raemer, Simulation in obstetrics and gynecology, *Obstetrics and Gynecology Clinics of North America*, 35, 97–127 (2008).

379. R. Moreau, M. T. Pham, R. Silveira, T. Redarce, X. Brun, and O. Dupuis, Design of a new instrumented forceps: Application to safe obstetrical forceps blade placement, *IEEE Transactions on Biomedical Engineering*, 54, 1280–1290 (2007).

380. R. Moreau, M. T. Pham, X. Brun, T. Redarce, and O. Dupuis, Assessment of forceps use in obstetrics during a simulated childbirth, *International Journal of Medical Robotics and Computer Assisted Surgery*, 4, 373–380 (2008).

381. R. Moreau, V. Ochoa, M. T. Phama, P. Boulanger, T. Redarce, and O. Dupuis, A method to evaluate skill transfer and acquisition of obstetric gestures based on the curvatures analysis of the position and the orientation, *Journal of Biomedical Informatics*, 41, 991–1000 (2008).

382. G. van Haasteren, S. Levine, and W. Hayes, Pediatric robotic surgery: Early assessment, *Pediatrics*, 224, 1642–1649 (2009).

383. P. Casale, Robotic pediatric urology, *Expert Review of Medical Devices*, 5, 59–64 (2008).

384. H. Nagar and N. J. Mabjeesh, Decision-making in pediatric varicocele surgery: Use of color Doppler ultrasound, *Pediatric Surgery International*, 16, 75–76 (2000).

385. J. H. Kaouk and J. S. Palmer, Single-port laparoscopic surgery: Initial experience in children for varicocoelectomy, *British Journal of Urology International*, 102, 97–99 (2008).

386. P. Casale, Robotic pyeloplasty in the pediatric population, *Current Urology Reports*, 10, 55–59 (2009).

387. P. Casale, Robotic pyeloplasty in the pediatric population, *Current Opinion in Urology*, 19, 97–101 (2009).

388. J. J. Meehan, S. Elliott, and A. Sandler, The robotic approach to complex hepatobiliary anomalies in children: Preliminary report, *Journal of Pediatric Surgery*, 42, 2110–2114 (2007).

389. D. Kondziolka (ed.), Radiosurgery: *The Seventh International Stereotactic Radiosurgery Society Meeting*, September 11–15, 2005, Brussels, Belgium, Vol. 6, S. Karger AG, Basel, Switzerland, 2006.

390. L. S. Chin and W. F. Regine (eds.), *Principles and Practice of Stereotactic Radiosurgery*, Springer Science and Business Media LLC, New York, 2008.

391. J. C. Chen, D. M. Bugoci, M. R. Girvigian, M. J. Miller, A. Arellano, and J. Rahimian, Control of brain metastases using frameless image-guided radiosurgery, *Neurosurgery Focus*, 27, E6 (2009).

392. A. Pennathur, G. Abbas, N. Christie, R. Landreneau, and J. D. Luketich, Video assisted thoracoscopic surgery and lobectomy, sublobar resection, radiofrequency ablation, and stereotactic radiosurgery: Advances and controversies in the management of early stage non-small cell lung cancer, *Current Opinion in Pulmonary Medicine*, 13, 267–270 (2007).

393. A. O. Dare, K. J. Gibbons, G. M. Proulx, and R. A. Fenstermaker, Resection followed by radiosurgery for advanced juvenile nasopharyngeal angiofibroma: Report of two cases, *Neurosurgery*, 52, 1207–1211 (2003).

394. G. Ambrosino, F. Polistina, G. Costantin, P. Francescon, R. Guglielmi, P. Zanco, F. Casamassima, A. Febbraro, G. Gerunda, and F. Lumachi, Image-guided robotic stereotactic radiosurgery for unresectable liver metastases: Preliminary results, *Anticancer Research*, 29, 3381–3384 (2009).

395. R. Krempien, H. Hoppe, L. Kahrs, S. Daeuber, O. Schorr, G. Eggers, M. Bischof, M. W. Munter, J. Debus, and W. Harms, Projector-based augmented reality for intuitive intraoperative guidance in image-guided 3D interstitial brachytherapy, *International Journal of Radiation Oncology, Biology, Physics*, 70, 944–952 (2008).

396. G. Y. Tan, R. K. Goel, J. H. Kaouk, and A. K. Tewari, Technological advances in robotic-assisted laparoscopic surgery, *Urologic Clinics of North America*, 36, 237–249 (2009).

397. G. W. Dachs II and W. J. Peine, A novel surgical robot design: Minimizing the operating envelope within the sterile field, in *Proceedings of the 28th Annual Conference of the IEEE Engineering in Medicine and Biology Society*, August 30-Sept. 3, 2006, *New York*, 1, 1505–1508 (2006).

398. M. F. McGee, M. J. Rosen, J. Marks, R. P. Onders, A. Chak, A. Faulx, V. K. Chen, and J. Ponsky, A primer on natural orifice transluminal endoscopic surgery: Building a new paradigm, *Surgical Innovation*, 13, 86–93 (2006).

399. J. Buyske, Natural orifice transluminal endoscopic surgery, *Journal of the American Medical Association*, 298, 1560–1561 (2007).

400. C. R. Tracy, J. D Raman, J. A Cadeddu, and A. Rane, Laparoendoscopic single-site surgery in urology: Where have we been and where are we heading? *Nature Clinical Practice Urology*, 5, 561–568 (2008).

401. W. M. White, G.-P. Haber, R. K. Goel, S. Crouzet, R. J. Stein, and J. H. Kaouk, Single-port urological surgery: Single-center experience with the first 100 cases, *Urology*, 74, 801–804 (2009).

402. D. W. Gee and D. W. Rattner, Natural orifice translumenal endoscopic surgery: Current status, *Advances in Surgery*, 43, 1–12 (2009).

403. J. Marescaux, B. Dallemagne, S. Perretta, A. Wattiez, D. Mutter, and D. Coumaros, Surgery without scars: Report of transluminal cholecystectomy in a human being, *Archives of Surgery*, 142, 823–826 (2007).

404. J. P. Isariyawongse, M. F. McGee, M. J. Rosen, E. E. Cherullo, and L. E. Ponsky, Pure natural orifice transluminal endoscopic surgery (NOTES) nephrectomy using standard laparoscopic instruments in the porcine model, *Journal of Endourology*, 22, 1087–1091 (2008).

405. T. Rösch, Who votes for NOTES? *Gut*, 57, 1481–1486 (2008).

406. A. C. Allori, I. M. Leitman, and E. Heitman, Natural orifice transluminal endoscopic surgery: Lessons learned from the laparoscopic revolution, *Archives of Surgery*, 143, 333–334 (2008).

407. F. Thele, M. Zygmunt, A. Glitsch, C.-D. Heidecke, and A. Schreiber, How do gynecologists feel about transvaginal NOTES surgery? *Endoscopy*, 40, 576–580 (2008).

408. L. A. DeCarli, R. Zorron, A. Branco, F. C. Lima, M. Tang, S. R. Pioneer, J. I. Sanseverino, R. Menguer, A. V. Bigolin, and M. Gagner, New hybrid approach for NOTES transvaginal cholecystectomy: Preliminary clinical experience, *Surgical Innovation*, 16, 181–186 (2009).

409. D. Canes, M. M. Desai, M. Aron, G. P. Haber, R. K. Goel, R. J. Stein, J. H. Kaouk, and I. S. Gill, Transumbilical single-port surgery: Evolution and current status, *European Urology*, 54, 1020–1030 (2008).

410. P. F. Escobar, A. N. Fader, M. F. Paraiso, J. H. Kaouk, and T. Falcone, Robotic-assisted laparoendoscopic single-site surgery in gynecology: Initial report and technique, *Journal of Minimally Invasive Gynecology*, 16, 589–591 (2009).

411. A. Menciassi, M. Quirini, and P. Dario, Microrobotics for future gastrointestinal endoscopy, *Minimally Invasive Therapy & Allied Technologies*, 16, 91–100 (2007).

412. D. Oleynikov, Minimally invasive and computer assisted surgery, *Surgical Clinics of North America*, 88, 1121–1130 (2008).

413. V. Karimyan, M. Sodergren, J. Clark, G.-Z. Yang, and A. Darzi, Navigation systems and platforms in natural orifice translumenal endoscopic surgery (NOTES), *International Journal of Surgery*, 7, 297–304 (2009).

414. D. Canes, A. C. Lehman, S. M. Farritor, D. Oleynikov, and M. M. Desai, The future of NOTES instrumentation: Flexible robotics and in vivo minirobots, *Journal of Endourology*, 23, 787–792 (2009).

415. M. Aron, G. P. Haber, M. M. Desai, and I. S. Gill, Flexible robotics: A new paradigm, *Current Opinion in Urology*, 17, 151–155 (2007).

416. H. H. Hopkins and N. S. Kapany, A flexible fibrescope using static scanning, *Nature*, 173, 39–41 (1954).

417. A. B. Slatkin and I. Burdick, The development of a robotic endoscope, in *Proceedings of the 1995 IEEE/RSJ International Conference on Intelligent Robots and Systems*, August 5–9, 1995, Pittsburgh, PA, 1995, pp. 162–171.

418. S. J. Phee, W. S. Ng, I. M. Chen, F. Seow-Choen, and B. L. Davies, Locomotion and steering aspects in automation of colonoscopy, *IEEE Engineering in Medicine and Biology Magazine*, 16, 85–96 (1997).

419. C. A. Mosse, T. N. Mills, M. N. Appleyard, S. S. Kadirkamanathan, and C. P. Swain, Electrical stimulation for propelling endoscopes, *Gastrointestinal Endoscopy*, 54, 79–83 (2001).

420. L. Phee, D. Accoto, A. Menciassi, C. Stefanini, M. C. Carrozza, and P. Dario, Analysis and development of locomotion devices for the gastrointestinal tract, *IEEE Transactions on Biomedical Engineering*, 49, 613–616 (2002).

421. I. Kassin, W. S. Ng, G. Feng, and S. J. Phee, Review of locomotion techniques for robotic colonoscopy, in *Proceedings of the 2003 IEEE International Conference on Robotics and Automation*, September 14–19, 2003, Taipei, Taiwan, 2003, pp.1086–1091 (2003).

422. B. Kim, Y. Jeong, H.-Y. Lim, J.-O. Park, A. Menciassi, and P. Dario, Functional colonoscope robot system, in *Proceedings of the 2003 IEEE International Conference on Robotics and Automation*, September 14–19, 2003, Taipei, Taiwan, 2003, pp. 1092–1097.

423. D. Glozman and M. Shoham, Flexible needle steering for percutaneous therapies, *Computer Aided Surgery*, 11, 194–201 (2006).

424. V. K. Zworkin, Radio pill, *Nature*, 179, 895–898 (1957).

425. R. S. Mackay and B. Jacobson, Endoradiosonde, *Nature*, 179, 1239–1240 (1957).

426. H. G. Noller, Die Endoradiosonde. Zur elektronischen pH-Messung im Magen und ihre klinische Bedeutung, *Deutsche Medizinische Wochenschrift*, 85, 1707–1712 (1960).

427. G. Iddan, G. Meron, A. Glukhovsky, and P. Swain, Wireless capsule endoscopy, *Nature*, 405, 417 (2000).

428. F. Gong, P. Swain, and T. Mills, Wireless endoscopy, *Gastrointestinal Endoscopy*, 51, 725–729 (2000).

429. G. G. Ginsberg, A. N. Barkun, J. J. Bosco, G. A. Isenberg, C. C. Nguyen, B. T. Petersen, W. B. Silverman, A. Slivka, and G. Taitelbaum, Wireless capsule endoscopy, *Gastrointestinal Endoscopy*, 56, 621–624 (2002).

430. A. C. Lehman, M. E. Rentschler, S. M. Farritor, and D. Oleynikov, The current state of miniature in vivo laparoscopic robotics, *Journal of Robotic Surgery*, 1, 45–49 (2007).

431. M. E. Rentschler and D. Oleynikov, Recent in vivo surgical robot and mechanism developments, *Surgical Endoscopy*, 21, 1477–1481 (2007).

432. M. E. Rentschler, S. R. Platt, K. Berg, J. Dumpert, D. Oleynikov, and S. M. Farritor, Miniature in vivo robots for remote and harsh environments, *IEEE Transactions on Information Technology in Biomedicine*, 12, 66–75 (2008).

433. D. Oleynikov, Robotic surgery, *Surgical Clinics of North America*, 88, 1121–1130 (2008).

434. M. Aron and M. M. Desai, Flexible robotics, *Urologic Clinics of North America*, 36, 157–162 (2009).

435. S. J. Bardaro and L. Swanström, Development of advanced endoscopes for natural orifice transluminal endoscopic surgery (NOTES), *Minimally Invasive Therapy & Allied Technologies*, 15, 378–383 (2006).

436. L. L. Swanström, M. Whiteford, and Y. Khajanchee, Developing essential tools to enable transgastric surgery, *Surgical Endoscopy*, 22, 600–604 (2008).

437. L. L. Swanström, Y. Khajanchee, and M. A. Abbas, Natural orifice transluminal endoscopic surgery: The future of gastrointestinal surgery, *The Permanente Journal*, 12, 42–47 (2008).

438. R. Guy Hudson, M. J. Conlin, and D. H. Bagley, Ureteric access with flexible ureteroscopes: Effect of the size of the ureteroscope, *British Journal of Urology International*, 95, 1043–1044 (2005).

439. B. H. Eisner, M. P. Kurtz, and S. P. Dretler, Ureteroscopy for the management of stone disease, *Nature Reviews Urology*, 7, 40–45 (2010).

440. M. M. Desai, M. Aron, I. S. Gill, G. Pascal-Haber, O. Ukimura, J. H. Kaouk, G. Stahler, F. Barbagli, C. Carlson, and F. Moll, Flexible robotic retrograde renoscopy: Description of novel robotic device and preliminary laboratory experience, *Urology*, 72, 42–46 (2008).

441. D. J. Abbott, C. Becke, R. I. Rothstein, and W. J. Peine, Design of an endoluminal NOTES robotic system, in *Proceedings of the 2007 IEEE/RSJ International Conference on Intelligent Robots and systems*, October 29–November 2, 2007, San Diego, CA, 2007, pp. 410–416.

442. S. J. Phee, S. C. Low, Z. L. Sun, K. Y. Ho, W. M. Huang, and Z. M. Thant, Robotic system for no-scar gastrointestinal surgery, *International Journal of Medical Robotics and Computer Assisted Surgery*, 4, 15–22 (2008).

443. C. C. Thompson, M. Ryou, N. J. Soper, E. S. Hungess, R. I. Rothstein, and L. L. Swanström, Evaluation of a manually driven, multitasking platform for complex endoluminal and natural orifice transluminal endoscopic surgery applications (with video), *Gastrointestinal Endoscopy*, 70, 121–125, (2009).

444. K. Xu, R. E. Goldman, J. Ding, P. K. Allen, D. L. Fowler, and N. Simaan, System design of an insertable robotic effector platform for single port access (SPA) surgery, in *The 2009 IEEE/RSJ International Conference on Intelligent Robots and Systems*, October 11–15, 2009, St. Louis, MO, 2009, pp. 5546–5552.

445. I. Kassim, L. Phee, W. S. Ng, F. Gong, P. Dario, and C. A. Mosse, A literature review of locomotion techniques for robotic colonoscopy, *IEEE Engineering in Medicine and Biology Magazine*, 25, 49–56 (2006).

446. S. H. Park, K. B. Lim, and Y. S. Yoon, Design of master console of surgical robot for NOTES, in *Proceedings of IFMBE World Congress on Medical Physics and Biomedical Engineering: Surgery, Minimal Invasive Interventions, Endoscopy and Image Guided Therapy*, Vol. 25, September 7–12, 2009, Munich, Germany, 2009, pp. 144–147.

447. P. Swain, Wireless capsule endoscopy, *GUT*, 52, iv48–iv50 (2003).

448. M. Q.-H. Meng, T. Mei, J. Pu, C. Hu, X. Wang, and Y. Chan, Wireless robotic capsule endoscopy: State-of-the-art and challenges, in *Proceedings of the Fifth World Congress on Intelligent Control and Automation*, June 15–19, 2004, Hangzhou, P. R. China, 2004, pp. 5561–5565.

449. M. E. Riccioni, R. Riccardo, E. Nista, C. Spada, and G. Costamagna, State of the art of capsule endoscopy in Europe, *Endoscopia Digestiva*, 18, 1732–1742 (2006).

450. R. de Franchisa, E. Rondonottia, and F. Villa, Capsule endoscopy—State of the art, *Digestive Diseases*, 25, 249–251 (2007).

451. C. Collins, Miniature passive pressure transensor for implanting in the eye, *IEEE Transactions in Biomedical Engineering*, 14, 74–83 (1967).

452. G. D. Meron, The development of the swallowable video capsule (M2A), *Gastrointestinal Endoscopy*, 52, 817–819 (2000).

453. G. J. Iddan and C. P. Swain, History and development of capsule endoscopy, *Gastrointestinal Endoscopy Clinics of North America*, 14, 1–9 (2004).

454. A. Glukhovsky and H. Jacob, The development and application of wireless capsule endoscopy, *International Journal of Medical Robotics and Computer Assisted Surgery*, 1, 114–123 (2004).

455. S. K. Lo and G. Y. Melmed, Capsule endoscopy: Practical applications, *Clinical Gastroenterology and Hepatology*, 3, 411–422 (2005).

456. G. S. Raju and S. K. Nath, Capsule endoscopy, *Current Gastroenterology Reports*, 7, 358–364 (2005).

457. J. A. Leighton, S. L. Triester, and V. K. Sharma, Capsule endoscopy: A meta-analysis for use with obscure gastrointestinal bleeding and Crohn's disease, *Gastrointestinal Endoscopy Clinics of North America*, 16, 229–250 (2006).

458. D. K. Christodoulou, G. Haber, U. Beejay, S. J. Tang, S. Zanati, R. Petroniene, M. Cirocco et al., Reproducibility of wireless capsule endoscopy in the investigation of chronic obscure gastrointestinal bleeding, *Canadian Journal of Gastroenterology*, 21, 707–714 (2007).

459. R. Eliakim, K. Yassin, Y. Niv, Y. Metzger, J. Lachter, E. Gal, B. Sapoznikov et al., Prospective multicenter performance evaluation of the second-generation colon capsule compared with colonoscopy, *Endoscopy*, 41, 1026–1031 (2009).

460. Z. Fireman, A. Glukhovsky, and E. Scapa, Future of capsule endoscopy, *Gastrointestinal Endoscopy Clinics of North America*, 14, 219–227 (2004).

461. Y. Kusuda, A further step beyond wireless capsule endoscopy, *Sensor Review*, 25, 259–260 (2005).

462. M. Sendoh, K. Ishiyama, and K.-I. Arai, Fabrication of magnetic actuator for use in a capsule endoscope, *IEEE Transactions on Magnetics*, 39, 3232–3234 (2003).

463. G. Ciuti, P. Valdastri, A. Menciassi, and P. Dario, Robotic magnetic steering and locomotion of capsule endoscope for diagnostic and surgical endoluminal procedures, *Robotica*, 28(2), 199–207 (2010), Published online by Cambridge University Press doi:10.1017/S0263574709990361 (2009).

464. A. Uehara and K. Hoshina, Capsule endoscope NORIKA system, *Minimally Invasive Therapy & Allied Technologies*, 12, 227–234 (2003).

465. S. Hwang, J. H. Oh, J. Cox, S. J. Tang, and H. F. Tibbals, Blood detection in wireless capsule endoscopy using expectation maximization clustering, *Proceedings of SPIE on Medical Imaging*, 6144, 577–587 (2006).

466. J. E. Pandolfino, J. E. Richter, T. Ours, J. M. Guardino, J. Chapman, and P. J. Kahrilas, Ambulatory esophageal pH monitoring using a wireless system, *The American Journal of Gastroenterology*, 98, 740–749 (2004).

467. J. M. Pritchett, M. Aslam, J. C. Slaughter, R. M. Ness, C. G. Garrett, and M. F. Vaezi, Efficacy of esophageal impedance/pH monitoring in patients with refractory gastroesophageal reflux disease, on and off therapy, *Clinical Gastroenterology and Hepatology*, 7, 743–748 (2009).

468. T. Ativanichayaphong, S. J. Tang, J. Wang, W.-D. Huang, H. F. Tibbals, S. J. Spechler, and J.-C. Chiao, An implantable, wireless and batteryless impedance sensor capsule for detecting acidic and non-acidic reflux, *Gastroenterology*, 134, A-63 (2008).

469. P. Dario, M. C. Corrozza, and A. Peitrabissa, Development and in vitro testing of a miniature robotic system for computer-assisted colonoscopy, *Computer Aided Surgery*, 4, 1–14 (1999).

470. D. Oleynikov, M. Rentschler, A. Hadzialic, J. Dumpert, S. Platt, and S. Farritor, In vivo camera robots provide improved vision for laparoscopic surgery, *International Congress Series*, 1268, 787–792 (2004).

471. D. Oleynikov, M. E. Rentschler, J. Dumpert, S. R. Platt, and S. M. Farritor, In vivo robotic laparoscopy, *Surgical Innovation*, 12, 177–181 (2005).

472. S. C. Low and L. Phee, A review on master-slave robotic systems for surgery, *International Journal on Humanoid Robotics*, 3, 547–567 (2006).

473. H. Li, G. Yan, and G. Ma, An active endoscopic robot based on wireless power transmission and electromagnetic localization, *International Journal of Medical Robotics and Computer Assisted Surgery*, 4, 355–367 (2008).

474. B. C. Shah, S. L. Buettner, A. C. Lehman, S. M. Farritor, and D. Oleynikov, Miniature in vivo robotics and novel robotic surgical platforms, *Urologic Clinics of North America*, 36, 251–263 (2009).

475. M. R. Marohn and E. J. Hanly, Twenty-first century surgery using twenty-first century technology: Surgical robotics, *Current Surgery*, 61, 466–473 (2004).

476. M. E. Rentschler, J. Dumpert, S. R. Platt, S. M. Farritor, and D. Oleynikov, Natural orifice surgery with an endoluminal mobile robot, *Surgical Endoscopy*, 21, 1212–1215 (2007).

477. A. C. Lehman, J. Dumpert, N. A. Wood, A. Q. Visty, S. M. Farritor, B. Varnell, and D. Oleynikov, Natural orifice translumenal endoscopic surgery with a miniature in vivo surgical robot, *Surgical Endoscopy*, 23, 1649 (2009).

478. J. A. Hawks, M. E. Rentschler, S. Farritor, D. Oleynikov, and S. R. Platt, A modular wireless in vivo surgical robot with multiple surgical applications, *Studies in Health Technology and Informatics*, 142, 117–121 (2009).

479. A. C. Lehman, K. A. Berg, J. Dumpert, N. A. Wood, A. Q. Visty, M. E. Rentschler, S. R. Platt, S. M. Farritor, and D. Oleynikov, Surgery with cooperative robots, *Computer Aided Surgery*, 13, 95–105 (2008).

480. Z. Nagy, M. Flückiger, R. Oung, I. K. Kaliakatsos, E. W. Hawkes, B. J. Nelson, K. Harada et al., Assembling reconfigurable endoluminal surgical systems: Opportunities and challenges, *International Journal of Biomechatronics and Biomedical Robotics*, 1, 3–16 (2009).

481. K. Harada, E. Susilo, A. Menciassi, and P. Dario, Wireless reconfigurable modules for robotic endoluminal surgery, in *2009 IEEE International Conference on Robotics and Automation, Kobe International Conference Center*, May 12–17, 2009, Kobe, Japan, 2009, pp. 2699–2704.

482. J. J. Abbott, K. E. Peyer, M. C. Lagomarsino, L. Zhang, L. Dong, I. K. Kaliakatsos, and B. J. Nelson, How Should Microrobots Swim? *International Journal of Robotics Research*, 28, 1434–1447 (2009).

483. B. Chen, Y. Liu, S. Chen, S. Jiang, and H. Wu, A biomimetic spermatozoa propulsion method for interventional micro robot, *Journal of Bionic Engineering*, 5, 106–112 (2008).

484. G. M. Wang, L. C. Shen, and Y. H. Wu, Research on swimming by undulatory long dorsal fin propulsion, *Frontiers of Mechanical Engineering in China*, 2, 77–81 (2007).

485. W. Khalil, G. Gallot, and F. Boyer, Dynamic modeling and simulation of a 3-D serial eel-like robot, *IEEE Transactions on Systems, Man, and Cybernetics, Part C: Applications and Reviews*, 37, 1259–1268 (2007).

486. G. Kósa, P. Jakab, F. Jólesz, and N. Hata, Swimming capsule endoscope using static and RF magnetic field of MRI for propulsion, in *2008 IEEE International Conference on Robotics and Automation*, May 19–23, 2008, Pasadena, CA, 2008, pp. 2922–2927.

487. G. Chen, M. T. Pham, and T. Redlace, Sensor-based guidance control of a continuum robot for a semi-autonomous colonoscopy, *Robotics and Autonomous Systems*, 57, 712–722 (2009).

488. S. Park, R. A. Bergs, R. Eberhart, L. Baker, R. Fernandez, and J. A. Cadeddu, Trocar-less instrumentation for laparoscopy: Magnetic positioning of intra-abdominal camera and retractor, *Annals of Surgery*, 245, 379–384 (2007).

489. I. S. Zeltser, R. Bergs, R. Fernandez, L. Baker, R. Eberhart, and J. A. Cadeddu, Single trocar laparoscopic nephrectomy using magnetic anchoring and guidance system in the porcine model, *Journal of Urology*, 178, 288–291 (2007).

490. D. J. Scott, S. Tang, R. Fernandez, R. Bergs, M. T. Goova, I. Zeltser, F. J. Kehdy, and J. A. Cadeddu, Completely transvaginal NOTES cholecystectomy using magnetically anchored instruments, *Surgical Endoscopy*, 21, 2308–2316 (2007).

491. I. S. Zeltser and J. A. Cadeddu, A novel magnetic anchoring and guidance system to facilitate single trocar laparoscopic nephrectomy, *Current Urology Reports*, 9, 62–64 (2008).

492. L. W. Fullerton and M. D. Roberts, Correlated magnetic coupling device and method for using the correlated coupling device, U.S. Patent Application Number 12/499,039, Cedar Ridge Research, LLC, New Hope, AL, 2009.

493. J. D. Raman, R. A. Bergs, R. Fernandez, A. Bagrodia, D. J. Scott, S. J. Tang, M. S. Pearle, and J. A. Cadeddu Jeffrey, Complete transvaginal NOTES nephrectomy using magnetically anchored instrumentation, *Journal of Endourology*, 23, 367–371 (2009).

494. J. D. Raman, D. J. Scott, and J. A. Cadeddu, Role of magnetic anchors during laparoendoscopic single site surgery and NOTES, *Journal of Endourology*, 23, 781–786 (2009).

495. J. Cadeddu, R. Fernandez, M. Desai, R. Bergs, C. Tracy, S.-J. Tang, P. Rao, M. Desai, and D. Scott, Novel magnetically guided intra-abdominal camera to facilitate laparoendoscopic single-site surgery: Initial human experience, *Surgical Endoscopy*, 23, 1894–1899 (2009).

496. G. M. Dominguez, Colecistectomía con un trócar asistida por imanes de neodimio: Reporte de un caso, *Revista Mexicana de Cirugía Endoscópica*, 8, 172–176 (2007).
497. A. G. Hunter, Avoidance of bile duct injury during laparoscopic cholecystectomy. *American Journal of Surgery*, 162, 71–76 (1991).
498. S. M. Strasberg, M. Herlt, and N. J. Soper, An analysis of the problem of biliary injury during laparoscopic cholecystectomy, *Journal of the American College of Surgeons*, 180, 101–125 (1995).
499. G. M. Dominguez, Magnetic surgical device to manipulate tissue in laparoscopic surgeries performed with a single trocar or via natural orifices, U. S. Patent Application, USPTO Applicaton No. 20,090,043,246, U.S Patent and Trade Mark Office, Washington, DC, 2009.
500. G. M. Dominguez, Magnetic surgical device to manipulate tissue in labroscopic surgeries or via natural holes performed with a single trocar, International Patent Application No. PCT/EP2008/060338, Pub. No. WO/2009/019288, Crowell & Moring LLP, Intellectual Property Group, Washington, DC, 2009.
501. L. Phee, J. Yuen, D. Xiao, C. F. Chan, H. Ho, C. H. Thng, P. H. Tan, C. Cheng, and W. S. Ng, Ultrasound guided robotic biopsy of the prostate, *International Journal on Humanoid Robotics*, 3, 463–483 (2006).
502. E. C. Pua, M. P. Fronheiser, J. R. Noble, E. D. Light, P. D. Wolf, D. von Allmen, and S. W. Smith, 3-D ultrasound guidance of surgical robotics: A feasibility study, *IEEE Transactions on Ultrasonics, Ferroelectrics and Frequency Control*, 53, 1999–2008 (2006).
503. J. Whitman, M. P. Fronheiser, N. M. Ivancevich, and S. W. Smith, Autonomous surgical robotics using 3-D ultrasound guidance: Feasibility study, *Ultrasonic Imaging*, 29, 213–219 (2007).
504. A. J. Rogers, E. D. Light, and S. W. Smith, 3-D ultrasound guidance of autonomous robot for location of ferrous shrapnel, *IEEE Transactions on Ultrasonics, Ferroelectrics and Frequency Control*, 56, 1301–1303 (2009).
505. C. Böhm, D. Newrzella, and O. Sorgenfrei, Laser microdissection in CNS research, *Drug Discovery Today*, 10, 1167–1174 (2005).
506. X. S. Guo, F. Bourgeois, T. Chokshi, N. J. Durr, M. Hilliard, N. Chronis, and A. Ben-Yakar, Femtosecond laser nanoaxotomy lab-on-a-chip for in-vivo nerve regeneration studies, *Nature Methods*, 5, 531–533 (2008).
507. M. W. Berns, J. Aist, J. Edwards, K. Strahs, J. Girton, P. McNeill, J. B. Rattner et al., *Laser microsurgery in cell and developmental biology, Science*, 505–513 (1981).
508. V. Magidson, J. Lon·arek, P. Hergert, C. L. Rieder, and A. Khodjakov, Laser microsurgery in the GFP era: A cell biologist's perspective, *Methods in Cell Biology*, 82, 237–266 (2007).
509. S. Ninomiya, N. Maeda, T. Kuroda, T. Fujikado, and Y. Tano, Comparison of ocular higher-order aberrations and visual performance between photorefractive keratectomy and laser in situ keratomileusis for myopia, *Seminars in Ophthalmology*, 18, 29–34 (2003).
510. F. W. Medeiros, W. M. Stapleton, J. Hammel, R. R. Krueger, M. V. Netto, and S. E. Wilson, Wavefront analysis comparison of LASIK outcomes with the femtosecond laser and mechanical microkeratomes, *Journal of Refractive Surgery*, 23, 880–887 (2007).
511. J. A. Werner, A. A. Dünne, B. J. Folz, and B. M. Lippert, Transoral laser microsurgery in carcinomas of the oral cavity, pharynx, and larynx, *Cancer Control*, 9, 379–386 (2002).

512. S. M. Shapshay (ed.), *Science and Practice of Surgery Series*: *Endoscopic Laser Surgery Handbook*, Vol. 10, Marcel Dekker, Basel, Switzerland, 1987.

513. M. S. Baggish (ed.), *Endoscopic Laser Surgery*, Elsevier, New York, 1990.

514. K. Hecher and B.-J. Hackelöer, Intrauterine endoscopic laser surgery for fetal sacrococcygeal teratoma, *Lancet*, 347, 470 (1996).

515. R. W. Ryan, T. Wolf, R. F. Spetzler, S. W. Coons, Y. Fink, and M. C. Preul, Application of a flexible CO2 laser fiber for neurosurgery: Laser-tissue interactions, *Journal of Neurosurgery*, 112, 434–443 (2010), online at http://thejns.org/toc/jns/112/2.

516. J. Colombelli, E. G. Reynaud, and E. H. Stelzer, Subcellular nanosurgery with a pulsed subnanosecond UV-A laser (Subzelluläre Nanochirurgie mit einem gepulsten Subnanosekunden UV-A Laser), *Medical Laser Application*, 17, 217–222 (2005).

517. N. Shen, D. Datta, C. B. Schaffer, P. LeDuc, D. E. Ingber, and E. Mazur, Ablation of cytoskeletal filaments and mitochondria in live cells using a femtosecond laser nanoscissor, *Mechanics and Chemistry of Biosystems*, 2, 17–25 (2005).

518. I. Maxwell, S. Chung, and E. Mazur, Nanoprocessing of subcellular targets using femtosecond laser pulses (Nano-Manipulation von subzellularen Strukturen mit dem Femtosekundenlaser), *Medical Laser Application*, 20, 193–200 (2005).

519. J.-C. Diels and W. Rudolph, *Ultrashort Laser Pulse Phenomenon*: *Fundamentals, Techniques and Applications on a Femtosecond Time Scale*, Academic Press, Boston, MA, 1996.

520. A. Shashurin, M. Keidar, S. Bronnikov, R. A. Jurjus, and M. A. Stepp, Living tissue under treatment of cold plasma atmospheric jet, *Applied Physics Letters*, 93, 181501 (2008).

521. M. G. Kong, G. Kroesen, G. Morfill, T. Nosenko, T. Shimizu, J. van Dijk, and J. L. Zimmermann, Plasma medicine: an introductory review, *New Journal of Physics*, 11, 115012 (2009), online at http://iopscience.iop.org/ 1367–2630/11/11/115012.

522. H. Lubatschowski, G. Maatz, A. Heisterkamp, U. Hetzel, W. Drommer, H. Welling, and W. Ertmer, Application of ultrashort laser pulses for intrastromal refractive surgery, *Graefe's Archive for Clinical and Experimental Ophthalmology*, 238, 33–39 (2000).

523. C. L. Hoy, N. J. Durr, P. Chen, W. Piyawattanametha, H. Ra, O. Solgaard, and A. Ben-Yakar, Miniaturized probe for femtosecond laser microsurgery and two-photon imaging, *Optics Express*, 16, 9996–10005 (2008).

524. A. Vogel, J. Noack, G. Hüttman, and G. Paltauf, Mechanisms of femtosecond laser nanosurgery of cells and tissues, *Applied Physics B*, 81, 1015–1047 (2005).

525. S. Chung and E. Mazur, Surgical applications of femtosecond lasers, *Journal of Biophotonics*, 2, 557–572 (2009).

526. R. A. Freitas, Nanotechnology, nanomedicine and nanosurgery, *International Journal of Surgery*, 2005, 1–4 (2005), published online: doi:10.1016/j.ijsu.2005.10.007.

527. D. B. Camarillo, T. M. Krummel, and J. K. Salisbury, Robotic technology in surgery: Past, present, and future, *American Journal of Surgery*, 188, S2–S15 (2004).

528. N. Jalili and E. Esmailzadeh, Vibration Control, in *Vibration and Shock Handbook*, Chap. 23, CRC Press, Boca Raton, FL, 2005, pp. 1047–1092.

529. S. N. Mahmoodi and N. Jalili, Piezoelectrically-driven microcantilevers: An experimental nonlinear vibration analysis, *Sensors and Actuators A*: *Physical*, 1–6 (2009).

530. A. Menciassi, A. Moglia, S. Gorini, G. Pernorio, C. Stefanini, and P. Dario, Shape memory alloy clamping devices of a capsule for monitoring tasks in the gastrointestinal tract, *Journal of Micromechanics and Microengineering*, 15, 2045–2055 (2005).

531. N. Liu, W. M. Huang, S. J. Phee, H. Fan, and K. L. Chew, A generic approach for producing various protrusive shapes on different size scales using shape-memory polymer, *Smart Materials and Structures*, 16, N47–N50 (2007).

532. T. G. Leong, C. L. Randall, B. R. Benson, N. Bassik, G. M. Stern, and D. H. Gracias, Tetherless thermobiochemically actuated microgrippers, *Proceedings of the National Academy of Sciences*, 106, 703–708 (2009).

533. A. M. Popov, Y. E. Lozovik, S. Fiorito, L. Yahia, Biocompatibility and applications of carbon nanotubes in medical nanorobots, *International Journal of Nanomedicine*, 2, 361–372 (2007).

534. I. Agnarsson, A. Dhinojwala, V. Sahni, and T. A. Blackledge, Spider silk as a novel high performance biomimetic muscle driven by humidity, *Journal of Experimental Biology*, 212, 1990–1994 (2009).

535. R. H. Baxter, C. I. Chang, Y. Chelliah, S. Blandin, E. A. Levashina, and J. Deisenhofer, Structural basis for conserved complement factor-like function in the antimalarial protein TEP1, *Proceedings of the National Academy of Sciences*, 104, 11615–11620 (2007).

536. P. Gorostiza and E. Isacoff, Optical switches and triggers for the manipulation of ion channels and pores, *Molecular BioSystems*, 3, 686–704 (2007).

537. R. Numano, S. Szobota, A. Y. Lau, P. Gorostiza, M. Volgra, B. Roux, D. Trauner, and E. Y. Isacoff, Nanosculpting reversed wavelength sensitivity into a photoswitchable iGluR, *Proceedings of the National Academy of Sciences*, 106, 6814–6819 (2009).

538. S. Weihe, M. Wehmöller, H. Schliephake, S. Haßfeld, A. Tschakaloff, J. Raczkowsky, and H. Eufinger, Synthesis of CAD/CAM, robotics and biomaterial implant fabrication: Single-step reconstruction in computer aided frontotemporal bone resection, *International Journal of Oral and Maxillofacial Surgery*, 29, 384–388 (2000).

539. M. J. Curet, Robotics: Past, present, and future considerations, *Seminars in Colon and Rectal Surgery*, 20, 156–161 (2009).

540. S. W. Guyton, Robotic surgery: The computer-enhanced control of surgical instruments, *Otolaryngologic Clinics of North America*, 35, 1303–1316 (2002).

541. W. Korb, R. Marmulla, J. Raczkowsky, J. Mühling, and S. Hassfeld, Robots in the operating theatre—Chances and challenges, *International Journal of Oral and Maxillofacial Surgery*, 33, 721–732 (2004).

7

Regeneration: Nanomaterials for Tissue Regeneration

In the body, the nanoscale structure of the extra-cellular matrix provides a natural web of intricate nanofibers to support cells and present an instructive background to guide their behaviour. Unwinding the fibers of the extra-cellular matrix reveals a level of detail unmatched outside the biological world. Each hides clues that pave the way for cells to form tissue as complex as bone, liver, heart, and kidney. The ability to engineer materials to a similar level of complexity is fast becoming a reality.

Nanomedicine—Nanotechnology for Health,
The European Technology Platform, November 2006

A fundamental issue in much of nanomedicine, and especially tissue regeneration, is to understand and to eventually control nano-structure–biomolecule interactions ... to elucidate the fundamental bases for changes of protein conformation and function on nano-structured surfaces, and hence select responses including those of stem cells...

Joseph H. Nuffer and Richard W. Siegel,
Rensselaer Nanotechnology Center,
Rensselaer Polytechnic Institute,
Troy, New York.

7.1 Introduction: The Role of Nanotechnology in Tissue Regeneration

Regenerative medicine is the practice of rebuilding and restoring function to damaged, diseased, or missing tissues and organs. It involves the promotion of wound healing in soft tissue; the regeneration of bone, cartilage, tendon, and skin tissues; and the replacement of defective proteins in tissue damaged by ischemia, degenerative diseases, or pathogens. Regenerative medicine in some respects encompasses the integration of pharmaceutical, surgical, and supportive care at the nanoscale.

The techniques employed in regenerative medicine include cell and tissue engineering, gene therapy, and delivery of chemical and physical stimuli for the body's own immune, defense, and growth mechanisms.

Cellular engineering includes recruitment or stimulation of endogenous cells to promote healing, as well as exogenous introduction of stem cells or other appropriate explants (Figure 7.1). Tissue engineering includes the application of tissue growth scaffolds and guides, with biochemical and nanosurface engineering to promote the recruitment, adhesion, and organization of cell growth. Gene therapy involves delivery of genetic materials into cells to replace missing or defective protein sources, growth promoters, cell signaling, or immunological components.

Tissue engineering and regenerative medicine can be used to heal tissue damage at its sources rather than treating symptoms. Nanotechnology plays a significant role with biotechnology in implementing regenerative cures that hold out the promise of prolonging and enhancing the quality of life. To develop these possibilities, a number of global research initiatives are in progress.

The Nanotechnology Center for Mechanics in Regenerative Medicine was established with funding from the United States National Institutes of Health. It is an international partnership of researchers at seven institutions: Columbia University; Mount Sinai Medical Center; New York University; the Weizmann Institute of Science in Israel; the University of Heidelberg in Germany; Max Planck Institut für Metallforschung; and ETH, the Swiss Federal Institute of Technology in Zurich.

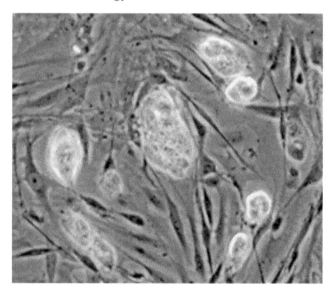

FIGURE 7.1
Stem cells: Nanotechnology is used to design vehicles for delivery, guidance, and tracking of stem cells for tissue regeneration. (Courtesy of Niels Geijsen, Massachusetts General Hospital/ National Science Foundation, Boston, MA.)

The European Commission has initiated a research and development program to create bioinert, bioactive, and resorbable materials for regenerative nanomedicine applications directed toward medical challenges like cancer, diabetes, Parkinson's disease, Alzheimer's disease, cardiovascular problems, and inflammatory and infectious diseases.

Advances in regenerative medicine, tissue engineering, and biomaterials are being pursued around the world. In 2009, the latest developments in Asia were highlighted in Hong Kong at an international conference, Biomaterials Asia 2009, showcasing many significant technological advances in healthcare, including stem cell science, nanomedicine and tissue engineering, and demonstrating that research laboratories and hospitals across Asia are making tremendous contributions in these areas.

Nanotechnology plays an integral role in creating materials and structures for tissue regeneration to match the nanoscale structures of biological cells and connective tissues. In addition, nanotechnology is valuable for the enhancement of surface properties for cell adhesion and protection. Nanotechnology is currently being applied to regenerative medicine with the potential to lead to clinical trials for arthritis, musculoskeletal diseases and disorders, and the renewal of bone, cartilage, disc, ligament, meniscus, muscle, tendon, and skin. Nanotechnology is also being used to monitor outcomes in tissue regeneration by tracking cell distribution, proliferation, and differentiation after cell transplantation [1].

7.2 Biomaterials for Tissue Regeneration

Since the 1970s, the field of biomaterials for tissue engineering has seen the replacement of inert materials with bioactive components capable of eliciting controlled actions and reactions to stimulate and guide cell growth. Bioactive material compositions include glasses, ceramics, glass-ceramics and composites, as well as a range of bioresorbable polymers. These advanced therapeutic materials are the basis for a shift from substitutive medicine to tissue engineering, where the purpose of the implant is to help the body to heal itself. The two technology drivers for these advances have been materials science and nanotechnology. Nanotechnology has opened new abilities for material science to synthesize nanoscale macromolecular structures with finely controlled composition and architecture, corresponding to extracellular matrices present in tissues [1].

Polymer nanoengineering has been a central technology for advancing tissue engineering; polymers can be formulated with high strength, toughness, biocompatibility, biodegradability, and recyclability. Polymers can be combined with each other and with functional biomolecules to tailor properties for specific biomedical applications. The surfaces of polymers can be fabricated with nanoscale features or patterned with nanoscale elements made from other materials to add functionality at the level of cellular membranes, for example, to transfer therapeutic material into cells with arrays of nanoscale fibers [2].

New polymer chemistries and formulations, combined with techniques such as electrospinning, phase separation, direct patterning, and self-assembly, are being used to fabricate structures such as nanofibers, porous scaffolds, nanowires, nanoguides, nanospheres, nano "trees" (dendrimers), nanocomposites, and other macromolecular structures for tissue engineering.

Natural biopolymers such as collagen or even cartilage structures like the larynx can be used with special pre-treatment to remove cells and antigens. Such decellularized materials can be used to form xenograft scaffolding, which can be revascularized and even enervated by the recipient's body.

Another class of important biomaterials for regenerative medicine is the bioreactive ceramics and glasses. In addition to bioactive glasses and glass-ceramics, these include dense hydroxylapatite ceramics and similar materials. These can be formed on the surfaces of strong metal implants to improve their biocompatibility, tissue adhesion, and durability using techniques like electrochemical deposition. They are especially useful in bone restoration and bone and joint implants to bond the implant more naturally to the adjoining tissue and significantly prolong its lifetime. Nanotechnology is guiding the design of nanocomposites with enhanced mechanical properties to reduce fatigue failures due to crack initiation and propagation in implants that undergo physiological loading [3,4].

Other materials that have been newly introduced for tissue engineering include various fibers, carbon nanotubes, diamond-like films, porous silicon, biomimetic materials, and so-called smart or intelligent materials [5–7].

Intelligent biomaterials are engineered at the molecular level to elicit cellular responses for tissue regeneration. These adaptive materials can react to changes in the immediate environment to stimulate specific cellular responses at the molecular level. Molecular modifications of resorbable polymers can direct cell proliferation, differentiation, and extracellular matrix production and organization. In addition, new generations of synthetic polymers can change their molecular conformation in response to changes in temperature, pH, electrical stimuli, or energetic status. Third-generation bioactive glasses and macroporous foams incorporate functionalization to activate genes that stimulate regeneration of living tissues.

Nanomaterials can improve the performance and durability of electrodes used to interface neural prostheses, with better biocompatibility and resistance to the build up of coatings and deposits. Improved electrical properties and better understanding of the interface to cells promise to increase efficiencies of electrical stimulation and lower risk of long term damage to neurons.

Another area in which nanofabricated materials have been applied is for barriers to surround implanted cells and tissues to protect them from the rejection mechanisms of the host, allowing a wider utilization of donated organs.

By contributing to the understanding of the fundamental properties of materials and tissues, nanotechnology is enabling rapid progress in the fabrication of more natural and useful biomaterials for regenerative medicine.

7.3 Nanotechnology and Tissue Engineering

Tissue engineering is the application of biomaterials, biomolecules, and cells to guide the construction, self-organization, and/or growth of renewed living material to replace tissues and functions in the body that have been lost or impaired [8,9]. Tissue engineering is successfully used in clinical applications for replacement of skin, cartilage, and bone, and is beginning to be tested for replacement of muscle and nerve tissue. Conceptual and experimental work is being done to replace and regenerate complex organs like the pancreas.

Tissue engineering can be considered a more advanced and natural approach to the aims of prosthetics for replacement of body parts. Traditionally, prosthetics has focused on replacement of functionality of mechanical, neuromuscular, and sensory organs, whereas tissue engineering has focused on tissue and organs with structural and biochemical functions. Tissue engineering in its current state of development can be considered to be in transition from the concept of substitution medicine, where a laboratory grown "spare part" is implanted in the body to compensate for lost tissue, toward the concept of guidance and stimulation of the body's own healing mechanisms.

The ultimate goal of tissue engineering is to support a fully capable regenerative medicine by initiating and controlling the regeneration of tissue by use of cell-signaling and cell programming. When realized, these capabilities would lead to treatments and prevention for chronic disabling diseases such as diabetes, osteoarthritis, cardiovascular disease, and degenerative disorders of the central nervous system.

Nanotechnology-assisted regenerative medicine promises a path for development of cost-effective therapies for in situ tissue regeneration, guidance of tissue growth, and halting or reversal of pathological processes. Nanotechnology is providing the tools to initiate and control the regenerative process by fabrication of scaffolds and delivery of signaling molecules and stem cells. These tools enable effective application of the growing understanding of the basic biology of tissue regeneration, which is being gained by elucidation of cellular and molecular mechanisms on the nanoscale.

Thus, nanotechnology-based tissue engineering is enabling the emergence of regenerative medicine through three interrelated areas: nanoengineering of biomaterials and scaffolds, controlled delivery of signaling biomolecules, and delivery and shepherding of cells, especially stem cells for tissue regeneration.

7.3.1 Bioactive Scaffold-Guided Tissue Regeneration

Tissue engineering uses techniques such as scaffold-guided tissue regeneration, with the seeding of porous, biodegradable scaffolds with donor cells, which become differentiated and replace the structure and function of naturally occurring tissues. These tissue-engineered constructs can be grown in place or outside the body, and then implanted into the patient. In successful tissue engineering, the bioengineered tissues are accepted by the host body and vascularized and enervated with the ingrowth of viable blood supplies and nerves. The scaffolds can be composed of inert materials, a natural biomaterial, or a biodegradable compound, which is resorbed over time and replaced by host tissues [10,11].

Scaffolding should have good properties for cell adhesion and binding to connective tissue and, if appropriate, bone material. Depending on the application, porosity-allowing cells and cell extensions to penetrate the material may be needed. Major areas for the application of tissue scaffolding are treatment of burns for regrowth of skin, guiding and stimulating regrowth of bone after surgery or injury, reconstruction and growth of ligaments and connective tissues, and guiding regrowth of nerves. This is a large field with many materials being developed and applied to many tissue types [12].

Artificial constructs or autologous material from the patient's own body may be borrowed for use in fabricating scaffolds and implants. The most recent advanced techniques use adult stem cells to seed scaffolds with regenerative cells. Scaffolds and implants are also being infused with cell-signaling molecules, which act as molecular regeneration messengers.

Cells in natural tissues are held in place by an extracellular matrix with exquisitely sophisticated nanostructures made up of adhesive and connective macromolecules, with connective and adhesive proteins, peptides and other biomolecules. By immobilizing these molecules onto a scaffold, it is possible to provide a cell-adhesive surface that mimics the natural extracellular environment. Polymer surfaces can be tailored with proteins that influence cell-specific interactions for endothelium, synaptic development, and neurite stimulation. Cellular recognition factors can be incorporated into resorbable polymers, including adhesive proteins, integrins, fibronectin, and functional domains of extracellular matrix components. Artificial cell growth environments are being developed with nanoengineered materials that incorporate natural polymers or with structures that combine synthetic molecules with extracellular matrix signaling cues.

7.3.2 Nanotechnology and Cellular Signaling

Signaling biomolecules control the growth and metabolism of cells. They include hormones, growth factors, receptors, cytokines, histamines, and other messenger molecules, which trigger regenerative activity. Regulation of growth, inflammation, calcium binding, healing, and other processes are controlled by a complex signaling network, with dynamic cascades of chemical interchanges and responses. Understanding the correct signaling sequences is necessary for the fabrication and repair of tissues.

Nanoengineering of techniques and materials will be required for the controlled delivery of proteins, peptides, and genes to guide tissue regeneration. Current techniques are moving beyond the release of single growth factors toward more sophisticated sequential delivery of signaling cascades that reproduce the processes followed by natural networks that control cell growth and healing. Nanotechnologies will be critical for the development of therapies involving the activation and spatiotemporal control of tissue regeneration.

Nanotechnologies will enable the development of bioactive materials, which release signaling molecules in controlled sequences and rates to activate cells and initiate a cascading growth process. This process will continue as multiple generations of cells release additional growth factors to guide self-assembly of functional new tissues in their environment.

7.3.3 Cell Transplants and Nanotechnology

Cells for use in tissue engineering can come from several types of sources. Tissue explants, consisting of sections of organized tissue containing large numbers of cells and supporting matrix, can be transplanted in surgical procedures. Examples are skin transplants for burn treatment and liver lobe transplants. Transplanted tissue can be harvested from a healthy part of the patient's body, or from a donor matched for tissue compatibility. Nanotechnology can play a role in this type of transplant through matrices, tools, and surgical glues (see Chapter 8). Smaller units of tissue can be useful as sources of new cells or structural material for restoration. Biopolymers such as heart valves, lenses, cartilage structures, and even nerve sheaths can be transplanted, sometimes after treatment to remove cells and immunogenic substances [13].

In terms of the uses of medical nanotechnology, we are interested primarily in cells. With cells, rather than merely substituting replacement parts, there is a greater potential to grow and regenerate new tissue. Cells for transplantation can be harvested from intact tissues of the same type as the tissue to be restored, from donors, or from stem cells. (Figure 7.1). Cells differ greatly in their potential to adapt and multiply. Stem cells are cells that are capable of multiplying to replace tissue. There are many types of stem cells, ranging from embryonic pluripotent stem cells, which have the potential to differentiate into any type of tissue found in the body, to somatic or progenitor stem cells, which give rise only to specialized differentiated tissues. A third source of stem cells comes from stimulating differentiated cells to revert to a progenitor-like state. These are called induced pluripotent stem cells (iPSCs); they have become more important as nanotechnology has opened possibilities for directing their growth in the restoration of tissues.

7.3.4 Stem Cell–Based Therapies

Cellular growth, differentiation, and apoptosis take place continually in mammals from embryological development to maturity. This process of cell turnover continues through adult life to maintain the body and to repair injury. Maintaining the homeostasis of the organism involves a continuous process of renewal that is fed by stem cells, which multiply and mature into progenitor and fully differentiated specialized cells (somatic stem cells). This has led to the strategy of using stem cells from various sources to seed the renewal of tissues.

Stem cells are most evidently present and active during the rapid stages of embryonic growth and development, but research has led to the understanding that some stem cells continue as the source of tissue renewal throughout the life cycle of an individual. As the mechanisms of cell growth and differentiation have become better understood, efforts are succeeding to harvest and culture fully potent stem cells from adult organs, and to reprogram mature cells into less differentiated, pluripotent stem cells. Autologous stem cells harvested or reverse programmed from an individual's own cells not only eliminate risks of rejection and transfer of pathologies, but make moot the very real moral objections to using human embryos as a source of stem cells for research and therapy.

Cellular turnover takes place at different rates in different types of tissue. Cellular turnover is relatively rapid, for example, in intestinal epithelium, blood, and epidermis, and slow in bone and cartilage. Tissue self-renewal was long considered limited or nonexistent in tissues such as the brain and the heart, but research in recent years has shown that these tissues not only can recover from injury, given the right conditions, but also undergo turnover and renewal to maintain normal health. This radical new perspective has refocused research into mechanisms for healing and renewal of vital organs following degeneration, disease, trauma, or ischemic injury.

These two new understandings—of the role and source of stem cells in the body, and of the plasticity of vital differentiated tissues—have raised hopes of harnessing the enormous self-repair potential of adult stem cells for therapeutic purposes and re-energized research into regenerative medicine.

Current tissue engineering therapies are largely based on harvesting autologous differentiated cells, and growing them in culture or fixing them in scaffolding for reimplantation. The potential use of endogenous undifferentiated stem cells opens the way toward a new generation of cell-based regeneration therapies. The use of stem cells to seed regeneration could reduce the complexity and amount of material needed to build scaffolding, and increase the potential for self-assembly and self-healing. Realizing this potential will require better understanding of the signaling systems that control stem cell development, differentiation, and organization into tissues.

7.3.5 Future Directions in Stem Cell–Based Tissue Engineering

Nanotechnology is playing a significant role in research to elucidate the molecular basis of cell growth, and in the design of biomaterials and scaffolds for tissue engineering that can provide for tissue regeneration and repair with minimally invasive surgery.

Research is ongoing to use nanotechnology for efficient harvesting, reprogramming, and delivery of adult stem cells, and for development of intelligent bioactive materials to serve as administration and growth support vehicles. An ultimate vision would be the development of implantable, cell-free, intelligent, bioactive materials that would provide signaling to initiate, promote, and guide self-healing by the patients own stem cells. This approach integrates the concepts of biomaterial scaffolding, cell signaling, and stem cell therapy into a single, unified nanotechnology-based therapy. Nanotechnology is both a disruptive and an integrative force in innovation.

A related goal is the use of bioactive stimuli to activate, silence, and regulate genes as a regenerative or even a preventative therapy. This would open the possibility of forestalling or preventing many diseases and degenerative processes, even maintaining the vigor of tissues that would otherwise undergo deteriorations associated with aging.

Any healing or treatment strategy based on genes carries the implication of therapy tailored to individual genomes and phenotypes. This opens an entire new vista of personalized medicine, which is being made possible by nanotechnology-driven improvements in the speed and cost of determining genotypes. All of our explorations of the impacts of nanotechnology—on diagnostics, drug delivery, and regenerative medicine—lead to the new potential of personalized medicine. We will come back to this subject later, but first we will survey some specific examples of biomaterials and tissue engineering.

7.3.6 Nanoencapsulation of Cells and Tissues

One of the important applications of nanoengineered biomaterials is for encapsulation of tissues to protect them from the action of the immune system and other disruptions. Encapsulation of cells and tissues is a special case of tissue scaffolding. The primary motivation for cell and tissue encapsulation is for immunoprotection. Transplantation of encapsulated or scaffolded cells is a promising therapy for the replacement of complex tissues, whether with stem cell therapies, or using normal or genetically engineered adult cells [14].

The loss of specialized differentiated tissues is a feature of many serious and difficult to treat conditions, including diseases of the endocrine system (diabetes, hypoparathyroidism, adrenal insufficiency), the central nervous system (Parkinson's, Alzheimer's, ALS, Huntington's), liver failure, kidney failure, heart disease, and cancer. In many cases, such as diabetes, the loss of the patient's tissues is severe or complete, involving highly specialized cells and tissues, so there is no opportunity for the transplantation of allogeneic cells of the same functional type.

In such cases, xenogeneic cell transplants are a potential therapy, provided rejection by the recipient's immune system can be avoided, suppressed, or managed. Tissue matching and immunosuppressive therapies have limitations of efficiency, cost, and effectiveness, especially for complex tissues. An alternative approach is the isolation of transplanted cells from the host immune system using semipermeable barriers, which allow nutrients and cell-signaling biomolecules to pass, but block antibodies and white blood cells. Research has been pursued for decades on immunoisolation devices capable of protecting transplanted allo- and xenogeneic cells from rejection, while facilitating adequate transport of oxygen, nutrients, and secreted therapeutic molecules [14–16]. In these systems, the capsules are sized in hundreds of micrometers to accommodate cells, but nanotechnology is highly relevant in the design of functional surfaces and pores and in their fabrication and assembly [17].

In Chapters 5 and 6, we reviewed the encapsulation of cells where the focus was on delivery of therapeutic biomolecules—insulin. For this purpose, a number of encapsulation materials and systems for live cells have been developed and tested, including alumina [18], silica [19,20], and various polymer materials. To date, the greatest success has been with alginate-based materials. In particular, alginate-based microencapsulation has been used successfully to implant human islets of Langerhans into immunocompetent diabetic mice [21–23]. Microencapsulation has been used to transplant individual insulin-producing beta cells as well as living islets of Langerhans. In both cases, many of the same technologies are used for encapsulation [21–26].

In addition to insulin-producing cells, development has also been carried out for implanting cells in immunoprotected biocapsules for the promotion of tissue replacement in the central nervous system. One application of this line of research is aimed at the potential treatment of Alzheimer's disease, Huntington's chorea, and other neurodegenerative diseases. The implants contain cells that are genetically engineered to secrete human nerve growth factor. The cells are encapsulated in a semipermeable polymer membrane and the device is surgically implanted into the target area of the brain, thus bypassing the blood–brain barrier, while isolating the foreign cells from the patient's immune system [27].

Cellular encapsulation has been used as a tool for fundamental cell signaling research. Polymer microcapsules were nanoengineered for permeability and biocompatibility to isolate different types of cells in order to separate and identify their signaling biomolecules. Different cell types are isolated in the capsules and grown in a common environment to study their signaling dynamics. This approach has been used to analyze drug metabolism, intercellular regulations, and metabolic pathways [28].

This technique was used to study the interactions between murine liver cells and adipocytes, measuring transaminase activity, urea synthesis, and protein secretion. The multicomponent polymer capsules were formed by polyelectrolyte complexation between sodium alginate, cellulose sulphate, and poly(methylene-*co*-guanidine) hydrochloride, for which the permeability was characterized. Absence of cytotoxicity and excellent biocompatibility of the capsules was demonstrated toward the hepatocytes, which are difficult to culture. Encapsulated hepatocytes retained their specific functions, and measurements confirmed identical profiles between free and embedded adipocytes [28].

Encapsulation has also been proposed for use in the establishment of a tissue bank for storage and supply of murine hepatocytes and other cells used in research [28].

An encapsulation device for study of molecules released from transplanted cells in the brain was developed, with a refillable capsule for introducing cells into the brain while keeping them physically isolated from contact with brain tissue by means of a semipermeable membrane. The cell-containing insert can be introduced or removed to study the influence of soluble factors released from transplanted cells over time. It has been used in a rat model of Parkinson's disease to study how implanted cells influence remodeling of central nervous system tissue, to better understand the dosing and mechanism of action of soluble factors released by the cells [29].

Encapsulation and immobilization of cells and enzymes have also been used in the fabrication of sensitive and selective biosensors for fundamental research, with potential for the development of medical monitors. This will be discussed in Chapter 9.

In tissue engineering, encapsulation is used as a technique for cell immobilization and assembly, in order to organize three-dimensional scaffold structures [30–32]. These three-dimensional encapsulation structures are used as research tools as well as for tissue regeneration. For example, an encapsulation framework allows mouse embryonic stem cells used for research to stay in the undifferentiated state longer than with conventional culture dishes, by providing an microenvironment similar to the in vivo extracellular matrix, but with isolation from cell signaling. This approach facilitates the study of stem cells without the disadvantages of growing them in live animal models.

For tissue regeneration scaffolds, temporary encapsulation in biodegradable or resorbable material is generally used. Alternatively, natural or biocompatible polymer or ceramic can be used to make a three-dimensional encapsulated scaffolding with pores for vascularization and enervation. Thus, our discussion of encapsulation leads into the consideration of tissue scaffolding.

From the nanomedicine drug delivery point of view reviewed in Chapter 5, the purpose of cellular encapsulation is to provide delivery of a therapeutic substance without regard to structural or other functionality of the encapsulated cells [33]. The goal is long-term delivery of the therapeutic substance without focus on the eventual integration of transplanted cells into the host organs. From the broader perspective of regenerative medicine, the focus is on protecting whole systems of tissues or even whole organs, with the possibility of their functioning permanently as a whole in the host body, or growing and integrating seamlessly. An intermediate viewpoint is the use of resorbable or discardable materials for the delivery of healing promoters during the regeneration process, after which the implant can be biodegraded, rejected, or removed.

Yet another approach is the engineering of artificial organs, which may or may not include living encapsulated cells, but which are designed to function as an entire replacement for complex units such as the pancreas, liver, kidney, or even the heart or eye. The design of artificial organs and artificial cells or bioreactors may be considered as a development of the prosthetics or substitutional medicine paradigm from the mechanical and neuromuscular arena into the biochemical and cell-signaling domain.

There are no sharp dividing lines between these various approaches just as there are none between tissue engineering, drug delivery, and surgery. The focus in medicine is on curing the patient rather than the technology strategy used. We will review the impact of nanotechnology on the artificial kidney and heart later in this chapter, and prosthetics later in Chapter 9. First, we will review a few examples of nanoguides and tissue scaffolds, and then look at artificial organs in the sense in which the term is generally used to refer to endocrine or ductal organs with primary biochemical functions, as opposed to structural implants, kidneys and hearts, or prostheses with neuromuscular or neurosensory functionality.

7.4 Tissue Engineering for Nerve Regeneration

In addition to encapsulating cells and tissues, nanostructures are used to guide and stimulate the growth of cells, serving as scaffolding for growing new tissues. Tissue scaffolding for use in surgery and wound healing is being given new options and opportunities by the development of nanomaterials and nanostructures. Some of the most striking advances in the application of tissue growth scaffolding have come in the regeneration of nerve cells and neural tissues. This is also an area with tremendous medical impact for the restoration of function following paralysis, spinal injury, and stroke. Exciting progress is being made in regeneration of tissues, which until relatively recent times were considered non-regenerating.

7.4.1 Guiding and Monitoring Nerve Growth

The technology of silicon microchips has been in use for several decades to make structures to guide cell growth on the microscale. The technique of growing cells on micropatterned and nanopatterned glass or silicon substrates has become important for evaluating nerve growth [34,35]. Nanotechnology is now available to fabricate more detailed and finer structures for use in sensor functionalization and cell growth patterning by fabricating microchannel cell growth guides with specific degrees of surface roughness and coatings nano-bioengineered to promote cell adhesion [36].

Micropatterned plates have been developed for use as a template for evaluating the growth of neurons in the presence of growth stimulators and inhibitors. This type of growth guide is used in evaluating the effects of different neuronal growth stimulants and inhibitors in the laboratory, with the goal of understanding how to promote regeneration or severed or damaged nerves [37]. Fabricated cell growth surfaces with patterns and coatings, and printing equipment to apply cells, adhesion agents, and reagents to plates is now readily available from a number of sources [38]. These techniques are supporting research into spinal cord injuries and other forms of paralysis.

Technology for neural growth guidance is now being taken from basic research laboratories into the clinical setting, where experiments are being conducted on promoting repair and growth of nerves, including the spinal cord. After injury, axonal regeneration occurs across short gaps in the peripheral nervous system, but regeneration across larger gaps remains a challenge. Cellular channels during development and after peripheral nerve injury have been shown to provide guidance cues to growing axons. The size scale for fabricating nerve growth conduits is in micrometers, but features such as patterning on the inside of the growth channels, porosity, and cross-linking of polymer structures involve nanoscale materials engineering. In the following section, we look at some examples of technologies aimed a bridging the nerve regeneration gap, which may one day be applied to restoring mobility to patients with spinal nerve column damage.

7.4.2 Promoting Nerve Repair

A number of research groups are obtaining promising results in animal studies using various types of micro- and nano-porous guides for nerve regeneration. In the complex biological system of nerve repair, early physiological intervention to minimize the spread of injury will always be the first line of defense in treating nerve damage. Devices and techniques based on nanotechnology may eventually contribute to such intervention.

Basic research in prevention and treatment of permanent nerve injury, especially of the spinal cord, include (1) reduction of edema and free radical production, (2) rescue of neural tissue at risk of dying in secondary processes such as abnormally high extracellular glutamate concentrations, (3) control of inflammation, (4) rescue of neuronal/glial populations at risk of apoptosis, (5) repair of demyelination and conduction deficits, (6) promotion of neurite growth through improved extracellular environment, (7) cell growth and replacement therapies, (8) transplantation approaches, (9) gene therapy to activate expression of growth factors, (10) rehabilitation to retrain and relearn motor tasks, (11) restoration of lost function by electrical stimulation, and (12) relief of chronic pain syndromes [39,40].

Nanotechnology will impact many of these areas, but it must be integrated into the entire therapeutic regimen. Possible benefits from nanotechnology capabilities will be in (1) rapid, efficient and minimally invasive surgical repair, (2) improved automation of rehabilitation through sensors and smart materials to provide feedback, (3) improved electrical stimulation devices for prostheses and pain relief, (4) nanoengineered microdevices to promote cell growth.

Certain cell, molecular, and bioengineering strategies for repairing the injured peripheral nerves and spinal cord are showing encouraging results (either alone or in combination) in animal models. The most promising route is the application of nanoengineered nerve growth guidance matrices in combination with (1) seeding of neuronal support cells such as glial and Schwann cells, and (2) molecular coatings and growth factors embedded into the matrix material.

Therapies based on stem cells and gene therapy are also being developed for nerve regeneration, and will be important for clinical application with bioactive growth scaffolds. We will look at gene and stem cell therapies later, some in combination with intelligent scaffolding. In the meantime, rapid progress is being made in developing implantable devices for neural growth promotion and support, some of which may be useful in delivering future gene and stem cell therapies.

There is a critical difference between regeneration in peripheral nerves and those of the central nervous system. In the peripheral nervous system, axons are myelinated by Schwann cells, which wrap around axons to form a myelin sheath. Myelination insulates the axons and provides a mechanism for speeding and strengthening the propagation of action potentials by which the nerves communicate with each other, and with sensory and motor cells. The Schwann cells promote axon repair by at least two mechanisms. After injury, the myelin sheath formed by Schwann cells can be retained and form a channel to guide the regrowth of a renewed axon. Schwann cells can also regress to an earlier developmental state as glial cells, which promote the regeneration of the axon. Schwann cells are absent from the central nervous system—the spinal cord and the brain. Therefore, research and clinical progress has tended to start with repair of peripheral nerves and progress to the spinal cord and brain.

This is a challenging and productive area with many multidisciplinary teams actively pursuing the goal of nerve repair with promising results. Here are some examples of the different materials and designs for neural conduits, focusing on repair of the spinal cord.

7.4.3 Polylactide Foams

A research team at the University of Liège in Belgium has made macroporous polylactide foams and assessed the ability of dorsal root ganglion (spinal ganglion) derived neurons to survive and adhere in vitro [41]. (Polylactides are biodegradable, aliphatic polyester thermoplastic polymers made from lactic acids in one of several chiral forms.) The foams were fabricated using a thermally induced polymer–solvent phase separation. Two types of pore structures were obtained: oriented or interconnected pores. The foams were coated with polyvinyl alcohol to improve the wettability for cell culture. Microscopic observations of the cells seeded onto the polymer foams showed that the interconnected pore networks were more favorable to cell attachment than the anisotropic ones.

The Liège group investigated the capacity of the highly oriented foams to support in vivo peripheral nerve regeneration in rats. A sciatic nerve gap of 5 mm length was bridged with a polymer implant showing macrotubes of 100 microns diameter. At four weeks postoperatively, the polymer implant was still present and well integrated anatomically. An abundant cell migration was observed at the outer surface of the polymer implant, but not within the macrotubes. This dense cellular microenvironment was found to be favorable for axogenesis.

7.4.4 Polylactide Filaments

A research project conducted jointly between the University of Texas at Arlington, the University of Texas Southwestern Medical Center, and the University of Kentucky is producing nerve guidance channels made from laminin-coated poly(L-lactide) filaments to induce directional axonal growth and to enhance the rate of axonal growth after injury [42]. Dorsal root ganglia grown on these filaments in vitro extend longitudinally oriented neurites in a manner similar to native peripheral nerves. The extent of neurite growth is significantly higher on laminin-coated filaments compared with uncoated and poly-L-lysine-coated filaments. Schwann cells were found to grow on all types of filaments, and were associated with greater neurite growth.

To improve regeneration across extended nerve defects, the team fabricated wet-spun microfilaments of different fiber densities, with the capability for drug release to support cellular migration and guide axonal growth across a lesion. In bundles that were not loaded with drug release, after 10 weeks, nerve cable formation increased significantly in the filament bundled groups when compared to empty-tube controls. At lower packing densities, the number of myelinated axons was more than twice that of controls or the highest packing density. In a consecutive experiment, PLLA bundles with lower filament-packing density were examined for nerve repair across 1.4 and 1.8 cm gaps. After 10 weeks, the number of successful regenerated nerves receiving filaments was more than twice that of controls. These initial results demonstrate that PLLA microfilaments enhance nerve repair and regeneration across large nerve defects, even in the absence of drug release. Ongoing studies are examining nerve regeneration using microfilaments designed to release neurotrophins or cyclic AMP.

7.4.5 Polylactide Tubules

A group at the University of Iowa have developed biodegradable conduits that provide a combination of physical, chemical, and biological cues at the cellular level to facilitate peripheral nerve regeneration [43]. The conduit consists of a porous poly(D,L-lactic acid) tubular support structure with a micropatterned inner lumen. Schwann cells were pre-seeded into the lumen to provide additional trophic support.

In evaluation experiments, tubular conduits with micropatterned inner lumens seeded with Schwann cells (MS) were compared with three types of conduits used as controls: M (conduits with micropatterned inner lumens without pre-seeded Schwann cells), NS (conduits without micropatterned inner lumens pre-seeded with Schwann cells), and N (conduits without micropatterned inner lumens, without pre-seeded Schwann cells).

The conduits were implanted in rats with 1 cm sciatic nerve transections and the regeneration and functional recovery were compared in the four different cases. The number or size of regenerated axons did not vary significantly among the different conduits. The time of recovery and the sciatic function index, however, were significantly enhanced using the MS conduits, based on qualitative observations as well as quantitative measurements using walking track analysis. This and other experiments indicated that the micropatterning and the Schwann cells provide a combination of physical, chemical, and biological guidance cues for regenerating axons at the cellular level. The patterned and seeded conduits performed significantly better than conventional biodegradable conduits.

7.4.6 Biosynthetic Nerve Implants

Another type of conduit for promoting nerve regeneration, the biomimetic biosynthetic nerve implant (BNI), was developed by a group based at the Texas Scottish Rite Hospital for Children [44]. The BNI is a hydrogel-based, transparent, multichannel matrix designed as a 3-D substrate for nerve repair. Polymer scaffold casting devices were designed for the reproducible fabrication of grafts containing several micro-conduits. A number of different polymers were evaluated for making the grafts, including cellulose, hydroxymethyl cellulose, hydroxyethyl cellulose, carboxymethyl cellulose, carboxymethyl chitosan, poly-2-hydroxyethyl-meth-acrylate, poly(R-3-hydroxybutyric acid-*co*-(R)-3-hydroxyvaleric acid)-diol (PHB), collagen, gelatin, glycinin, both neat and as mixtures.

The grafts have been tested in vivo using a sciatic nerve animal model for repair of the adult hemitransected spinal cord. At 16 weeks post-injury of the sciatic nerve, empty tubes formed a single regenerated nerve cable. In contrast, animals that received the multi-luminal BNI showed multiple nerve cables within the available microchannels, better resembling the multi-fascicular anatomy and ultrastructure of the normal nerve. In the injured spinal cord, the BNI loaded with genetically engineered Schwann cells were able to demonstrate survival of the grafted cells with robust axonal regeneration through the implant up to 45 days after repair.

7.4.7 Carbon Nanotubes Enhance Cell Adhesion Surfaces

In a related series of experiments, the Texas Scottish Rite group tested electrodeposited, photolithographic, and micromachined gold microelectrodes for nerve cell stimulation [45]. The gold microprobe interface was modified by the addition of conductive polymers and carbon nanotubes. It was observed that the addition of carbon nanotubes favors the formation of nodules and increases the surface roughness. Also, electrochemical impedance spectroscopy revealed that conductive polymer composites lower the impedance of gold microelectrodes by three orders of magnitude. The carbon nanotube/polymer composite–coated electrodes maintain intimate contact with axons, enabling high-quality nerve spike signals and electrical stimulation of neurons.

7.4.8 Carbon Nanotube Sheets as Neuron Growth Support

In cooperation with the University of Texas Southwestern Medical Center and the University of Texas at Dallas Nanotech Institute, the Texas Scottish Rite group used sheets and yarns made from multiwalled carbon nanotubes to support the long-term growth of a variety of cell types ranging from skin fibroblasts and Schwann cells to postnatal cortical and cerebellar neurons [46]. The study found that the carbon nanotube sheets stimulate fibroblast cell migration compared to plastic and glass culture substrates, entice neuronal growth to the level of those achieved on polyornithine-coated glass, and can be used for directed cellular growth. The carbon nanotube yarns were recently developed at the Nanotech Institute [47]. These findings have positive implications for the use of this type of material in applications such as nerve growth channels, as well as for tissue engineering, wound healing, neurostimulation, and biosensors.

7.4.9 Biocompatibility Issues with Carbon Nanotubes

Many published studies on biocompatibility of carbon nanotube materials have been contradictory [48]. A number of recent studies found that neural cells adhere to multiwall carbon nanotubes [49,50]. Studies with cardiac cells found some short-term effects attributed to physical rather than chemical interactions, but no long-term toxicity [51]. Studies on toxicity in the lung have produced some ambiguous results; these appear to be related to absorption of other nanoparticles on the carbon nanotubes [52,53]. Biocompatibility issues for nonspecific protein absorption onto single-walled carbon nanotubes can be circumvented by co-adsorption of a surfactant and poly(ethylene glycol), whereas specific binding is achieved by the cofunctionalization of nanotubes with biotin and protein-resistant polymers, thus making the nanotubes essentially inert to most forms of interaction with biological systems, and providing a substrate that can be used as a base for preparing protein-specific molecular recognition systems [54].

The Texas Scottish Rite studies used multiwalled carbon nanotubes produced with a minimal residual content of catalytic transition materials to obtain good cell growth. The sheets were found to stimulate fibroblast cell migration, and neuronal growth was enticed to the level achieved on polyornithine-coated glass, which is the standard used for directed cellular growth.

7.4.10 Natural Material Scaffolds from Agarose and Laminin

One way to avoid issues of biocompatibility is to use a well-characterized natural material and coat it with laminin. Researchers at the Cell and Tissue Engineering Laboratory of Case Western Reserve University made hydrogels from agarose and loaded the gel structure with laminin and nerve growth factors to create a three-dimensional scaffold for neurite growth [55]. The agarose hydrogel scaffolds were engineered to stimulate and guide neuronal process extension in three dimensions in vitro. The extracellular matrix protein laminin was covalently bound to agarose hydrogel using the bifunctional cross-linking reagent 1,1'-carbonyldiimidazole. Compared to unmodified agarose gels, laminin-modified gels significantly enhanced neurite extension in chick dorsal root ganglia cells. The Case Western team used inhibitors to study which types of receptors on the surfaces of the ganglia cells were active in the adhesion and growth process on the laminin. They also embedded nerve growth factors into the hydrogels. The resulting trophic factor gradients stimulated directional neurite extension. As a result of this and similar research, agarose hydrogel scaffolds may find application as biosynthetic three-dimensional bridges that promote regeneration across severed nerve gaps.

7.4.11 Natural Material Scaffolds with Collagen

Another natural connective material used for nanoengineered nerve growth guides is collagen. For this purpose, collagen polymer can be cross-lined chemically or with microwave radiation. Collagen polymers thus made can incorporate peptides to promote nerve growth. A number of research groups around the world have fabricated collagen tube and fiber microdevices with nanoengineered substructures and demonstrated their ability to support nerve regeneration.

The Institute for Frontier Medical Science at Kyoto University in Japan made tubeless grafts with 2000 collagen filaments in each to bridge 20 mm defects in rat sciatic nerve. Effective growth of myelinated axons was observed in the collagen filament nerve guides [56,57].

At the Bio-Organic and Neurochemistry Laboratory of the Central Leather Research Institute in Chennai, India, researchers fabricated multilayered collagen tubes by a lamellar evaporation technique and successfully used 14 mm tubules for regeneration of 10 mm nerve gaps in a rat model. Fourier transform infrared spectra of the collagen films showed that the native triple helicity of collagen was unaltered during the multilayered preparation process. Several different means of inducing cross-linking in the fibers were studied, including treatment with glutaraldehyde (GTA) and microwave radiation [58,59].

Scanning electron microscopy of cross-linked tubes showed porous, fibrillar structures of collagen filaments in the matrices. Microscopic histology analysis showed that the tubule surfaces provide for good adherence and proliferation for the sprouting axons from the cut proximal nerve stumps. Among the two types of cross-linking, the microwave irradiated collagen conduits result in ample myelinated axons compared with the GTA group, where more unmyelinated axons were observed. Solute diffusion studies indicated that the tubes are highly porous to a wide range of molecular sizes during regeneration.

Functional evaluations of the regenerated nerves were performed by measuring the sciatic functional index (SFI), nerve conduction velocity (NCV), and electromyography (EMG). The conduction velocity and recovery index improved significantly after 5 months, reaching the normal values in the autograft and microwave induced cross-linked collagen groups compared to GTA and non-cross-linked collagen tubes.

Studies were conducted with nerve growth–promoting peptides incorporated into the collagen matrix. Immunofluorescence studies demonstrated the staining of S100 proteins in the peripherally located cells indicating the proliferation of Schwann cells in the early days of regeneration. The staining pattern of integrin-αV was observed mostly in the perineurial regions in close proximity to the peptide-incorporated collagen tubes. Evaluation of the SFI and conduction velocity at 90 days postoperatively showed regeneration of lesioned nerves with the peptide-incorporated collagen implants [60,61].

Extensive evaluations were carried out for different cross-linking methods, including microwave, GTA, di-tertiary butyl peroxide, and dimethyl suberimidate. The physical properties of collagen-based biomaterials are profoundly influenced by the method and extent of cross-linking. Cross-linking density, swelling ratio, thermo-mechanical properties, stress–strain characteristics, and resistance to collagenase digestion were determined to evaluate the physical properties of cross-linked matrices. The spatial orientation of amino acid side-chain residues on collagen plays an important role in determining the cross-linking density and consequent physical properties of the collagen matrix. The microwave cross-linked matrices gave the best result for nerve regeneration [62].

Tendon autografts have been shown capable of providing a source of collagen that can support nerve regeneration across a gap in the sciatic nerve in rats. It is known that a dual laminin/collagen receptor present in regenerating nerve cells aids their growth and adhesion in laminin-coated scaffolds, and laminin–fibronectin-coated biodegradable collagen grafts have been used to demonstrate the promotion of peripheral nerve growth [13,63–65]. Citicoline, a derivative of the B-vitamin choline, has been shown to improve functional recovery, promote nerve regeneration, and reduce postoperative scarring in a rat model [66]. Research continues to advance the understanding of neuron cell regeneration factors and develop technology aids to guide the regrowth of severed nerves.

7.4.12 Polymer Hydrogels

A research team at MIT, Harvard, and Children's Hospital, Boston, used an injectable, biodegradable biogel formulation with trophic nerve growth promoters to enhance axonal rewiring following spinal cord injury in an adult rat model. The hydrogel for growth scaffolding and trophic factor delivery was made with a cross-linked acrylated copolymer of polylactic acid and polyethylene glycol (PEG) [67]. The injectable hydrogel provided a minimally invasive means of delivering the growth-promoting molecules, with sustained release over a 2 week period.

Researchers at the Toronto Western Research Institute in Canada used hydrogel guidance channels to promote the regrowth of severed axons from motor neurons in the brain stem of adult rats. Hydrogel tubes were surgically implanted to link the gap between stumps of completely severed spinal cords in rats. The hydrogel guidance tubes were composed of poly(2-hydroxyethyl methacrylate-*co*-methyl methacrylate), and the spinal cord stumps were inserted with fibrin glue. This research was the first to show that axons from brain stem motor neuron nuclei can regenerate in unfilled synthetic hydrogel guidance channels after complete spinal cord transaction, although functional recovery was not observed.

This study was unique in that the hydrogel channels were not prefilled with matrix or cells, and animals were not treated with adjuvant drugs or neurotrophic factors. Achieving regeneration of brain stem motor nuclei in simple unfilled channels after complete cord transection is promising and suggests that combination therapies that include bioactive compounds could yield results that could lead to effective therapies.

The superior results compared to other spinal axon guides may be due in part to the match of mechanical properties between the hydrogel and the spinal cord, which maximizes tissue regeneration and minimizes the formation of necrotic tissue at the interface. Another factor is the permeability of the channels to small nutrient molecules such as glucose and oxygen. The channels also confine the nerve growth factors endogenously secreted by neurites and maintain optimal alignment of growth within a tissue cable.

The hydrogel tubes are molded at low temperatures and do not contain any potentially toxic solvents, making them very suitable for incorporation of bioactive compounds such as neurotrophic factors, enzymes such as chondroitinase, and antibodies such as IN-1 to neutralize the inhibition of axonal regeneration or loading with cells. The interior of the channels can be engineered with networks of microchannel scaffolding for optimal axon growth and organization.

Entubulation has been used extensively in peripheral nerve regeneration both experimentally and clinically; this study suggests that intubation with bioengineered gels may be a viable therapeutic strategy for spinal cord injury [68,69].

7.4.13 Bioengineered Bridges for Neuron Growth

Researchers at the NIH National Heart, Lung and Blood Institute and the Cambridge Centre for Brain Repair have analyzed the behavior of neurons growing in polymer grafts, and designed sophisticated bridge grafts for neuron regeneration with "on-ramps" and "off-ramps" for enhancing the interfaces where growing axons enter the graft, are guided along the graft, and exit at their destinations. Using sophisticated matrices containing axon chemoattractants and matrix compounds containing molecules such as laminin, tenascin, and chondroitin, and heparan sulfate proteoglycans to encourage axon growth, the "on-ramps" recruit growing neuronal axons into the graft matrix, where growth-stimulating and adhesive-signaling molecules guide extended growth across an injury gap. At the "off-ramp," the scaffolding must be engineered to assist the growing axons to exit the scaffold matrix and penetrate any glial scar tissue to link up with nerve cells on the other side of the injury [70].

The design principles for bridge grafts apply equally to any matrix material: polymers, polysaccharides, collagens, polypeptides, or fibronectin nets. The most important factors for the matrix material are biocompatibility, biodegradability, and the ability to functionalize the matrix for bioactive signaling. Polypeptides made by chemical synthesis or genetic engineering can have neural adherence, guidance, and growth-promoting motifs engineered directly into the polymer backbone. In all cases, materials must be selected to avoid challenges to the host immune system. Peptide matrices will be particularly useful for regeneration within the central nervous system.

7.4.14 Summary of Progress in Peripheral and Spinal Nerve Regeneration

Research on nerve regeneration being conducted around the world offers possible solutions for the need to sacrifice a healthy nerve to make a graft, and for the shortage of graft material available, for the repair of severed peripheral and spinal nerves [69–71]. This work is progressing toward clinical treatments for the repair of spinal cord injuries and cures for paralysis. More than 50 clinical trials are in progress worldwide on various treatments for spinal cord injury. Consequently, in this millennium, unlike in the last, no spinal cord injury patient will have to hear "nothing can be done" [39]. Nanoengineering of tissues will have played a significant part in making such cures possible.

7.5 Nanotechnology for Regeneration of the Brain

Even more formidable than peripheral and spinal nerve regrowth is the challenge of regeneration of the brain. Attempting to restore even part of the daunting complexity of the structures in the brain has required a step-change in thinking. Functional regeneration after serious injury to the mammalian brain has been found to be extremely poor, especially in the nonpermissive growth environment of the mature brain. Daunting barriers to the repair process include formation of scar tissue, gaps in nerve tissue formed during phagocytosis of dying cells, biochemical factors that inhibit axon growth, and the inability of many mature neurons to initiate axonal extension [71].

To overcome these barriers has required first of all an increasing understanding of the detailed functional organization and structure of the brain. This insight continues to be developed with tools such as functional magnetic resonance imaging and mapping with molecular and electronic probes. At the same time, advances in molecular biology, genetic engineering, proteomics, and genomics have increased the detailed knowledge necessary to treat or reverse the underlying pathology of disease processes. Advances in cell-based therapeutics, regenerative medicine, and tissue engineering raise the possibility of replacing damaged neurons or coaxing neuronal circuits to regenerate. Encouragement has come from discoveries of previously unexpected plasticity in the mature brain following injury. In many cases, capability has been demonstrated to at least reorganize and remap brain functions following injury, if not regenerate original structures completely.

It is easy to focus on the neurons, with their electrical activity and complex interconnections, to the exclusion of the many supporting cells in the central nervous system, termed glial cells. The glial cells (from the Greek for "glue") were originally considered merely space fillers providing structural support to the neurons in the brain and spinal cord. Research in neuron cell culture and regeneration has led to a more complete appreciation of the many essential roles of glial cells in maintaining healthy neuron function. It is now known that glial cells participate in calcium channel signaling with neurons and regulate growth, plasticity, and neurotransmitter management in neurons. Star-shaped glial cells called astrocytes perform many functions, including biochemical support of endothelial cells, which form the blood–brain barrier, provision of nutrients to the nervous tissue, and maintenance of extracellular ion balance and repair and scar formation following nerve damage.

Glial cells have an essential supporting role in the growth, development, and regeneration of nerve tissue. In the brain and spinal cord, only the axons, which provide relatively long distance connections, are myelinated. Many axons in the brain are unmyelinated, as their primary function is to communicate with neighboring neurons in complex networks, rather than carry signals to distant locations. Thin, unmyelinated axons are the most common axonal type in the mammalian cortex—they are also the part of the brain that we have least knowledge about, mainly due to their tiny dimensions, below the light microscopic resolution [72,73]. Where myelation is needed in the central nervous system, it is provided by glial cells called oligodendrocytes. Unlike the Schwann cells of the peripheral system, which are dedicated to a single axon, each oligodendrocyte can extend its processes to wrap myelin sheath over as many as 50 axons.

Oligodendrocytes do not provide the regeneration functions performed by the Schwann cells found in the peripheral system, so regeneration in the central nervous system is inhibited. This is a key distinction between the response to injury in the peripheral nervous system and in the brain. Upon injury to nerve cells within the central nervous system, astrocytes become phagocytic to ingest the injured nerve cells, forming a glial scar which replaces the neurons that cannot regenerate. The glial scar tissue significantly inhibits subsequent axonal elongation and repair.

Trauma or infarction in the brain causes cell death, followed by necrosis with delayed cell death in adjacent tissue and formation of a lesion cavity surrounded by glial scar tissue. Biomaterial scaffolds are being evaluated for placement into damaged areas of the brain to provide support for the surrounding tissue, to act as a substrate for cell growth, axon regeneration and neurite formation, and to promote cell infiltration into the lesion. A number of different types of scaffolding are being investigated; most provide delivery of growth-promoting factors, cells, or both to the site of injury. Neurons or stem cells may be isolated from the host and incorporated into three-dimensional scaffoldings for transplantation.

The fully developed human brain is a complex hierarchy of many different interacting subsystems, from the medulla to the cerebral cortex, each with its own organization and function. There are many different sources and types of injury and disease that can affect the brain. Regeneration must restore neurons with their interconnections as well as the extracellular environment including supportive glial cells. Vascularization and the integrity of the blood–brain barrier must also be restored. Because of this complexity, treatments to mitigate global or diffuse forms of brain damage such as that resulting from hypoxia are the most challenging of long-term goals. Any global restorative therapy must somehow stimulate, protect, and harness the brain's own ability for regrowth and reorganization.

A nearer-term possibility is the treatment of damage that is more limited and localized to specific neuronal populations or brain circuits. Examples of these types of damage include the loss of dopaminergic neurons in Parkinson's disease or the compartmentalized trauma that occurs following a traumatic contusion or penetrating brain injury.

7.5.1 Strategies for Brain Regeneration

Neuroscientists and medical specialists in brain health have developed strategies for regeneration based on four principles: preservation, permissivity, promotion, and plasticity. Ellis Behnke, a leading neuroscientist at MIT, quoted in a recent interview in *The Lancet Neurology* [74], explained these principles: "First, when the brain is injured you want to keep the neurons alive, or preserve them, second, you want to create a permissive environment for axon growth. Third, you want to promote the growth of the preserved axons through the permissive environment. Finally, for the axons to reconnect to the target tissue you want to increase plasticity, which will help the brain to repair itself."

The guidelines for the preservation of neurons following injury to the spinal cord are also applicable in the more complex environment of the brain. The first goal of therapy is to prevent permanent nerve injury due to edema, free radical production, and high concentrations of extracellular glutamate and other damaging by-products of disruption. Inflammation must be controlled to prevent or minimize a cascade of apoptosis and other spreading damage. A supportive extracellular environment must be established to permit and promote the growth of axons, neurites, and glial cells. Plasticity can be increased by growth-initiating and growth-stimulating biomolecules, by gene therapy, and other cell growth promotion and replacement therapies, including stem cells. Finally, plasticity and restoration of function can be accelerated by stimulation therapies, including neuromuscular exercises, sensory stimulation, and electromagnetic stimulation relevant to the disordered portion of the brain. Just as with spinal and peripheral nerve regeneration, nanotechnology is an important source of tools and therapeutic techniques [75,76].

As we saw in the previous chapter on drug delivery, nanotechnology can help deliver therapies across the blood–brain barrier to control edema, free radicals, and inflammation. Nanoengineered scaffolds can serve as permissive and supportive substrates for cell growth, differentiation, and biological function. On the leading edge of research, nanomaterials can provide active signaling cues for guided axon growth in brain regeneration therapies. In the meantime, research with scaffolds for brain regeneration is producing promising results [77,78].

7.5.2 Nanoengineered Materials for Brain Regeneration

Nanoengineered materials for the treatment of brain lesions is an active area of research being pursued by multidisciplinary teams of neuroscientists, neurosurgeons, and neurologists in close collaboration with physical scientists and engineering colleagues. Nanoengineered biomaterials and structures for the protection and regeneration of injuries in the central nervous system are being investigated for potential clinical applications. Here, we will survey a few examples of recent promising developments.

Nanomaterials have been found to be especially good platforms for free radical scavengers that can protect the brain from immediate and secondary cell death caused by superoxides, nitric oxide, and other free radical excitotoxins, which can be produced in ischemia associated with stroke or injury to the brain or spinal cord. Elimination of these toxins can reduce edema and infarction. Fullerenes, for example, have been functionalized to serve as effective catalysts for the destruction of free radicals in injured brain tissue [79–81].

Nanoengineered scaffolds are designed to guide and regulate tissue growth and allow the transport of nutrients, metabolites, and signaling molecules. The goal is to mimic the environment present in brain development to promote the regeneration of functional tissue. Every aspect of the interaction of the scaffolds with the cells must be carefully engineered: mechanical support and compliance, degradation rate, release of growth-promoting factors and/or DNA incorporated in the material, and surface control of adhesion by ligand-receptor mechanisms [82].

Materials being investigated include gels, polymer sponges, and other materials with various degrees of rigidity and biodegradation rates. Much of the knowledge of materials for the effective regeneration of brain tissue is based on experience with spinal cord regeneration, and many of the same technologies are being applied. The main difference is that tubes or channels are applicable to the repair of spinal cord trauma, whereas three-dimensional gels and networks are more suited to brain regeneration.

In experiments, cortical cavities are formed surgically in rats, and porous biomaterial scaffolds are implanted into the lesions. Scaffolds have been shown to decrease local cell death, secondary cell loss and lesion growth, and support neuron growth. A reduced inflammatory response has been found with some ingrowth of neurons into the periphery of the scaffolds.

7.5.3 Physical and Biochemical Cues for Regeneration

Research with rat models has shown that cortical regeneration is highly dependent on the microstructure, surface properties, and material composition of the scaffolding. Orientation of microscopic pores and grooves in the scaffold guides cellular migration and neuronal alignment [82]. Gels are particularly good at inducing the ingrowth of the endothelial, astroglial, and microglial cells that are important in guiding the organization and function of the neurons. Vascular endothelial growth factor (VEGF), which promotes growth of blood vessels, has been found to increase the formation of new brain tissue when incorporated into gel scaffolds [84].

Small molecule chemical messengers play an important role in the cell communication that takes place during development and regeneration. Experiments with bioactive polymers that have surface functionality based on the neurotransmitter dopamine have shown increased attachment and growth. A biodegradable polymer with pendant dopamine functional groups demonstrated more vigorous neurite outgrowth on the polymer surface than on tissue culture polystyrene, laminin, and poly(D-lysine). The dopamine functional polymer promoted distinctive patterned organization or the neurites that was absent on the control materials. Addition of dopamine or its precursor tyrosine to cell cultures on nonfunctionalized polymers had comparatively little effect, indicating the importance of the surface interactions in guiding cell growth. Further research is investigating the effects of small-molecule chemical messengers on regeneration [85].

Electrical properties have been found to be important in the growth of nerve cells. Studies have demonstrated enhanced neural tissue regeneration in electrical fields applied through conductive and piezoelectric materials, which generate a transient electrical potential when mechanically deformed. Because of surface-to-volume ratios, nanoparticles made from piezoelectric material are more sensitive to stress from small forces. Researchers at Brown University investigated what effect piezoelectric zinc oxide (ZnO) nanoparticles embedded in a flexible polymer scaffold had on the growth of neural tissue. They evaluated the adhesion and proliferation of astroglial cells using x-ray photoelectron spectroscopy and scanning electron microscopy to characterize the scaffolding and measure cell growth. Astrocyte adhesion was significantly reduced on nanocomposite polymer containing ZnO [86].

The physical and chemical surface properties of the scaffold are critical for cell attachment, adhesion, and spreading to ensure survival and integration into tissue. Factors for neuron differentiation and growth include surface roughness, surface chemistry, surface charge, mechanical properties, addition of extracellular matrix proteins, and seeding with cells pre-attached to the scaffold [87,88]. One of the most promising approaches is the modification of the scaffold's surface with adhesive peptides such as laminin and fibronectin, which are known to play a key role in cell adhesion, development, and regeneration [89–91].

Fibronectin is a large glycoprotein that forms a major component of the extracellular matrix in combination with other extracellular matrix proteins such as laminin, collagen, and fibrin. Fibronectin fixes cells to the extracellular matrix by binding to the transmembrane receptor proteins called integrins in a complex process mediated by cell growth, migration, and adhesion factors. The peptide amino acid sequence, RGD (arginine (R), glycine (G), and aspartate (D)), has been identified as the region that is key to identification and adhesion of fibronectin and other extracellular matrix proteins. Integrin receptors on neurons and other cells selectively bind to this sequence, and this binding modulates cell differentiation and migration. Using simpler peptides that contain the RGD sequence in scaffold materials has been shown to facilitate neuron migration, adhesion, and differentiation following injury, as well as increasing angiogenesis and reducing necrosis. Fibronectin contains other peptide sequences that function synergistically with RGD to enhance cell binding. Artificial peptide polymers that contain the same sequences separated by inert spacers to approximate the distance on fibronectin can mimic the functionality of the native fibronectin glycoprotein. Understanding the function and structure relationships of cell-binding factors such as fibronectin makes possible the development of cellular engineering for the control of specific aspects of cell growth and regeneration. This includes inhibition of cell binding in cases where it is associated with pathology, as in cancer or in formation of scar tissue in eye diseases [92,93].

The laminins are another family of glycoproteins that form an important bioactive component of the extracellular matrix, influencing cell migration, adhesion, and differentiation. Laminins are known as a substrate for nerve growth and have been widely used in neuron repair scaffolds, as described in some previous examples. The cell-binding domains of laminin have been identified and found to consist of two 5-amino acid sequences. One sequence facilitates cell binding and the other facilitates neurite extension. The binding affinity of laminin has been duplicated by the conjugation of these peptide sequences to polymer scaffolds, which were used to demonstrate neurite extension and spinal cord regeneration [94,95]. Synthetic-peptide-functionalized surfaces presenting combinations of the laminin and fibronectin adhesion-promoting sequences have been used in experiments in which the binding affinity approached that observed on laminin-coated tissue culture plates. The result showed that a synergistic peptide motif in an artificial matrix can approach the efficacy of a natural material, pointing to future directions for enhancing biomaterial scaffolds for neural regeneration.

7.5.4 Morphologies of Porous Scaffolds

In addition to surface cues from biomolecular motifs, subtle changes in the physical surface morphology of porous scaffolds can also influence neuronal growth patterns. Recent research has shown that scaffolds incorporating nanotubes and nanofibers seem to create a superior permissive environment for axonal growth while minimizing the formation of scar tissue. Porous networks of nanoscale fibers would seem to reproduce the natural environment of the extracellular matrix with its microtubules, axons, and dendrites. Three main approaches have been used to fabricate nanofiber nerve growth scaffolds: functionalized carbon nanotubes, electrospun polymers, and self-assembled peptides [42–47,96,97].

Carbon nanotubes have been used as the basis for neural growth scaffolds [42–47]. Their size, relative inertness, and electrical conductivity make them useful as growth substrates, although they can affect neural function by interaction with ion channels. They can be readily functionalized by the attachment of biological compounds and other chemical groups to promote neural interaction and increase solubility and biocompatibility [98]. The electrical properties of functionalized carbon nanotubes can affect the growth and branching of neuronal processes. Patterned arrays of carbon nanotubes have been used for studying the growth and organization of neural networks. The electrical conductivity of nanotubes can be exploited to monitor or stimulate neurons through the substrate itself [99].

An interdisciplinary team in Australia produced nanofibrous scaffolds by electrospinning, using an electrical charge to draw nanofibers from liquid polymers (poly(L-lactide), PLLA and poly(lactide-co-glycolide), PLGA). Mouse embryonic cortical neurons were cultured on the randomly orientated scaffolds. The scaffolds were surface treated with a strong base to partially hydrolyze the surface, changing the surface tension to increase hydrophilicity. The degree of hydrophilicity did not significantly influence the number of primary and secondary nerve branches, but had a considerable effect on neurite extension: less hydrophillic scaffolds had greater overall neurite length. A most interesting finding was that the distance between fibers influenced how the neurites extended. When the fibers were greater than approximately 15 μm apart, the neurites followed the fibers and avoided regions of higher fiber density. At smaller separations, the neurites traversed between the fibers [100].

The interactions of astrocyte neural cells cultured in vitro with electrospun nanofiber scaffolds have been investigated by researchers in Germany [101]. Scaffolds were based on aligned polycaprolactone nanofibers with and without blended collagen. Growth on the scaffolds was assessed for astrocytes derived from human neural progenitor stem cells and for two cell lines from brain tumors. Both the normal astrocytes and tumor cells aligned and grew on the scaffolds. Migration and adhesion of the normal cells was increased on the collagen blended nanofibers, but the collagen had no effect on the cancer cells, which proliferated indiscriminately on both types of scaffold compared to the normal cells. Morphology and alignment of cell growth was influenced strongly by the nanofibers.

An international research team with members from the Nanoscience and Nanotechnology Initiative, National University of Singapore, the Department of Textile Engineering, Isfahan University of Technology, and other Isfahan institutes has used polymer blending to make electrospun nanofibrous scaffolds using mixtures of polycaprolactone and gelatin type A from porcine skin. Aligned and randomized nanofiber scaffolds of varying compositions were characterized and evaluated by scanning electron microscopy (SEM), attenuated total reflectance Fourier transform infrared (ATR-FTIR) spectrometry, capillary flow porometry, and contact angle and tensile strength measurements. Neonatal mouse cerebellum stem cells were incubated with the scaffolds and growth and morphology were examined by SEM. A blend of 70% polycaprolactone with 30% gelatin was found to have the most balanced properties for enhancing the nerve differentiation and proliferation, and providing cues for neurite outgrowth, compared to polycaprolactone fibers. Gelatin, a natural biopolymer derived from collagen by controlled hydrolysis, increased the hydrophilicity and biodegradability of the scaffold, and improved cell adhesion, migration, proliferation, and differentiation [102].

A recent study led by Rutledge Ellis-Behnke of Massachusetts Institute of Technology is an example of the versatility of self-assembly for neural scaffolds. In this research, a peptide-based nanofiber scaffold was used to enable the regeneration of the severed optic tract in the hamster brain. This represented a significant milestone for in vivo brain regeneration. Ellis-Behnke and his colleagues used a self-assembling peptide scaffold material that had been shown to be permissive for cell attachment in previous in vitro experiments. Synthetic peptide polymers have the following advantages: they form a network of nanofibers similar to the natural extracellular network in scale and composition; they biodegrade into natural L-amino acids potentially usable by the surrounding tissue; they are free of chemical and biological contaminants that typically are present in animal-derived biomaterials such as collagens; and they appear relatively immunologically inert. The peptide sequences are synthesized to present targets for cell attachment, such as arginine-alanine-aspartate-alanine (RADA), which is known to promote neuron growth. Visual ability was regained in 75% of the treated animals [103]. The scaffolds were also used to reknit spinal cord injuries in rats [104].

This same type of self-assembling peptide nanofiber scaffold has recently been used at the University of Hong Kong in experiments to reconstruct severe brain injuries in rats. The lesion cavity was filled with the scaffold immediately after surgically induced brain damage. The scaffold integrated well with the host tissue with no obvious gaps, and there were relatively few astrocytes and macrophages around the lesion site in the treated rats. In untreated controls, there were many macrophages but few cells tested positive with stain for DNA fragmentation, indicating that secondary tissue loss was due mainly to necrosis rather than apoptosis. These experiments indicate that such scaffolds help reduce glial reaction and inflammation in brain injuries, and are another step toward eventual use of self-assembling peptide scaffolds to regenerate acutely injured brain tissue [105].

Researchers at Northwestern University used solutions of amphiphilic peptide molecules to form a self-assembling three-dimensional network of nanofibers. The amino acid sequence of the peptides incorporated the five-member epitope isoleucine–lysine–valine–alanine–valine (IKVAV), which is one of the domains found in laminin that is known to promote neurite sprouting and to direct neurite growth. Neural stem cells suspended in the solution were surrounded and enclosed in the scaffolding, so that they were presented with the neurite-promoting epitope at close quarters. This scaffold arrangement produced very rapid differentiation of cells into neurons, while discouraging the development of astrocytes (which would correspond to the formation of scar tissue) [106].

The nanostructured IKVAV scaffolds were tested on rat spinal cord injuries, where they promoted the regeneration of both descending motor fibers and ascending sensory fibers through the lesion site, with reduced astrogliosis, reduced cell death, and increased oligodendroglia. Because the peptide polymer self-assembles when exposed to the ionic environment of the cerebrospinal fluid, the scaffold can be administered by a simple injection [107].

Together, these and other examples demonstrate how close research has come to producing nanoscaffolds that can structurally mimic portions of the extracellular matrix to provide precise control over cell development. To be most effective, and to deal with large lesions, nanoengineered tissue scaffolding must be able to deliver live cells into the damaged area and support their growth. Artificial three-dimensional scaffolds that are capable of attracting or storing cells, and then directing cell proliferation and differentiation, will be of critical importance in regenerative medicine.

7.6 Use of Nanoengineered Scaffolding with Cells for Central Nervous System Regeneration

Being able to support the regrowth of new cells into regenerated tissue is a major challenge of regenerative medicine—a challenge for which nanotechnology is offering answers. Finding sources of compatible and adaptable cells for use in regenerating tissues has been another major goal. Researchers have turned to stem cells as a possible solution but, until recently, faced many obstacles. Nanotechnology is now becoming an enabling factor in overcoming many of these obstacles.

Neural stem cells have great potential for brain repair; they can differentiate into neurons and glia that integrate into the injured brain to replace lost cells. But in order to produce and maintain the differentiated gene expressions and functions of a mature cell phenotype, stem cells must be provided with an environment that sends the appropriate signals for development and growth. The ability of neural stem cells to grow and differentiate is affected by the surface morphology of their substrate matrix, the presence of the correct neurotropic factors, and interactions with neighboring cells.

Scaffolds with directive components and nanotextured surfaces can provide chemical, physical, and spatial cues to promote natural growth and development. The factors that promote stem cell differentiation and growth are not unlike those that promote regeneration of native neurons following injury. Seeding a scaffold with neural stem cells is potentially a means of accelerating and improving nerve tissue regeneration in a lesion. Achieving this potential depends on the properties of the scaffold [106].

Simply injecting neural stem cells into a brain injury does not yield therapeutic results: the stem cells migrate away from the lesion into healthy tissue, or they fail to differentiate and succumb to cytotoxic factors in the injured tissue. Therefore, advances in nanoengineering of scaffolds are critical to the successful application of stem cells for brain regeneration [108].

Ongoing research is investigating the use of many types of scaffolds for brain regeneration with stem cells [109]. Promising results in animal studies have been achieved using various approaches including self-assembling peptide scaffolds that present growth-directing functional epitope sites [107], fibrin scaffolds [110], and stem cell–impregnated carbon nanotubes [108].

Stem cell growth has been evaluated and compared for both endogenously and exogenously derived stem and progenitor nerve cells [111]. Effects on the growth and differentiation of cells have been evaluated for biodegradable matrices and scaffolds incorporating collagen-hyaluronan [112], collagen [113], chitosan [114], and a number of polymer substrates [114,115]. Stem cell differentiation has been studied on three-dimensional polymer scaffolds with release of cell growth and differentiation factors such as retinoic acid, transforming growth factor β, activin-A, or insulin-like growth factor. These growth factors induced differentiation into three-dimensional structures with the characteristics of developing neural tissues, cartilage, or liver, respectively. In addition, the formation of a vessel-like network was observed. When transplanted into severe combined immunodeficient mice, the scaffolds continued to express specific human proteins in defined differentiated structures and appeared to recruit and integrate with the host vasculature [116].

Polymer hydrogels seeded with stem cells for spinal nerve repair have been evaluated by clinical researchers in the Czech Republic, using bone marrow cells and with gels made from derivatives of 2-hydroxyethyl methacrylate and 2-hydroxypropyl methacrylamide. There, researchers treated rats with induced spinal cord injuries and a small number of human patients. Treatment in animals with different bone marrow cell populations had a positive effect on behavioral outcome and histopathological assessment. The human clinical study showed no complications following cell administration, and produced positive effects in a small sample of treated patients with subacute and chronic spinal cord injuries [117].

Neural regeneration with stem cells continues to be pursued with many innovative strategies. In work supported by NASA at Cornell University, researchers addressed the recapitulation of the unique combinations of matrix, growth factor, and cell adhesion cues in the microenvironments that control stem cell differentiation and growth. They preassembled cells and neural growth factor (NGF) in a controlled release matrix into neo-tissue modules to mimic the chemical and physical microenvironment of developing tissue. The characteristics of the synthetic microenvironment were programmable in the sense that the release of NGF can be controlled by changing conditions during formation so as to vary the concentration of particles in the modules or the rate of the release of NGF. When the neo-tissues were transplanted into the brains of rats, the cells remained in place at the site of injection in the striatum (in the basal ganglia of the cerebrum, which is involved in Parkinson's disease). The cells remained aggregated, and elevated levels of NGF were observed for modules programmed for its release. This work demonstrated an approach by which the extracellular microenvironment necessary for therapeutic application of stem cells can be synthetically controlled [118].

In studies conducted by the Yonsei University College of Medicine, Seoul, Korea, with participation from Harvard Medical School, neural stem cells supported by a biodegradable polymer scaffold were transplanted into infarction cavities caused by hypoxia-ischaemia in mice. The mice were subjected to a type of infarction that is a model for cerebral palsy. New brain parenchyma (functional tissue, as opposed to stroma, structural tissue) was regenerated as the PGA scaffolding degraded, while the amount of damaged brain tissue shrank. Multiple spontaneous reciprocal interactions ensued between the implanted stem cells and the brain tissue surrounding the infarction. An intricate meshwork of highly branched neurites emerged from both donor and host cells, and some anatomical structures appeared to be reconstituted. Donor neurons exhibited directed, target-appropriate neurite outgrowth without specific external guidance or genetic manipulation of host or donor cells, while the trajectory and complexity of host neurites was altered, forming "biobridges" between host and renewing brain tissue. Thus, the reparative response of host and donor appeared to take place via a series of reciprocal interactions, which facilitated neuronal differentiation, the elaboration of neural processes, and the reformation of cortical tissue with connectivity. Inflammation and scarring were also reduced, with significant improvement in survival and function as measured by a spatial learning task. These experiments demonstrated the effectiveness of polymer scaffolds with stem cells in reducing secondary brain tissue loss and supporting organized regeneration [119].

Researchers at Georgia Tech and Emory University used laminin- and fibronectin-based scaffolds to enhance the survival and integration of stem cells transplantated into the traumatically injured brains of mice. In designing the scaffolds, they sought to mimic key aspects of developing fetal brain tissue: three dimensionality, cell–cell and cell–matrix support, and enrichment with extracellular matrix proteins such as fibronectin and laminin, which are known to be involved in neural development. The matrix proteins provide adhesive support for donor cells and mediate subsequent cell-signaling events. They achieved significant improvement for cell distribution into surrounding tissue and in long-term cell survival and behavioral recovery. Laminin was found to be more effective than fibronectin as a base for scaffolding in promoting long-term recovery [120–122].

7.6.1 Translation of Nanoscaffold Neural Cell Therapy toward Clinical Application

Nanoengineered scaffolds for supporting neural cell regeneration have shown significant enhancements to the efficacy of stem cell therapy for brain regeneration. As a result, there has been great interest in the technology development required for the translation of this research to clinical use [123–126]. One of the challenges to successful translation of the large body of preclinical work is the development of clinically useful means of delivery of scaffold-supported stem cells into targeted tissue sites.

Researchers in the United Kingdom designed a scaffolding system on which neural stem cells can attach and grow, and which can be injected into the brain through a fine needle to fill lesion cavities, with imaging guidance. They developed a scaffold system using individual small particles of scaffold material, which when coated with cells could fit through a needle for delivery, and which have the added advantage of being able to fill lesion cavities of arbitrary shape and size. As the particles pack into the cavity, the cells maintain contact with cells on neighboring particles to create tissue connections [127].

This modular approach also reduces the risk of a collagen-like response that tends to seal off the graft from surrounding host tissue. Gaps between the particles enhance interaction with host cells and provide spaces for ingrowth of axons and blood vessels. As the particles biodegrade, more space is created for the growing tissue to become established. In a series of experiments, the researchers demonstrated delivery of large numbers of supported cells into lesions and confirmed that the transplants integrated efficiently within host tissue. This study provides a substantial step toward the translation of this approach into clinical application. Intensive developmental and translational research continues to make advances in this area [128,129].

7.6.2 Regeneration for Chronic and Neurodegenerative Disorders

In our discussion so far, we have focused on regeneration of nerve tissue following injury or infarction, but nanotechnology-enhanced tissue engineering and stem cell technologies are equally applicable to the restoration of tissues damaged or disabled in cases of Parkinson's, Alzheimer's, Huntington's, lateral sclerosis, and other debilitating and incurable diseases and disorders of the central nervous system.

7.6.3 Preventing Oxidative Stress

Many degenerative brain conditions are associated with oxidative stress. Derivatives of buckminsterfullerene have been synthesized to create unique types of compounds with potent antioxidant properties, capable of countering the peroxides and free radicals known to cause stress-induced tissue damage. A class of malonic acid C_{60} derivatives, carboxyfullerenes, can consume superoxide anions and hydrogen peroxide, and inhibit lipid peroxidation. Fullerene derivatives have been shown to delay motor deterioration and death in a mouse model of familial amyotrophic lateral sclerosis (ALS). Studies with systemic administration of fullerene antioxidants have shown neuroprotective activity in animal models of other neurodegenerative disorders, including Parkinson's disease [130]. Other types of antioxidants and free radical scavengers are being found to modulate the assembly and toxicity of amyloid fibrils, which are involved in the formation of plaques associated with Alzheimer's, Parkinson's, Huntington's, and Creutzfeldt-Jakob diseases. (More recently, amyloid has been found to have many non-pathological functional roles as well.) Nanotechnology methods are being employed to study the structure and roles of these nanoscale fibrils, which could lead to better understanding and treatment strategies [131].

7.6.4 Polymer-Encapsulated Cells Engineered to Secrete Neural Regulation Factors

Implantation of cells in immunoprotective encapsulations is being developed as a means of treating some of the most devastating and intractable neurological disorders such as Parkinson's disease, Alzheimer's disease, Huntington's disease, ALS, and cerebral ischemia. In many cases, delivery of neurotransmitters or neurotrophic factors into the brain can alleviate symptoms and even halt progression of the disease. The delivery of neurotropic factors can stimulate reconstruction of lost neuron circuits, offering a potential route to a cure. Direct injection of neurotropic factors, by osmotic pumps or by peripheral administration, is not very effective, and is associated with undesirable side effects (on heart rate, blood pressure, temperature, sedation). An alternative that has been the subject of much research is delivery of neurotropic factors by cell modification and/or transplantation [132].

Many types of neurotrophic factor-secreting cells can be created using biotechnology techniques for genetic engineering, but immunological reaction and tumorigenesis of genetically engineered cells have presented formidable barriers to their use in therapy. Even where host-compatible cells are available for the production of neurotrophic factors, delivering cells and keeping them in the most effective locations in the brain is a challenge. Encapsulation in nanoengineered polymer carriers can protect transplanted cells from immunological rejection while protecting the host brain from inflammatory reactions. Encapsulation can also prevent tumorigenesis of donor cells and keep implanted cells from migrating away from the most effective target areas in the brain; it can also inhibit the modification of specially engineered implanted cells by influences and signaling from neighboring host cells and the surrounding extracellular matrix [133].

7.6.5 Huntington's Disease

Encapsulation of cells for neurotrophic factor delivery has been used experimentally in treatment of Huntington's disease [134]. Huntington's is a genetic disease with severe impacts on cognitive, psychological, and motor functions. It is associated with the progressive loss of efferent neurons of the striatum responsible for the release of the neurotransmitter gamma-aminobutyric acid (GABA), the chief inhibitory neurotransmitter in the vertebrate central nervous system. There is no clinical treatment to date. The development of the condition is protracted over many years after onset, and the genetic marker is known, so there is a possibility that a strategy of protecting neurons would be effective. Neurotrophic factors such as ciliary neurotrophic factor (CNTF) have been shown to protect striatal neurons in experimental animal models of Huntington's disease [135].

Experimental treatment programs for Huntington's disease have been conducted in France and Switzerland; microcapsules containing cultured cells genetically engineered to produce human CNTF were implanted into the right lateral cerebral ventricle in six patients. The semipermeable capsules contained up to around 100 cells, for continuous release from 0.15 to 0.5 µg of CNFT per day. The microcapsules were replaced every 6 months over a period of 2 years. The procedure was found to be safe and well-tolerated. Improvements in electrophysiological results were observed and positively correlated with the amount of CNTF released. Further work is ongoing to improve the technique, focused on ensuring longer term survival of the encapsulated cells [136,137].

7.6.6 Parkinson's Disease

Microsphere capsules engineered to deliver bone marrow–derived progenitor cells and growth factors are showing promise as a means of treating Parkinson's disease. Stem cells have been demonstrated to reverse dopaminergic degeneration in a Parkinsonian rat model [138,139].

7.6.7 Alzheimer's Disease

Microspheres engineered to release NGF are being investigated in animal models of Alzheimer's disease, which is characterized by a loss of cholinergic neurons in the basal forebrain. Sustained targeted release of NGF by the microspheres has been shown to promote the survival of cholinergic neurons [140,141].

7.6.8 Multiple Sclerosis

Demyelinating autoimmune diseases in the central nervous system, such as multiple sclerosis (MS), have been the target of many therapeutic research strategies based on gene therapy [142]. The use of encapsulation to deliver genetically modified cells for neuroprotection is a possible, but little explored, therapy for MS, characterized by loss of myelinating cells. In animal studies, non-replicative viruses have been used to deliver genes within the central nervous system that code for anti-inflammatory and/or neurotrophic molecules. The production of these molecules within the central nervous system can inhibit the detrimental function of blood-borne mononuclear effector cells and foster proliferation and differentiation of surviving oligodendrocytes within demyelinated areas. Administration of these molecules systemically outside of the central nervous system has minimal effect, probably because of limited ability to penetrate the blood–brain barrier. Molecular targets for leucocyte activation, cytokines, and nerve growth factors have shown some promising benefit in animal models of MS. Work is continuing to develop possible clinical applications of these techniques [143,144].

7.6.9 Canavan Disease

At the CNS Gene Therapy Center of Thomas Jefferson University in Philadelphia, researchers are working toward the goal of developing safe and effective in vivo gene therapy for the treatment of Canavan disease and other neurological disorders. Canavan disease is a leukodystrophy caused by a deficiency in the enzyme aspartoacylase that breaks down aspartic acid. The CNS Gene Therapy Center has developed gene therapy based on nonviral plasmids in a lipid-entrapped, polycation-condensed delivery system for gene transfer into the central nervous system. This is an effective system that avoids the proliferative and immunological problems associated with virus and cell-based gene therapies. Toxicity and gene expression were tested in human cell cultures, showing effective transfer of genes for aspartoacylase and high levels of activity for the enzyme. The gene transfer system was then tested in rodents and primates before initial clinical tests on two children, with no significant adverse effects. The biochemical, radiological, and clinical changes in human patients are being assessed. If successful, this trial would have implications for Canavan disease, for which there is currently no treatment, and for other types of leukodystrophy [145].

7.6.10 Metachromatic Leukodystrophy

Other researchers in Italy have used gene therapy to reverse neurological damage and deficits in a mouse model of metachromatic leukodystrophy by transplanting gene-corrected hematopoietic stem progenitor cells [146]. Microencapsulation is a potential means of enhancing cell transplant therapy for this and other leukodystrophies.

7.6.11 Amyotrophic Lateral Sclerosis

Extensive research, including gene therapy, is devoted to the treatment of ALS, a neurodegenerative disease of motor neurons in the spinal cord [147–149]. Encapsulated delivery of cells genetically engineered to produce CNTF has been evaluated for the treatment of ALS in Phase I and II trials on 12 patients [150,151]. CNTF delivery was delivered in the cerebrospinal fluid of nine patients and persisted for up to 20 weeks in two patients. Some immune response occurred in three patients, which was determined to be caused by traces of bovine fetuin antigen, which came from the culture medium used to prepare the cell capsules before implantation. The study showed no adverse side effects in the implanted patients [152]. Other studies are continuing [153].

7.6.12 Ocular Neurodegeneration: Glaucoma, Retinitis Pigmentosa, and Macular Degeneration

Neuroprotection with nanoengineered encapsulation is also being evaluated as a therapeutic strategy for degenerative conditions of ocular neurons, including retinitis pigmentosa, macular degeneration, and glaucoma [134,154–160]. One such approach uses cells encapsulated into polymers with coaxially situated poly(ethylene terephthalate) strands of yarn as a matrix. The sustained-release polymer capsules contain human retinal epithelial cells, which have been genetically transfected to produce CNTF. This study is an important demonstration of stable, long-term delivery of CNTF using genetically modified cells transplanted into the vitreous humor [161]. CNTF is a potent protective factor for retinal neurons, but until recently, there has been no way to provide slow steady release to the human retina. The drug cannot be taken orally because it is too big to cross the blood–retinal barrier. This research has progressed through a Phase I trial and, as of 2009, was undergoing Phase II trials to evaluate efficacy for macular degeneration and retinitis pigmentosa.

7.6.13 Severe and Chronic Pain

Gene therapy is also being investigated for the treatment of severe and chronic pain that cannot be satisfactorily managed with conventional therapies. In one approach, immunoisolated xenogeneic neuroendocrine chromaffin cells for the production of adrenaline and other hormone regulators are implanted for the treatment of chronic pain. Chromaffin cells from the adrenal gland secrete a mixture of compounds, such as histogranin [162–165], that have a strong analgesic effect, especially when administered into the intrathecal space of the spinal canal [165,166]. In a number of animal and human studies, encapsulated bovine chromaffin cells have been implanted in the subarachnoid space containing the spinal fluid [167–169]. The human-scale capsules were implanted with minimally invasive surgery, and the device design allowed retrieval after weeks or months. Results indicate survival of cells and raised levels of analgesic compounds such as catecholamines and metenkephalin. Reductions in morphine intake and improvement in pain ratings were observed in some patients. Immunoprotected allo- or xenogeneic chromaffin cells acting as "mini pumps" continuously delivering neuroactive substances could eventually be a useful therapy for patients suffering from neuropathic pain [170].

7.6.14 Epilepsy

Implantation of cell-derived implants is also a potential therapy in epilepsy. Some epileptic seizures are associated with a lack of adenosine, an inhibitor of neuronal activity in the brain and, thus, an endogenous anticonvulsant. The release of adenosine from implanted encapsulated cells is being evaluated as an approach to suppress synchronous discharges and epileptic seizures. In these studies, fibroblast cells are genetically engineered to release adenosine by inactivating the adenosine-metabolizing enzymes adenosine kinase and adenosine deaminase. After encapsulation into semipermeable polymers, the cells were grafted into brain ventricles in a rat model of epilepsy. Grafted rats showed nearly complete protection from behavioral seizures and a near-complete suppression of after-discharges in electroencephalogram recordings, while control rats remained unaltered. Thus, the local release of adenosine from implanted encapsulated cells is a potential therapeutic strategy for the treatment of drug-resistant partial epilepsies. These studies have been the results of a series of investigations starting with the team led by surgeon Patrick Aebischer, president and professor at the Swiss Federal Institute of Technology in Lausanne, Switzerland. This group has been especially active in pursuit of in vivo encapsulation of exogeneous cells for central nervous system therapies in neurodegenerative diseases. The work on epilepsy has been carried forward by research at the University of Zurich, and at the Robert Stone Dow Neurobiology Laboratories at Legacy Health in Portland, Oregon, led by Dr. Detlev Boison [171–178].

7.6.15 Summary of Translational Development of Nanoengineered Regenerative Neural Therapy

The biological restoration of the central nervous system architecture and function is becoming a conceivable possibility, thanks to the convergence of nanoengineered scaffolding, cell and tissue engineering, and stem cell advances. Many approaches are emerging that extend beyond modifying disease symptoms to protecting, repairing, and regenerating complex neural tissues.

In the areas we have briefly reviewed—advanced bioactive materials for targeted drug delivery, directive materials to help growing cells integrate into the brain, and scaffolding to support, protect, and guide transplanted cells from various sources—nanotechnology is accelerating development by enabling control over interactions at the cell–cell and receptor–ligand level. Knowledge of the dynamic sequences on the map of cell differentiation and tissue development is especially important. Each advance in understanding these interactions opens powerful new therapeutic opportunities. One area of advancement, which is complementary to the development of nanoengineered scaffolding and encapsulation, is new types and sources of stem cells. This area is also being accelerated by nanoscience and nanotechnology.

7.7 New Developments in Cell Therapy Accelerated by Nanoscience and Nanotechnology

The growing realization of the potential for the regeneration of the central nervous system has launched a new tide of research in ways to use multipotent cells in treatments of neurological disorders. Nanotechnology has spurred both the development of new encapsulation and delivery techniques and the understanding of new sources of stem cells.

Stem cells include the pluripotent embryonic cells that support organ development in utero, as well as more specialized multipotent stem cells that form a regenerative reserve in the developing and mature body. As the organism matures, stem cells differentiate into more sets of limited numbers of multipotent progenitor cells, each with the capacity to repopulate specialized niches for the renewal of particular tissues. For example, hematopoietic stem cells under normal conditions give rise to blood cells. Adult multipotent stem cells are a potential resource for regenerative therapy, but their populations are limited and typically require extraction and culture procedures to obtain quantities of cells for populating tissue implants.

7.7.1 Sources of Stem Cells

For nanoscaffold-supported tissues to be truly useful as a therapy, there must be a source of usable cells to be delivered and nurtured. Until recently, sources of stem cells were problematic for a number of reasons: moral, technical, and biological. Ideally, cells for regeneration should come from the patient's own tissues, thus eliminating objections and obstacles, including immune rejection, transfection, the logistics of transplantation, and other problems. But as the body matures, more and more cells are programmed into differentiated phenotypes. This differentiation is apparently irreversible, and is accompanied in most cases by a cessation of cell division and growth. This has been the greatest problem where we have the greatest need—the brain and neural tissues that are so central to our identity and existence. Neurons have long appeared to be the least amenable to regrowth and to have the fewest sources of native stem cells. But as we have learned more about the processes of cell differentiation and development, cell signaling, and the control of gene expression, more opportunities have opened to find usable stem cells in many parts of the body.

There is turnover in most tissues of the body to varying degrees. Blood and epithelial tissue like skin and intestinal lining are at one extreme, neurons and bone are at the other. In many ways, blood cells undergo an even more drastic and irreversible transformation than nerve cells, as they develop. Blood cells are constantly renewed in the body from a source of ever-growing and dividing stem cells, buried deep within the bone marrow, spleen, and a few other secreted and protected places.

The bone marrow is one widely used source of multipotent progenitor cells for research and for autologous transplant. A stem cell taken from bone marrow is variously referred to as a marrow stem cell, marrow stromal cell, multipotent stromal cell or MSC. (MSC also can refer to any stem cell originating from mesenchyme, embryonic connective tissue.) MSCs are multipotent adult (somatic) stem cells that can differentiate into a variety of cell types. MSCs have been induced to differentiate into osteoblasts, chondrocytes, myocytes, adipocytes, endothelia, beta-pancreatic islet cells, and nerve cells [179].

Researchers have looked at many other sources of stem cells. The cell with the greatest, or at least the most irrefutably obvious and accessible, potential for differentiation into any mature tissue is the fertilized egg, which divides and differentiates ultimately into every tissue of the body. When regenerative medicine was focused mainly on finding replacement parts, a straightforward source would be to grow new parts by co-opting growing cells from an embryo. This has obvious moral problems, which, as is generally the case, turn out to be practical and economic problems as well. Other sources of stem cells include umbilical cord tissue and pulp from baby teeth [180,181].

A more complete and subtle understanding of the nanoscale mechanisms of cell growth, gene expression, metagenomics, and proteomics is revealing many other sources of multipotent and even pluripotent stem cells, and showing how to reprogram some types of stem cells that are committed to a specialized growth path, and redirect their development [182–189].

Experiments to evaluate implants of cell-loaded scaffolding for brain regeneration have used cells from many sources other than nerve progenitor or stem cells. Bone marrow cells injected into the brain have been shown to survive and migrate toward injury sites in rats, and produced evidence of differentiation into brain cells, expressing proteins characteristic of glial cells and neurons [190]. Cells from postnatal bone marrow and umbilical cord blood have been induced to proliferate and differentiate into glia and neuron lineages in vitro, opening possible new sources of cells for central nervous system regeneration [191]. Transplantation of MSCs has been shown to promote endogenous cellular proliferation in the injured brains of rats through the secretion of bioactive factors in response to the local environment, stimulating the brain to amplify its own restorative processes [113,192–194]. However, definitive evidence does not exist for full differentiation of MSCs into functional neurons in vivo, so bone marrow as a source of replacement cells for the brain is an exciting but controversial issue [195–197]. If MSCs could be used for regenerative brain transplants, they could be harvested from the host, bypassing the issues of availability, transfection, and immune rejection.

Other sources of stem cells that have been investigated for central nervous system therapy include the umbilical cord [198], adipose tissues [199], traumatized muscle [200], and somatic cells (mesenchymal stem cells) [201]. It is beginning to be apparent that mesenchymal stem cells can be found in nearly all tissues of the body [202].

As research uncovers more details of the development and sustaining processes of the brain, new sources of regenerative cells are being found in the adult brain itself. The discovery of neurogenesis and neural stem cells existing in the mature central nervous system presents potential new sources of cells for regenerative therapy. Adult neural stem cells that were previously thought to be irreversibly committed to the production of a single specialized type of neuron in the brain have now been found capable of producing more generalized types of nerve cells [203–205].

Researchers in Germany led by Professor Magdalena Götz in Munich discovered that a type of adult neural stem cell in the olfactory bulb of the mouse brain could be reprogrammed. These stem cells were thought to be capable of producing only specialized neurons dedicated to sensory functions in the olfactory bulb. But Professor Götz's team took notice of previously known dendritic connections in adult olfactory cells, and identified them as resembling axons found in other parts of the brain. Through painstaking research, they mapped the sequential expression of transcription factors characteristic of the olfactory cells and found them duplicated in cells of the cerebral cortex and adult hippocampus. Based on these clues, they designed and performed experiments showing that the stem cells from the olfactory bulb could be recruited into the cerebral cortex after a lesion was induced, and regenerate cerebral cortex neurons [206]. This was accomplished without resort to scaffolding or genetic manipulation—the stem cells were capable of interacting with the novel environment of the cerebral cortex and adapting accordingly, responding to signals and directions from the other cells and extracellular matrix. If this type of process can take place in humans, it would provide a source of readily adaptable neural cells to regenerate damage from injury, strokes, or degenerative diseases like Alzheimer's.

7.7.2 Nanoscience- and Nanotechnology-Based Understanding of Cell Function

Thus, we see that adult stem cells from many different tissues can be induced to take on the capacities of less differentiated stem cells for regeneration of the brain, where until recently this was commonly thought impossible. This development was recently accelerated with the discovery of more and more ways to induce the refined and controlled reprogramming of differentiated cells, without genetic modification. Equally important has been the growing understanding of the mechanisms by which cell therapy is effective in regeneration [209–212]. Previously, it was thought that cell therapy might work by a "cell replacement" mechanism, but the emerging view is that cell therapy works by providing trophic or "chaperone" support to the injured tissue and brain. Appreciation of the coupled role of angiogenesis and neurogenesis regeneration of brain tissue is also growing. All of these developments have been assisted by advances in nanoscience and nanotechnology. The ability to map stem cell differentiation and fates is due to advances in proteomics coupled with nanotechnology tools such as live cell chips used to monitor cell differentiation processes and nanoparticles used to track the migration and fate of stem cells [213,214].

Nanoscience has underpinned developments in molecular genetics, physiology, proteomics, and epigenetics by providing more powerful tools for examining phenomena on the scale between biochemistry and cell biology, thereby opening new insights into mechanisms of macromolecular interactions that carry out life processes. With the aid of nanoscience insights and nanotechnology tools, the macromolecular nanomachinery that performs essential functions of cell growth and differentiation are being studied, analyzed, understood, and ultimately influenced and controlled. This knowledge and capability are the basis for a new generation of therapeutics.

The scientific and technical advances upon which the new nanomedical therapeutics are based encompass molecular genetics, proteomics, epigenetics, and environmental influences on cell development. These advances start with more detailed understanding of the mechanisms by which genetic encoding in the cell nucleus specifies the fate of the cell in its development and differentiation, and how that fate can be influenced and even reprogrammed [215]. The complex network of proteins and their interactions to implement cell development and differentiation form an intricate informatic web of interactions whose study forms the new field of proteomics [216,217]. And the final piece of this foundation is the understanding of how development is guided by epigentic factors within the cell and by interactions with other cells and the environment [217,218].

7.7.3 Gene Therapy

The breakthroughs in cellular reprogramming have removed many previous obstacles faced by gene therapy. Gene therapy for regeneration has been a promising strategy for many years, based on research with transgenic cells and animals. Using genetically altered cell cultures and mice, it has been shown that switching on just two genes can induce considerable regeneration of damaged nerve fibers in the spinal cord. This suggested that genetic therapy or drugs that activate perhaps only a handful of genes might be enough to induce regeneration of spinal cord in humans. This result was surprising but promising because of the large number of different genes known to be involved in nerve growth.

For example, in experiments at Duke University, researchers inserted genes that expressed the two nerve-growth regulatory proteins, GAP-43 and CAP-23, in cells of mice. After spinal cord damage, regeneration was increased by as much as 60 times in transgenic mice as compared to controls [219].

Further research has been stimulated by these and similar discoveries, but several obstacles remain to using gene therapy for nerve regeneration. Transgenic animals used in the experiments expressed the axon growth promoter genes throughout life, whereas normally they turn off after the development of the spinal cord is complete. For the process to be used therapeutically, there would have to be some means of turning the genes on after an accident (and turning off other genes that suppress neuron growth) in a safe and rapid procedure.

Other questions to be answered include how long the genes need to be expressed to get an effect, and what would be the side effects (such as neural cancer) of leaving them turned on in adults, and how to turn them off at the right time [220–223]. Because of the potential for treatments using gene therapy for intractable congenital and degenerative diseases, these questions have been pursued actively in research programs [224,225].

Based on extensive preclinical research, the probability of introduction and activation of cancer-causing genes associated with gene therapy was expected to be very low [226]. Animal experiments and limited human trials have been conducted using gene therapy for the treatment of congenital degenerative blindness (Leber's congenital amaurosis) [227], and adrenoleukodystrophy [228].

Experience with clinical trials of gene therapy treatments has resulted in cancer in a small but unacceptable percentage of cases [229,230]. Oncogenesis has been a serious roadblock for developing the potential of gene therapy, which has spurred much assessment and further research directed at finding solutions [231,232]. These challenging problems are beginning to yield to new research efforts in molecular and cell biology, genomics, and proteomics, with a key role being played by nanoengineered protein tools for reprogramming cells.

7.7.4 Induced Pluripotent Stem Cells

A completely new source of autologous stem cells is possible through the reprogramming of differentiated cells. If adult cells from a patient's own body could be readily and safely reprogrammed, they would provide a source of cells for regeneration of tissue, avoiding most of the difficulties involved with transplanted stem cells.

Reprogrammed cells, called induced pluripotent stem cells (iPSCs), were first produced in 2006, in a significant breakthrough by Yamanaka's research group, based in Kyoto, using biotechnology techniques in mice [233,234]. Previously, the only demonstrated reprogramming of adult cells relied on transplant of a cell nucleus (cloning), or fusion of an adult cell with an embryonic stem cell [235]. The Yamanaka group in Japan and others at Wisconsin, MIT, and elsewhere soon demonstrated reprogramming a number of types of cells using lentiviral or retroviral vectors, which inserted genetic modifications into the target cells [236–239]. Subsequent improvements in reprogramming protocols yielded iPSCs that more closely resembled embryonic stem cells and included human cells. This work advanced with several groups showing that viral reprogramming can be achieved using fewer inserted genes and other efficiencies. Only four transcription factors were sufficient to reprogram somatic cells into a stem cell-like state [240–245].

But viral transgenic techniques carried the potential to introduce cancer causing oncogenes and other harmful mutations to the DNA. Techniques were developed to remove viral-introduced oncogenes from reprogrammed cells, possibly removing one barrier to use of iPSCs in therapy [246]. But finding and removing cancer-causing genes and other mutagenic defects after the fact was an involved and complex process, which still carried some risks.

In a rapid series of developments in 2009, a number of research groups reported methods to induce pluripotency without permanent modification of the host cell genome [247]. A Harvard University group employed adenoviruses, which redirect host gene expression without inserting their genes into the host DNA [248]. Yamanaka's group used plasmids to effect transient expression of reprogramming factors without disturbing the host genome [249]. Both these methods were inherently slow (requiring prolonged expression of the factors to turn on reprogramming) and inefficient (requiring a separate nonintegrating vector for each reprogramming factor).

The problem of multiple vector delivery was solved in an efficient manner by the Kyoto group, using the 2A oligopeptide sequence discovered originally in the foot and mouth virus, and now used in genetic engineering. The self-splicing 2A sequence is used to link several DNA codons, allowing transcription of multiple peptides in one step, and it is removed from the peptide following transcription [250–252]. The 2A sequence technique has since been widely used to create multi-protein expression vectors with other cell-programming delivery mechanisms.

Another group based in Madison, Wisconsin, produced human iPSCs completely free of vector and transgene sequences with a single transfection using Epstein–Barr nuclear antigen-based episomal vectors [253].

Other studies, carried out by researchers based in Toronto and Edinburgh, and in Cambridge England, showed an elegant and efficient alternative, using a technique in which genes that reprogrammed adult cells back into a pluripotent stem cell–like state could be temporarily inserted by easily removable genetic modifications [254–256]. They used a transposon/transposase system, which was originally discovered in Baculoviruses; the transposon protein expression vector is easily removed from the host DNA by the transposase enzyme, which is transiently expressed after the other inserted genes have done their work. No trace of the inserted genes is permanently left in the host. The single transposon incorporated all of the four genes needed to reprogram mouse somatic cells. The transposon, named piggyBac, has been in use in transgenic research. The Baculoviruses are used in insect control, and its transposon has been employed to generate vaccines and for genetic engineering of fluorescent proteins in mice. The piggyBac transposon has much higher efficiency than the transient transduction achieved with adenoviruses [257].

These techniques had different efficiencies and advantages, but as a group, they were much more effective and easier to apply than classical genetic engineering technology. They open up a huge opportunity to create custom stem cells for patients from their own cells without resort to exogenous cells, human embryonic cells, or laborious harvesting and culturing of scarce autologous somatic stem cells.

Even more recently, methods have been demonstrated for reprogramming adult cells without viruses or other classical genetic engineering technology. Cells have been induced to revert to a stem cell state using nanoengineered cell-penetrating peptides to deliver proteins into the cells to effectively reprogram gene expression.

7.7.5 Peptide-Induced Pluripotent Stem Cells

The year 2009 was a watershed in research toward regenerative therapy, with breakthrough advances in cell reprogramming. After the initial publication of multiple papers reporting the first ability to create pluripotent cells without permanent foreign gene insertion, an avalanche of developments ensued. A number of independent techniques were brought together in concert with newly developed methods and integrated into powerful new capabilities for cell reprogramming. Perhaps the most striking advance was the reprogramming of adult cells to sustained pluripotent states, using cell-penetrating peptides to deliver recombinant proteins, without viral vectors or genetic alteration. This was accomplished on mouse cells in cultures by a team at Scripps Research Institute led by Dr. Sheng Ding, with a team that included Prof. Hans Robert Schöler and students from the Max Plank Institute for Molecular Biomedicine at Münster, Germany, and with funding from Fate Therapeutics [259].

Ding and his group devised a strategy based on the previously demonstrated ability of certain peptides to deliver proteins into cells. Conjugation of the proteins with these cell-penetrating peptides mediated their transduction through the cell membrane. His group had the capability to produce needed quantities of the four protein reprogramming factors used, by genetic engineering of *E. coli* in their own laboratory. They reprogrammed mouse cells in culture by seeding the cell cultures with conjugated proteins in four cycles alternating with incubation periods of 36 h between treatments. The resulting cells were stable and essentially indistinguishable from mouse embryonic stem cells in morphology, genetic tests, and growth of embryoid bodies in culture. They named the cells produced by their peptide transduction technique "protein-induced pluripotent stem cells" or piPSCs.

This achievement was a major step toward creating therapeutic iPSCs, which are easier to produce, less controversial, are free of induced mutations and oncogenes, and can originate from the patient's own cells to avoid immunological and transfection risks. The ability to create such cells presents unprecedented opportunities for biomedical research and clinical applications. In order to realize these potentials, much work must still be done to evaluate risks and effectiveness, improve techniques and kinetics of induction, and establish production and treatment protocols. This work was widely seen as a key breakthrough, and brought new energy and attention to the already intense efforts aimed at producing usable regenerative cell therapies.

7.7.6 Cell-Penetrating Transduction Peptides

The plasma membrane of cells presents a barrier to passage of most substances, except where transmembrane gates of other special mechanisms exist. The ability for certain peptides to translocate through the membrane into live cells has been known since the first example was found: a peptide produced by the HIV virus, which carries its Tat transcription factor into cells and releases it to activate infection. Since then, many other natural examples have been found, and the mechanisms have been studied (Figure 7.2). It appears that to function as a cell-penetrating peptide (or transduction peptide), a protein must be small, amphiphilic, and highly charged, typically due to a high number of arginine amino acid residues in its sequence [259,260].

Based on the characterization of natural transduction peptide examples, a number of synthetic versions have been made and evaluated as drug delivery vehicles and research tools. Different protein structures can be optimal for conjugating and carrying different cargoes through the membrane, and releasing them into the cytoplasm. Much research and development in the domain of physiology, pharmacology, and biochemistry has been carried out, aimed at producing effective drug delivery vehicles, which has laid a foundation of knowledge and technique that is now available for producing cell-reprogramming vectors [261–263].

Research to understand the exact mechanisms of transduction and the delivery of cargoes into cell compartments continues as insights are gained

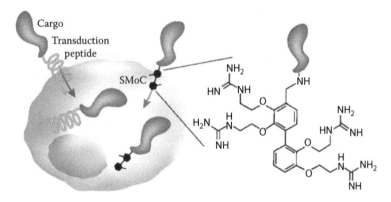

FIGURE 7.2
Cell-penetrating transduction peptides are used as drug delivery vehicles. They can also deliver epigenetic factors to reprogram adult differentiated cells into stem cell–like states or into different cell types. (From Prochiantz, A., *Nat. Methods*, 4, 119, 2007, With permission.)

into the external membrane and internal endoplasmic reticular structures of the cellular architecture. The field of bionanotechnology is elucidating the detailed structure and function of molecular machines such as ion gating channels and transmembrane shuttle proteins that operate to control the transfer of ions and small molecules across the membrane. For larger proteins, internalization occurs by an intricate mechanism of endocytosis, resulting in the uptake of the macromolecule into endocytic vesicles. Subsequent steps are then needed for release into the cytoplasm [264–266].

Research is continuing at an intensive pace on three fronts: new transduction enhancement factors, both proteins and other molecules that are more stable and effective for practical therapeutic delivery [267]; new proteins for reprogramming different target cells into specific differentiated types for therapy, and new techniques for their discovery and generation [268]; and new, more efficient and safer methodologies and protocols for the administration of programming factors into cells with cell-penetrating promotion factors [269].

7.7.7 Translational Research for iPSC Therapy

Translational research for the application of cell-penetrating peptides to the delivery of advanced cell-reprogramming factors is a challenging program, requiring collaboration of multiple disciplines and the integration of the results of many years of research in all aspects of molecular and macromolecular biology and chemistry. This diverse multidisciplinary effort is giving greater importance to the integrated approach of nanobiology and nanomedicine to address the broad conceptual and technical scope required. Stem cells are important as models in the study of human development and disease, and could lead to revolutionary new therapies [270–273].

Much work remains to be done to answer open questions about the eventual efficacy of regenerative therapies based on cell-penetrating peptide methods (such as piPSC) and their future refinements and enhancements. The space that can potentially be addressed by safe, readily available, and easily programmable cells for tissue regeneration is vast, in terms of the many types of diseases, disorders, protocols, and delivery methodologies. There are many challenges, both technical and medical, remaining [274,275]. The first step toward the translation of the newest and most powerful cell-reprogramming technology to clinical practice is to ensure safety. Although the cell-penetrating technology is still in an early stage of development, it has such enormous potential that attention is already being given to ensure that development will avoid safety pitfalls. Analysis and evaluation are being actively undertaken on many fronts [276,277].

It will be necessary to thoroughly characterize the iPSC cell lines that are produced by each variant of the latest techniques to produce programmed stem cells, in order to establish stability and potency of derived cells to produce the functions required of fully differentiated adult tissues, as well as their safety [278]. It should be determined how well iPSCs replicate the state of native embryonic cells and whether they generate differentiated progeny as efficiently and faithfully as embryonic stem cells. Methods employed to generate iPSCs need to be adapted to their use in a clinical environment. To answer these questions, it is necessary to analyze the underlying differences between induced and native stem cells at the molecular, genetic, and functional levels.

Early studies to characterize human iPSCs generated without viral vectors or genomic insertions reveal that these cells are, in general, similar to normal human stem cells, but with significant differences. The evaluation of iPSCs produced by an episomal methodology has so far shown a normal transcriptional signature, indicating that the episomal reprogramming strategy represents a safe way to generate human iPSCs for clinical purposes and basic research [279].

A thorough study of four lines of induced human pluripotent stem cells was conducted at the University of California at Los Angeles [280]. The conclusion was that iPSCs are distinctly different from normal cells in a number of statistically significant measures, as determined by genetic and molecular analysis. However, the induced cells were stable; the differences were primarily in degree of expression of genes, particularly those responsible for division, differentiation, and growth. The induced cells retained some expression signatures or patterns of the original cells. This extensive study began before the availability of quantities of peptide-induced pluripotent stem cell lines, so it reflects cells induced by earlier techniques. Much similar research is needed to learn more about the mechanisms of induced pluripotency in order to understand the nature and causes of differences between normal and induced stem cells [281]. This is an enormous area for further research that has only begun to be addressed [282–285].

7.7.8 Advances toward Clinical Therapies

The rapid advances being made in cell reprogramming are driving intensive preparations for new therapeutic modalities. Clinical researchers are now actively interested and involved in thinking about and planning for the potential application of readily available pluripotent cells, with all of their implications and possibilities. The notion of reprogramming nature cells into pluripotent stem cells has progressed from a fantastic conceptual idea into its current position, where it is appreciated as a mainstream research initiative with broad applications among all divisions of medicine. The impact covers many clinical disciplines focused on specific medical treatment modalities, treatments, and diseases [286].

One of the greatest near-term impacts of programmable autologous cells would be in the area of hematology, for the treatment of congenital disorders such as sickle cell anemia and cancers such as leukemia [287]. Here, the potential would be for the replacement of diseased stem cells in the bone marrow and other sources of rapidly replenished blood cells. For this therapy, tissue scaffolding is less of an issue than for many other tissues.

The availability of new sources of new types of cells for transplantation will have an impact on procedures, protocols, and standards for transplant immunology, for which implications and requirements are being analyzed [288].

As we have seen in the review of regenerative implants for treatment of nerve damage, the availability of cells suitable for regenerative therapies is a major issue, with relevance to research in the fields of neurology and neurosurgery. Because of this, much attention and study is being given to the implications of iPSC for design of new methodologies in neurosurgery, and to reviews alerting and informing practitioners of new developments [289–293]. In light of the potential implications of new sources of stem cells, new therapeutic approaches are being considered for treatment of peripheral nerve injury [294], pediatric motility disorders [295], Parkinson's disease [296], MS [297], ALS [298], and other types of nerve damage and neurodegenerative disorders.

The implications for diabetes are immediate and of great potential, calling for research into how cells can be reprogrammed into the complex differentiated beta cells that provide insulin and related regulatory hormones, and how they can be supported to overcome the causes of degeneration [299]. Among the major impacts of research into cell reprogramming will be insights into the mechanisms of degeneration, which in itself may be considered a kind of induced reprogramming. This aspect of cell reprogramming has similar implications for liver and kidney diseases, and for many other tissue disorders and cancers.

The impact for replacement of heart, vascular, and other muscle tissue is also important and relatively immediate for the repair of tissue following cardiovascular infarctions, progressive heart failure, and vascular disorders [300]. There is potential for the treatment of MS and other muscular disorders as well.

Stem cell therapies have potential application in the enteric nervous system for the treatment of gastroenteritic diseases such as Hirschsprung's disease and other aganglionic gut disorders and functional gastrointestinal disorders [301]. They could also be used in the repair and rescue of sphincter and other muscle function in gastroenterology, gynecology, and other areas.

Another focus in regeneration of hard tissues, including bone and teeth. Both of these areas could benefit from the availability of therapeutic cell reprogramming. There is virtually no area of medicine, from pediatrics to aging, in which the prospect of the ability to reprogram cells safely and efficiently would not be revolutionary, including infectious diseases and cancer.

The potential of new stem cell production methodologies has led to a wave of investments and start-up companies specifically focused on cell reprogramming as a source of stem cells [302,303]. Some existing companies that were formed to pursue the development of earlier stem cell technologies (such as Advanced Cell Technology) have added reprogramming research to their research base, as have major pharmaceutical companies. New companies created by the latest breakthroughs in cell reprogramming include BioQuark, Fate Therapeutics, Cellular Dynamics International, LD Biopharma, Inc., ProteomTech, iPierian (formerly iZumi), and others.

Perhaps to temper the impacts that we might imagine from stem cell technologies, we should consider that science and technology already possess comparable capabilities to reprogram the genomes of plants and bacteria. The results have indeed produced revolutionary impact for food supply and biotechnology for drug and materials production. But no technology, no matter how fundamentally disruptive, will cure all problems. The work to cure disease and disorders and provide care for their effects will continue with better and more powerful therapies, but not end.

7.8 Conclusion: Toward Clinical Therapies Based on Integrated Medical Nanoscience

In this chapter, we have reviewed developments in nanoengineered materials, cellular signaling, tissue encapsulation, and cellular programming, and how they are being brought together to realize a new medical technology for tissue regeneration and treatment in some of the most challenging and intractable diseases and disorders. The developments currently taking place are promising and exciting, but much work remains before the effectiveness of these approaches can be proven.

The potential availability of new sources of hindrance-free stem cells is a very promising prospect. But as we have seen in our earlier review of transplantation of cells, it is necessary to provide the right kind of supportive environment if stem cells are to be successfully used in therapy, even with the most suitable cell types. In order for new cell programming and stem cell research to develop toward potential therapies, translational research efforts are involving interdisciplinary efforts of cell and molecular biology, genetics, materials science and chemistry, physiology, and physics, with approaches that are aware of and take advantage of the latest insights provided by nanoscience and tools provided by nanotechnology. And in order for these new therapies to be usable, translational medicine will involve medical researchers, disease specialists, clinicians, and practitioners. These developments are taking place very rapidly.

The evident potential of these new technologies is already sufficiently promising that it is enlisting the interest and participation of the clinical medicine community. Translational research, clinical trials, and the development of protocols and therapeutics have already begun. New, effective, and safe therapies available to the practitioner can now be envisioned as a realistic possibility in the near future.

References

1. J. B. Thomas, N. A. Peppas, M. Sato, and T. J. Webster, Nanotechnology and biomaterials, in Y. Gogotsi (ed.), *Nanomaterials Handbook*, Chap. 22, CRC Press, Boca Raton, FL, 2006, pp. 605–636.
2. L. J. Lee, Polymer nanoengineering for biomedical applications, *Annals of Biomedical Engineering*, 34, 75–88 (2006).
3. T. Yamamuro, L. L. Hench, and J. Wilson-Hench, *CRC Handbook of Bioactive Ceramics*, Vol. I, CRC Press, Boca Raton, FL, 1990.
4. K.-Y. Lee, M. Park, H.-M. Kim, Y.-J. Lim, H.-J. Chun, H. Kim, and S.-H. Moon, Ceramic bioactivity: Progresses, challenges and perspectives, *Biomedical Materials*, 1, R31–R37 (2006).
5. B. D. Ratner, A. S. Hoffman, F. J. Schoen, and J. E. Lemons (eds.), *Biomaterials Science: An Introduction to Materials in Medicine*, Academic Press, London, U.K., 1996.
6. S. Y. Chew and T. G. Park, Nanofibers in regenerative medicine and drug delivery, *Advanced Drug Delivery Reviews*, 61, 987 (2009).
7. A. Atala and R. Lanza, *Methods of Tissue Engineering*, Academic Press, London, U.K., 2002.
8. W. T. Godbey and A. Atala, In vitro systems for tissue engineering, *Annals of the New York Academy of Sciences*, 961, 10–26 (2002).
9. L. G. Griffith and G. Naughton, Tissue engineering—Current challenges and expanding opportunities, *Science*, 295, 1009–1014 (2002).
10. R. S. Greco, F. B. Prinz, and R. L. Smith (eds.), *Nanoscale Technology in Biological Systems*, CRC Press, Boca Raton, FL, 2005.
11. G. Xiao-dong, Z. Qi-xin, D. Jing-yuan, Y. Shu-hua, W. Hong, S. Zeng-wu, and S. En-jie, Molecular tissue engineering: Concepts, status and challenge, *Journal of Wuhan University of Technology—Materials Science Edition*, 17, 30–34 (2002).
12. L. Zhang and T. J. Webster, Nanotechnology and nanomaterials: Promises for improved tissue regeneration, *NanoToday*, 4, 66–80 (2009).
13. J. B. Graham, Q.-S. Xue, D. Neubauer, D. Muir, A chondroitinase-treated, decellularized nerve allograft compares favorably to the cellular isograft in rat peripheral nerve repair, *Journal of Neurodegeneration and Regeneration*, 2, 19–30 (2009).
14. H. Uludag, P. De Vos, and P. A. Tresco, Technology of mammalian cell encapsulation, *Advanced Drug Delivery Reviews*, 42, 29–64 (2000).
15. A. Murua, A. Portero, G. Orive, R. M. Hernández, M. de Castro, and J. L. Pedraz, Cell microencapsulation technology: Towards clinical application, *Journal of Controlled Release*, 132, 76–83 (2008).
16. J. T. Wilson and E. L. Chaikof, Challenges and emerging technologies in the immunoisolation of cells and tissues, *Advanced Drug Delivery Reviews*, 60, 124–145 (2008).
17. F. Amato, C. Cosentino, S. Pricl, M. Ferrone, M. Fermeglia, M. M.-C. Cheng, R. Walczak, and Mauro Ferrari, Multiscale modeling of protein transport in silicon membrane nanochannels. Part 2. From molecular parameters to a predictive continuum diffusion model, *Biomedical Microdevices*, 8, 291–298 (2006).
18. K. E. La Flamme, K. C. Popat, L. Leoni, E. Markiewicz, T. J. La Tempa, B. B. Roman, C. A. Grimes, and T. A. Desai, Biocompatibility of nanoporous alumina membranes for immunoisolation, *Biomaterials*, 28, 2638–2645 (2007).

19. B. Gimi, T. Leong, Z. Gu, M. Yang, D. Artemov, Z. M. Bhujwalla, and D. H. Gracias, Self-assembled three dimensional radio frequency (RF) shielded containers for cell encapsulation, *Biomedical Microdevices*, 7, 341–345 (2005).
20. C. Smith, R. Kirk, T. West, M. Bratzel, M. Cohen, F. Martin, A. Boiarski, and A. A. Rampersaud, Diffusion characteristics of microfabricated silicon nanopore membranes as immunoisolation membranes for use in cellular therapeutics, *Diabetes Technology & Therapeutics*, 7, 151–162 (2005).
21. S. Schneider, P. J. Feilen, F. Brunnenmeier, T. Minnemann, H. Zimmermann, U. Zimmermann, and M. M. Weber, Long-term graft function of adult rat and human islets encapsulated in novel alginate-based microcapsules after transplantation in immunocompetent diabetic mice, *Diabetes*, 54, 687–693 (2005).
22. H. Zimmermann, S. G. Shirley, and U. Zimmermann, Alginate-based encapsulation of cells: Past, present, and future, *Current Diabetes Reports*, 7, 314–320 (2007).
23. C. G. Thanos, R. Calafiore, G. Basta, B. E. Bintz, W. J. Bell, J. Hudak, A. Vasconcellos et al., Formulating the alginate-polyornithine biocapsule for prolonged stability: Evaluation of composition and manufacturing technique, *Journal of Biomedical Materials Research Part A*, 83A, 216–224 (2007).
24. T. A. Desai, W. H. Chu, G. Rasi, P. Sinibaldi-Vallebona, E. Guarino, and M. Ferrari, Microfabricated biocapsules provide short-term immunoisolation of insulinoma xenografts, *Biomedical Microdevices*, 1, 131–138 (1999).
25. P. de Vos and P. Marchetti, Encapsulation of pancreatic islets for transplantation in diabetes: The untouchable islets, *Trends in Molecular Medicine*, 8, 363–366 (2002).
26. P. de Vos, A. F. Hamel, and K. Tatarkiewicz, Considerations for successful transplantation of encapsulated pancreatic islets, *Diabetologia*, 45, 159–173 (2002).
27. M. I. Cockett, CRIB (Cellular replacement by immunoisolatory biocapsule), *IDrugs*, 1, 362–367 (1998).
28. L. Canaple, N. Nurdin, N. Angelova, D. Hunkeler, and B. Desvergne, Development of a coculture model of encapsulated cells, *Annals of the New York Academy of Sciences*, 944, 350–361 (2006).
29. Y.-T. Kim, R. Hitchcock, K. W. Broadhead, D. J. Messina, and P. A. Tresco, A cell encapsulation device for studying soluble factor release from cells transplanted in the rat brain, *Journal of Controlled Release*, 102, 101–111 (2005).
30. F. J. Xu, S. P. Zhong, L. Y. L. Yung, Y. W. Tong, E. T. Kang, and K. G. Neoh, Collagen-coupled poly(2-hydroxyethyl methacrylate)–Si(111) hybrid surfaces for cell immobilization, *Tissue Engineering*, 11, 1736–1748 (2005).
31. R. Yao, Design and evaluation of a cell microencapsulating device for cell assembly technology, *Journal of Bioactive and Compatible Polymers*, 24, S48–S62 (2009).
32. X. Zhang, Y. Xie, C. G. Koh, and L. J. Lee, A novel 3-D model for cell culture and tissue engineering, *Biomedical Microdevices*, 11, 795–799 (2009).
33. F. J. Martin and C. Grove, Microfabricated drug delivery systems: Concepts to improve clinical benefit, *Biomedical Microdevices*, 3, 97–108 (2001).
34. G. W. Gross, W. Wen, and J. Lin, Transparent indium-tin oxide patterns for extracellular, multisite recording in neuronal culture, *Journal of Neuroscience Methods*, 15, 243–252 (1985).
35. U. Egert, B. Schlosshauer, S. Fennrich, W. Nisch, M. Fejtl, T. Knott, T. Muller, and H. Hammerle, A novel organotypic long-term culture of the rat hippocampus on substrate-integrated multielectrode arrays, *Brain Research Protocols*, 2, 229–242 (1998).

36. M. Bani-Yaghoub, R. Tremblay, R. Voicu, G. Mealing, R. Monette, C. Py, K. Faid, and M. Sikorska, Neurogenesis and neuronal communication on micropatterned neurochips, *Biotechnology and Bioengineering*, 92, 336–345 (2005).

37. M. D. Benson, M. I. Romero, M. E. Lush, Q. R. Lu, M. Henkemeyer, and L. R. Parada, Ephrin-B3 is a myelin-based inhibitor of neurite outgrowth, *Proceedings of the National Academy of Sciences*, 102, 10694–10699 (2005).

38. Application Note 111, Versatile biomolecular printing on a variety of surface types, BioForce Nanosciences, Inc., Ames, IA 50010 USA (2007).

39. C. E. Hulsebosch, Recent advances in pathophysiology and treatment of spinal cord injury, *Advances in Physiology Education*, 26, 238–255 (2002).

40. M. E. Schwab, Repairing the injured spinal cord, *Science*, 295, 1029–1031 (2002).

41. V. Maquet, D. Martin, B. Malgrange, R. Franzen, J. Schoenen, G. Moonen, and R. Jérôme, Peripheral nerve regeneration using bioresorbable macroporous polylactide scaffolds, *Journal of Biomedical Materials Research*, 52, 639–651 (2000).

42. T.-T. B. Ngo, P. J. Waggoner, A. A. Romero, K. D. Nelson, R. C. Eberhart, and G. M. Smith, Poly(L-lactide) microfilaments enhance peripheral nerve regeneration across extended nerve lesions, *Journal of Neuroscience Research*, 72, 227–238 (2003).

43. G. E. Rutkowski, C. A Miller, S. Jeftinija, and S. K. Mallapragada, Synergistic effects of micropatterned biodegradable conduits and Schwann cells on sciatic nerve regeneration, *Journal of Neural Engineering*, 1, 151–157 (2004).

44. M. Romero-Ortega and P. Galvan-Garcia, A biomimetic synthetic nerve implant, United States Patent 20070100358, Texas Scottish Rite Hospital for Children, Dallas, TX (2007).

45. T. Kmecko, G. Hughes, L. Cauller, J.-B. Lee, and M. Romero-Ortega, Nanocomposites for neural interfaces, in *Electrobiological Interfaces on Soft Substrates*, in J. P. Conde, B. Morrison III, and S. P. Lacour (eds.), Materials Research Society Symposium Proceedings 926E, Warrendale, PA, 926-CC04-06 (2006).

46. P. Galvan-Garcia, E. W. Keefer, F. Yang, M. Zhang, S. Fang, A. A. Zakhidov, R. H. Baughman, and M. I. Romero, Robust cell migration and neuronal growth on pristine carbon nanotube sheets and yarns, *Journal of Biomaterials Science, Polymer Edition*, 18, 1245–1261 (2007).

47. M. Zhang, K. R. Atkinson, and R. H. Baughman, Multifunctional carbon nanotube yarns by downsizing an ancient technology, *Science*, 306, 1358–1361 (2004).

48. S. K. Smart, A. I. Cassady, G. Q. Lua, and D. J. Martin, The biocompatibility of carbon nanotubes, *Carbon*, 44, 1034–1047 (2006).

49. J. Chłopek, B. Czajkowska, B. Szaraniec, E. Frackowiak, K. Szostak, and F. Béguin, In vitro studies of carbon nanotubes biocompatibility, *Carbon*, 44, 1106–1111 (2006).

50. M. A. Correa-Duarte, N. Wagner, J. Rojas-Chapana, C. Morsczeck, M. Thie, and M. Giersig, Fabrication and biocompatibility of carbon nanotube-based 3D networks as scaffolds for cell seeding and growth, *Nano Letters*, 4, 2233–2236 (2004).

51. S. Garibaldi, C. Brunelli, V. Bavastrello, G. Ghigliotti, and C. Nicolini, Carbon nanotube biocompatibility with cardiac muscle cells, *Nanotechnology*, 17, 391–397 (2006).

52. A. Magrez, S. Kasas, V. Salicio, N. Pasquier, J. W. Seo, M. Celio, S. Catsicas, B. Schwaller, and L. Forró, Cellular toxicity of carbon-based nanomaterials, *Nano Letters*, 6, 1121–1125 (2006).

53. J. M. Wörle-Knirsch, K. Pulskamp, and H. F. Krug, Oops they did it again! Carbon nanotubes hoax scientists in viability assays, *Nano Letters*, 6, 1261–1268 (2006).

54. M. Shim, N. Wong S. Kam, R. J. Chen, Y. Li, and H. Dai, Functionalization of carbon nanotubes for biocompatibility and biomolecular recognition, *Nano Letters*, 2, 285–288 (2002).

55. X. Yu, G. P. Dillon, and R. V. Bellamkonda, A laminin and nerve growth factor-laden three-dimensional scaffold for enhanced neurite extension, *Tissue Engineering*, 5, 291–304 (1999), doi:10.1089/ten.1999.5.291 (2008).

56. S. Yoshii and M. Oka, Peripheral nerve regeneration along collagen filaments, *Brain Research*, 888, 158–162 (2001).

57. S. Yoshii, M. Oka, M. Shima, A. Taniguchi, and M. Akagi, 30 mm regeneration of rat sciatic nerve along collagen filaments, *Brain Research*, 949, 202–208 (2002).

58. M. R. Ahmed and R. Jayakumar, Peripheral nerve regeneration in RGD peptide incorporated collagen tubes, *Brain Research*, 993, 208–216 (2003).

59. M. R. Ahmed, U. Venkateshwarlu, and R. Jayakumar, Multilayered peptide incorporated collagen tubules for peripheral nerve repair, *Biomaterials*, 25, 2585–2594 (2004).

60. V. Charulatha and A. Rajaram, Cross-linking density and resorption of dimethyl suberimidate-treated collagen, *Journal of Biomedical Materials Research*, 36, 478–486 (1997).

61. V. Charulatha and A. Rajaram, Influence of different cross-linking treatments on the physical properties of collagen membranes, *Biomaterials*, 24, 759–767 (2003).

62. M. R. Ahmed, S. Vairamuthu. M. Shafiuzama, S. H. Basha, and R. Jayakumar, Microwave irradiated collagen tubes as a better matrix for peripheral nerve regeneration, *Brain Research*, 1046, 55–67 (2005).

63. J. Brandt, L. B. Dahlin, M. Kanje, and G. Lundborg, Spatiotemporal progress of nerve regeneration in a tendon autograft used for bridging a peripheral nerve defect, *Experimental Neurology*, 160, 386–393 (1999).

64. S. Yoshii, M. Oka, N. Ikeda, M. Akagi, Y. Matsusue, and T. Nakamura, Bridging a peripheral nerve defect using collagen filaments, *Journal of Hand Surgery*, 26A, 52–59 (2001).

65. L. Cen, W. Liu, L. Cui, W. Zhang, and Y. Cao, Collagen tissue engineering: Development of novel biomaterials and applications, *Pediatric Research*, 63, 492–496 (2006).

66. R. Özay, A. Bekar, H. Kocaeli, N. Karlı, G. Filiz, and İ. H. Ulus, Citicoline improves functional recovery, promotes nerve regeneration, and reduces postoperative scarring after peripheral nerve surgery in rats, *Surgical Neurology*, 68, 615–622 (2007).

67. J. Piantino, J. A. Burdick, D. Goldberg, R. Langer, and L. I. Benowitz, An injectable, biodegradable hydrogel for trophic factor delivery enhances axonal rewiring and improves performance after spinal cord injury, *Experimental Neurology*, 201, 359–367 (2006).

68. E. C. Tsai, P. D. Dalton, M. S. Shoichet, and C. H. Tator, Synthetic hydrogel guidance channels facilitate regeneration of adult rat brainstem motor axons after complete spinal cord transection, *Journal of Neurotrauma*, 21, 789–804 (2004).

69. H. Nomura, C. H. Tator, and M. S. Shoichet, Bioengineered strategies for spinal cord repair, *Journal of Neurotrauma*, 23, 496–507 (2006).

70. H. M. Geller and J. W. Fawcett, Building a bridge: Engineering spinal cord repair, *Experimental Neurology*, 174, 125–136 (2002).
71. G. Orive, E. Anitua, J. L. Pedraz, and D. F. Emerich, Biomaterials for promoting brain protection, repair and regeneration, *Nature Reviews Neuroscience*, 10, 682–692 (2009).
72. G. M. G. Shepherd, M. Raastad, and P. Andersen, General and variable features of varicosity spacing along unmyelinated axons in the hippocampus and cerebellum, *Proceedings of the National Academy of Sciences*, 99, 6340–6345 (2002).
73. A. F. Soleng, K. Chiu and M. Raastad, Unmyelinated axons in the rat hippocampus hyperpolarize and activate an H current when spike frequency exceeds 1 Hz, *The Journal of Physiology*, 552, 459–470 (2004).
74. L. Thomas, Nano neuro knitting repairs injured brain, *The Lancet Neurology*, 5, 386 (2006).
75. R. G. Ellis-Behnke, L. A. Teather, G. E. Schneider, and K.-F. So, Using nanotechnology to design potential therapies for CNS regeneration, *Current Pharmaceutical Design*, 13, 2519–2528 (2007).
76. J. M. Provenzale and G. A. Silva, Uses of nanoparticles for central nervous system imaging and therapy, *American Journal of Neuroradiology*, 30, 1293–1301 (2009).
77. G. A. Silva, Nanotechnology approaches for the regeneration and neuroprotection of the central nervous system, *Surgical Neurology*, 63, 301–306 (2005).
78. G. A. Silva, Neuroscience nanotechnology: Progress, opportunities and challenges, *Nature Reviews Neuroscience*, 7, 65–74 (2006).
79. N. M. Gervasi, J. C. Kwok, and J. W. Fawcett, Role of extracellular factors in axon regeneration in the CNS: Implications for therapy, *Regenerative Medicine*, 3, 907–923 (2008).
80. S. S. Ali, J. I. Hardt, K. L. Quick, J. S. Kim-Han, B. F. Erlanger, T. T. Huang, C. J. Epstein, and L. L. Dugan, A biologically effective fullerene (C60) derivative with superoxide dismutase mimetic properties, *Free Radical Biology and Medicine*, 37, 1191–202 (2004).
81. J. Yin, F. Lao, P. P. Fu, W. G. Wamer, Y. Zhao, P. C. Wang, Y. Qiua et al., The scavenging of reactive oxygen species and the potential for cell protection by functionalized fullerene materials, *Biomaterials*, 30, 611–621 (2009).
82. Y. Zhong and R. V. Bellamkonda, Biomaterials for the central nervous system, *Journal of the Royal Society Interface*, 5, 957–975 (2008).
83. D. Y. Wong, P. H. Krebsbach, and S. J. Hollister, Brain cortex regeneration affected by scaffold architectures. *Journal of Neurosurgery*, 109, 715–722, (2008).
84. H. Zhang, T. Kamiya, T. Hayashi, K. Tsuru, K. Deguchi, V. Lukic, A. Tsuchiya et al., Gelatin-siloxane hybrid scaffolds with vascular endothelial growth factor induces brain tissue regeneration, *Current Neurovascular Research*, 5, 112–117 (2008).
85. J. Gao, Y. M. Kim, H. Coe, B. Zern, B. Sheppard, and Y. Wang, A neuroinductive biomaterial based on dopamine, *Proceedings of the National Academy of Sciences*, 103, 16681–16686 (2006).
86. J. T. Seil and T. J. Webster, Decreased astroglial cell adhesion and proliferation on zinc oxide nanoparticle polyurethane composites, *International Journal of Nanomedicine*, 3, 523–531 (2008).
87. A. Teixeira, J. K. Duckworth, and O. Hermanson, Getting the right stuff: Controlling neural stem cell state and fate in vivo and in vitro with biomaterials, *Cell Research*, 17, 56–61 (2007).

88. W. Potter, R. E. Kalil, and W. J. Kao, Biomimetic material systems for neural progenitor cell-based therapy, *Frontiers in Bioscience*, 13, 806–821 (2008).

89. R. Pankov and K. M. Yamada, Fibronectin at a glance, *Journal of Cell Science*, 115, 3861–3863 (2002).

90. G. L. Hornyak, H. F. Tibbals, J. Dutta, and J. J. Moore, Adhesive processes in the immune response, in *Introduction to Nanoscience and Nanotechnology*, CRC Press, Boca Raton, FL, 2009, pp. 558–565.

91. S. Woerly, E. Pinet, L. de Robertis, D. Van Diep, and M. Bousmina, Spinal cord repair with PHPMA hydrogel containing RGD peptides (NeurogelTM), *Biomaterials*, 20, 2213–2221 (2001).

92. Y. Chen, X. Xu, S. Hong, J. Chen, N. Liu, C. B. Underhill, K. Creswell, and L. Zhang, RGD-tachyplesin inhibits tumor growth, *Cancer Research*, 61, 2434–2438 (2001).

93. R. Hershkoviz, S. Melamed, N. Greenspoon, and O. Lider, Nonpeptidic analogues of the Arg-Gly-Asp (RGD) sequence specifically inhibit the adhesion of human tenon's capsule fibroblasts to fibronectin, *Investigative Ophthalmology & Visual Science*, 35, 2585–2591 (1994).

94. T. T. Yu and M. S. Shoichet, Guided cell adhesion and outgrowth in peptide-modified channels for neural tissue engineering, *Biomaterials*, 26, 1507–1514 (2005).

95. S. Itoh, M. Suzuki, I. Yamaguchi, K. Takakuda, H. Kobayashi, K. Shinomiya, and J. Tanaka, Development of a nerve scaffold using a tendon chitosan tube, *Artificial Organs*, 27, 1079–1088 (2003).

96. L. Brindley, Nanofibres reconnect nerves, *Chemistry World*, 5, 24–24 (2008).

97. H. Q. Cao, T. Liu, and S. Y. Chew, The application of nanofibrous scaffolds in neural tissue engineering, *Advanced Drug Delivery Reviews*, 61, 1055–1064 (2009).

98. P. A. Tran, L. Zhang, and T. J. Webster, Nanofibers in regenerative medicine and drug delivery, *Advanced Drug Delivery Reviews*, 61, 1097–1114 (2009).

99. E. B. Malarkey and V. Parpura, Applications of carbon nanotubes in neurobiology, *Neurodegenerative Diseases*, 4, 292–299 (2007).

100. D. R. Nisbet, S. Pattanawong, N. E. Ritchie, W. Shen, D. I. Finkelstein, M. K. Horne, and J. S. Forsythe, Interaction of embryonic cortical neurons on nanofibrous scaffolds for neural tissue engineering, *Journal of Neural Engineering*, 4, 35–41 (2007).

101. J. Gerardo-Nava, T. Führmann, K. Klinkhammer, N. Seiler, J. Mey, D. Klee, M. Möller, P. D. Dalton, and G. A. Brook, Human neural cell interactions with orientated electrospun nanofibers in vitro, *Nanomedicine*, 4, 11–30 (2009).

102. L. Ghasemi-Mobarakeh, M. P. Prabhakaran, M. Morshed, M.-H. Nasr-Esfahani, and S. Ramakrishna, Electrospun poly(-caprolactone)/gelatin nanofibrous scaffolds for nerve tissue engineering, *Biomaterials*, 29, 4532–4539 (2008).

103. R. G. Ellis-Behnke, Y. Liang, S. You, D. K. C. Tay, S. Zhang, K. So, and G. E. Schneider, Nano neuro knitting: Peptide nanofiber scaffold for brain repair and axon regeneration with functional return of vision, *Proceedings of the National Academy of Sciences*, 103, 5054–5059 (2006).

104. J. Guo, H. Su, Y. Zeng, Y. Liang, W. M. Wong, R. G. Ellis-Behnke, K. So, and W. Wu MD, Reknitting the injured spinal cord by self-assembling peptide nanofiber scaffold, *Nanomedicine: Nanotechnology, Biology and Medicine*, 3, 311–321 (2007).

105. J. Guo, K. K. G. Leung, H. Su, Q. Yuan, L. Wang, T.-H. Chu, W. Zhang et al., Self-assembling peptide nanofiber scaffold promotes the reconstruction of acutely injured brain, *Nanomedicine: Nanotechnology, Biology and Medicine*, 5, 345–351 (2009).

106. G. A. Silva, C. Czeisler, K. L. Niece, E. Beniash, D. A. Harrington, J. A. Kessler, and S. I. Stupp, Selective differentiation of neural progenitor cells by high-epitope density nanofibers, *Science*, 303, 1352–1355 (2004).

107. V. M. Tysseling-Mattiace, V. Sahni, K. L. Niece, D. Birch, C. Czeisler, M. G. Fehlings, S. I. Stupp, and J. A. Kessler, Self-assembling nanofibers inhibit glial scar formation and promote axon elongation after spinal cord injury, *Journal of Neuroscience*, 28, 3814–3823 (2008).

108. J. E. Lee, D. Khang, Y. E. Kim, and T. J. Webster, Stem cell impregnated carbon nanofibers/nanotubes for healing damaged neural tissue, *Materials Research Society Symposium Proceedings*, 915, 17–22 (2006).

109. S. Liao, C. K. Chan, and S. Ramakrishna, Stem cells and biomimetic materials strategies for tissue engineering, *Materials Science and Engineering: C*, 28(8), 1189–1202 (2008).

110. S. M. Willerth, K. J. Arendas, D. I. Gottlieb, and S. E. Sakiyama-Elbert, Optimization of fibrin scaffolds for differentiation of murine embryonic stem cells into neural lineage cells, *Biomaterials*, 27, 5990–6003 (2006).

111. I. Kulbatski, A. J. Mothe, H. Nomura, and C. H. Tator, Endogenous and exogenous CNS derived stem/progenitor cell approaches for neurotrauma, *Current Drug Targets*, 6, 111–126 (2005).

112. K. Brännvall, K. Bergman, U. Wallenquist, S. Svahn, T. Bowden, J. Hilborn, and K. Forsberg-Nilsson, Enhanced neuronal differentiation in a three-dimensional collagen–hyaluronan matrix, *Journal of Neuroscience Research*, 85, 2138–2146 (2007).

113. D. Lu, A. Mahmood, C. Qu, X. Hong, D. Kaplan, and M. Chopp, Collagen scaffolds populated with human marrow stromal cells reduce lesion volume and improve functional outcome after traumatic brain injury, *Neurosurgery*, 61, 596–602 (2007).

114. C. H. Hung, Y. L. Lin, and T. H. Young, The effect of chitosan and PVDF substrates on the behavior of embryonic rat cerebral cortical stem cells, *Biomaterials*, 27, 4461–4469 (2006).

115. T. H. Young and C. H. Hung, Behavior of embryonic rat cerebral cortical stem cells on the PVA and EVAL substrates, *Biomaterials*, 26, 4291–4299 (2005).

116. S. Levenberg, N. F. Huang, E. Lavik, A. B. Rogers, J. Itskovitz-Eldor, and Robert Langer, Differentiation of human embryonic stem cells on three-dimensional polymer scaffolds, *Proceedings of the National Academy of Sciences*, 100, 12741–12746 (2003).

117. E. Syková, P. Jendelová, L. Urdzíková, P. Lesný, and A. Hejcl, Bone marrow stem cells and polymer hydrogels—Two strategies for spinal cord injury repair, *Cellular and Molecular Neurobiology*, 26, 1113–1129 (2006).

118. M. J. Mahoney and W. M. Saltzman, Transplantation of brain cells assembled around a programmable synthetic microenvironment, *Nature Biotechnology*, 19, 934–939 (2001).

119. K. I. Park, Y. D. Teng, and E. Y. Snyder, The injured brain interacts reciprocally with neural stem cells supported by scaffolds to reconstitute lost tissue, *Nature Biotechnology*, 20, 1091–1093 (2002).

120. M. C. Tate, D. A. Shear, S. W. Hoffman, D. G. Stein, D. R. Archer, and M. C. LaPlaca, Fibronectin promotes survival and migration of primary neural stem cells transplanted into the traumatically injured mouse brain, *Cell Transplantation*, 11, 283–295 (2002).

121. D. A. Shear, M. C. Tate, D. R. Archer, S. W. Hoffman, V. D. Hulce, M. C. Laplaca, and D. G. Stein, Neural progenitor cell transplants promote long-term functional recovery after traumatic brain injury, *Brain Research*, 1026, 11–22 (2004).

122. C. C. Tate, D. A. Shear, M. C. Tate, D. R. Archer, D. G. Stein, and M. C. LaPlaca, Laminin and fibronectin scaffolds enhance neural stem cell transplantation into the injured brain, *Journal of Tissue Engineering and Regenerative Medicine*, 3, 208–217 (2009).

123. L. Longhi, E. R. Zanier, N. Royo, N. Stocchetti, and T. K. McIntosh, Stem cell transplantation as a therapeutic strategy for traumatic brain injury, *Transplant Immunology*, 15, 143–148 (2005).

124. S. Bajada, I. Mazakova, J. B. Richardson, and N. Ashammakhi, Updates on stem cells and their applications in regenerative medicine, *Journal of Tissue Engineering and Regenerative Medicine*, 2, 169–183 (2008).

125. P. Singh and D. J. Williams, Cell therapies: Realizing the potential of this new dimension to medical therapeutics, *Journal of Tissue Engineering and Regenerative Medicine*, 2, 307–319 (2008).

126. M. T. Harting, J. E. Baumgartner, L. L. Worth, L. Ewing-Cobbs, A. P. Gee, M.-C. Day, and C. S. Cox Jr., Cell therapies for traumatic brain injury, *Neurosurgical Focus*, 24, E17 (2008).

127. E. Bible, D. Y. S. Chau, M. R. Alexander, J. Price, K. M. Shakesheff, and M. Modo, The support of neural stem cells transplanted into stroke-induced brain cavities by PLGA particles, *Biomaterials*, 30, 2985–2994 (2009).

128. P. A. Walker, K. R. Aroom, F. Jimenez, S. K. Shah, M. T. Harting, B. S Gill, and C. S. Cox Jr., Advances in progenitor cell therapy using scaffolding constructs for central nervous system injury, *Stem Cell Reviews and Reports*, 5, 283–300 (2009).

129. Y. Xiong, A. Mahmood, and M. Chopp, Emerging treatments for traumatic brain injury, *Expert Opinion on Emerging Drugs*, 14, 67–84 (2009).

130. L. L. Dugan, E. G. Lovett, K. L. Quick, J. Lotharius, T. T. Lin, and K. L. O'Malley, Fullerene-based antioxidants and neurodegenerative disorders, *Parkinsonism and Related Disorders*, 7, 243–246 (2001).

131. J. Dong, J. M. Canfield, A. K. Mehta, J. E. Shokes, B. Tian, W. S. Childers, J. A. Simmons, Z. Mao, R. A. Scott, K. Warncke, and D. G. Lynn Engineering metal ion coordination to regulate amyloid fibril assembly and toxicity, *Proceedings of the National Academy of Sciences*, 104, 13313–13318 (2007).

132. D. F. Emerich and H. C. Salzberg, Update on immunoisolation cell therapy for CNS diseases, *Cell Transplantation*, 10, 3–24 (2001).

133. I. Date, T. Shingo and T. Ohmoto, Neurotrophic factor delivery by encapsulated cell grafts, in International Congress Series (*Molecular Mechanism and Epochal Therapeutics of ischemic Stroke and Dementia*. Invited papers from the International Symposium held in Okayama, Japan, October 18–20, 2002), 1252, 247–251 (2003).

134. D. F. Emerich and C. G. Thanos, Intracompartmental delivery of CNTF as therapy for Huntington's disease and retinitis pigmentosa, *Current Gene Therapy*, 6, 147–159 (2006).

135. V. Mittoux, J. M. Joseph, F. Conde, S. Palfi, C. Dautry, T. Poyot, J. Bloch et al., Restoration of cognitive and motor functions by ciliary neurotrophic factor in a primate model of Huntington's disease, *Human Gene Therapy*, 11, 1177–1187 (2000).

136. A. C. Bachoud-Levi, N. Déglon, J. P. Nguyen, J. Bloch, C. Bourdet, L. Winkel, P. Rémy et al., Neuroprotective gene therapy for Huntington's disease using a polymer-encapsulated BHK cell line engineered to secrete human CNTF, *Human Gene Therapy*, 11, 1723–1729 (2000).

137. J. Bloch, A. C. Bachoud-Levi, N. Déglon, J. P. Lefaucheur, L. Winkel, S. Palfi, J. P. Nguyen et al., Neuroprotective gene therapy for Huntington's disease, using polymer-encapsulated cells engineered to secrete human ciliary neurotrophic factor: Results of a phase I study, *Human Gene Therapy*, 15, 968–975 (2004).

138. E. Garbayo, C. N. Montero-Menei, E. Ansorena, J. L. Lanciego, M. S. Aymerich, and M. J. Blanco-Prieto, Effective GDNF brain delivery using microspheres— A promising strategy for Parkinson's disease, *Journal of Controlled Release*, 135, 119–126 (2009).

139. A. Glavaski-Joksimovic, T. Virag, Q. A. Chang, N. C. West, T. A. Mangatu, M. P. McGrogan, M. Dugich-Djordjevic, and M. C. Bohn, Reversal of dopaminergic degeneration in a Parkinsonian rat following micrografting of human bone marrow-derived neural progenitors, *Cell Transplantation*, 18, 804–814 (2009).

140. J. M. Péan, P. Menei, O. Morel, C. N. Montero-Menei, and J. P. Benoit, Intraseptal implantation of NGF-releasing microspheres promote the survival of axotomized cholinergic neurons, *Biomaterials*, 20, 2097–2101 (2000).

141. H. Gu, D. Long, C. Song, and X. Li, Recombinant human NGF-loaded microspheres promote survival of basal forebrain cholinergic neurons and improve memory impairments of spatial learning in the rat model of Alzheimer's disease with fimbria-fornix lesion, *Neuroscience Letters*, 453, 204–209 (2009).

142. R. Furlan, S. Pluchino, and G. Martino, Gene therapy-mediated modulation of immune processes in the central nervous system, *Current Pharmaceutical Design*, 9, 2002–2008 (2003).

143. R. Furlan, S Pluchino, and G. Martino, The therapeutic use of gene therapy in inflammatory demyelinating diseases of the central nervous system, *Current Opinion in Neurology*, 16, 385–392 (2003).

144. D. Baker and D. J. Hankey, Gene therapy in autoimmune, demyelinating disease of the central nervous system, *Gene Therapy*, 10, 844–853 (2003).

145. P. Leone, C. G. Janson, L. Bilaniuk, Z. Wang, F. Sorgi, L. Huang, R. Matalon et al., Aspartoacylase gene transfer to the mammalian central nervous system with therapeutic implications for Canavan disease, *Annals of Neurology*, 48, 27–38 (2000).

146. A. Biffi, A. Capotondo, S. Fasano, U. del Carro, S. Marchesini, H. Azuma, M. C. Malaguti et al., Gene therapy of metachromatic leukodystrophy reverses neurological damage and deficits in mice, *Journal of Clinical Investigation*, 116, 3070–3082 (2006).

147. P. Aebischer and A. C. Kato, Treatment of amyotrophic lateral sclerosis using a gene therapy approach, *European Neurology*, 35, 65–68 (1995).

148. J. D. Mitchell and G. D. Borasio, Amyotrophic lateral sclerosis, *The Lancet*, 369, 2031–2041 (2007).

149. C. O'riordan, Catherine, and S. Wadsworth, Gene therapy for amyotrophic lateral sclerosis and other spinal cord disorders, United States Patent Application 20090286857, Genzyme Corporation, Cambridge, MA (2009).

150. N. A.-M. Pochon, B. Heyd, N. Déglon, J.-M. Joseph, A. D. Zurn, E. E. Baetge, J. P. Hammang et al., Therapy for amyotrophic lateral sclerosis (ALS) Using a polymer encapsulated xenogenic cell line engineered to secrete hCNTF, *Human Gene Therapy*, 7, 851–860 (1996).

151. P. Aebischer, M. Schluep, N. Déglon, J.-M. Joseph, L. Hirt, B. Heyd, M. Goddard et al., Intrathecal delivery of CNTF using encapsulated genetically modified xenogeneic cells in amyotrophic lateral sclerosis patients, *Nature Medicine*, 2, 696–699 (1996).

152. A. D. Zurn, H. Henry, M. Schluep, V. Aubert, L. Winkel, B. Eilers, C. Bachmann, and P. Aebischer, Evaluation of an intrathecal immune response in amyotrophic lateral sclerosis patients implanted with encapsulated genetically-engineered xenogeneic cells, *Cell Transplantation*, 9, 471–484 (2000).

153. M. Azzouz, Gene therapy for ALS: Progress and prospects, *Biochimica et Biophysica Acta (BBA)—Molecular Basis of Disease*, 1762, 1122–1127 (2006).

154. S. C. Borrie, J. Duggan, and M. F. Cordeiro, Retinal cell apoptosis, *Expert Review of Ophthalmology*, 4, 27–45 (2009).

155. S. Kaushik, S. S. Pandav, and J. Ram, Neuroprotection in glaucoma, *Journal of Postgraduate Medicine*, 49, 90–95 (2003).

156. A. Bird, How to keep photoreceptors alive, *Proceedings of the National Academy of Sciences*, 104, 2033–2034 (2007).

157. C. Rowe-Rendleman and R. D. Glickman, Possible therapy for age-related macular degeneration using human telomerase, *Brain Research Bulletin*, 62, 549–553 (2004).

158. P. T. V. M. de Jong, Age-related macular degeneration, *New England Journal of Medicine*, 355, 1474–1485 (2006).

159. X. Cai, S. Conley, and M. Naash, Nanoparticle applications in ocular gene therapy, *Vision Research*, 48, 319–324 (2008).

160. V. Enzmann, E. Yolcu, H. J. Kaplan, and S. T. Ildstad, Stem cells as tools in regenerative therapy for retinal degeneration, *Archives of Ophthalmology*, 127, 563–571 (2009).

161. P. A. Sieving, R. C. Caruso, W. Tao, H. R. Coleman, D. J. S. Thompson, K. R. Fullmer, and R. A. Bush, Ciliary neurotrophic factor (CNTF) for human retinal degeneration: Phase I trial of CNTF delivered by encapsulated cell intraocular implants, *Proceedings of the National Academy of Sciences*, 103, 3896–3901 (2006).

162. S. Lemaire, V. K. Shukla, C. Rogers, I. H. Ibrahim, C. Lapierre, P. Parent, and M. Dumont, Isolation and characterization of histogranin, a natural peptide with NMDA receptor antagonist activity, *European Journal of Pharmacology*, 245, 247–256 (1993).

163. S. Lemaire, C. Rogers, M. Dumont, V. K. Shukla, C. Lapierre, J. Prasad, and I. Lemaire, Histogranin, a modified histone h4 fragment endowed with N-methyl-D-aspartate antagonist and immunostimulatory activities, *Life Sciences*, 56, 1233–1241 (1995).

164. J. B. Siegan, A. T. Hama, and J. Sagen, Suppression of neuropathic pain by a naturally-derived peptide with NMDA antagonist activity, *Brain Research*, 755, 331–334 (1997).

165. I. D. Hentall, W. A. Hargraves, and J. Sagen, Inhibition by the chromaffin cell-derived peptide serine-histogranin in the rat's dorsal horn, *Neuroscience Letters,* 419, 88–92 (2007).
166. S. W. Cramer, C. Baggott, J. Cain, J. Tilghman, B. Allcock, G. Miranpuri, S. Rajpal, D. Sun, and D. Resnick, The role of cation-dependent chloride transporters in neuropathic pain following spinal cord injury, *Molecular Pain,* 4, 36 (2008).
167. E. Buchser, M. Goddard, B. Heyd, J. M. Joseph, J. Favre, N. de Tribolet, M. Lysaght, and P. Aebischer, Immunoisolated xenogeneic chromaffin cell therapy for chronic pain, Initial clinical experience, *Anesthesiology,* 5, 1005–1112 (1996).
168. I. Décosterd, E. Buchser, N. Gilliard, J. Saydoff, A. D. Zurn, and P. Aebischer, Intrathecal implants of bovine chromaffin cells alleviate mechanical allodynia in a rat model of neuropathic pain, *Pain,* 76, 159–166 (1998).
169. Y. Jeon, K. Kwak, S. Kim, Y. Kim, J. Lim, and W. Baek, Intrathecal implants of microencapsulated xenogenic chromaffin cells provide a long-term source of analgesic substances, *Transplantation Proceedings,* 38, 3061–3065 (2006).
170. J. Sagen, D. Castellanos, and S. Gajavelli, Transplants for chronic pain, in *Cellular Transplants: From Lab to Clinic,* C. Halberstadt and D. Emerich (eds.), Chap. 26, pp 455–475, Elsevier, New York, 2007.
171. A. Huber, V. Padrun, N. Déglon, P. Aebischer, H. Möhler, and D. Boison, Grafts of adenosine-releasing cells suppress seizures in kindling epilepsy, *Proceedings of the National Academy of Sciences,* 98, 7611–7616 (2001).
172. J. A. Ribeiro, A. M. Sebastião, and A. de Mendonça, Adenosine receptors in the nervous system: Pathophysiological implications, *Progress in Neurobiology,* 68, 377–392 (2002).
173. M. Güttinger, D. Fedele, P. Koch, V. Padrun, W. F. Pralong, O. Brüstle, and D. Boison, Suppression of kindled seizures by paracrine adenosine release from stem cell-derived brain implants, *Epilepsia,* 46, 1162–1169 (2005).
174. D. Boison, Adenosine and epilepsy: From therapeutic rationale to new therapeutic strategies, *Neuroscientist,* 11, 25–36 (2005).
175. O. Pagonopoulou, A. Efthimiadou, B. Asimakopoulos, and N. K. Nikolettos, Modulatory role of adenosine and its receptors in epilepsy: Possible therapeutic approaches, *Neuroscience Research,* 56, 14–20 (2006).
176. D. Boison, Adenosine-based cell therapy approaches for pharmacoresistant epilepsies, *Neurodegenerative Diseases,* 4, 28–33 (2007).
177. D. Boison, Engineered adenosine-releasing cells for epilepsy therapy: Human mesenchymal stem cells and human embryonic stem cells, *Neurotherapeutics,* 6, 278–283 (2009).
178. D. Boison, Adenosine augmentation therapies (AATs) for epilepsy: Prospect of cell and gene therapies, *Epilepsy Research,* 85, 131–141 (2009).
179. Stem Cell Basics: Introduction. In *Stem Cell Information* (World Wide Web site). Bethesda, MD: National Institutes of Health, U.S. Department of Health and Human Services, 2009 (cited Tuesday, April 28, 2009), Available at <http://stemcells.nih.gov/info/basics/basics1>
180. S. C. Zhang, Embryonic stem cells for neural replacement therapy: Prospects and challenges, *Journal of Hematotherapy and Stem Cell Research,* 12, 625–634 (2003).
181. G. A. Silva and D. Yu, Stem cell sources and therapeutic approaches for central nervous system and neural retinal disorders, *Neurosurgical Focus,* 24, E11 (2008).

182. T. Shimazaki, Biology and clinical application of neural stem cells, *Hormone Research*, 60(Suppl 3), 1–9 (2003).
183. D. J. Webber and S. L. Minger, Therapeutic potential of stem cells in central nervous system regeneration, *Current Opinion in Investigational Drugs*, 5, 714–719 (2004).
184. D. A. Peterson, Stem cell therapy for neurological disease and injury, *Panminerva Medica*, 46, 75–80 (2004).
185. S. Goldman, Stem and progenitor cell-based therapy of the human central nervous system, *Nature Biotechnology*, 23, 862–871 (2005).
186. S. A. Goldman, M. S. Windrem, Cell replacement therapy in neurological disease, *Philosophical Transactions of the Royal Society B: Biological Sciences*, 361, 1463–1475 (2006).
187. J. Imitola, Prospects for neural stem cell-based therapies for neurological diseases, *Neurotherapeutics*, 4, 701–714 (2007).
188. Y. Uyanikgil and H. A. Balcioglu, Neural stem cell therapy in neurological diseases, *Archives of Medical Science*, 3, 296–302 (2009).
189. S. U. Kim and J. de Vellis, Stem cell-based cell therapy in neurological diseases: A review, *Journal of Neuroscience Research*, 87, 2183–2200 (2009).
190. A. Mahmood, D. Lu, L. Yi, J. L. Chen, and M. Chopp, Intracranial bone marrow transplantation after traumatic brain injury improving functional outcome in adult rats, *Journal of Neurosurgery*, 94, 589–595 (2001).
191. J. R. Sanchez-Ramos, Neural cells derived from adult bone marrow and umbilical cord blood, *Journal of Neuroscience Research*, 69, 880–893 (2002).
192. A. Mahmood, D. Lu, and M. Chopp, Marrow stromal cell transplantation after traumatic brain injury promotes cellular proliferation within the brain, *Neurosurgery*, 55, 1185–1193 (2004).
193. Y. Xiong, C. Qu, A. Mahmood, Z. Liu, R. Ning, Y. Li, D. L. Kaplan, T. Schallert, and M. Chopp, Delayed transplantation of human marrow stromal cell-seeded scaffolds increases transcallosal neural fiber length, angiogenesis, and hippocampal neuronal survival and improves functional outcome after traumatic brain injury in rats, *Brain Research*, 1263, 183–191 (2009).
194. C. Qu, Y. Xiong, A. Mahmood, D. L. Kaplan, A. Goussev, R. Ning, and M. Chopp, Treatment of traumatic brain injury in mice with bone marrow stromal cell-impregnated collagen scaffolds: Laboratory investigation, *Journal of Neurosurgery*, 111, 658–665 (2009).
195. Y. Li and M. Chopp, Marrow stromal cell transplantation in stroke and traumatic brain injury, *Neuroscience Letters*, 456, 120–123 (2009).
196. M. Opydo-Chanek, Bone marrow stromal cells in traumatic brain injury (TBI) therapy: True perspective or false hope? *Acta Neurobiologiae Experimentalis*, 67, 187–195 (2007).
197. J. J. Ross and C. M. Verfaillie, Evaluation of neural plasticity in adult stem cells, *Philosophical Transactions of the Royal Society B: Biological Sciences*, 363, 199–205 (2008).
198. S. Ruhil, V. Kumar, and P. Rathee, Umbilical cord stem cell: An overview, *Current Pharmaceutical Biotechnology*, 10, 327–334 (2009).
199. Y. Zhu, T. Liu, K. Song, X. Fan, X. Ma, and Z. Cui, Adipose-derived stem cell: A better stem cell than BMSC, *Cell Biochemistry and Function*, 26, 664–675 (2008).
200. W. M. Jackson, A. B. Aragon, F. Djouad, Y. Song, S. M. Koehler, L. J. Nesti, and R. S. Tuan, Mesenchymal progenitor cells derived from traumatized human muscle, *Journal of Tissue Engineering and Regenerative Medicine*, 3, 129–138 (2009).

201. Y. Chen, J.-Z. Shao, L.-X. Xiang, X.-J. Dong, and G.-R. Zhang, Mesenchymal stem cells: A promising candidate in regenerative medicine, *International Journal of Biochemistry and Cell Biology*, 40, 815–820 (2008).

202. M. L. da Silva, P. C. Chagastelles, and N. B. Nardi, Mesenchymal stem cells reside in virtually all post-natal organs and tissues, *Journal of Cell Science*, 119, 2204–2213 (2006).

203. M. Wernig and O. Brüstle, Fifty ways to make a neuron: Shifts in stem cell hierarchy and their implications for neuropathology and CNS repair, *Journal of Neuropathology and Experimental Neurology*, 61, 101–110 (2002).

204. E. Kokovay, Q. Shen, and S. Temple, The incredible elastic brain: How neural stem cells expand our minds, *Neuron*, 60, 420–429 (2008).

205. J. Sharp and H. S. Keirstead, Stem cell-based cell replacement strategies for the central nervous system, *Neuroscience Letters*, 456, 107–111 (2009).

206. M. S Brill, J. Ninkovic, E. Winpenny, R. D. Hodge, I. Ozen, R. Yang, A. Lepier et al., Adult generation of glutamatergic olfactory bulb interneurons, *Nature Neuroscience*, 12, 1351–1474 (2009).

207. A. V. Kabanov and H. E. Gendelman, Nanomedicine in the diagnosis and therapy of neurodegenerative disorders, *Progress in Polymer Science*, 32, 1054–1082 (2007).

208. Z. Wang, J. Ruan, and D. X. Cui, Advances and prospect of nanotechnology in stem cells, *Nanoscale Research Letters*, 4, 593–605 (2009).

209. R. H. Miller, The promise of stem cells for neural repair, *Brain Research*, 1091, 258–264 (2006).

210. B. K. Ormerod, T. D. Palmer, and M. A. Caldwell, Neurodegeneration and cell replacement, *Philosophical Transactions of the Royal Society, B Biological Sciences*, 153–170 (2008).

211. D. C. Hess and C. V. Borlongan, Stem cells and neurological diseases, *Cell Proliferation*, 41 Suppl 1, 94–114 (2008).

212. D. M. Suter and K. H. Krause, Neural commitment of embryonic stem cells: Molecules, pathways and potential for cell therapy, *The Journal of Pathology*, 215, 355–368 (2008).

213. C. Maercker, T. Rogge, H. Mathis, H. Ridinger, and K. Bieback, Development of live cell chips to monitor cell differentiation processes, *Engineering in Life Sciences*, 8, 33–39 (2008).

214. P. Jendelová, V. Herynek, J. DeCroos, K. Glogarová, B. Andersson, M. Hájek, and E. Syková, Imaging the fate of implanted bone marrow stromal cells labeled with superparamagnetic nanoparticles, *Magnetic Resonance in Medicine*, 50, 767–776 (2003).

215. C. W. Lederer and N. Santama, Neural stem cells: Mechanisms of fate specification and nuclear reprogramming in regenerative medicine, *Biotechnology Journal*, 3, 1521–1538 (2008).

216. S. Beyer, E. Mix, R. Hoffrogge, K. Lünser, U. Völker, and A. Rolfs, Neuroproteomics in stem cell differentiation, *Proteomics—Clinical Applications*, 1, 1513–1523 (2007).

217. R. L. Gundry, K. R. Boheler, J. E. Van Eyk, and B. Wollscheid, A novel role for proteomics in the discovery of cell-surface markers on stem cells: Scratching the surface, *Proteomics—Clinical Applications*, 2, 892–903 (2008).

218. L. Migliore and F. Coppedè, Genetics, environmental factors and the emerging role of epigenetics in neurodegenerative diseases, *Mutation Research—Fundamental and Molecular Mechanisms of Mutagenesis*, 667, 82–97 (2009).

219. H. M. Bomze, K. R. Bulsara, B. J. Iskandar, P. Caroni, and J. H. P. Skene, Spinal axon regeneration evoked by replacing two growth cone proteins in adult neurons, *Nature Neuroscience*, 4, 38–43 (2001).
220. J. B. Opalinska and A. M. Gewirtz, Nucleic-acid therapeutics: Basic principles and recent applications, *Nature Reviews Drug Discovery*, 1, 503–514 (2002).
221. U. P. Davé, N. A. Jenkins, and N. G. Copeland, Gene therapy insertional mutagenesis insights, *Science*, 303, 333 (2004).
222. M. Sadelain, Insertional oncogenesis in gene therapy: How much of a risk? *Gene Therapy*, 11, 569–573 (2004).
223. M. Themis, S. N. Waddington, M. Schmidt, C. von Kalle, Y. Wang, F. Al-Allaf, L. G. Gregory et al., Oncogenesis following delivery of a nonprimate lentiviral gene therapy vector to fetal and neonatal mice, *Molecular therapy*, 12, 763–771 (2005).
224. N. Korin and S. Levenberg, Engineering human embryonic stem cell differentiation, *Biotechnology and Genetic Engineering Reviews*, 24, 243–262 (2007).
225. J. B. Gurdon and D. A. Melton, Nuclear reprogramming in cells, *Science*, 322, 1811–1815 (2008).
226. L. Naldini, A comeback for gene therapy, *Science*, 326, 805–806 (2009).
227. A. M. Maguire, K. A High, A. Auricchio, J. F. Wright, E. A. Pierce, F. Testa, F. Mingozzi et al., Age-dependent effects of RPE65 gene therapy for Leber's congenital amaurosis: A phase 1 dose-escalation trial, *Lancet*, 374, 1597–1605 (2009).
228. N. Cartier, S. Hacein-Bey-Abina, C. C. Bartholomae, G. Veres, M. Schmidt, I. Kutschera, M. Vidaud et al., Hematopoietic stem cell gene therapy with a lentiviral vector in X-linked adrenoleukodystrophy, *Science*, 326, 818–823 (2009).
229. S. Hacein-Bey-Abina, A. Garrigue, G. P. Wang, J. Soulier, A. Lim, E. Morillon, E. Clappier et al., Insertional oncogenesis in 4 patients after retrovirus-mediated gene therapy of SCID-X1, *Journal of Clinical Investigation*, 118, 3132–3142 (2008).
230. S. J. Howe, M. R. Mansour, K. Schwarzwaelder, C. Bartholomae, M. Hubank, H. Kempski, M. H. Brugman et al., Insertional mutagenesis combined with acquired somatic mutations causes leukemogenesis following gene therapy of SCID-X1 patients, *Journal of Clinical Investigation*, 118, 3143–3150 (2008).
231. M. Cavazzana-Calvo, Gene therapy trials: Lessons and remaining questions—Basic research tries to decrease the risks of translational medicine, *Gene Therapy*, 16, 309–310 (2009).
232. O. S. Kustikova, B. Schiedlmeier, M. H Brugman, M. Stahlhut, S. Bartels, Z. Li, and C. Baum, Cell-intrinsic and vector-related properties cooperate to determine the incidence and consequences of insertional mutagenesis, *Molecular Therapy*, 17, 1537–1547 (2009).
233. K. Takahashi and S. Yamanaka, Induction of pluripotent stem cells from mouse embryonic and adult fibroblast cultures by defined factors, *Cell*, 126, 663–76 (2006).
234. R. Alberio, K. H. Campbell, and A. D. Johnson, Reprogramming somatic cells into stem cells, *Reproduction*, 132, 709–720 (2006).
235. K. Hochedlinger, R. Blelloch, C. Brennan, Y. Yamada, M. Kim, L. Chin, and R. Jaenisch, Reprogramming of a melanoma genome by nuclear transplantation, *Genes and Development*, 18, 1875–1885 (2004).
236. K. Takahashi, K. Tanabe, M. Ohnuki, M. Narita, T. Ichisaka, K. Tomoda, and S. Yamanaka1, Induction of pluripotent stem cells from adult human fibroblasts by defined factors, *Cell*, 131, 861–872 (2007).

237. J. Yu, M. A. Vodyanik, K. Smuga-Otto, J. Antosiewicz-Bourget, J. L. Frane, S. Tian, J. Nie et al., Induced pluripotent stem cell lines derived from human somatic cells, *Science*, 318, 1917–1920 (2007).

238. M. Wernig, A. Meissner, R. Foreman, T. Brambrink, M. Ku, K. Hochedlinger, B. E. Bernstein, and R. Jaenisch, In vitro reprogramming of fibroblasts into a pluripotent ES-cell-like state, *Nature*, 448, 318–324 (2007).

239. K. Okita, T. Ichisaka, and S. Yamanaka, Generation of germline-competent induced pluripotent stem cells, *Nature*, 448, 260–262 (2007).

240. G. Vogel and C. Holden, Developmental biology—Field leaps forward with new stem cell advances, *Science*, 318, 1224–1225 (2007).

241. N. Maherali and K. Hochedlinger, Guidelines and techniques for the generation of induced pluripotent stem cells, *Cell Stem Cell*, 3, 595–605 (2008).

242. R. H. Brown Jr., Neuron research leaps ahead, *Science*, 321, 1169 (2008).

243. I.-H. Park and G. Q. Daley, Debugging cellular reprogramming, *Nature Cell Biology*, 9, 871–873 (2007).

244. D. Hockemeyer, F. Soldner, E. G. Cook, Q. Gao, M. Mitalipova, and R. Jaenisch, A drug-inducible system for direct reprogramming of human somatic cells to pluripotency, *Cell Stem Cell*, 3, 346–353, (2008).

245. C. Li, J. Zhou, G. Shi, Y. Ma, Y. Yang, J. Gu, H. Yu et al., Pluripotency can be rapidly and efficiently induced in human amniotic fluid-derived cells, *Human Molecular Genetics*, 18, 4340–4349 (2009).

246. F. Soldner, D. Hockemeyer, C. Beard, Q. Gao, G. W. Bell, E. G. Cook, G. Hargus et al., Parkinson's disease patient-derived induced pluripotent stem cells free of viral reprogramming factors, *Cell*, 136, 964–977 (2009).

247. M. F. Pera, Stem cells: Low-risk reprogramming, *Nature*, 458, 715–716 (2009).

248. M. Stadtfeld, M. Nagaya, J. Utikal, G. Weir, and K. Hochedlinger, Induced pluripotent stem cells generated without viral integration, *Science*, 322, 945–949 (2008).

249. K. Okita, M. Nakagawa, H. Hyenjong, T. Ichisaka, and S. Yamanaka, Generation of mouse induced pluripotent stem cells without viral vectors, *Science*, 322, 949–953 (2008).

250. K. Hasegawa, A. B. Cowan, N. Nakatsuji, and H. Suemori, Efficient multicistronic expression of a transgene in human embryonic stem cells, *Stem Cells*, 25, 1707–1712 (2007).

251. S. Furler, J.-C. Paterna, M. Weibel, and H. Büeler, Recombinant AAV vectors containing the foot and mouth disease virus 2A sequence confer efficient bicistronic gene expression in cultured cells and rat substantia nigra neurons, *Gene Therapy*, 8, 864–873 (2001).

252. G. A. Luke, P. de Felipe, A. Lukashev, S. E. Kallioinen, E. A. Bruno, and M. D. Ryan, Occurrence, function and evolutionary origins of '2A-like' sequences in virus genomes, *Journal of General Virology*, 89, 1036–1042 (2008).

253. J. Yu, K. Hu, K. Smuga-Otto, S. Tian, R. Stewart, I. I. Slukvin, and J. A. Thomson, Human induced pluripotent stem cells free of vector and transgene sequences, *Science*, 324, 797–801 (2009).

254. K. Woltjen, I. P. Michael, P. Mohseni, R. Desai, M. Mileikovsky, R. Hämäläinen, R. Cowling et al., piggyBac transposition reprograms fibroblasts to induced pluripotent stem cells, *Nature*, 458, 771–775 (2009).

255. K. Kaji, K. Norrby, A. Paca, M. Mileikovsky, P. Mohseni, and K. Woltjen, Virus-free induction of pluripotency and subsequent excision of reprogramming factors, *Nature*, 458, 771–775 (2009).

256. K. Yusa, R. Rad, J. Takeda, and A. Bradley, Generation of transgene-free induced pluripotent mouse stem cells by the piggyBac transposon, *Nature Methods*, 6, 363–369 (2009).
257. M. Stadtfeld and K. Hochedlinger, Without a trace? PiggyBac-ing toward pluripotency, *Nature Methods*, 6, 329–330 (2009).
258. H. Zhou, S. Wu, J. Y. Joo, S. Zhu, D. W. Han, T. Lin, S. Trauger et al., Generation of induced pluripotent stem cells using recombinant proteins, *Cell Stem Cell*, 4, 381–384 (2009).
259. Ü. Langel (ed.), *Handbook of Cell Penetrating Peptides*, 2nd edn., CRC Press, Boca Raton, FL, 2007.
260. A. Joliot and A. Prochiantz, Transduction peptides: From technology to physiology, *Nature Cell Biology*, 6, 189–196 (2004).
261. K. M. Wagstaff and D. A. Jans, Protein transduction: Cell penetrating peptides and their therapeutic applications, *Current Medicinal Chemistry*, 13, 1371–1387 (2006).
262. M. Okuyama, H. Laman, S. R. Kingsbury, C. Visintin, E. Leo, K. L. Eward, K. Stoeber, C. Boshoff, G. H. Williams, and D. L. Selwood, Small-molecule mimics of an α-helix for efficient transport of proteins into cells, *Nature Methods*, 4, 153–159 (2007).
263. A. Prochiantz, For protein transduction, chemistry can win over biology, *Nature Methods*, 4, 119–120 (2007).
264. K. M. Stewart, K. L. Horton, and S. O. Kelley, Cell-penetrating peptides as delivery vehicles for biology and medicine, *Organic and Biomolecular Chemistry*, 6, 2242–2255 (2008).
265. C. Foerg and H. P. Merkle, On The biomedical promise of cell penetrating peptides: Limits versus prospects, *Journal of Pharmaceutical Sciences*, 97, 144–162 (2008).
266. F. Heitz, M. C. Morris, and G. Divita, Twenty years of cell-penetrating peptides: From molecular mechanisms to therapeutics, *British Journal of Pharmacology*, 157, 195–206 (2009).
267. B. Feng, J.-H. Ng, J.-C. D. Heng, and H.-H. Ng, Molecules that promote or enhance reprogramming of somatic cells to induced pluripotent stem cells, *Cell Stem Cell*, 4, 301–312 (2009).
268. C. A. Lyssiotis, R. K. Foreman, J. Staerk, M. Garcia, D. Mathur, S. Markoulaki, J. Hanna et al., Reprogramming of murine fibroblasts to induced pluripotent stem cells with chemical complementation of Klf4, *Proceedings of the National Academy of Sciences*, 106, 8912–8917 (2009).
269. D. Kim, C.-H. Kim, J. I. Moon, Y.-G. Chung, M.-Y. Chang, B.-S. Han, S. Ko et al., Generation of human induced pluripotent stem cells by direct delivery of reprogramming proteins, *Cell Stem Cell*, 4, 472–476 (2009).
270. M. W. Lensch, Cellular reprogramming and pluripotency induction, *British Medical Bulletin*, 90, 19–35 (2009).
271. K. Hochedlinger and K. Plath, Epigenetic reprogramming and induced pluripotency, *Development*, 136, 509–523 (2009).
272. S. Yamanaka, A fresh look at iPS cells, *Cell*, 137, 13–17 (2009).
273. C. Mason, The development of developmental neuroscience, *The Journal of Neuroscience*, 29, 12735–12747 (2009).
274. K. Saha and R. Jaenisch, Technical challenges in using human induced pluripotent stem cells to model disease, *Cell Stem Cell*, 5, 584–595 (2009).

275. A. Rolletschek and A. M. Wobus, Induced human pluripotent stem cells: Promises and open questions, *Biological Chemistry*, 390(9), 845–849 (2009).

276. M. K. Carpenter, J. Frey-Vasconcells, and M. S. Rao, Developing safe therapies from human pluripotent stem cells, *Nature Biotechnology*, 27, 606–613 (2009).

277. M. Jalving and H. Schepers, Induced pluripotent stem cells: Will they be safe? *Current Opinion in Molecular Therapeutics*, 11, 383–393 (2009).

278. A. Colman and O. Dreesen, Induced pluripotent stem cells and the stability of the differentiated state, *EMBO Reports*, 10, 714–721 (2009).

279. M. C. N. Marchetto, G. W. Yeo, O. Kainohana, M. Marsala, F. H. Gage, and A. R. Muotri, Transcriptional signature and memory retention of human-induced pluripotent stem cells, *PLoS ONE*, 4, e7076 (2009).

280. M. H. Chin, M. J. Mason, W. Xie, S. Volinia, M. Singer, C. Peterson, G. Ambartsumyan et al., Induced pluripotent stem cells and embryonic stem cells are distinguished by gene expression signatures, *Cell Stem Cell*, 5, 111–123 (2009).

281. W. Scheper and S. Copray, The molecular mechanism of induced pluripotency: A two-stage switch, *Stem Cell Reviews and Reports*, 5, 204–223 (2009).

282. P. Koch, Z. Kokaia, O. Lindvall, and O. Brüstle, Emerging concepts in neural stem cell research: Autologous repair and cell-based disease modeling, *The Lancet Neurology*, 8, 819–829 (2009).

283. J. O'Malley, K. Woltjen, and K. Kaji, New strategies to generate induced pluripotent stem cells, *Current Opinion in Biotechnology*, 20, 516–521 (2009).

284. S. Pei, Medecine régénérative: Nouvelles percées pour les cellules souches pluripotentes induites, *Biofutur*, 2009, 11 (2009).

285. L. Chen and L. Liu, Current progress and prospects of induced pluripotent stem cells, *Science in China, Series C: Life Sciences*, 52, 622–636 (2009).

286. D. A. Williams, Rapid development of pluripotent stem cells as a potential therapeutic modality, *Molecular Therapy*, 17, 929–930 (2009).

287. D. S. Kaufman, Toward clinical therapies using hematopoietic cells derived from human pluripotent stem cells, *Blood*, 114, 3513–3523 (2009).

288. P. J. Fairchild, Transplantation tolerance in an age of induced pluripotency, *Current Opinion in Organ Transplantation*, 14, 321–325 (2009).

289. S. P. Leary, C. Y. Liu, and M. L. Apuzzo, Toward the emergence of nanoneurosurgery: Part II–nanomedicine: Diagnostics and imaging at the nanoscale level, *Neurosurgery*, 58, 805–823 (2006).

290. S. P. Leary, C. Y. Liu, and M. L. Apuzzo, Toward the emergence of nanoneurosurgery: Part III–nanomedicine: Targeted nanotherapy, nanosurgery, and progress toward the realization of nanoneurosurgery, *Neurosurgery*, 58, 1009–1026 (2006).

291. J. B. Elder, C. Y. Liu, and M. L. Apuzzo, Neurosurgery in the realm of 10(-9): Part 1: Stardust and nanotechnology in neuroscience, *Neurosurgery*, 62, 1–20 (2008).

292. J. B. Elder, C. Y. Liu, and M. L. Apuzzo, Neurosurgery in the realm of 10(-9): Part 2: Applications of nanotechnology to neurosurgery–Present and future, *Neurosurgery*, 62, 269–284; discussion, 284–285 (2008).

293. A. Farin, C. Y. Liu, I. A. Langmoen, and M. L. J. Apuzzo, Biological restoration of central nervous system architecture and function: Part 3: Stem cell-and cell-based applications and realities in the biological management of central nervous system disorders: Traumatic, vascular, and epilepsy disorders, *Neurosurgery*, 65, 831–859 (2009).

294. Y. Amoh, M. Kanoh, S. Niiyama, Y. Hamada, K. Kawahara, Y. Sato, R. M. Hoffman, and K. Katsuoka, Human hair follicle pluripotent stem (hfPS) cells promote regeneration of peripheral-nerve injury: An advantageous alternative to ES and iPS cells, *Journal of Cellular Biochemistry*, 107, 1016–1020 (2009).

295. R. Hotta, D. Natarajan, and N. Thapar, Potential of cell therapy to treat pediatric motility disorders, *Seminars in Pediatric Surgery*, 18, 263–273 (2009).

296. K. M. Fitzpatrick, J. Raschke, and M. E. Emborg, Cell-based therapies for Parkinson's disease: Past, present, and future, *Antioxidants and Redox Signaling*, 11, 2189–2208 (2009).

297. L. Fugger, M. A. Friese, and J. I. Bell, From genes to function: The next challenge to understanding multiple sclerosis, *Nature Reviews Immunology*, 9, 408–417 (2009).

298. J. T. Dimos, K. T. Rodolfa, K. K. Niakan, L. M. Weisenthal, H. Mitsumoto, W. Chung, G. F. Croft et al., Induced pluripotent stem cells generated from patients with ALS can be differentiated into motor neurons, *Science*, 321, 1218–1221 (2008).

299. R. Maehr, S. Chen, M. Snitow, T. Ludwig, L. Yagasaki, R. Goland, R. L. Leibel, and D. A. Melton, Generation of pluripotent stem cells from patients with type 1 diabetes, *Proceedings of the National Academy of Sciences*, 106, 15768–15773 (2009).

300. T. J. Kamp and G. E. Lyons, On the road to iPS cell cardiovascular applications, *Circulation Research*, 105, 617–619 (2009).

301. L. Becker and H. Mashimo, Further promise of stem cells therapies in the enteric nervous system, *Gastroenterology*, 136, 2055–2058 (2009).

302. S. Webb, The gold rush for induced pluripotent stem cells, *Nature Biotechnology*, 27, 977–979 (2009).

303. M. Baker, Stem cells: Fast and furious, *Nature*, 458, 962–965 (2009).

8

Restoration: Nanotechnology in Tissue Replacement and Prosthetics

> Thanks to nanotechnology, a cellular and molecular basis has been established for the development of third generation biomaterials that will provide the scientific foundation for the design of scaffolds for tissue engineering, and for in situ tissue regeneration and repair, needing only minimally-invasive surgery.
>
> **Nanomedicine: European Technology Platform, November 2006 [1]**

> At this unique moment in the history of technical achievement, improvement of human performance becomes possible. … Better understanding of the human body and development of tools for direct human-machine interaction have opened completely new opportunities.
>
> **M.C. Roco and W.S. Bainbridge, U.S. National Science Foundation, June, 2002 [2]**

8.1 Introduction

In this chapter, we look at nanomaterials for implants and for tissue and organ replacement—the impact of nanotechnology on materials for tissue engineering, implants, and prosthetics. Nanotechnology enables the creation of new types of biocompatible and biodegradable materials and systems for reconstructing and replacing damaged tissue with implants and prostheses.

As we saw in Chapter 7, damaged tissues can be encouraged to regenerate with the aid of new programmed cells and scaffolding that stimulates cell recruitment and growth. But there are still many types of damage and conditions where tissue loss cannot be replaced by cellular growth or transplantation of living tissue. For these cases, medical treatment requires advanced artificial materials.

In many cases, relatively static structural or functional tissue must be replaced, such as teeth, bones, or connective tissue. In other cases, the loss of natural neuronal or hormonal functions needs to be remedied, as for the cardiac pacemaker or insulin delivery device. Temporary replacement of vital organs such as the kidney or heart is achievable, and permanent replacement with artificial devices is at least conceivable at present. Artificial limbs—feet, legs, arms and hands—have been the subject of intensive research in recent years resulting in remarkable improvements. Articulated prostheses can interface with the body's neuromuscular control system. Finally, the performance of prostheses for sensory perception—especially hearing and sight—is making rapid progress.

In this chapter, we will review these areas and show how fundamental progress in nanoscience, with its strong convergences of many disciplines, is an enabling factor for progress in medical biomaterials and prosthetics. Tissue engineering overlaps and interacts with surgery, drug release, and prosthetics. For the purposes of this chapter, we will take a broad view of tissue engineering, including aspects of surgery, devices, materials, and methods for wound healing, reconstructive surgery, tissue scaffolding, implants, transplantation, and artificial organs. Overlap with prosthetics begins with implants and tissue replacements, and progresses fully into prosthetics with implanted neurostimulation devices, artificial limbs, and neuroprostheses.

8.2 Nanoscale Biomaterials and Technologies for Tissue Engineering

Materials for applications in biology and medicine must meet complex needs—host biocompatibility, biodegradation, mechanical strength requirements for load bearing and impact resistance, elasticity and conformability, porosity, and many other properties. We have noted that nanotechnology is bringing insights into how properties of materials depend on their structure at the nanoscale. This knowledge is being used to create new materials for tissue repair and replacement [3–8]. Biomimetic designs are yielding nanomaterials with compatibility in strength, weight, and other properties for biomedical implants, devices, and artificial organs [9]. Natural biopolymers are also an excellent source of material for tissue scaffolding, but they must be sterile and free of cells and antigens [10]. Biodegradable materials are used when cell ingrowth can be promoted to replace the implant, or when the device is used for temporary support until weakened tissue can recover, as with stents. Biodegradation can also be used to provide measured release of bioactive molecules [11].

8.2.1 Materials Composition and Methods of Fabrication

Nanotechnology allows control over surface properties such as wettability, porosity, roughness, chemical affinities, and textures at the micro- and nanoscale, for optimizing interaction with proteins for cell adhesion. Examples of nanostructured materials for implants include aluminum and titanium oxides, hydroxyapatite, carbon nanofibers and nanotubes, titanium metal and various alloys, polymers, bioactive glasses, and ceramic polymer composites [12–22].

These and other nanostructured ceramics, metals, polymers, and composites can be synthesized using gas-phase chemical synthesis, chemical vapor deposition, severe plastic deformation, electrochemical anodization, chemical etching, and other techniques for evaluation as implants and tissue scaffolding.

Nanotechnology methods help fabricate customized materials for compatibility with specific cells and tissues. Different cell types respond to different chemical signals for migration, growth, differentiation, and adhesion. What works for endothelial cells might not work for chondrocytes.

8.2.2 Fabrication of Nanofibrous Scaffolding

The extracellular matrix of many tissues is characterized by bundles of collagen and elastin nanofibers (Figure 8.1). Nanofibrous materials made from biocompatible polymers have been shown to support cell attachment and

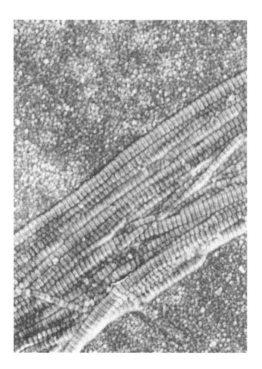

FIGURE 8.1
An atomic force microscopy image of collagen fibrils in a collagen fiber. (From Structure of protein collagen seen at unprecedented level of detail, U.S. Department of Energy, Argonne National Laboratory, *Science Daily*, Science News, online at: http://www.anl.gov/Media_Center/News/2008/APS080222.html, 2008.)

proliferation. Cells grown without suitable supporting matrices tend to lose their differentiation, but nanofibrous scaffolds have been synthesized on which seeded cells maintain their phenotypic shape and growth patterns, following the orientation of the fibers.

To emulate the nanofibrous extracellular matrix of epithelial, bone, and connective tissue, a number of nanotechnology techniques and materials are being adapted. Currently, three basic techniques are used to generate nanofibrous scaffolding for tissue engineering: electrospinning, molecular self-assembly, and thermally induced phase separation. These scaffolds can then be further treated by various surface modification techniques to more precisely emulate the native extracellular matrix. Even without modification, synthetic nanofibrous scaffolds support cell growth and tissue formation better than more traditional types of scaffolding [23].

Each of the three commonly used methods for generating nanofibrous scaffolding has its own advantages and limitations. For example, nanofibers of different size ranges are produced by each. Natural extracellular matrix collagen fibrils are about 1.5 nm in diameter and from 300 to 500 nm long [24]. Electrospinning yields nanofibers in the upper part of this diameter range or larger (typically >3 nm or greater). Most self-assembly techniques can only generate small diameter nanofibers in the lowest end of the range. Phase separation produces nanofibers in the same size range as natural extracellular matrix collagens, and lends itself to the design of macropore structures that allow for in-migration of cells. However, phase separation is a complex multistep process involving freeze drying and is limited to certain polymers [25–28]. Self-assembly processes are promising because they offer a route to incorporation of customized cell signaling peptide sequences. Thus, all of these methods and more continue to be investigated.

8.2.3 Carbon Nanotubes in Tissue Scaffolding

A number of novel materials and methods are being developed and evaluated for nanofibrous and thin-film scaffolds to be used in tissue engineering. As was discussed in Chapter 7, carbon nanotubes have been evaluated experimentally as additions to nerve growth scaffolding. Incorporation of carbon nanotubes has been proposed for more general and larger scale tissue scaffolding for other tissues such as bone, to provide structural reinforcement and impart properties such as electrical conductivity to aid and direct cell growth [28,29].

8.2.4 Titanium Dioxide Nanoporous Films

Nanostructured thin films of titanium dioxide have been fabricated as nanoporous cellular scaffolding. Titanium is a good bioscaffold component because of its low toxicity and nonhemorrhagic properties. Titanium dioxide, like alumina, can be formulated into nanoporous oxide layers that can be lifted off the metal substrate to form stable films. Electrochemical techniques can be used to precisely control the pore size and density and the thickness of the film, and the oxide can be coated with bioactive materials [28,30].

8.2.5 Viral and Virus-Like Particles for Tissue Scaffolds

One of the most versatile and innovative means of fabricating tissue engineering scaffolds is by using viral capsids, genetically engineered viruses, and virus-like protein supramolecular assemblies. Viral capsids can be assembled using layer-by-layer techniques and used to control growth of fibroblasts [28,31]. Control of protein sequence is important in promoting cell growth and adhesion, as we saw in Chapter 7 on tissue regeneration. With genetic engineering, viral RNA and DNA can be programmed to synthesize desired growth-promoting peptides, incorporated into a long-chain structural protein matrix. Display of high densities of cell signaling peptide motifs can be engineered with phage coat protein building blocks, due to their long rod shape and monodispersity. These proteins self-assemble into well-organized structures, enabling the construction of nanofiber scaffolds that support cell proliferation and differentiation as well as directional orientation of growth in three dimensions [32].

Virus-like supramolecular proteins are generated using a limited set of 20 amino acids, with functionalites determined by the sequence of amino acids and their presentation on the surface of the macromolecular particles due to their conformation into three-dimensional secondary and tertiary structures. These systems include viruses, virus-like particles, ferritins, enzyme complexes, cellular microcompartments, and other supramolecular protein assemblies. They self-assemble into precise arrangements that can be used for nucleic acid packaging, metal sequestration, catalysis, or other reactions on the nanometer scale. These bionanoparticles can be used independently or incorporated into tissue scaffolding to give functional and smart material properties for cell protection and proliferation, drug delivery, and other therapeutic applications [33].

8.2.6 Large-Scale Fabrication of Nanostructured Materials

For tissue reconstruction and wound healing, relatively large amounts of nanostructured material may be required for medical treatment. Researchers are developing ways to scale up fabrication of nanostructured biomaterials, creating large volumes or areas of nanostructured materials using techniques that maintain control of the nanoenvironment.

Some techniques used to create nanoscale topographies for cell scaffolding are borrowed from the nanotechnologies used for electronics and other inorganic nanomaterials. These techniques are contrasted between "top-down" approaches with high degrees of ordered control, as in electron beam lithography and photolithography, and inherently unordered surface patterning processes such as polymer demixing, phase separation, colloidal lithography, and chemical etching [34–36]. These latter "bottom-up" approaches depend upon self-assembly of the molecular components to produce their nanostructured topography.

Although self-organization of materials on the macroscale would have to overcome huge entropy costs and is therefore infeasible, on the nanoscale spontaneous processes driven by surface interactions between nanomaterials with suitable complementary properties can be exploited for bottom-up nanofabrication by indirect and relatively efficient techniques.

8.2.7 Layer-by-Layer Self-Assembly of Membranes and Composite Materials

The classic method for fabricating self-assembled thin films is the formation of planar supported bilayers from phospholipids and other bipolar macromolecules by Langmuir and Blodgett methods and their extensions using layer-by-layer fabrication [34–38]. Nanocolloids can be self-assembled into a variety of complex superstructures using micellular and surfactant molecule assemblies as templates. Multilayer thin-film structures can be seeded with a variety of types of nanoparticles to provide reinforcement and other properties. Carbon nanotubes, nanodiamonds, mineral and clay platelets, silica nanostructures, bacterial filaments, viral capsids, macromolecular peptides, graphemes, and magnetic nanoparticles have been incorporated into bioinorganic nanocomposites to produce thin-film materials for a variety of applications, including tissue scaffolding [39–44]. Study of the mechanisms by which special proteins control the mineralization of biopolymer scaffolds in the growth of shell and bone have led to new insights, techniques, and materials [28,41–44].

8.2.8 Nanoskiving

A technique that combines some of the features of top-down and bottom-up approaches is "nanoskiving," which involves thin-film deposition of metal on a topographically contoured substrate to make nanostructure assemblies, which can be used as arrays or separated into individual nanodevices by sectioning using an ultramicrotome. Although this technique cannot be used to produce nanodevices integrated into electronic circuits, it has the advantage of not requiring expensive clean rooms, photolithography, or electron beam equipment. It is a useful way to make quantities of simple nanostructures quickly and inexpensively in the 30 nm regime using metals or other materials that can be deposited by physical vapor methods. It provides a route to fabrication of nanostructures with high aspect ratios and other geometries that are difficult to prepare by other methods [45].

8.2.9 Self-Assembly of Nanomaterials on the Macromolecular Level

The natural extracellular matrix is comprised mainly of fibrillar proteins, collagen, and elastin. These biopolymers are synthesized as monomers, and

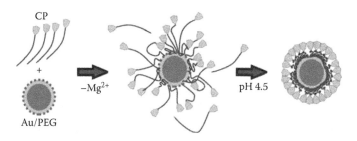

FIGURE 8.2
Self-assembly process. (From Chen et al., *Nano Lett.*, 6(4), 611, 2006. Copyright 2006 American Chemical Society. With permission.)

undergo hierarchical self-organization into well-defined nanoscaled structural units. Complex macromolecules can undergo self-assembly processes to form well-defined structures such as layered particles, fibers, and matrices (Figure 8.2).

Self-assembly is the process in which a system's components organize into ordered and/or functional structures without explicit external guidance. Self-assembly of atoms and molecules results from surface, chemical, electronic, and steric interactions between molecular particles and their surrounding solvents and ligands. The process and the resulting structures are the result of the chemical, electronic, and physical profiles presented to neighboring molecules, and depend on the chemical composition and shape of the molecules [46].

By understanding and manipulating these forces, researchers can exploit natural self-organizing materials or synthesize new ones. As polymer science expands the repertoire of materials and geometries available for scaffolding, theory and computation are providing design tools. Heuristic rules can be formulated that guide the design of self-assembling materials under various conditions and thermodynamic constraints, but a general strategy for programming materials to undergo a desired form of self-assembly based on their molecular formula is very complex and elusive [47].

Self-assembly of macromolecules, like chemical synthesis, can be driven by a combination of forces and influences: energy, entropy, templates, and electromagnetic fields, any one or group of which can predominate in a particular environment. Living cells and organisms represent highly complex hierarchies of self-organizing nonequilibrium systems and subsystems, organized by and organizing flows of materials and energy. On the nanoscale, self-assembly takes place at a level that can be understood and manipulated relatively simply, in order to make functional nanoparticles, films, and scaffoldings [48].

Self-assembly processes can be understood by modeling the structure and force interactions of macromolecules—something that has been made possible by advances in electronics at the nanoscale for powerful computing, storage, and display of information. For well-characterized classes of compounds with a limited set of building blocks, such as proteins, design rules can be formulated for sequence-structure and sequence-assembly relationships. For natural proteins, these rules are of course the same ones that govern the foldings and interactions that make tertiary and quaternary structures. Thus, for example, certain amino acid sequences can be recognized as β-sheet fibrillizing peptides of varying stiffness, others will result in alpha helix structures, etc. Thus, we have the concept of a coding or programming of structure in the amino acid sequence. But these codes exert subtle influences on structure in concert with other factors; it is only the complete structure of the molecule and its context that give rise to the full complexities of three-dimensional interactions [49,50].

Thus, it is a major challenge to predict what structures will result from the aggregation of a large number of complex molecules, even if they are identical. Some general design rules apply. For example, amphiphilic molecules that have both hydrophilic and hydrophobic subgroups tend to form structures in which the hydrophilic parts interact with the aqueous environment, while the hydrophobic parts interact with each other. But this type of simple rule does not determine which of the many possible assemblies can result when the molecules aggregate, particularly under different pH and salt concentrations. Often only one structure results, but the factors that determine which one will dominate must be determined by systematic study [51].

Using insights from conceptual models, design rules, and computer modeling, researchers seek to design peptide sequences that result in scaffold structures that elicit specific desired behaviors in cells. This is done by producing self-assembled arrangements that display cell signaling ligands in accessible external surfaces of the complex macromolecule. This is ideally achieved without inadvertently compromising the other important physicochemical properties of the scaffold, such as viscoelasticity [52]. Using design rules and knowledge, researchers are producing self-assembled tissue scaffolding materials in a variety of forms, such as complex multifunctional particles, fibers, films, amphiphiles, hierarchically ordered sacs and membranes, and toroidal triblock copolymers [53–56].

In a sense, classical chemical synthesis induces the self-assembly of chemical bonds by providing conditions such as concentrations, catalyzing templates, and energy to bring molecules into proximity and overcome barriers to reaction—since we do not actually assemble the bonds of the individual molecules. In much the same way, researchers are learning how to induce self-assembly processes at macromolecular levels; these nanoscale self-assembly processes involve fewer chemical covalent and ionic bonds and depend more on weaker intramolecular and conformational forces. Thus, despite describing these processes as "self-assembly," we have a number of ways to coach them into occurring by mixing components and providing various kinds of templates and energy inputs—just as in molecular synthesis [57–60]. When we think of self-assembly in these terms, it takes a lot of the mystery out of the process—or conversely, it makes us appreciate more the mystery of a chemical reaction, or a soap bubble!

As nanotechnology matures and interacts with biology and chemistry, strict concepts of externally programmed top-down assembly are tending to converge with concepts of synthesis, orchestrating and coaching material to allow it to assemble itself atom by atom and molecule by molecule, as we learn to appreciate and respect the intrinsic and peculiar propensities for self-assembly that are unique to every species of atom and molecule in relation to every other, in other words—*chemistry.*

8.3 Application of Tissue Engineering in Medicine

By whatever means we obtain our tissue engineering scaffolding, in medicine we are ultimately interested in how well it works to promote healing or at least to restore function. In looking at applications of tissue engineering assisted by nanotechnology, we will start with particles, and then consider fibers and higher dimensional nanomaterials, before moving to complex nanodevices, then to micro- and macroscale devices whose operation and properties are derived directly or indirectly from nanotechnology.

A key area that illustrates how nanotechnology is improving tissue engineering is in biocompatibility of implant materials. Improved materials are needed: the average lifetime of orthopedic implants was less than 15 years in the first decade of this century. Bone, vascular, and bladder implants, and implants for other organs, frequently failed due to insufficient integration of the implant with surrounding tissues. Nanotechnology offers the capability of fabricating implants with nanostructured components that promote cell growth and attachment, by tailoring pores and surfaces to match natural tissue environments, such as hydroxyapatite nanofibers dispersed in supporting collagen that characterize bone [61,62]. Nanostructured cell environments in which the scaffold surfaces provide localized signaling can promote cell migration and guide the directions and dimensions of cell growth by emulating the signaling and membrane trafficking of cells and their extracellular matrices [63].

Increased synthesis of bone, cartilage, vascular, bladder, and nerve tissue has been observed on nanophase compared to conventional materials for a wide variety of structures with different compositions and preparations. Nanostructured materials have also been found to result in decreased scar tissue formation. In tissue growth experiments, nanostructured inorganic materials that most closely resemble bone in structure and surface chemistry were found to function best in bone replacement and repair. But a hierarchy of structure is needed in addition to nanofeatures on surfaces; cell infiltration, bone growth, and vascularization were promoted best for substances with pores and interconnections larger than 100 μm in diameter [12–16].

Nanoscale surface features are important in creating more natural cell growth and function. Therefore, for all the fabrication techniques and materials, the goal is the presentation of a microenvironment to growing cells that mimics the nanoscale topographical features of extracellular matrix proteins such as collagen, with its nanofibrous and microporous topography. It is important to understand the biochemical as well as the topographic environment for each type of tissue into which the implant or tissue scaffolding is to be integrated. Intercellular adhesion can be promoted in tissue repair scaffolding using the same techniques that we reviewed in Chapter 7 for neural tissue regeneration, with special variations for different types of tissue. Growth promoting factors such as peptides and cations can be incorporated as copolymers in the matrix or engineered for sustained progressive release [17–22].

8.3.1 Experimental Evaluations of Nanoengineered Tissue Scaffolding

In experiments demonstrating these concepts, polymer sponge tissue scaffolds coated with gelatin (collagen) impregnated with bioactive growth-promoting molecules have been found experimentally to encourage the growth of human fibroblasts. The fibroblasts adhered to the scaffold matrix and had good morphology and spreading activity. Biochemical testing confirmed that the cells were able to produce extracellular matrix molecules such as type I collagen, fibronectin, and laminin, not observed in unsupported cell cultures. The cells also produced growth factor TGF-beta1 and the intracellular signal transduction molecule RhoA [64,65].

Another example of experimental work demonstrating the potential of nanoengineered bioactive scaffolds used a dorsal skinfold model to evaluate the effectiveness of supramolecular nanofibers formed by self-assembly of a heparin-binding peptide amphiphile and heparan sulfate-like glycosaminoglycans heparin-binding peptides. The heparin compounds were designed to promote angiogenesis, and thus have great potential in regenerative medicine for rapid revascularization of damaged tissue, survival of transplanted cells, and healing of chronic wounds. Dynamic monitoring of the interaction between the nanofiber gel and the microcirculation of the host tissue showed excellent biocompatibility. As the nanofibers biodegraded over 30 days, striking formation of new vascularized connective tissue was observed. Nanofiber-based bioactive gels of this type are being developed as angiogenesis-promoting materials for a number of wound repair and regenerative applications [66].

Delivery of peptide growth factors to promote wound repair is challenged by premature inactivation of the bioactive compounds in the wound environment. Studies of growth factors conjugated with polymer nanoparticles led to the concept of Polymer-masking-UnMasking-Protein Therapy (PUMPT) as a methodology for generating bioresponsive nanomedicines to promote tissue repair. Succinoylated dextrin polymer conjugated with recombinant human epidermal growth factor (rhEGF) was evaluated for effectiveness in promoting proliferation in cell culture assays, designed to simulate the degradation environment in wounds. The conjugate was able to protect the growth factor, enabling observed stimulation of cell growth. The PUMPT approach uses polymer conjugation to protect the bioactivity of the covalently bound drug, until triggered polymer degradation occurs to regenerate protein bioactivity at a target site. Drug release occurs as dextrin is degraded by α-amylase in the wound fluid, releasing the rhEGF [67]. This study illustrates the potential usefulness of nanomedicines for topical as well as systematic administration, with drug targeting based on specific stimuli found in wound sites.

Carbon nanodiamond particles have been found to bind extremely well with therapeutic proteins such as insulin, which acts as a growth hormone in wound healing. It encourages skin cells to proliferate and divide, restores blood flow to the wound, suppresses inflammation, and fights infection. Nanodiamond-insulin clusters have been synthesized and evaluated for wound healing applications, which could be formulated in gels, ointments, bandages, or suture materials. Skin pH levels can reach very basic levels at wound sites during the repair and healing process. Researchers have found that insulin bound to nanodiamonds is released at basic pH levels significantly greater than the physiological pH level of 7.4. These levels are commonly observed in bacterially infected wounds. Diamond nanoparticles can carry a substantial load of insulin due to their high surface area and organic carbon surface chemistry. Further work could lead to treatments for severe burns and traumatic bone fractures [68].

A number of different electrospun polymeric nanofibers have been evaluated as tissue scaffolding. Scaffolds made from electrospun biocomposite polymer nanofibers have been seeded with osteoblasts, mesenchymal stem cells, glioma cells, and silver nanoparticles by different research groups. These so-called "one-dimensional" fibrous nanomaterials have been evaluated for cell growth and promotion of wound healing in a number of experimental studies [69–71]. As an example, one study has developed and characterized electrospun poly(lactic acid) (PLLA) nanofibers containing multiwalled carbon nanotubes [72].

Two-dimensional nano-thin sheets have been fabricated and tested as alternatives to sutures in surgery and wound healing. The nanosheets are made from PLLA, a polyester that is used clinically in drug delivery and for biodegradable stitches. But only recently have sheets been produced with thicknesses on the order of nanometers. The mechanical properties of the nanosheets are very different from conventional thin films of the same polymer. The nanofilm combines high strength, adhesiveness, flexibility, and transparency, making it usable in place of conventional sutures, ligations, and surgical webbing. It can be fabricated in sheets of 20 nm thickness with dimensions on the order of centimeters. Besides being biodegradable, it has been effective in tests at sealing and holding tissues after surgical incisions, and was found to produce significantly less scarring than conventional methods. The PLLA nanosheet has been demonstrated in experiments to seal gastric incisions [73].

A number of other types of cross-linked fibers, sheets, and mats have been developed for tissue engineering based on different types of biodegradable polymers and composites, including PLLA, silk fibroin, and chitosan–poly(ethylene oxide) composites [74–76]. Two-dimensional sheets are useful for many purposes in wound repair and surgery, but three-dimensional scaffolding is needed for many types of tissue repair [77].

Scaffolds based on hydrogels of self-assembled peptides are a promising route to tissue engineering because of the three-dimensional structure of the gel and because custom peptide sequences can be synthesized and presented to tailor promotion of growth in different types of tissue [78,79].

A major challenge in choosing an appropriate scaffold for tissue repair is the identification of a material that can simultaneously stimulate high rates of cell division and high rates of cell synthesis of extracellular matrix macromolecules for specific types of cells and tissues. Self-assembled peptides can be synthesized with phenotype-specific signaling and form hydrogel scaffolds customized to promote growth with encapsulated cells for different types of tissue [80].

Three-dimensional hydrogel scaffolds based on self-assembling peptides have been synthesized and have been shown to be excellent biological material for cell culture. In animal experiments, the peptide nanofibers stimulate cell migration into the scaffold for repairing tissue defects. Several such peptide nanofiber scaffolds have been designed and tested in cultures and animals for osteoblasts, cartilage, aortic, epithelial, and other specific tissues [81].

Gels and liquid suspensions of nanoparticulate materials have the advantage of being fluid and thus formable to fit into any lesion cavity, or to form a layer between two sections of tissue of arbitrary shape, and to fill in any gaps caused by mismatch of the tissues. Fluid scaffolding can be injected laparoscopically into cavities and wounds to form the volume and geometry required. This can be a particularly desirable characteristic for surgical adhesives and glues.

Nanotechnology has been used to produce new surgical glues and hemostat coatings based on the interaction of nanoparticles with platelets and the use of natural and biomimetic adhesive proteins, for example fibrin, and to provide methods for their rapid and inexpensive custom production [82,83].

Research teams are developing photo-controlled polymer scaffolds with the capability for dynamic control of the properties of the biomaterial by the application of light-direct photochemical changes in structure, surface composition, and release of growth-directing biomolecules. This could provide the useful ability to alter the properties of a tissue scaffold in situ or as it is being applied [84].

Photodegradable polymer hydrogels have been developed whose functionality and physical properties can be altered photochemically. Photopolymerization and photoreactions can be done by remote manipulation with lasers and/or fiber optics to set the gel by cross-linking polymer chains, to open channels or cages by photodegradation, or perform other operations, such as photoactivation for the release of bioactive molecules or drugs. Photosculpting can be used to shape the scaffold. Photochemical changes allow for temporal variation of the surface properties of fibers to influence cell migration or chondrogenic differentiation of encapsulated cells. This is an area of biomaterial nanomanipulation that is just beginning to be explored [84].

An example that illustrates the potential of synthetic photochemical alterations possible for functional nanoscale structures in biological materials is the design of photoswitchable gates for cell membrane channels [85,86]. Another example of the potential for photo-manipulation for tissue engineering at the level of individual cells is the use of optical tweezers, optical traps, and dielectrophoresis to manipulate cells [28]. Optical trapping, also called optical tweezers, is a technique that utilizes the momentum transferred by refracted light to manipulate an object [87]. For macroscale bodies, this momentum transfer is negligible in comparison with the inertial mass of the object, but for microscopic and nanoscale objects such as cells and molecules, the momentum transferred by a suitably focused laser or radiofrequency field is sufficient to manipulate the object. Laser beams with wavelengths that are refracted rather than scattered by an object can trap the object in the center of a force field gradient, and the object can be moved with the beam. The intensity of the laser beam required to move a cell is enough to damage the cell in most cases. But recently a new method was developed, focusing a polarized laser beam so that a vortex of low light intensity is formed at the center of the gradient force field. This technique, called polarization-shaped optical vortex trapping, exerts less photodamage on trapped cells than a conventional optical trap [88].

Using polarization-shaped optical vortex traps, laser micromanipulation could be performed on cell scaffolding, moving cells to seed the scaffold matrix, reposition or remove cells from the matrix, or perform other microsurgical manipulations, perhaps in combination with laser nanosurgery for alterations on subcellular structures.

Dielectrophoresis is another technique that can selectively move cells based on their polarizability, using dynamic patterning of radiofrequency fields [89]. Dielectrophoresis has been used to separate cancer cells from normal cells and to concentrate bacteria for detection in water supplies. Dielectrophoresis can be operated in modes that do not harm cells, or can be used to lyse selected cells [28]. Using dielectrophoresis, it would conceivably be possible to select cells for seeding a scaffold, pull cells into the scaffold from adjacent healthy tissues, or selectively add and remove cells en masse for tissue engineering.

8.3.2 Smart Materials: Adaptive Nanostructured Materials for Medical Applications—The Future

The incorporation of photoswitchable functionality into tissue scaffolding is just one possibility in a range of potential biomedical applications for active and smart nanomaterials in tissue engineering. Biocompatible nanoscale MEMS and NEMS are now being developed, and it is only a matter of time before they will be integrated into tissue scaffolding, to measure and report physiological changes by wireless communication links.

Smart materials in implants will soon be capable of adjusting a number of parameters for bioactive material release, electrical stimulation, adjustments in elasticity, porosity, shape, and other parameters [36,90–98]. Devices will be powered by efficient nanogenerators that harvest power from light, radio waves, or mechanical motion, so batteries will be unnecessary, especially as their circuitry will be nanoengineered to perform functions with minimal energy consumption.

Although these visionary devices are still on the horizon, the prototypes are already being demonstrated. For example, an electric power generator based on piezoelectric zinc nanowires has a mechanical to electrical energy conversation efficiency of up to 30%, is small enough to be embedded in implantable devices or prostheses, and had been demonstrated as a prototype [99,100].

These nanodevices, nanosensors, and adaptive materials are leading to a convergence between drug delivery devices, implants, tissue engineering, and prosthetics. As implants and tissue scaffolding become more multifunctional, they begin to resemble nanoscale prostheses. As we will see later in the chapter, as prostheses become more miniaturized and capable of more subtle functions, they begin to resemble artificial tissues.

8.3.3 Translation of Nanoengineered Biomaterials into Clinical Applications

In the previous section we looked at nanoengineered biomedical materials in development and experiment for tissue engineering. Now we will survey some actual applications.

8.3.3.1 Nanoparticle Materials for Wound Healing

Tissues have the potential to regenerate from damage or wounds; maintenance of the body is a constant dynamic process on the cellular level. When a major wound is incurred, application of medical help makes a great difference in facilitating timely recovery without complications. The major principles of wound care include stopping of bleeding, prevention of infection, and support of the rejoining of tissues for healing. Surgical wounds and transplants must be treated to encourage healing just like any other wound, although random wounds such as abrasions and burns are typically much more complex and traumatic.

Ideally, we seek a dressing material that supports the tissue around the lesion, fights infection and inflammation, and promotes cell migration and proliferation, until repair evolves into natural steady-state tissue maintenance. Biofunctional nanomaterials and systems are being developed to meet these needs.

Nanotechnology is providing surface treatments of wound dressings to accelerate blood clotting and kill bacteria, as well as tissue glues and adhesives for dressings. Silver nanoparticles are one of the antimicrobial treatments used to impart antiseptic properties to dressings and sutures. These are used as nanoporous silver powders, with particle sizes of between 50 and 100 nm, which can be encapsulated for gradual release. Preparations that provide slow release of silver nanoparticles can kill bacteria as effectively as organosilver compounds, and the nanoparticles are not as readily absorbed into tissues, where they can be toxic to human cells, although there is some evidence that their toxicity is far greater to bacteria [101].

A dressing formulated of single-walled carbon nanotubes coated with an iodine-releasing compound has been designed for use as an antiseptic coating for wound application. It is promising for its antiseptic properties, combined with allowing oxygen to reach the wound through micron-sized pores. In addition, since the dressing is conductive, it facilitates the application of electrostimulation therapy to promote nerve and tissue regeneration [102].

Nitric oxide-releasing silica nanoparticles have been shown to be more effective as antiseptics than molecular sources of nitric oxide. Nitric oxide is one of the few means of combating the growth of biofilms in wounds and dressings; the biofilms resist the penetration of most antibiotics. Nitric oxide is released naturally by infection fighting cells, and is not as toxic to human cells as silver. Another advantage of nanoparticles over small molecules is that their physicochemical properties (e.g., hydrophobicity, charge, and size) may be tuned synthetically to maximize penetrating power into biofilms [103].

Peptide growth factors are known to promote wound repair, but topical application is not clinically effective because of premature inactivation of the peptides in the wound environment. Polymer conjugates of growth factors have been developed and shown to be effective in promoting bioresponsive wound repair, by masking the peptide from deactivating factors until it enters the tissue [67]. This application is completely analogous to the use of conjugate nanomedicines in oral and percutaneous administration of peptide drugs, as we saw in Chapter 5.

8.3.3.2 Nanomaterials in Tissue Scaffolding for Cartilage and Bone

Musculoskeletal disorders and injury affect millions of people throughout the world. Nanotechnology research is being pursued for prevention and treatment for joint disease, osteoporosis, osteoarthritis, low back pain, spinal disorders, fractures, trauma to the extremities, and crippling disease and deformities in children. As populations age, the prevalence of chronic bone and joint diseases and conditions will increase, consuming more resources and resulting in more human suffering. The WHO estimates that several hundred million people already suffer from bone and joint disease and injuries around the world.

Tissue scaffolding is especially important for repair of bone and cartilage. These supportive and connective tissues depend on a relatively low density of living cells to maintain relatively large structures that are predominantly mineral and polymer in composition. When cartilage or bone is damaged, broken, or lost, cells must be given support and guidance to undertake the task of first rebuilding a cartilage scaffold, and then re-mineralizing it with calcium and phosphate building blocks.

The structure of bone is very complex, dynamic, and adaptable. Bone shares some structural features with the carbonate mineral shells of sea creatures: it is a complex composite of nanoscale mineral building blocks held in a resilient polymer matrix. Vertebrate bone has a multi-hierarchal micro- and nanostructure composed of lipids, proteins, and polysaccharides and inorganic mineral components containing hydroxyapatite, calcium carbonate, and silica.

Unlike the exoskeleton of sea shells, the endoskeleton of vertebrate bone contains living cells—osteoblasts—which renew deposits of mineral from within the structure. Bony skeletons must perform a varied and complex set of functions; bones have to bear complex loads of moving bodies, provide a protective cage for vital organs, anchor tendons and muscles, and act as joints, fulcrums, and levers. Because of this functional complexity, the nano- and microstructure of bone is more complex than the carbonate nanostructure of shells. Different parts of the same skeleton must have different directional, compression, and tension strengths to prevent fracture and distortion under stresses, loads, impact, and fatigue [104].

Medical nanotechnologies for bone contribute to artificial replacement, scaffolding for bone repair and growth, and interfaces between bone and implants. Bone is a challenging material to duplicate artificially. Its combination of strength and resilience with light weight is the result of its nanocomposite structure composed of mineral and hydrated organic macromolecules [28]. Its structure consists of layers of mineral crystals (hydroxylapatite) interspersed with protein and biopolymers that add resilience to the compression-bearing strength of the mineral component. Special proteins control the deposition of mineral salts and determine orientation and crystalline structure [105]. The active peptide sequences in these proteins should be important in the design of scaffolding.

8.3.3.2.1 Nanomaterials for Bone Implants

Nanotechnology research for implants has been directed toward new nanocomposite materials and toward coatings and surface treatments for conventional implant materials [106–108]. Coating of metal or Bioglass® orthopedic implants with nanoparticles has been studied as a strategy to improve adhesion and fusion with bone, and has in many cases been shown to improve adhesion, joint strength, and lifetime of the implant. Coating technologies include bioactive composite layers of Bioglass® with carbon nanotubes [109], formation of nanostructured oxide layers on titanium by anodization [110], and growth of nanoscale hydroxyapatite onto titanium oxide nanotubes formed by anodization of the metal surface [111].

8.3.3.2.2 Nanomaterials for Bone Scaffolding

The approach to promoting the growth and healing of bone is based on the same principles as for other tissues: to provide scaffold material into which bone-forming cells can migrate, leading to the fusion of new bone growth with the scaffold.

Bone forms by mineralization of precursor cartilage tissues [112]. Successful growth, maintenance, and healing of bone depend on each portion of the structure matching the types of forces to which it is subjected in the body. Much work is being done to understand how precursor cells are programmed and influenced to promote mixtures of mineralization and organic fibers that optimally match the compressing and tension loads that must be borne by the skeleton, and how this can be mimicked and encouraged by scaffolds, growth-promoting substances, and electromagnetic stimulation.

Researchers in Beijing, China have developed a bone scaffold by biomimetic synthesis of nanohydroxyapatite and collagen assembled into mineralized fibrils [113]. This material shows some features of natural bone in composition and hierarchical microstructure, with three-dimensional porous scaffold materials that mimic the microstructure of cancellous bone. In cell culture and animal tests, bone-forming osteoblast cells from rats adhered, spread, and proliferated throughout the pores of the scaffold material within a week. This scaffold composite has promise for the clinical repair of bone defects. This and similar work being done elsewhere shows how biomimetic structures can integrate with natural tissues [114,115].

Nanostructured inorganic, polymer, and peptide scaffolding have all been evaluated as bone scaffolding, including ceramics with macroporous structures for cell ingrowth and vascularization [114], biodegradable and bioactive porous polymer/inorganic composites [116], electrospun biodegradable nanofiber scaffolds [117], and biodegradable polymer nanocomposites containing single-walled carbon nanotubes for strength reinforcement [118].

Phosphate-based glasses formulated into nanoporous foam-like scaffolds have been fabricated as bone scaffolding. The addition of zinc was found to significantly increase bone growth [119,120].

Certain peptides and proteins presented on the surfaces of scaffolds promote bone regrowth by activating signaling pathways that direct osteoblast survival, cell-cycle progression, gene expression, and matrix mineralization. Integrin adhesion receptors for extracellular matrix components, such as fibronectin and type I collagen, are particularly effective in this regard. Other peptide sequences have been found that promote bone growth and can be incorporated into synthetic peptide scaffolds [121–123].

Novel techniques have been developed for the fabrication of strong fibrous scaffolding for bone growth, including laser spinning of bioactive glass nanofibers, and the use of ultrasonication to prepare nanohydroxyapatite [124,125].

For repair of bone structure in complex tissues such as the craniofacial area, injectable biomaterial scaffolds have been developed and evaluated [126,127].

Nanomaterial-based treatments for osteoporosis are being actively researched, including use of nanostructured biodegradable ceramics, and magnetic nanoparticles as drug-carriers for delivery of hydroxyapatite [128,129].

8.3.3.2.3 Impact of Nanotechnology on Medical Devices for Bone Healing

Fixation devices are incorporating nanoengineered materials such as carbon nanotubes to make strong, lightweight, resilient materials to aid bone healing, especially for complex fractures on bone structures such as the pelvis.

A bone healing therapy that has benefited from advances in microelectronics and materials is electromagnetic stimulation of bone growth. Bone is a piezoelectric material, and its growth has been demonstrated to respond to ultrasound and electromagnetic fields [130,131]. It is possible that bone growth in response to stress and loading is mediated by a piezoelectric-initiated signaling that stimulates osteoblaths. Electromagnetic stimulation devices are now part of the orthopedist's armamentarium for the care of delayed union, nonunion, and fresh fractures. Advances in microelectronics, antenna materials, and power sources will continue to contribute to improvements in this area of biomedical technology.

8.3.4 Nanotechnology for Cardiac and Vascular Tissue Repair

Nanofabricated materials are being used for vascular grafts, vascular tissue scaffolds, ventricular replacement materials, and coatings on stents and heart valves [132].

In one study, vascular stents coated with nanolayers of the polysaccharides, hyaluronan, and chitosan reduced platelet adhesion in vitro by 38%, but did not prevent fouling by neutrophils. The coatings were also assessed for delivery of the nitric oxide-donor drug sodium nitroprusside to further reduce platelet adhesion. The enhanced thromboresistance of the self-assembled polysaccharide multilayer together with the anti-inflammatory and wound healing properties of hyaluronan and chitosan are expected to reduce the complications associated with stent implantation [132]. In another study, alkanethiol self-assembled monolayers on 316 L stainless steel were evaluated in coronary artery stents for stability and drug delivery [133].

In general, drug eluting stents have made a major impact in the treatment of occlusive coronary artery disease by producing a marked reduction of in-stent restenosis [134].

Nanotechnology continues to have an evolving impact on the design and use of stents. Microfabrication and nanotechnology strategies offer new opportunities for improving stent technology for the treatment of more extensive and complex lesions. Stents with microfabricated reservoirs for controlled temporal and spatial drug release have already been successfully applied to coronary lesions. Microfabricated needles to pierce lesions and deliver therapeutics deep within the vascular wall represent an additional microscale approach. At the nanoscale, investigators have primarily sought to alter the strut surface texture or coat the stent to enhance endothelialization and host artery integration. Nanotechnology research is also identifying promising strategies to limit restenosis through targeted drug delivery after angioplasty and stenting [135].

The discovery that heart muscle is less static and more capable of regeneration than was previously realized has led to new interest in ways to promote regeneration of heart tissue after infarctions [136–138]. Induced pluripotent stem cells with supporting bioactive substances and tissue matrix support material are being investigated for these applications, which hold great promise for treatment of heart attacks [139,140].

Revascularization is important for rescue of muscle tissue damaged after ischemia, especially for continually hard working tissues of the heart. Vascular support for transplanted stem cells and in-migrating cells can be provided by scaffolds and/or injectable gels for controlled release of basic fibroblast growth factor, bFGF. Therapeutic angiogenesis by bFGF-releasing hydrogels has been found effective in animal experiments for heart and limb ischemia [141,142].

8.3.5 Nanoengineered Encapsulation and Implantation of Cells and Tissues

Cell encapsulation devices have been developed as research vehicles for studying the release of growth factors, neurotransmitters, and other signaling molecules from cells [143]. Various types of nanotechnology-assisted bioencapsulations have been developed for uses in medicine, biotechnology, tissue regeneration, stem cell therapy, nanorobotics, and artificial cells [144]. Here, we see the convergence of drug delivery, tissue scaffolding, and MEMS microdevices. The boundaries between these types of medical nanotechnology have become somewhat arbitrary.

In Chapter 5, on nanotechnology for drug delivery, we encountered nanoengineered encapsulation for delivery of drugs and for protection of peptide drugs such as insulin from the immune system, including use of encapsulated cells, nanodevices, and micro-pumps for delivery of insulin. Encapsulation of tissues for protection from the immune system is also a strategy used generally for transplanted tissues, especially tissues that produce therapeutic agents, such as insulin-producing islets [145–147].

8.3.5.1 Encapsulation and Implantation Techniques

Extensive efforts for the development of encapsulation techniques have been directed toward protection of transplanted cells and tissues. A challenge for transplanting encapsulated cells is delivery of oxygen and nutrients to the cells inside the capsule, and outward diffusion of therapeutic agents and waste products such as carbon dioxide. Delivery of sufficient oxygen and glucose is especially critical, since suboptimal supply will impair the production of insulin or other metabolites, even if the cells survive [147,148].

Effective diffusion of oxygen and nutrients into microcapsules can occur up to a distance of about 200 µm, so research has been directed at finding ways to increase transport to encapsulated cells. Advances in nanotechnology have enabled the design of capsules with high surface areas and high permeability for oxygen and diffusion of therapeutic agents, while still giving protection to encapsulated cells. Experiments been done to enhance vascularization of the outside surfaces of capsules by incorporating angiogenic factors into the membranes, such as vascular endothelial growth factor (VEGF) or bFGF. However, continuous delivery of biochemical growth factors may be necessary to support growth and sustain vasculature. Sustained release of angiogenic substances can be provided by incorporating microspheres impregnated with slowly released growth factor into the capsules, or by also encapsulating vascular endothelial TMNK-1 cells, which provide continuous biochemical support for vasculature, along with the therapeutic-generating cells [148,149].

Instead of inducing vascularization of the immunoisolation capsule, another approach is to use tissue engineering to generate highly vascularized subcutaneous, intramuscular, or intraperitoneal sites for cell transplantation using metal or polymer mesh. Generation of such sites may allow microencapsulated cells to be removed and replaced, and may potentially circumvent complications associated with the transplantation of encapsulated cells into native tissue. These artificial cell-recipient beds for implanted capsules can be engineered by localized delivery of angiogenic factors [148].

Transplanting encapsulate cells such as islets into prevascularized sites dramatically improves graft survival and function relative to transplantation into non-modified tissue, but it remains difficult to create and maintain such sites. It is challenging to create and maintain recipient sites with sufficient vascularization to accommodate conventional microencapsulation devices effectively. Reducing the size of the encapsulation device would make this task easier, but would reduce the volume of graft cells and therapy factor delivered by each site.

8.3.5.1.1 Microfabrication Technologies for Cell and Tissue Encapsulation

Microfabrication technologies using silicon and metal based capsules have been designed and tested for cell and tissue encapsulation [148–151]. Sophisticated self-closing devices have been fabricated on planar silicon, and folded by chemical and thermal treatment into boxes with pores to capture and isolate cells [146,152,153].

Silica gel encapsulation of islets has been evaluated for immunoisolation [154]. Other techniques used include prevascularized expanded polymer support systems [155] and nanomat-reinforced amphiphilic co-networks deposited on perforated metal scaffolds [156]. Nanoporous alumina membranes have also been evaluated for potential use in bioencapsulation [157].

8.3.5.1.2 Long-Term Support of Transplanted Islets and Development of Artificial Pancreas

The development of replacement therapy for the pancreas, with its insulin-providing islets, has been a long-term goal for researchers seeking a transplantation approach to diabetes treatment [158–160]. Advances in tissue engineering and encapsulation techniques are bringing such a development close to clinical usefulness. The survival of encapsulated islets is being demonstrated in laboratory experiments for weeks to months by researchers using several different approaches.

In one promising development, alginate-based microcapsules have been fabricated and used to demonstrate long-term support of survival for transplanted adult rat and human islets into immunocompetent mice [161].

Other researchers achieved survival for several weeks in canine models with islets encapsulated in polymer membranes, without prevascularization or immunosuppression. The membrane is an amphiphilic co-network reinforced with electrospun nanomat. It has extraordinarily high oxygen permeability and small hydrophilic channel dimensions (3–4 nm) [162].

Another approach uses a 20×20 mm bag-type device with two layers of polymer membranes; the outer membrane functions as an immunoisolation layer, and the inner layer is a scaffold for islet cells. Vascularization around the devices was increased by coating with a fibroblast growth factor gel. The device is designed so that new cells can be injected into it after implantation [163].

Another approach uses an encapsulation layer composed of live cells, with immunodelusive cell sheet engineering. Donor islet cells were incorporated between chondrocyte cell sheets grown and prepared by a tissue-responsive culture technique from canine cartilage. The cell sheet engineered islets survived, with a gradually decreased insulin secretion for 3 months [164,165].

8.3.5.1.3 Artificial Microdevices for Insulin Delivery and Other Organ Support

Artificial pumps for heart assist or delivery of insulin, kidney dialysis machines, and other biomechanical devices for organ support or replacement take us to the boundary between tissue engineering and prosthetics. Biomedical engineering of assistive devices, especially artificial means of insulin delivery, has benefited from advances in nanoengineering of materials, microelectronics, and microfluidics. Delivery through the skin by arrays of microneedles is now an option to implantation of an insulin pump [166]. Several new devices have recently been approved for release [167,168]. (See also Chapter 5, Sections 5.5.7 and 5.5.8 on insulin drug delivery.)

8.4 Nanotechnology and Prosthetics

Nanotechnology has impacted prosthetics indirectly in the same ways that it has impacted medical and surgical robotics. Nanodevices and nanotechnology enabled microdevices are accelerating performance and functionality of computing, communication, sensors, actuators, and controllers, which are at the heart of automated feedback loops and real-time control strategies for both robotics and advanced prosthetics [28].

Prostheses include artificial devices for neural stimulation, replacement of lost motor function, replacement of lost sensory function, or combinations of all three.

8.4.1 Neuronal Stimulation and Monitoring

The cardiac pacemaker is one of the best known and most widely used neuroprostheses. Since 2001, the number implanted in the United States has approached 200,000 per year. Other pacemakers are not implanted permanently but are used during cardiac catheterization and other procedures [169,170]. Other types of electronic stimulators include cardiac defibrillators, cochlear implants, bone growth stimulators, and neural stimulators for deep brain, spinal cord, vagus, sacral, and other nerve stimulators [171].

Nanotechnology advances these devices with improved battery technologies, biocompatible materials, surface treatments for enclosures and leads, electrode miniaturization and efficiency improvements, and smaller sized integrated circuits for control and power, while speed and processing capabilities increase. These improvements made possible the accessible, inexpensive emergency cardiac defibrillators in public places and on transportation such as aircraft, with control systems safe to use by nonspecialists.

An area in which nanotechnology is likely to benefit cardiac pacemakers directly is in improvements in electronic lead and electrode biocompatibility and durability. The leads have been a weak link for cardiac pacemakers while size, power, and battery life have improved, thus requiring longer life service for the wires and electrodes. Cardiac pacemaker leads must be biocompatible with tissue, but unlike surgical implants, the internal portion near the heart must not promote tissue adhesion and growth which would make them difficult to remove. In addition they must heal to skin and surface tissues and seal to prevent becoming a channel for infection. They must resist the growth of bacterial and fungal biofilms. These are challenges taken up by nanoengineering of materials, along with long-term factors affecting cell growth and adhesion to leads.

8.4.1.1 Neurostimulation for Pain and Nervous Disorders

Nanofabrication is increasing the resolution and capabilities of neurostimulation devices. Neurostimulation is used medically for cardiac pacemaking, deep brain stimulation to control tremors in Parkinson's disease, management of chronic pain, stimulation of tissue healing, prevention and reversal of nerve degeneration, and other conditions and therapies, including chronic neuropathy, diabetic neuroarthropathy, and cardiomyoplasty.

Integrated micro- and nanoscale devices make it possible to apply much finer resolution with many more electrode stimulation points, which can be dynamically programmed. Every advance in computer and signal processing power resulting from electronics nanoengineering contributes directly to the power and sophistication of programmable medical devices such as neurostimulation systems. These advantages may appear in new generations of cochlear implants, cardiac pacemakers, deep brain stimulation, and in new types of devices.

An important aspect of the development of neural prostheses is the enhancement of suitable implantable micro-electrode arrays for chronic neural recording as well as stimulation. A promising approach to this function is use of implantable silicon-substrate micromachined probes. Work on these probes has improved their reliability and signal quality. In rodent models, the probes provide high-quality spike recordings over extended periods of time lasting up to 127 days. More than 90% of the probe sites consistently record spike activity with signal-to-noise ratios sufficient for amplitude- and waveform-based discrimination. Histological analysis of the tissue surrounding the probes generally indicated the development of a stable interface sufficient for sustained electrical contact [172]. Surface treatments, new electronic circuit materials, and other advances contributed by nanotechnology will result in continual improvements in making such probes resistant to the challenging environment of implantation. In addition to the general improvements in size, power, and mobility made possible by nanotechnology, we have seen in Chapter 7 examples of how nanoengineering of the surfaces of electrodes, including the use of carbon fiber nanotubes, is contributing to improved interfaces between neurons and electrostimulation devices.

Electrical stimulation of neural tissue by surgically implanted neuro-electronic devices is now an approved modern therapy. The reduction of the size and power requirements with integrated microelectronic devices makes it feasible in many cases to energize an implanted device by radiofrequency electromagnetic transmission of power, eliminating wires and batteries. Implanted neurostimulation devices such as pacemakers are already available that receive power from radiofrequency energy, thus eliminating transcutaneous wires that are a source of infection and complications [173]. The question of radiofrequency interference becomes an important design consideration for such devices.

Improvements in energy storage through nanoengineered supercapacitors and hypercapacitors, aerocapacitors, and conductive polymers [174], coupled with lower power requirements for nanoengineered electronics, allow room for great improvements in size and capability of embedded devices, allowing very small implantable devices to perform electrostimulation in selected points of the nervous, sensory, and neuromuscular system. Such devices may make it practical for increased use of implanted electrostimulation for bone and tissue grafts, and to stimulate function in the endocrine system and other organs.

8.4.2 Neuroprosthetics

Neural interfaces to nano- and microelectronic devices open new opportunities to design more powerful neurostimulators for prosthetics. Broadly defined, a neural prosthesis is a device implanted to restore a lost or altered neural function [175]. The Greek word "prostheses" originally refers to the addition of a syllable to the beginning of a word. In classical medicine, it means an artificial replacement for a missing part of the body [176]. The term "prosthetics" denotes the medical art of providing prostheses to improve the life of patients.

8.4.3 Assistive Devices

Neuroprostheses are distinct from "assist devices" such as heart ventricular assist pumps, which do not interface to the voluntary nervous system [177]. Neuroprostheses are also distinguished from assistive devices that translate or amplify movement, for example systems that enable paralyzed persons to control computers or devices by eye, tongue, or small muscle movement [178]. Nanotechnology is a key driver advancing the state of the art for assistive devices, and most dramatically for neuroprosthetics. Nanotechnology is improving the electrodes that interface to nerves, and it is providing smaller and more powerful sensors, actuators, and distributed control systems to make prosthetics more natural and effective.

8.4.4 Types of Neural Prostheses

Neural prostheses are of two types: motor and sensory. Sensory neuroprostheses are devices that translate external stimuli such as sound or light into signals that are interfaced to the brain either directly of via neural pathways, to restore lost or damaged perception ability. Eyeglasses and external hearing aids are prostheses, but a sensory neuroprosthesis is an active device that delivers electrical stimulus to the nervous system, such as a cochlear implant or artificial retina.

8.4.4.1 Motor Neuroprostheses

Motor neuroprosthetic devices take signals from the brain or motor nerve pathway and convert that information into control of an acuator device to execute the user's intentions. Motor neuroprosthetics work in one of two ways, either by (1) translating motor nerve impulses to electrical stimulation that excites or inhibits neuromuscular paths to paretic or paralyzed organs and limbs (functional electrical stimulation), or (2) picking up electricity generated by the brain or nerves and interpreting it to control prostheses or assistive devices (device control). In both cases, nerve signals can be interfaced to the neuroprosthesis by recording electrical impulses externally through the surface of the skin (myoelectric control) or through implanted electrodes.

Functional stimulation enables neural command signals to control muscle movement where native motor nerve function is paretic or impaired. Device control collects and maps nerve impulses to control electronic or electromechanical aids—actuated braces, artificial limbs or hands, synthetic speech generators, devices to allow control of bowel or bladder sphincter function, etc. Nerve signals interfaced to an active neuroprosthesis, or brain–computer interface, can be used to drive assistive technologies such as computer-based communication programs, environmental controls, and assistive robots [179,180].

For a motor neuroprosthesis to restore function, it must be integrated with the human owner's nervous system. The signals picked up by the electrodes from the nerves or brain must be translated into smooth and controlled actuation of the prosthesis. This involves some combination of learning and adapting by the user and some sophisticated electromechanical control strategies to decode signals from either (1) the remaining peripheral nerves, or (2) the brain, and translate them into actions [181].

The design and implementation of a device capable of complex motor tasks—such as grasping, manipulation, and walking with smooth gait, coordinating movement with vision and balance, responding with appropriate force and velocity—all require that the prosthesis have a sophisticated distributed network of control, actuation, and feedback. Limb and hand prostheses also need a high degree of fidelity to mechanical and dynamic properties of the natural limb. Otherwise the task of learning to use the device will be difficult. Therefore to be effective, the nanotechnical design of nanoactuators and nanosensors must be fully integrated with the control systems from design to implementation, including the very special ergonomic interface between patient and device [182].

There is a high degree of overlap between prosthetics, robotics, virtual reality, design of space suits, and other human augmentation technologies [183–185]. These highly multidisciplinary fields present many opportunities for application of nanotechnologies in materials as well as electronics. Nanotechnology is already enabling more natural prostheses by providing (1) smaller (and more affordable) sensors, processor elements, and the wiring and interconnections to network them into distributed control systems [186–189]; (2) smaller, more powerful, efficient, and responsive scaleable actuators whose mode of movement is natural and smooth because it is based on molecular forces, similar to those in natural muscle [190,191]; and (3) engineered materials that match the strength/weight ratios, elasticity/rigidity, and mechanical energy storage characteristics of key components of natural extremities [3,192].

Nanomaterials such as conductive polymers and carbon nanotubes offer routes to nanosensors, and nanoscale distributed-computing elements, as well as to modular, lightweight, and strong artificial muscles that can be ganged in parallel to match force requirements. Nanoscale magnetometers, accelerometers, pressure sensors, and gyroscopic devices will be able to more precisely detect even minute movements and angle changes; these will support the design of internal device rotation mechanisms that feature smooth, accurate movement as well as accurate transmittance of control and feedback information for human operation [193].

Nanotechnology will have its greatest impact on medicine not with tiny mobile robots, but with assemblies of cooperating interconnected networks of computing, communicating, and sensing nanoprocessors, driving assemblies of modular interworking nanoactuators to make up a micro or macro device like a powerful but subtle motor neuroprosthesis.

To see the current state of the art in prosthetics for limbs, and how integrated nanotechnology can be harnessed by distributed control to enable their design, consider some examples of artificial limbs.

8.4.4.2 Leg, Knee, and Foot Prostheses

Loss of a foot or leg is one of the most common amputations, due to war, civilian encounters with land mines, accidents, and complications of diabetes. Before the 1990s, artificial legs, knees, and feet were difficult to use, and required more energy for movement than normal walking.

Without a control and feedback system that reproduces the natural interaction of the limb with the body of the wearer and the external environment, amputees walking with a leg prosthesis consume more energy than a non-amputee at comparable walking velocities. The elastic tendons of the foot and leg store and release energy with each step, and artificial limbs have been designed to reproduce this spring mechanism, with improved results.

Designs with distributed microprocessor control in a complex prosthesis have given improved usability, but until recently, processors, sensors, and actuators have been too large, power-hungry, and expensive to offer a practical solution. The most challenging function to reproduce was the proprioception or kinesthetic sense that provided virtually unconscious and autonomous feedback to the body, enabling us to keep our balance through all types of movement and terrain. This requires low-power, rugged, fast sensors, processors, and actuators that have only recently become available through advances in micro- and nanotechnology.

Advanced strong and lightweight materials, including smart materials with built-in sensors, are also necessary to achieve the full potential of the electromechanical control system. As these prerequisites have become available, being able to build and test prototypes has led to better understanding of how the limb interacts with its physical environment as well as with the body and the nervous system.

Laboratories and companies around the world working on the leading edge of nanotechnology and control have now produced highly advanced artificial feet, knees, and legs that are giving life-like restoration of function to amputees. A walk through a few step cycles with a leading commercial prosthesis shows how it uses highly miniaturized but powerful accelerometers, processors, and actuators, with an optimized control strategy that reproduces essential features of the natural gait and posture. A prosthesis like the Proprio Foot [194] for example, might use adaptive neural network algorithms to learn from the user's movements and stride to optimize its response. Such a system would use fuzzy logic feedback algorithms to ensure smooth reactions and avoid overshooting responses. Distributed parallel processing enables the system to plan the positioning of parts of the limb for the next movement in real time while executing a step. Force sensors and accelerometers provide feedback for adjustment to slope, speed, and sudden off-balance movements by making thousands of measurements per second.

Distributed and embedded artificial intelligence and electrophysical feedback control the autonomous functions involved in walking that we do not have to think about—like keeping the leg positioned relative to the center of gravity of the body, rotating the ankle, and controlling the angle of the foot to the ground, with compensation for forward speed, slope, and other factors. At the same time, the prosthesis interfaces to the user's nervous system to respond to motor commands and execute voluntary movements. A requirement for success of the system is that it should interface, interact, and adapt to the forces and patterns of movement from the physical environment and the rest of the body, as well as to the nerve impulses, just like a natural limb would do. Thus we see that our definition of a motor neuroprosthesis was somewhat limited: it has to interact appropriately with its entire environment, not just with the nervous system.

8.4.4.3 Hand Prostheses

The hand has one of the highest densities of motor nerves and sensory nerve endings of any part of the human body, serving its highly developed tactile and sensory capabilities with 22 degrees of freedom in its four fingers and thumb. Prostheses to replace a lost hand are one of the oldest forms of prosthetics: the surgeon Ambroise Paré designed an anthropomorphic hand for wounded soldiers in the sixteenth century. Modern motor neuroprostheses provide considerable functionality, thanks to advances in microelectronics, microactuators, and robotics [195].

Like the lower extremity, the hand interacts with its environment as well as with the nervous system, but the hand is much more intimately and intricately connected with the brain in the performance of voluntary planned and executed tasks. A number of prosthetic hands have been developed with embedded controls. Much has been learned about hand movement from development of robotic hands for industry and space, as well as prosthetic use. As in the case of the artificial foot, the most recent and advanced designs use distributed control and sensors with local feedback rather than requiring the user to decide and communicate how much force is exerted by each finger at a given time [28,196–199].

Artificial hands with advanced capabilities can be used for robotics or human augmentation aids as well as prosthetics. Devices for robotics and prosthetics have been developed with 20 degrees of freedom, using shape memory alloy actuators. Some advanced designs implement the complex degrees of freedom of the fingers and thumb and employ sensitive microphones to detect vibration when a grasped object is slipping [200–202].

On-going progress toward more natural artificial hands is making use of MEMS accelerometers, as well as force and pressure sensors (and hence more nanotechnology). Designs have been proposed for smart artificial skin with embedded nanosensors, which will give more options for designers of prostheses.

Prosthetics, like other medicine, is human oriented, and thus seeks to adapt an assistive device to the unique needs of each patient, within inevitable constraints of cost, technical, and rehabilitative learning feasibility. With the advance of nanotechnology making devices adaptable as well as affordable, this ideal becomes more realizable. The range of options for fitting a pirate hook was much narrower than with a modern nanosensor and processor enhanced prosthesis.

A number of research centers are working on biomechatronic hands that aim to approach natural dexterity, speed, and strength with normal weight and appearance. A challenge is to minimize power requirements, operate noiselessly, and be resistant to water, oils, food, and be easily cleanable. The goal is to have an intelligent, adaptable self-programming control system that makes it easy for the user to develop skill. Some current designs have excellent dexterity, but are lacking in some of the other requirements.

Examples of several recent projects in artificial hand development include the Touch Bionics i-LIMB [203,204], the ARMin [205,206], the Modular Prosthetic Limb (MPL) [207], the EU/Rome LifeHand and Southhampton hand projects, and others [208,28]. Reviews and additional references can be found in Zecca et al. [208] and in [28].

This is a very active and exciting area for application of new nanotechnology. In the case of actuators, miniature electronic motors or pneumatic muscles have yet to be replaced by nanoengineered artificial muscles in an integrated design for an artificial hand. Lifelike, durable, soil-resistant skin coverings have yet to be developed and evaluated (perhaps using some of the nanosurface soil and water shedding features learned from the lotus petal).

8.4.5 Brain–Machine Interface

The control of physical objects by the power of thought alone has long captured the human imagination. Using our thoughts to control a computer or robot used to be the realm of science-fiction writers. Now, with the aid of new technology and years of study of neural activity in the brain, the control of machines and computers by the brain is becoming a reality [209–211]. Systems are being made in which patterns of neuronal firing in the brain can be translated into electronic controls to support communication, mobility, and independence for paralyzed people [211,212]. Nanoengineered electronic and magnetic detection devices are helping brain–machine interfaces reach a level of speed and responsiveness that will make a brain interface a usable prosthesis that does not require long and difficult concentration and training for the user.

8.4.5.1 Motor and Sensory Interfaces

To fully interface with the brain, a neuroprosthesis must not only receive signals from the brain, but must also return sensory information for feedback. This feedback is visual, auditory, kinesthetic, and haptic. In later sections, we will discuss sensor neuroprostheses as important topics on their own, but first we will examine aspects of motor control.

8.4.5.2 Promising Breakthroughs in Brain–Machine Prostheses

Many research groups have been working for decades to integrate sensors, computers, and knowledge of the patterns of nerve firing with which the brain controls movement, in order to help people who have brain or spinal cord damage to communicate and interact with the outside world. The goal is to use prostheses to replace or restore lost motor functions in paralyzed humans by routing movement-related signals from the brain, around damaged parts of the nervous system, to external effectors.

Much remains to be done before neuroprostheses that can respond to the brain become a clinical reality, but in experiments, paralyzed patients with electrodes implanted in the part of the brain that controls movement, the cerebral motor cortex, have been able to control computers and televisions, open e-mail, and move objects using a robotic arm [28].

8.4.5.3 Challenges to Be Overcome

Control of prosthetic devices is made possible by extracellular recordings from the cortical neurons in the brain, where movement control originates. To design a system, years of preclinical experimentation with implanted neurosensor electrodes has been necessary; the pattern of neuron firing has to be at least approximated in order to map signals onto movement in the prosthesis. Thus, the development of smaller and faster neuroelectrodes has been important in laying the foundations for current success in patients [213–216].

To make a brain–machine interface requires the estimation of a mapping from neural spike trains collected in motor cortex areas onto the kinematics of a normal limb—but fortunately, this mapping does not have to be absolutely accurate—otherwise the task would be impossible. Imagine that someone ripped the dashboard and steering column out of a car, or the cockpit out of an airplane, and handed it to you and asked you to reconnect all of the wires and controls back together so that it worked again. That would be an extremely simple task compared to mapping the connections between the brain and muscles after a spinal cord injury. That a brain–machine neuroprosthesis can work is as much as tribute to the adaptive and regenerative power of the brain and nervous system as it is to the years of patient experimentation and intricate deciphering by neuroscientists. If the brain is presented with an interface that is at all workable and predictable, the cortex can adapt in most cases, to learn how to associate patterns with movement [217].

There are purely clinical factors and obstacles for success of a brain neuroprosthesis. Firing patterns and maps from brain to motor effector neurons must be measured in intact animals and human subjects, to establish a baseline for translation from brain to machine. Movement signals in the motor cortex of the brain may not persist after nerve paths to a limb are cut off. ("Use it or lose it" holds true in the brain.)

But given the clinical obstacles, early experiments give indications that workable prostheses may be possible. There are worthy engineering challenges to be solved in both materials and control system architectures. The systems for recognizing and interpreting brain signals to movement must be robust and adaptable enough to deal with changes in pattern presented after injury, during learning, and due to individual differences. Current experimental systems typically sample ensembles of 100–200 cortical neurons. Advances in nanotechnology will allow denser and larger arrays to be implemented. The neural interfaces must be compatible with nerve cells and their environment, so that the transmission of signals does not fade over time due to build up of plaques on the electrodes or withering away of the neurons in contact with the surfaces. In the opinion of many scientists, "most of these difficulties are now engineering challenges, rather than problems of principle." [209]

8.4.5.4 Design of Control Algorithms

Much work by neuroscientists has been done to tell us what part of the cortex controls which limbs, and how control spreads out down the neural networks. If a control system could simply be "hard-wired" for the brain to talk to a prosthesis, the paradigm would be to interface electrodes to the appropriate part of the brain's motor cortex or motor pathway, and analyze the relationship between the cortical activity and measured arm or hand movements; this relationship would then map cortical activity to similar prosthetic arm movements. However, the pathway to the brain is not so simple, and there is the clinical problem that measured limb movements are not feasible for amputees or patients with physical mobility limitations [214,215].

The firing patterns of the nerves controlling natural neuromuscular systems are very complex, and are modulated by chemical neurotransmitters and inhibitors, so a purely electronic interface can never be completely natural. The motor signals spread out, and sensory feedback returns, over a network of dendritic paths in patterns that can be mapped experimentally to the musculature and sensory surfaces of the body. The areas of the cortex that control particular motor movements set up predictable patterns prior to initiating motor commands. For a neuroprosthesis, we merely want to provide the brain a tool to work with, rather than try to duplicate its operation [216].

We know from neuroscience that, to a large degree, the brain is adaptable and can learn new control tasks by response to feedback presented to it. If we can present the cortex cells with a coding system of responses that activate the prosthesis, then the brain can learn to exercise control. Hopefully, this learning can be automatic, implemented by feedback loops within the cortex that are similar to natural control mechanisms for the original limb. Otherwise control of the prosthesis will require extra effort and conscious attention to execute. Thus, getting the control coding right is as important as the weight, power, and agility of the robotics in the prosthesis. Fortunately, progress is being made in designing workable control schemes that enable the brain to successfully map intent onto movements of prostheses. And the brain has shown itself to be remarkably adaptable in learning to control devices by neural stimulation [217].

8.4.5.5 Adaptive Coding and Training

Recent research has shown that adaptive control strategies shorten the learning time and increase the effectiveness of brain–machine interfaces. A number of coding and training methods have been used to interface such neuroprostheses. These coding techniques compute statistical scores to match patterns in the cortex with movements of the limb or prosthesis. Adaptive methods can automatically improve their performance with practice, by iterative computation that optimizes the correlation between nerve firing patterns and movements with practice.

8.4.5.6 Distributed Control Networks of Nanocomputers

Because the brain is more universal than any specialized branch of the neural pathways connecting it to the extremities, and is the starting point for voluntary control signals, one might assume that the neuroprosthetic interface could be controlled largely and directly by the brain, bypassing the functions of the spinal cord, ganglia, motor nerves, etc. But distribution of function, especially motor functions, serves to prevent overload of the brain; much preprocessing of stimuli takes place along the pathways.

In the case of the leg, a great many of the control feedback loops are automatic, and can be implemented entirely within the limb. But for the hand or for speech, a complex mixture of voluntary initiation and automatic cascades of control must take place, with the option for voluntary control to override the automatic function at any point playing a much greater role. To match the learning and adaptive power of neural networks that control complex tasks like manipulation or speech, the control systems must be adaptive.

Analysis of such control systems reveals that they are best implemented with distributed, communicating networks of processing elements. Thus, a network of nanofabricated small processors with communication links, sensors, and actuators will be an optimal platform for implementing agile and responsive control systems for prosthetics (as well as robotics) that can adapt to external conditions and to the stimuli from the user's brain. Such a network also has the advantage of requiring less energy for the same computation capability of one or two fast processors for controlling prostheses.

8.4.5.7 Noninvasive Brain–Machine Interfaces

Noninvasive or minimally invasive methods of communicating between brain and prosthesis would be highly desirable—eliminating surgery, electrodes, and wires. Some obvious minimally invasive techniques, such as using finger, toe, or eye movements, have the disadvantage of requiring a high degree of the patient's attention, even if muscle movement is possible. One way to avoid the disadvantages of wires through the skull and skin would be to communicate with an implanted electrode via wireless radiofrequency signals—but this raises many technical problems and still requires an implant.

In principle, it is also possible to control computer cursors through noninvasive electrodes monitoring the brain from outside the head. The electrical potential of neurons collectively firing is detectable on the scalp. Its recording is termed the *electroencephalogram* (EEG), whereas the pattern of signals measured by electrodes on the surface of the cerebral cortex is called the *electrocortiogram* (ECoG). The EEG shows an average of many neurons firing in a broad region of the cortex, filtered through the skull and scalp, but a number of patterns can be detected nevertheless. Considerations for control programming are similar to those for ECoG, but mapping is more arbitrary. The lower interface resolution of the EEG makes it difficult to provide a wide range of subtle and distinct movement controls, and requires long training periods. EEG-based systems have generally been too slow for controlling rapid and complex sequences of movements, so this type of interface remains a less desirable option [216,217].

8.4.6 Magnetic Neural Stimulation and Monitoring

Advances in micro- and nanotechnology are on the cusp of giving an alternative to low-performance EEG interfaces and invasive electrode implants. With advances in materials and electronic nanosensors, it is becoming feasible to use magnetic fields to stimulate and monitor the brain. Magnetic stimulation is noninvasive; focused magnetic fields can stimulate nerves deep within the body and brain without implanted electrodes or shocks through the skin [218].

8.4.6.1 Basic Principles

The firings of neurons and the travel of ion currents along axon membranes generate magnetic fields. A steady current induces a static magnetic field, and any change in current creates a change in the magnetic field. Thus, magnetism is a second-order effect of the movement of an electrical charge: the magnetic field is proportional to the velocity of the charge and the change in magnetic field is proportional to the acceleration or deceleration of the charge. This indirectness makes magnetic fields more difficult to use, but it also creates the possibility of noninvasive communication with nerves, without implanted electrodes or painful transcutaneous shocks.

High intensity changes or pulses in strong magnetic fields can induce electrical fields in the nervous system that can exceed the firing threshold for neurons (*the action potential*). The induced electrical currents are proportional to the rate of change of magnetic field (dB/dt). Thus, magnetic stimulation can induce electrical currents in the neuron cell membranes like those induced by implanted electrodes, but without physical contact [219].

8.4.6.2 Magnetic Stimulation

The induction of nerve firing by application of strong focused magnetic fields is a new medical technique used to stimulate motor nerves in the limbs (*functional stimulation*) or neurons in the brain (*transcranial magnetic stimulation*). Magnetic stimulation requires strong magnetic fields, which must vary or pulse in order to generate an electric field—generation of an electrical field requires movement of an electrical charge relative to a magnetic field. Electrical stimulation of nerves could be obtained with a simple voltaic jar or electrostatic spark, but magnetic stimulation requires equipment that can generate short, intense pulsed, and focused magnetic fields of very high strength, about 0.5 T at the surface of the cortex, which typically requires a 2 T magnetic coil outside of the body.

To localize the stimulation, arrays of magnetic coils are positioned outside of the head to focus the combined fields inside the brain. Relatively low frequency magnetic fields can be used (typically a few kHz) that are not absorbed by the skull or spinocerebral fluid. The electromagnets are controlled so that the strength of the magnetic pulse exceeds the excitation threshold only at the focal point. The resolution that can be achieved is less than with electrodes, but the noninvasive advantage is spurring efforts to increase the precision of the magnetic focus [220].

8.4.6.3 Development of Medical Applications

Electric and magnetic fields are complementary: electrical currents generate magnetic fields, and changes in magnetic fields induce electrical fields. There were a number of early attempts to stimulate the brain and motor nerves using magnetic fields, but the technical challenges are formidable for either stimulation or monitoring with magnetism.

The first successful development of technology for magnetic stimulation was conducted at the University of Sheffield in England starting in 1976. The repetitive stimulator (rTMS), which can generate up to 30 pulses per second, became available in the 1990s. Since then the field has expanded rapidly, with several companies producing clinical equipment and obtaining regulatory approvals for experimental and some clinical uses. One use of magnetic stimulation is to temporarily shut down portions of the neural network. This allows connections to be mapped, and is being studied for treating conditions such as Parkinson's disease [221–223].

8.4.6.4 Magnetic Monitoring

The magnetic fields produced by nerve currents are weak but can be detected with sensitive magnetic field detectors (*magnetometers*) [224,225]. Extremely sensitive magnetometers are needed to detect the fields produced within the brain. Fortunately, a great deal of development has been invested toward high-performance magnetic sensors for many applications such as computer disk drives, oil exploration, and security detection. With current state of the art, *magnetoencephalography* (MEG) can map brain activity on a one millimeter grid or less. With powerful signal processing and statistical analysis, magnetoencephalographs can be co-registered with MRI scans with good accuracy. Because magnetic fields are induced perpendicular to the direction of current flow, MEG gives orthogonal information to EEG in terms of the types of neural tissue and direction of nerve impulses that are revealed.

The first generation of MEG equipment was typically bulky, requiring shielded rooms, high power consumption, cryogenic cooling of detectors, and significant processing times to deconvolute data from relatively few sensors. Thus, MEG has until recently been limited to research and highly specialized diagnostic applications for life threatening conditions. This is a rapidly developing area that is being accelerated by applying nanofabrication to existing types of magnetic sensors and entirely new concepts made possible by nanotechnology.

The results are thousand-fold improvements in sensitivity and reductions in size and power requirements by factors of ten to one hundred [226].

8.4.6.5 Devices for Magnetic Stimulation and Monitoring

The improvements in performance necessary to make noninvasive magnetic communication with the brain a practical reality are already being delivered by nanotechnology. For stimulation, the impacts of nanotechnology are largely indirect; nanofabrication of interstitial compounds and alloys is producing better high-temperature superconducting materials to reduce the size and cryogenic environmental constraints for high-performance superconducting magnets, and nanoparticle thin films are being used to fabricate magnetic shielding materials.

In the area of magnetic sensors, many older types of magnetic measurement devices can be sub-miniaturized with nanofabrication, but nanotechnology is also making new designs possible based on previously inaccessible physical phenomena. Both types of development are producing concrete results, and applications are expanding.

Historically, three classes of magnetic sensors have been developed: mechanical, electronic, and quantum. Researchers are reexamining magnetic sensing to find opportunities for enhancement based on phenomena that appear at the nanoscale, with very small masses and volumes.

Mechanical magnetic sensors include geometric magnetometers, where the sensor is moved or deformed by interaction with the magnetic field, and resonance sensors, whose vibration rate is influenced by field forces [227]. Electronic sensors include Hall effect sensors [228], which measure the resistance to flow of electrons caused by their deflection in a magnetic field; magnetoresistive, giant magnetoresistive, and colossal magnetoresistive sensors, based on thin-film conduction effects (the 2007 Nobel Prize in Physics was awarded to the discoverers of giant magnetoresistance, Albert Fert and Peter Grünberg) [229], and flux-gate devices, which compare the difference in current required to magnetize a coil in two directions. Some sensor designs utilize more than one physical effect in the same device for enhanced performance. Quantum sensors include the *superconducting quantum interference device* (SQUID), based on *Josephson junction* currents—the magnetically sensitive tunneling of electrons through a thin insulating barrier separating two superconductors [230].

The SQUID is the highest sensitivity magnetometer commercially available. Magnetic scanning systems approved for mapping neural activity are based on SQUID sensors. Although the first generation was bulky, it has been used successfully for brain and cardiac imaging. A second-generation design has been optimized with highly sophisticated software and good engineering to increase resolution and reduce the size and weight of the cooling and shielding systems. Applications include diagnostic imaging for neonatal brain assessment, liver susceptometry, and gastric ischemia, difficult to diagnose and serious conditions [231,232].

8.4.6.6 *Nanotechnology-Based Advances in Magnetic Sensor Design*

A number of new nanoscale magnetometer designs are being developed that approach or exceed the sensitivity of SQUID, without cryogenic cooling, and with less power consumption, lower cost, and smaller size. One, the *optical atomic magnetometer*, reported by the U.S. National Institute of Standards and Technology, with the University of Colorado and Sandia Laboratories, is based on the interaction of laser light with atoms oriented in a magnetic field in the gas phase [233]. Workers at Princeton University, Berkeley, and elsewhere are also developing optical atomic magnetometers, and improvements in performance continue to be published [234,235]. Another promising new magnetometer is a nanoscale cantilever design developed at Lucent Technologies' Bell Labs [236]. These and other designs may open new possibilities for magnetic medical imaging.

8.4.6.6.1 *Optical Atomic Magnetometers*

The NIST optical atomic magnetometer measures the change in alignment when atoms with a magnetic spin moment interact with a beam of laser light. In the absence of an external magnetic field, the atoms will align with the laser beam's crossed electric and magnetic fields. Any perturbation by a magnetic field will disorient the alignment with the laser light, reducing the amount of light transmitted through the gas. Magnetic shielding is used to make the detector selective and directional. The fabrication of a cell containing the gas, a small solid-state laser, and a detector for the transmitted light can be scaled down to microchip form, with nanoscale geometries, to make an extremely small, sensitive, and economical sensor element.

At NIST, a prototype, millimeter-scale microfabricated rubidium vapor cell with a low-power laser was able to detect the heartbeat of a rat. In Berkeley, researchers used the atomic magnetometer to detect magnetic particles flowing through water. Princeton researchers using a high-sensitivity atomic magnetometer based on potassium vapor performed MEG experiments [237]. Physicists at the University of Wisconsin and elsewhere are refining optical atomic magnetometer designs to reduce noise for biomedical applications [238].

The millimeter-scale prototype at NIST contains about 100 billion atoms of rubidium gas in a vial the size of a grain of rice. The change in spin alignment was easily detectable, and scalable down to much smaller sizes. The atomic magnetometer is about 1000 times more sensitive than previous devices of a similar size. With sensitivity below 70 fT (femto Tesla) per root Hertz, it is comparable to, or even exceeds SQUID sensors. It can be made much smaller than a SQUID, and operates at much higher temperatures, at around 150°C.

Currently, the complete NIST device is a few millimeters on each side. Developers predict that with the small size and high performance, such sensors could lead to magnetocardiograms that provide similar information to an electrocardiogram (ECG), without requiring electrodes on the patient's body, even from outside clothing. The current versions of the atomic detector are sensitive enough to detect alpha waves from the human brain, which produce magnetic fields of about 1000 fT just outside the skull.

To pick up the full range of magnetic fields emanating from the human head, the atomic optical devices would need to be more sensitive—down to 10 fT or less, which is projected to be feasible. The thermal magnetic noise level generated by the human brain is on the order of 0.1 fT. A sensitivity of 0.2 fT is projected for the Princeton potassium-based atomic magnetometer, if supercooled shielding were used to reduce the noise level at the detector. This would enable imaging of individual cortical modules in the brain, which have a size of 0.1–0.2 mm. This could provide an alternative to MRI and PET imaging, without injection of contrast enhancement agents or tracers.

Previous atomic magnetometers and SQUIDs are larger and require much more power than the gas laser design. Even with the laser and heating components, the new devices use relatively low power and can be extremely small. Thus, they could be used in high-resolution arrays of distributed sensors. The small size allows the sensor to get close to the heart or brain for magnetic measurements. Developers project that the sensors could even be used to make portable MEG helmets for brain–machine interfaces. They could also be used to identify markers for specific chemicals by measuring nuclear quadrupole resonance of excited atoms, opening further possibilities for monitoring and research.

8.4.6.6.2 Nanoscale Electromechanical Resonator Magnetometers

Mechanical magnetometers can be made using nanoscale cantilevers or bridges, coated or implanted with magnetic materials, to harness the sensitivity of nanoscale resonance vibrations. Fundamental breakthroughs in nanotechnology made in the past few years by Bell Labs and the New Jersey Nanotechnology Center (NJNC) have led to a new nanomechanical magnetometer design with performance that is potentially 100 to 1000 times greater than existing commercial devices, at extremely low cost based on silicon lithographic fabrication [236].

The new Bell Labs MEMS magnetometers employ a silicon resonator carrying an electric circuit. Oscillation of the resonator in a magnetic field generates a current around a closed-loop circuit damped by a resistor. Variations in magnetic field strength alter the amplitude and frequency of the resonator. This mechanical sensitivity can be used to measure the magnetic field by coupling the mechanical motion of a silicon bar or paddle to the ambient magnetic field.

In order to give a sensitive measure of a magnetic field, this nonlinear resonator must have negligible internal damping—a high Q-factor. Nanoscale crystalline oscillators made from quartz or silicon can be made with much higher Q numbers than all but superconducting electronic oscillators.

Magnetometers that use electronic detection (Hall, magnetoresistance, or flux-gate devices) have sensitivity limited by their electronic Q-factor, which depends on the resistance to electrons traveling through the metal in the circuit; it is difficult to reduce this factor (and increase sensitivity) without resorting to superconducting materials (which is why SQUIDs remain the ultimate purely electronic detector). A tuning fork resonator made from single-crystal silicon (with less internal friction than that of the hardest metal) will vibrate almost a thousand times longer than the best room-temperature electronic oscillators.

Researchers are working to optimize resonator magnetometer designs to achieve substantial improvements in sensitivity by modifying the microscale geometries with nanoscale features. Nanoscale mechanical resonators with mechanical Q-factors approaching 10,000 or more at room temperature can be made from semiconductor-grade silicon and similar single-crystal materials. This is a huge improvement over electronic detectors, without cryogenic cooling for superconductivity. Electromechanical resonator magnetometers should be up to 100–1000 times more sensitive than existing commercial devices.

In the meantime, improved designs using nanotechnology continue to be applied to optical atomic magnetometers, as well as to devices based on the Hall effect, magnetoresistance, and SQUID [239–242]. Advances in signal processing are being applied to provide capacity to extract, analyze, and efficiently present magnetic sensing data for medical use [243].

The MEG signals measured on the scalp surface must be interpreted and converted into information about the distribution of currents within the brain. This task is complicated by the fact that such inversion is nonunique. Additional mathematical simplifications, constraints, or assumptions must be employed to obtain useful source images, along with sophisticated signal extraction algorithms [244]. Beam forming techniques such as synthetic-aperture magnetometry beamformers can also reduce extraneous signals and focus the detector into the body [245].

8.4.6.7 Future Opportunities in Medical Magnetic Sensing

Imaging systems based on the newest sensors have not yet been built, but they will undoubtedly bring wider use of MEG, perhaps taking the portable non-invasive, efficient brain–machine interface closer to reality. In the meantime, other techniques for brain stimulation are being explored, such as the stimulation of neural tissue by light [246,247], and vibrotactile or acoustic stimulation [248]. And the possibilities of feedback with MEG and other modalities for brain–machine interfaces are being explored [249]. So, there are entirely new paths that the development of neuroprostheses could take. Whatever they are, nanotechnology will play a key role in implementing them.

8.4.7 Sensory Neuroprosthetics: Haptics

Haptics refers to the sense of touch, and more generally to the sense of pressure and force feedback from the body to the brain [250]. This brings us to the area of sensory neuroprosthetics, of which haptic sensors are a special case, since they are usually an integral part of motor prostheses. We discussed the importance of haptics and kinesthetics in the sections above on control and feedback of motor prostheses, and for brain–machine interfaces in general.

Haptics, along with vision, hearing, and balance, is an essential component of the stream of feedback that the nervous system sends to the brain [251]. A deficit in the haptic sense is usually the result of loss of the sensory nerve endings due to injury or amputation, but in rare and more difficult cases it can be due to brain injury. Haptics is a diffuse sense, so there is no one prosthetic device that satisfies the brain's requirement. It has been less well-understood than more obvious senses, even taste and smell, which are more localized and less intuitive.

Because tactile feedback is so important to the fine motor control necessary for dexterous and delicate tasks, as well as athletic performance, it is becoming an important research area. Nanotechnology-based haptic sensors are having an impact on robotics, design of spacesuits, and in medicine—not only for neuroprosthetics, but in the design of robotics assisted surgery systems [252,253]. It is extremely important in design of prosthetic strategies and in rehabilitation. Surgical connection of sensory as well as motor nerves to a prosthesis can give dramatically improved results [254,255]. So-called smart materials and embedded nanosensors will provide many options for implementing haptics in medical devices and surgical tools, and will assist in improving the quality of telemedicine.

8.4.8 Cognitive Prosthetics

The concept of a *cognitive prosthesis*, a system developed to support and augment the cognitive abilities of its user, has only been made possible recently with the advances in computing and interface technologies [256,257]. To the extent that cognitive prosthetics includes augmentative and alternative communication for people with impaired communication, and virtual reality systems, there is not a sharp dividing line between the term and the functions provided by other sensory–motor augmentation modes such as implants to relieve seizures, hearing prostheses, and brain–computer interfaces in general. However, the concept does raise the possibilities of powerful augmentation of human capabilities, as well as treatment for mental deficits, both small and profound. The idea raises many psychological, social, ethical, and medical concerns, as well as research issues.

8.4.9 Future Directions for Brain–Machine Interfaces

The progress that has been made is remarkable, but many obstacles must still be overcome. Without invasive implants, current experimental brain–machine prostheses require the patient to be tethered to bulky equipment, which needs tuning and maintaining by a team of technicians. Prototype implants have wires that penetrate the skull and skin, with the risk of infection. Wireless signal transmission for brain implants is still in the future, along with wearable magnetic brain–machine interfaces.

A more difficult obstacle is that the performance of microelectrodes recording from neurons tends to fall off over time; better engineering of interfaces using nanoengineered materials is needed to improve biocompatibility and allow lower stimulation potentials. Even if implants are supplanted by non-invasive magnetic communication, there is still research to be done in neurocognition and how to interface learning systems.

Although patterns of control for hands and arms have been mapped, individual differences are not fully explored—some experimental patients are able to control prostheses much more easily than others. Concerted efforts are developing adaptive learning systems that require less effort from the patient by embedding neural networks and adaptive filters into the control system of the prosthesis, with impressive results.

Paths and mechanisms for feedback is another area where more research is needed. To succeed in duplicating or restoring limb function instead of merely controlling machines, researchers have to work out how the body tells the brain where its limbs are positioned in space—proprioception. Better pressure and vibration sensors, accelerometers, actuators, and force sensors are needed in order to develop improved artificial proprioception, haptics, and kinesthetics. All of these pieces need to be integrated seamlessly in intelligent control systems that respond precisely and adapt over time to changes in their environment. Nanotechnology is playing an important role in sensors, actuators, communications, and computing elements to make the brain–machine interface a clinical reality. Most of the difficulties for motor neuroprosthetics are now engineering challenges, rather than problems of principle. They will be solved by closely knit interdisciplinary teams that include doctors, engineers, rehabilitation specialists, and patients.

8.4.10 Neuroprosthetics for the Ear

Restoring sensory pathways is as important for neural prosthetics as restoring motor function. Sight and hearing are valuable not only because of their role in performing tasks, but because they are the bridges for social communication. Hearing loss is the most common form of sensory impairment. Electronic aids for hearing have a long history intertwined with the telecommunications inventions that shape the modern world. Alexander Graham Bell was an audiologist; the telephone was a by-product of his interest in making an electronic hearing aid [258–260].

The study of how the human ear distinguishes sounds is important in design and optimization of large-scale telephone networks sending usable speech over long distances. Voice compression, recognition, and synthesis are modeled largely on an understanding of how the ear and brain process speech. The study of how hearing works—how information is encoded and decoded in sounds by the brain—has been essential in developing telephony, and in turn has helped to develop aids to ameliorate hearing disorders [261]. Research to optimize telecommunications led to signal processing technology that made advanced hearing aids possible. Artificial stereocilia MEMS, modeling the resonators in the cochlea, are being fabricated in nanotechnology laboratories in order to understand the mechanisms of hearing [262–268].

Cochlear implants for hearing disorders are one of the most mature and best established areas of any electronic neuroprostheses. Nanotechnology has enhanced microelectronics, batteries, and micromechanical transducers in cochlear implant devices and thus has contributed significantly to the quality of life of persons with hearing impairment. Patients with cochlear implants benefit from improved understanding of speech in noise, sound quality, and localization of sounds compared to patients with acoustic hearing aids, without the ear canal occlusion, acoustic feedback, and inconvenience and cosmesis of external devices [269–271].

Cochlear prostheses are implanted in the middle ear, where they stimulate the ossicles electromechanically, rather than acoustically, through either electromagnetic or piezoelectric transducers. Sound signals transduced by an externally worn microphone are sent to the implant by wireless transmission. Cochlear implants achieve an average threshold improvement of 10 dB from 500 to 4000 Hz. At 6000 Hz, the gain is about 20 dB compared with conventional fitted acoustic hearing aids [272].

Another type of hearing neuroprosthesis, the auditory brainstem implant, uses electrodes placed over the cochlear nucleus or inserted into the brainstem. This direct interface is capable of restoring some residual hearing in many patients who have lost both hearing nerves [273,274].

Because the organ to which the prosthesis connects the brain is inside the skull, neuroprostheses for hearing can bypass many of the problems faced in getting signals from the ear and its prosthesis to the relevant part of the brain. Cochlear implants (like cardiac pacemakers or spinal stimulators or deep brain stimulators) can be self-contained, with power transmitted through the skull by electromagnetic induction. Thus, the main problems are long-term biocompatibility (build up of biofilms and plaques) and refinement of the signal processing to improve performance by attempting to match the natural function of the ear. Challenges include recognition of pitch for understanding and enjoyment of music, and preventing bacterial and fungal infections. The latter is an area that has prospects of being improved through nanomaterials [275–279].

8.4.10.1 Neuroprosthesis for Balance

Besides the sensory organ for hearing, the inner ear contains the vestibular arches, filled with fluid and cilia which can sense microscopic inertial fluid flows caused by head and body movements. Disruption of this function can cause severe dizziness, loss of balance, inability to walk or even sit upright, and sensations of sea-sickness or air-sickness. Some research is being pursued to develop an implantable MEMS neuroprosthesis that could restore or compensate for loss or disturbance of this sensory organ [280–284].

8.4.10.2 Neuroprosthesis for Tinnitus

Tinnitus is a condition that results in a constant sensation of sound, regardless of whether an audial stimulus is present. It is difficult to treat, and can be very troubling. Most treatment seeks to modulate the patient's response, rather that treating the tinnitus itself. One alternative development is an implantable device to deliver electrical stimulation in the middle ear, close to the cochlea; the goal is to turn off the nerve pathway, similar to stimulators for relief of pain and tremor [285].

8.4.10.3 Anatomy of the Ear

In order to see the relevance of nanotechnology to cochlear implants, consider the neuroanatomy of the inner ear and how it is stimulated.

Mechanoacoustical pressure is delivered to the membrane that seals off the inner ear, the cochlea, by an extremely delicate linkage from the eardrum to the malleus, incus, and stapes (hammer, anvil, and stirrup) bones. Sound is collected by the eardrum, causing the stapes to vibrate against the membrane that separates the cochlea from the outer ear, transmitting pressure waves to fluids in the interior. This linkage is a powerful mechanical amplifier: the human ear can detect motions of the eardrum on the order of a picometer—smaller than the diameter of an atom.

The cochlea is a hollow tapering helix supported by a bony spiral shelf, the *osseous spiral lamina*, which winds around a central core, the *modiolus*. The cochlea's spiral cone geometry, like a French horn or conch shell, acts as a mechanical acoustical transform to select for different vibration frequencies along its interior. The interior of the cochlea is separated into two fluid-filled chambers (the *scala vestibuli* and *scala tympani* or upper and lower ducts) by a thin sac, called the *cochlear duct*, filled with gelatinous material. The large end of the spiral is sealed from the outer ear by two membranes, the oval and round windows, on either side of the cochlear duct. The duct separates the two chambers all the way up the spiral to its apex, where there is a small opening between them. The sensory hair cells are inside the cochlear duct adjacent to a thin layer of tissue (the *tectorial membrane*). Each hair cell has a group of stereocilia projecting into the viscous gelatin, which resonate with sound [286,287].

The chambers on either side of the cochlear duct are filled with an electrolyte solution that conducts sound from the oval window, to which the stapes is attached, into the scala vestibuli. When pressure waves travel through the upper side of the cochlear duct to the apex of the spiral, and down the lower side, the duct is compressed by the fluid, causing movements of the cell hairs. The shearing movement of the hair cells opens potassium ion channels in hair cell membranes, depolarizing the cells and initiating an electrical signal.

The mechanical stress is transmitted to the ion channels in hair cells via tiny filaments that connect neighboring hairs in a bundle. The hairs are about 500 nm in diameter and tip links are on the order of 2 nm in diameter.

The stereocilia are linked in a complex network, with an inner and outer layer. The cochlea contains about 28,000 hair cells in humans. The absolute number of cells does not directly relate to auditory acuity: cats have 39,000; bats, rats, and dolphins about 15,000. In human, the interior linear extent of the cochlea is about 3.5 cm. So the density of sense cells is about 800 per millimeter (spaced at about 1.25 μm along the cochlea).

Behind the hair cells is a layer of neurons, the spiral ganglion, which contains four or five times more cells than the sensory cell layers. The network of auditory neurons in the spiral ganglion lies close to the interior or modiolar wall of the cochlear duct. The spiral ganglion neurons control the selection and organization or stimuli that are sent to the auditory cortex in the brain.

The hair cells are extremely sensitive to acoustical vibrations, and vulnerable to damage. Up to one third of the sensory hair cells typically die with age and damage by intense or chronic sound overload, chemicals, and disease. Unlike disorders in the mechanical acoustical path, nerve damage cannot be compensated by external devices.

8.4.10.4 Design of Cochlear Implants

Cochlear implants serve to bypass damaged inner ear hair cells and transfer auditory information to the brain. A cochlear implant takes sound from an external microphone and converts it into electrical impulses to stimulate the cochlea. The microphone and signal processing module are worn outside the head, and the stimulator is implanted behind the ear, with wires inserted into the cochlea. Stimulation is usually applied to the ganglion layer, which is accessed by inserting electrodes into the scala tympani, the lower cochlear chamber next to the modiolus where it can be placed close to the spiral ganglion.

Coding of sound and mapping stimulation onto the cochlea is guided by neurocognitive research in how the cochlea receives and processes sound. Early cochlear implants used a single electrode and encoded sounds by converting sound frequencies into electronic pulse frequencies, which are perceived as sound when applied to the ganglion. This encoding is oversimplified and does not reproduce fine details of sound perception. Newer cochlear implants map different frequencies spatially along the cochlea, from lower to higher frequencies. This improved mapping is closer to the natural perception of sound by the ganglion, and is the coding used by most current cochlear implant devices.

Current devices have from 16 to 100 electrodes. While it may never be necessary to approximate the number of discrete stimulation points on the spiral ganglion that are presented by the 20,000 or more hair cells, clearly there is plenty of room at the bottom for delivery of sound-coded impulses with higher resolution along the cochlear duct.

Researchers and developers are working to overcome a number of challenges in what is called the *electroneural bottleneck*. Currently, the voltage required to stimulate the neurons in the spiral ganglion is not localized—it stimulates a relatively large area. The electrodes cannot be placed very close together because it would result in cross talk. The electrodes cannot be too conforming or embedded in the cochlea because the device may have to be removed without damage to the tissues. The electrodes are currently hand-made assemblies; integrated device electrode assemblies have been proposed and used experimentally in the lab, but performances in electrode resistance, durability, reliability, and biocompatibility are still not sufficient for clinical use. Currently, the signal processing power available to fit into a low-power wearable package is not sufficient to process received sound into many more channels for discrete delivery, and a large number of channels would present a wiring challenge.

Work has been done on designs using nested wiring with electrode contacts that can be de-insulated by laser, which may resolve some obstacles. Electrode coatings and treatment with platinum, iridium, gold, platinum black, and alloys have been studied to lower resistance and reduce corrosion. Shape metal alloys have been proposed to produce better conformance to the modiolus and spiral ganglion. Designs with quadrupolar electrodes, with contact points on various places in the modiolus have been proposed, which might help to focus the excitation area. Coating of electrodes with brain-derived growth factors has been studied experimentally in an effort to reduce long-term atrophy of spiral ganglion cells [288–290]. Surface treatment of electrodes with carbon nanotubes is another technique that is being investigated for improved interfaces to neurons [291].

Long-term wear of cochlear implants has given rise to biofilm contamination and infection; the ear is particularly vulnerable to infection since it is open to the mouth and throat.

Nanotechnology may in future offer solutions to some or all of theses challenges with better materials, circuits, signal processing arrays, and stimulation methods. Application of nanotechnology may even come up with convenient, low-cost nanoengineered smart acoustical materials that could filter out damaging frequencies and noise levels when foamed or inserted into the ear, while allowing the wearer to hear normal sounds in comfort, thus preventing hearing loss.

8.4.11 Vision Prosthetics

Loss of sight has profound psychological as well as social and physical consequences; some 30% of the sensory input to the brain comes from the eye [292,293]. The sense of sight involves highly parallel processing of image data from light focused onto a surface. Vision involves the process by which the eye and the optical nerves gather light, extract image data by sampling areas on the projection, detect features in the image, and send the information to the brain for further processing, recognition, and analysis.

The brain is very plastic, especially with respect to the pathways to the visual cortex; with a prosthesis that maps pixels onto the surface of a suitable area of skin, with dense nerve receptors, it is possible for the brain to map the signals to the visual cortex so that the patient learns to visualize from the haptic inputs. The adaptability of the brain gives a good prognosis for development of a number of types of visual prostheses, whether mapping light images to haptic nerve endings or stimulating some level in the layers of processing that lead from the eye to the brain, all the way up to direct stimulation of the visual cortex.

Any of these routes is a formidable undertaking from both technical and neurological viewpoints. If the ear is the foot of sensory prosthetics, then the eye is the hand. Both are difficult, but hearing is a mapping onto a one-dimensional sensory cell space, the linear array of cilia, whereas vision is a mapping onto a two-dimensional space of rods and cones in the retina. Additional dimensionality for both hearing and sight is added by parallelism in time—sensation from millions of cells is simultaneous over the sensing space rather than serial. One of the jobs of the layers of neurons behind the retina is to organize a sampling scheme for transmitting images to the brain. Vision is not totally asynchronous; somewhere on the path to the brain the incoming data is organized into periodic sampling or refresh cycles, which is why the visual cortex can be satisfied to generate images from strobed motion picture and television screens, so long as their output rate exceeds the sampling rate of the brain's optical system. The latter is not a simple scanning process, but in practice a frame rate of about 30 frames per second is perceived as continuous [294–296].

8.4.11.1 The Retina

The retina is the point at which light is converted into neural impulses, which are processed into images by networked layers of neurons carrying information to the visual cortex. The retina samples images with photoreceptor cells (rods and cones) whose overall size is on the order of microns. Cones are color sensitive. Rods have a sharper acuity than cones, but do not discriminate colors [297–299].

The human retina contains approximately 120 million rod and 6 million cone cells. The densely packed cones in the center of the retina where vision is most acute, the fovea, have a center-to-center spacing of about 2.5 microns. Cone density in the fovea is between 100,000 and 300,000/mm^2, but rods and cones are both present in surrounding periphery of the retina. Rods are absent in the fovea, and are packed at a density of 80,000–100,000/mm^2 in the periphery.

8.4.11.2 Fovea

The area of the fovea, where rods are absent, has a radius of from 200 to 300 μm; the central part of the fovea where cones are packed most densely is only about 50 × 50 μm. The total number of cones in the fovea is approximately

200,000. The total number of cones in the entire retina is approximately 6,400,000. The total number of rods in the retina is 110,000,000–125,000,000.

The peak rod density is located in a ring around the fovea between 1.5 and 5 mm from the center, where the rod density is between 100,000 and 160,000 rods/mm². In terms of the radius of the field of vision, the peak is between 5° and 18° from the center. The rod-free area of the fovea is only 1° or 2° of the visual field.

The photoreceptors communicate with ganglion neurons located in a tissue layer 150 to 300 μm behind the retina, and separated from it by a layer of support cells, the retinal pigment epithelium. There are one or two cones and about 20 rods for each ganglion cell. A network of interconnected neurons process the information from the more than six million receptors in the retina down to where it is carried by approximately one million axons in the optic nerve to the brain.

8.4.11.3 Bypassing the Retina

Retinal degeneration or detachment is one of the main causes of vision loss. Therefore, most efforts to develop a visual neuroprosthesis have attempted to stimulate the ganglia cell layer behind the retina, as the simplest strategy to interface to the visual signal processing that is in place on the optical nerve path. Some prostheses have been designed and tested that stimulate the visual cortex directly, producing a low-resolution pattern of visual sensation, and some have mapped digitized imaging onto touch sensors in the back or other skin areas, in a kind of transposed Braille that delivers images rather than encoded letters.

8.4.11.4 Artificial Retinas

Most recent research in visual neuroprosthetics has been focused on artificial retina replacements or bypasses converting visual information into patterns of electrical stimulation onto inner retinal neurons. More than a dozen projects around the world are aimed at using advances in nanotechnology and high-density integrated microelectronics to develop an implant analogous to the cochlear implant for the ear, to restore lost vision. Like the cochlear implant, an eye implant is not anticipated to fully restore all lost function. Research devices are expected to provide enough visual perception of contours, outlines, and shades of light to allow a blind person to move freely in unfamiliar environments.

Treatment of diseases such as retinitis pigmentosa is focused on growing knowledge of affected biochemical pathways, development of animal models, and possible gene therapy, especially for genetically defined subsets of patients, based on newly identified genes [300]. As is the case with many other parts of the nervous system, vision, its development, and its degeneration are controlled by a large number of different genes, and this approach is still in early stages of development. Another possible approach being investigated is transplantation of cells to the retina [301]. Visual neuroprostheses will probably still be needed, even when other therapies become available, because of the large number and diversity of causes of vision loss.

In the remainder of this section, we look at some of the projects for developing prostheses that can be implanted in the visual cortex, around the optic nerve, or in the eye. Some of these approaches have shown promise for useful visual perception to patients with visual impairments [302–306].

A large-scale project has been undertaken for a number of years by the U.S. Department of Energy (DOE) National Laboratories and the National Science Foundation, with a team that includes a number of universities, institutes, and private industry. The artificial retina device bypasses nonfunctioning retinal cells to transmit signals directly to the optic nerve. The device consists of a tiny camera and microprocessor mounted in eyeglasses, a receiver implanted behind the ear, and an electrode-studded array that is tacked to the retina. Power is provided by a wireless battery pack worn on the belt.

A microprocessor converts the camera image and transmits information to an implanted wireless receiver. The receiver sends the signals through a tiny cable to the electrode array to generate stimulating pulses. The pulses are perceived as patterns of light and dark spots corresponding to the electrodes stimulated. Patients have learned to interpret the visual patterns produced, enabling them to detect when lights are on or off, describe an object's motion, count individual items, and locate objects. To evaluate the long-term effects of the retinal implant, five devices have been approved for home use.

The DOE project has produced three successively more sophisticated models, which are being tested and evaluated. Surgical time was reduced from the 6h required for the first model to 2h for the second version, which has 60 electrodes. The third model will have more than 200 electrodes, and will use more advanced materials than previous ones. A special coating, only a few microns thick, will replace the bulky sealed package used in previous models. The new model will use flexible conductive materials for the electrode array so that it will conform to the shape of the inner eye. The latest model will be many times smaller than earlier models. Engineering goals include enhancing the resolution with more electrodes, and decreasing the size of the device and complexity of the surgical procedure. A prototype is being developed as a product, named the Argus II [307–311].

Other retinal prostheses systems have been developed including subretinal versions, and versions with high pixel density, in Australia, Europe, Japan, and elsewhere including international teams [312–317].

Researchers face numerous challenges in developing retinal prosthetic devices that are effective, safe, and durable enough to last for the lifetime of the individual. Materials must be biocompatible with delicate eye tissue, yet able to withstand corrosion. The device must remain fixed to a precise area of the retina and not compress or pull the tissue. The apparatus also needs to deliver enough power to stimulate electrodes, without generating excess heat to damage the remaining functional nerve tissue. Image processing needs to be performed in real time so there is no delay in interpreting an object in view. In addition, effective surgical approaches are critically important to ensure a successful implant.

8.4.11.5 Other Research on Vision Prosthetics

A number of interdisciplinary research teams are looking at the effect of implant surgery on the retina, the sensitivity of the retina to electronic charge, spatial resolution in relation to stimulation, the best patterns and locations for nerve stimulation, and evaluating the learning and adaptation of patients with early versions of the devices [318–340]. One approach uses an implantable miniature telescope for restoring sight in cases of macular degeneration by focusing the plane of vision onto undamaged portions of the retina [341].

The possibility of electrode or tissue damage limits excitation schemes to those that may be employed with electrodes that have relatively low charge densities. The excitation thresholds that have been required to achieve vision have been found to be relatively high. This may result in part from poor apposition between neurons and the stimulating electrodes, and is confounded by the effects of the photoreceptor loss, which initiates other pathology in the surviving retinal tissue. The combination of these and other factors imposes a restriction on the pixel density that can be used for devices that actively deliver electrical stimulation to the retina. The resultant use of devices with relatively low pixel densities presumably will limit the degree of visual resolution that can be obtained with these devices. Further increases in pixel density, and therefore increased visual acuity, will necessitate either improved electrode–tissue biocompatibility or lower stimulation thresholds. To meet this challenge, innovations in materials and devices are needed, as well as experiments on the factors and functional parameters relevant to the designing of implants, such as thresholds and electrical point spread functions [342–344].

Nanotechnology offers a potential way to avoid the obstacles with electrical stimulation, by using nanofabricated microfluidics to inject chemical neurotransmitter stimulants into the subretinal ganglion. Researchers at Stanford University have developed a prototype test system to study the possibility, by characterizing the stimulus produced with a microfluidics system fabricated on a 500 nm thick silicon nitride membrane, with a single 5 or 10 μm aperture overlaying a microfluidic delivery channel in a silicone elastomer. Controlled excitation based on picoliter amounts of neurotransmitter delivered was obtained in rat neurons grown in culture on the surface of the apparatus. In the experiments, the stimulation radius was as small as 10 μm, comparable to what has been achieved in electrical stimulation experiments with a micrometer-size electrode. This experimental study shows how future neurostimulation systems, scaled up with arrays of delivery channels, might be possible with advances in integrated nanofabrication and cell engineering [345,346].

8.5 Summary of Nanoengineered Restorative Tissue Engineering and Prosthetics

The restoration of tissue structure and function by artificial engineered materials and techniques is gaining new possibilities through the application of nanotechnology. As nanoscale methods are applied, a convergence is taking place between drug delivery, implants, tissue engineering, and prosthetic devices. Interaction with tissue at the nanoscale involves signaling on the biomolecular level, as well as unique surface and energetic nanoscale effects.

Nanotechnology is making significant impacts in the area of nanoengineered bioactive materials for implants, encapsulation of living cells and tissue implants for immunoprotection, and miniaturization and power engineering for prosthetic devices.

A large amount of work remains before the effectiveness and safety of many of these approaches can be proven. But many are nearing successful translation into clinical practice as their potential is borne out in clinical trials and experience.

References

1. European Commission, Nanomedicine: Nanotechnology for health, European Technology Platform Strategic Research Agenda for Nanomedicine, online at: http://cordis.europa.eu/nanotechnology/nanomedicine.htm (2009).
2. M. C. Roco and W. S. Bainbridge (eds.), *Converging Technologies for Improving Human Performance: Nanotechnology, Biotechnology, Information Technology, and Cognitive Science (NBIC)*, U.S. National Science Foundation/Department of Commerce Report of a Workshop, World Technology Evaluation Center (WTEC), Arlington, VA, June 2002.
3. Y. Gogotsi, *Nanomaterials Handbook*, CRC Press, Boca Raton, FL, 2006.
4. H.-J. Fecht and Y. Champion, *Nano-Architectured and Nanostructured Materials: Fabrication, Control and Properties*, Wiley-VCH, Weinheim, Germany, 2006.
5. H. S. Nalwa, *Handbook of Nanostructured Biomaterials and Their Applications in Nanobiotechnology*, 2 Vols., American Scientific Publishers, Valencia, CA, 2005.
6. P. M. Taylor, Biological matrices and bionanotechnology, *Philosophical Transactions of the Royal Society B*, 362, 1313–1320 (2007).
7. G. B. Wei and P. X. Ma, Nanostructured biomaterials for regeneration, *Advanced Functional Materials*, 18, 3568–3582 (2008).
8. S. P. Adiga, C. Jin, L. A. Curtiss, N. A. Monteiro-Riviere, and R. J. Narayan, Nanoporous membranes for medical and biological applications, *Wiley Interdisciplinary Reviews: Nanomedicine and Nanobiotechnology*, 1, 568–581 (2009).
9. O. Shoseyov and I. Levy (eds.), *Nanobiotechnology: Bioinspired Devices and Materials of the Future*, Springer Verlag, Berlin, Germany, 2007.

10. J. F. Mano, G. A. Silva, H. S. Azevedo, P. B. Malafaya, R. A. Sousa, S. S Silva, L. F. Boesel et al., Natural origin biodegradable systems in tissue engineering and regenerative medicine: Present status and some moving trends, *Journal of the Royal Society Interface*, 4, 999–1030 (2007).

11. S. K. Mallapragada and B. Narasimhan (eds.), *Handbook of Biodegradable Polymeric Materials and Their Applications*, 2 Vols., American Scientific Publishers, Valencia, CA, 2005.

12. M. O. Riehle, Biocompatibility: Nanomaterials for cell- and tissue engineering, *NanoBioTechnology*, 1, 308–309 (2005).

13. J. K. Leach, Multifunctional cell-instructive materials for tissue regeneration, *Regenerative Medicine*, 1, 447–455 (2006).

14. L. J. Lee, Polymer nanoengineering for biomedical applications, *Annals of Biomedical Engineering*, 34, 75–88 (2006).

15. A. R. Boccaccini and J. E. Gough (eds.), *Tissue Engineering Using Ceramics and Polymers*, CRC Press, Boca Raton, FL, 2007.

16. A. R. Boccaccini (ed.), *Tissue Engineering Using Ceramics and Polymers*, Woodhead Publishing, Abington, Cambridge, U.K., 2009.

17. M. M. Stevens and J. H. George, Exploring and engineering the cell surface interface, *Science*, 310, 1135–1138 (2005).

18. H. J. Chung and T. G. Park, Surface engineered and drug releasing pre-fabricated scaffolds for tissue engineering, *Advanced Drug Delivery Reviews*, 59, 249–262 (2007).

19. D. Leckband, Beyond structure: Mechanism and dynamics of intercellular adhesion, *Biochemical Society Transactions*, 36, 213–220 (2008).

20. S. Pokutta, F. Drees, S. Yamada, W. J. Nelson, and W. I. Weis, Biochemical and structural analysis of α-catenin in cell–cell contacts, *Biochemical Society Transactions*, 36, 141–147 (2008).

21. K. S. Straley and S. C. Heilshorn, Independent tuning of multiple biomaterial properties using protein engineering, *Soft Matter*, 5, 114–124 (2009).

22. V. P. Shastri, In vivo engineering of tissues: Biological considerations, challenges, strategies, and future directions, *Advanced Materials*, 21, 3246–3254 (2009).

23. P. A. Madurantakam, C. P. Cost, D. G. Simpson, and G. L. Bowlin, Science of nanofibrous scaffold fabrication: Strategies for next generation tissue-engineering scaffolds, *Nanomedicine*, 4, 193–206 (2009).

24. J. P. R. O. Orgel, T. C. Irving, A. Miller, and T. J. Wess, Microfibrillar structure of type I collagen in situ, *Proceedings of the National Academy of Sciences*, 103, 9001–9005 (2006).

25. W.-J. Li, C. T. Laurencin, E. J. Caterson, R. S. Tuan, and F. K. Ko, Electrospun nanofibrous structure: A novel scaffold for tissue engineering, *Journal of Biomedical Materials Research Part A*, 60, 613–621 (2002).

26. L. A. Smith and P. X. Ma, Nano-fibrous scaffolds for tissue engineering, *Colloids and Surfaces B: Biointerfaces*, 39, 125–131 (2004).

27. L. A. Smith, X. Liu, and P. X. Ma, Tissue engineering with nano-fibrous scaffolds, *Soft Matter*, 4, 2144–2149 (2008).

28. G. L. Hornyak, H. F. Tibbals, J. Dutta, and J. J. Moore, *Introduction to Nanoscience and Nanotechnology*, CRC Press, Boca Raton, FL, 2009.

29. B. S. Harrison and A. Atala, Carbon nanotube applications for tissue engineering, *Biomaterials*, 28, 344–353 (2007).

30. A. S. Zuruzi, B. C. Butler, N. C. MacDonald, and C. R. Safinya, Nanostructured TiO$_2$ thin films as porous cellular interfaces, *Nanotechnology*, 17, 531–535 (2006).

31. Y. Lin, Z. Su, Z. Niu, S. Li, G. Kaur, L. A. Lee, and Q. Wang, Layer-by-layer assembly of viral capsid for cell adhesion, *Acta Biomaterialia*, 4, 838–843 (2008).

32. A. Merzlyak, S. Indrakanti, and S.-W. Lee, Genetically engineered nanofiber-like viruses for tissue regenerating materials, *Nano Letters*, 9, 846–852 (2009).

33. L. A. Lee, Z. Niu, and Q. Wang, Viruses and virus-like protein assemblies— Chemically programmable nanoscale building blocks, *Nano Research*, 2, 349–364 (2009).

34. J. J. Norman and T. A. Desai, Methods for fabrication of nanoscale topography for tissue engineering scaffolds, *Annals of Biomedical Engineering*, 34, 89–101 (2006).

35. G. Cao, *Nanostructures and Nanomaterials: Synthesis, Properties, and Applications*, Imperial College Press, London, U.K., 2004.

36. M. J. Schulz, A. D. Kelkar, and M. J. Sundaresan, *Nanoengineering of Structural, Functional and Smart Materials*, CRC Press, Boca Raton, FL, 2005.

37. G. M. Whitesides and M. Boncheva, Beyond molecules: Self-assembly of mesoscopic and nanoscopic components, *Proceedings of the National Academy of Sciences*, 99, 4769–4774 (2006).

38. B. S. Shim, P. Podsiadlo, D. G. Lilly, A. Agarwal, J. Lee, Z. Tang, S. Ho et al., Nanostructured thin films made by dewetting method of layer-by-layer assembly, *Nano Letters*, 7, 3266–3273 (2007).

39. S. Srivastava, V. Ball, P. Podsiadlo, J. Lee, P. Ho, and N. A. Kotov, Reversible loading and unloading of nanoparticles in "exponentially" growing polyelectrolyte LBL films, *Journal of the American Chemical Society*, 130, 3748–3749 (2008).

40. A. K. Geim and K. S. Novosolov, The rise of graphene, *Nature Materials*, 6, 183–191 (2007).

41. D. Green, D. Walsh, S. Mann, and R. O. C. Oreffo, The potential of biomimesis in bone tissue engineering: Lessons from the design and synthesis of invertebrate skeletons, *Bone*, 30, 810–815 (2002).

42. A. Lin and M. A. Meyers, Growth and structure in abalone shell, *Materials Science and Engineering A*, 390, 27–41 (2005).

43. L. J. Bonderer, A. R. Studart, and L. J. Gauckler, Bioinspired design and assembly of platelet reinforced polymer films, *Science*, 319, 1069–1073 (2008).

44. P. K. Hansma, P. J. Turner, and R. S. Ruoff, Optimized adhesives for strong, lightweight, damage-resistant, nanocomposite materials: New insights from natural materials, *Nanotechnology*, 18, 044026 (2007).

45. Q. Xu, R. M. Rioux, M. D. Dickey, and G. M. Whitesides, Nanoskiving: A new method to produce arrays of nanostructures, *Accounts of Chemical Research*, 41, 1566–1577 (2008).

46. G. M. Whitesides and B. Grzybowski, Self-assembly at all scales, *Science*, 295, 2418–2421 (2002).

47. H. J. Kong, T. Boontheekul, and D. J. Mooney, Quantifying the relation between adhesion ligand-receptor bond formation and cell phenotype, *Proceedings of the National Academy of Sciences*, 103, 18534–18539 (2006).

48. B. A. Grzybowski, C. E. Wilmer, J. Kim, K. P. Browne, and K. J. M. Bishop, Self-assembly: From crystals to cells, *Soft Matter*, 5, 1110–1128 (2009).

49. L. C. Palmer, Y. S Velichko, M. Olvera de la Cruz, and S. I. Stupp, Supramolecular self-assembly codes for functional structures, *Philosophical Transactions of the Royal Society A*, 365, 1417–1433 (2007).

50. D. Papapostolou, A. M. Smith, E. D. T. Atkins, S. J. Oliver, M. G. Ryadnov, L. C. Serpell, and D. N. Woolfson, Engineering nanoscale order into a designed protein fiber, *Proceedings of the National Academy of Sciences*, 104, 10853–10858 (2007).

51. G. C. Schatz, Using theory and computation to model nanoscale properties, *Proceedings of the National Academy of Sciences*, 104, 6885–6892 (2007).

52. J. P. Jung, A. K. Nagaraj, E. K. Fox, J. S. Rudra, J. M. Devgun, and J. H. Collier, Co-assembling peptides as defined matrices for endothelial cells, *Biomaterials*, 30, 2400–2410 (2009).

53. M. C. Branco and J. P. Schneider, Self-assembling materials for therapeutic delivery, *Acta Biomaterialia* 5, 817–831 (2009).

54. H. Hosseinkhani, M. Hosseinkhani, and H. Kobayashi, Design of tissue-engineered nanoscaffold shrough self-assembly of peptide amphiphile, *Journal of Bioactive and Compatible Polymers*, 21, 277–296 (2006).

55. R. M. Capito, H. S. Azevedo, Y. S. Velichko, A. Mata, and S. I. Stupp, Self-assembly of large and small molecules into hierarchically ordered sacs and membranes, *Science*, 319, 1812–1816 (2008).

56. H. Cui, Z. Chen, S. Zhong, K. L. Wooley, and D. J. Pochan, Block copolymer assembly via kinetic control, *Science*, 317, 647–650 (2007).

57. A. M. Hugh and S. I. Stupp, Understanding factors affecting alignment of self-assembling nanofibers patterned by sonication-assisted solution embossing, *Langmuir*, 25, 7084–7089 (2009).

58. Y. Liu, S. Wang, J. W. Lee, and N. A. Kotov, A floating self-assembly route to colloidal crystal templates for 3D cell scaffolds, *Chemistry of Materials*, 17, 4918–4924 (2005).

59. B. B. Koleva, T. Kolev, R. W. Seidel, M. Spiteller, H. Mayer-Figge, and W. S. Sheldrick, Self-assembly of hydrogen squarates: Crystal structures and properties, *Journal of Physical Chemistry A*, 113, 3088–3095 (2009).

60. J. Chen and A. J. McNeil, Analyte-triggered gelation: Initiating self-assembly via oxidation-induced planarization, *Journal of the American Chemical Society*, 130, 16496–16497 (2008).

61. S. Weiner and H. D. Wagner, The material bone: Structure-mechanical function relations, *Annual Review of Materials Science*, 28: 271–298 (1998).

62. M. Ferrari, T. Desai, and S. Bhatia (eds.), *BioMEMS and Biomedical Nanotechnology: Therapeutic Micro/Nanotechnology*, Vol. 3, Springer Science and Business Media, LLC, New York, 2006.

63. R. J. Petrie, A. D. Doyle, and K. M. Yamada, Random versus directionally persistent cell migration, *Nature Reviews Molecular Cell Biology*, 10, 538–549 (2009).

64. L. Lazzeri, M. G. Cascone, S. Danti, L. P. Serino, S. Moscato, and N. Bernardini, Gelatine/PLLA sponge-like scaffolds: Morphological and biological characterization, *Journal of Materials Science, Materials in Medicine*, 18, 1399–1405 (2007).

65. S. Moscato, L. Mattii, D. D'Alessandro, M. G. Cascone, L. Lazzeri, L. P. Serino, A. Dolfi, and N. Bernardini, Interaction of human gingival fibroblasts with PVA/gelatine sponges, *Micron*, 39, 569–579 (2008).

66. S. Ghanaati, M. J. Webber, R. E. Unger, C. Orth, J. F. Hulvat, S. E. Kiehn, M. Barbeck, A. Rasic, S. I. Stupp, and C. J. Kirkpatrick, Dynamic in vivo biocompatibility of angiogenic peptide amphiphile nanofibers, *Biomaterials*, 30, 6202–6212 (2009).

67. J. Hardwicke, E. L. Ferguson, R. Moseley, P. Stephens, D. W. Thomas, and R. Duncan, Dextrin-rhEGF conjugates as bioresponsive nanomedicines for wound repair, *Journal of Controlled Release*, 130, 275–283 (2008).
68. R. A. Shimkunas, E. Robinson, R. Lam, S. Lu, X. Xu, X.-Q. Zhang, H. Huang, E. Osawa, and D. Ho, Nanodiamond–insulin complexes as pH-dependent protein delivery vehicles, *Biomaterials*, 30, 5720–5728 (2009).
69. Q. P. Pham, U. Sharma, and A. G. Mikos, Electrospinning of polymeric nanofibers for tissue engineering applications: A review, *Tissue Engineering*, 12, 1197–1211 (2006).
70. J.-H. Song, H.-E. Kim, and H.-W. Kim, Electrospun fibrous web of collagen–apatite precipitated nanocomposite for bone regeneration, *Journal of Materials Science: Materials in Medicine*, 19, 2925–2932 (2008).
71. X. Lu, C. Wang, and Y. Wei, One-dimensional composite nanomaterials: Synthesis by electrospinning and their applications, *Small*, 5, 2349–2370 (2009).
72. S. D. McCullen, K. L. Stano, D. R. Stevens, W. A. Roberts, N. A. Monteiro-Riviere, L. I. Clarke, and R. E. Gorga, Development, optimization, and characterization of electrospun poly(lactic acid) nanofibers containing multi-walled carbon nanotubes, *Journal of Applied Polymer Science*, 105, 1668–1678 (2007).
73. Y. Okamura, K. Kabata, M. Kinoshita, D. Saitoh, and S. Takeoka, Free-standing biodegradable poly(lactic acid) nanosheet for sealing operations in surgery, *Advanced Materials*, 21, 4388–4392 (2009).
74. C. Vaquette, C. Frochot, R. Rahouadj, and X. Wang, An innovative method to obtain porous PLLA scaffolds with highly spherical and interconnected pores, *Journal of Biomedical Materials Research Part B: Applied Biomaterials*, 86B, 9–17 (2008).
75. A. Alessandrino, B. Marelli, C. Arosio, S. Fare, M. C. Tanzi, and G. Freddi, Electrospun silk fibroin mats for tissue engineering, *Engineering in Life Sciences*, 8, 219–225 (2008).
76. J. L. Vondran, W. Sun, and C. L. Schauer, Crosslinked, electrospun chitosan–poly(ethylene oxide) nanofiber mats, *Journal of Applied Polymer Science*, 109, 968–975 (2008).
77. E. Cukierman, R. Pankov, D. R. Stevens, and K. M. Yamada, Taking cell-matrix adhesions to the third dimension, *Science*, 294, 1708–1712 (2001).
78. J. Kisiday, M. Jin, B. Kurz, H. Hung, C. Semino, S. Zhang, and A. J. Grodzinsky, Self-assembling peptide hydrogel fosters chondrocyte extracellular matrix production and cell division: Implications for cartilage tissue repair, *Proceedings of the National Academy of Sciences*, 99, 9996–10001 (2002).
79. S. Zhang, F. Gelain, and X. Zhao, Designer self-assembling peptide nanofiber scaffolds for 3D tissue cell cultures, *Seminars in Cancer Biology*, 15, 413–420 (2005).
80. E. Genové, C. Shen, S. Zhang, and C. E. Semino, The effect of functionalized self-assembling peptide scaffolds on human aortic endothelial cell function, *Biomaterials*, 26, 3341–3351 (2005).
81. H. Meng, L. Chen, Z. Ye, S. Wang, and X. Zhao, The effect of a self-assembling peptide nanofiber scaffold (peptide) when used as a wound dressing for the treatment of deep second degree burns in rats, *Journal of Biomedical Materials Research Part B: Applied Biomaterials*, 89B, 379–391 (2009).
82. S. M. Alston, K. A. Solen, F. Mohammad, and S. Sukavaneshvar, A rapid inexpensive method to make autologous fibrin glue, *ASAIO Journal*, 51, 5A (2005).

83. R. G. Ellis-Behnke, Y.-X. Liang, D. K. C. Tay, P. W. F. Kau, G. E. Schneider, S. Zhang, W. Wu, and K.-F. So, Nano hemostat solution: Immediate hemostasis at the nanoscale, *Nanomedicine: Nanotechnology, Biology and Medicine*, 2, 207–215 (2006).

84. A. M. Kloxin, A. M. Kasko, C. N. Salinas, and K. S. Anseth, Photodegradable hydrogels for dynamic tuning of physical and chemical properties, *Science*, 324, 59–63 (2009).

85. P. Gorostiza and E. Isacoff, Optical switches and triggers for the manipulation of ion channels and pores, *Molecular BioSystems*, 3, 686–704 (2007).

86. R. Numano, S. Szobota, A. Y. Lau, P. Gorostiza, M. Volgraf, B. Roux, D. Trauner, and E. Y. Isacoff, Nanosculpting reversed wavelength sensitivity into a photo-switchable iGluR, *Proceedings of the National Academy of Sciences*, 106, 6814–6819 (2009).

87. A. Ashkin, History of optical trapping and manipulation of small-neutral particle, atoms, and molecules, *IEEE Journal of Selected Topics in Quantum Electronics*, 6, 841–856 (2000).

88. G. D. M. Jeffries, J. S. Edgar, Y. Zhao, J. P. Shelby, C. Fong, and D. T. Chiu, Using polarization-shaped optical vortex traps for single-cell nanosurgery, *Nano Letters*, 7, 415–420 (2007).

89. J. Vykoukal and P. R. C. Gascoyne, Particle separation by dielectrophoresis, *Electrophoresis*, 23, 1973–1983 (2002).

90. R. S. Greco, F. B. Prinz, and R. L. Smith, *Nanoscale Technology in Biological Systems*, CRC Press, Boca Raton, FL, 2004.

91. N. H. Malsch (ed.), *Biomedical Nanotechnology*, CRC Press, Boca Raton, FL, 2005.

92. J. D. Bronzino (ed.), *Biomedical Engineering Handbook*, IEEE Press/CRC Press, Boca Raton, FL, 2005.

93. M. Ferrari, A. P. Lee, and L. J. Lee (eds.), *BioMEMS and Biomedical Nanotechnology: Biological and Biomedical Nanotechnology*, Vol. 1, Springer, New York, 2006.

94. H. H. Park, A. C. Jamison, and T. T. Lee, Rise of the nanomachine: The evolution of a revolution in medicine, *Nanomedicine*, 2, 425–439 (2007).

95. T. Vo-Dinh (ed.), *Nanotechnology in Biology and Medicine: Methods, Devices, and Applications*, CRC Press, Boca Raton, FL, 2007.

96. T. J. Huang and B. K. Juluri, Biological and biomimetic molecular machines, *Nanomedicine*, 3, 107–124 (2008).

97. C. M. Puleo, H.-C. Yeh, and T.-H. Wang, Applications of MEMS technologies in tissue engineering, *Tissue Engineering*, 13, 2839–2854 (2008).

98. D. Ho, A. O. Fung, and C. D Montemagno, Engineering novel diagnostic modalities and implantable cytomimetic nanomaterials for next-generation medicine, *Biology of Blood and Marrow Transplantation*, 12, 92–99 (2006).

99. Z. L. Wang, Towards self-powered nanosystems: From nanogenerators to nano-piezotronics, *Advanced Functional Materials*, 18, 1–15 (2008).

100. R. Yang, Y. Qin, C. Li, G. Zhu, and Z. L. Wang, Converting biomechanical energy into electricity by a muscle-movement-driven nanogenerator, *Nano Letters*, 9, 1201–1205 (2009).

101. B. S. Atiyeh, M. Costagliola, S. N. Hayek, and S. A. Dibo, Effect of silver on burn wound infection control and healing: Review of the literature, *Burns*, 33, 139–148 (2007).

102. T. J. Simmons, S.-H. Lee, T.-J. Park, D. P. Hashim, P. M. Ajayan, and R. J. Linhardt, Antiseptic single wall carbon nanotube bandages, *Carbon*, 47, 1561–1564 (2009).

103. E. M. Hetrick, J. H. Shin, H. S. Paul, and M. H. Schoenfisch, Anti-biofilm efficacy of nitric oxide-releasing silica nanoparticles, *Biomaterials*, 30, 2782–2789 (2009).

104. N. A. Kotov, *Nanoparticle Assemblies and Superstructures*, CRC Press, Boca Raton, FL, 2005.

105. M. Stoneham, How soft materials control harder ones: Routes to bioorganiza- tion, *Reports on Progress in Physics*, 70, 1055 (2007).

106. H. Liua and T. J. Webster, Nanomedicine for implants: A review of studies and necessary experimental tools, *Biomaterials*, 28, 354–369 (2007).

107. A. Hertz and I. J. Bruce, Inorganic materials for bone repair or replacement applications, *Nanomedicine*, 2, 899–918 (2007).

108. M. Mazzocchi and A. Bellosi, On the possibility of silicon nitride as a ceramic for structural orthopaedic implants. Part I: Processing, microstructure, mechani- cal properties, cytotoxicity, *Journal of Materials Science: Materials in Medicine*, 19, 2881–2887 (2008).

109. J. Cho, M. Cannio, and A. R. Boccaccini, The electrophoretic deposition of bio- glass®/carbon nanotube composite layers for bioactive coatings, *International Journal of Materials and Product Technology*, 35, 260–270 (2009).

110. C. Yao and T. J. Webster, Anodization: A promising nano-modification tech- nique of titanium implants for orthopedic applications, *Journal of Nanoscience and Nanotechnology*, 6, 2682–2692 (2006).

111. S.-H. Oh, R. R. Finõnes, C. Daraio, L.-H. Chen, and S. Jin, Growth of nano-scale hydroxyapatite using chemically treated titanium oxide nanotubes, *Biomaterials*, 26, 4938–4943 (2005).

112. M. K. El Tamer and R. L. Reis, Progenitor and stem cells for bone and cartilage regeneration, *Journal of Tissue Engineering and Regenerative Medicine*, 3, 327–337 (2009).

113. S. S. Liao, F. Z. Cui, W. Zhang, and Q. L. Feng, Hierarchically biomimetic bone scaffold materials: Nano-HA/collagen/PLA composite, *Journal of Biomedical Materials Research B: Applied Biomaterials*, 69B, 158–165 (2004).

114. G. Heness and B. Ben-Nissan, Innovative bioceramics, *Materials Forum*, 27, 3–21 (2004).

115. D. Vashishth, K. E. Tanner, and W. Bonfield, Experimental validation of a micro- cracking-based toughening mechanism for cortical bone, *Journal of Biomechanics*, 36, 121–124 (2003).

116. K. Rezwan, Q. Z. Chen, J. J. Blaker, and A. R. Boccaccini, Biodegradable and bioactive porous polymer/inorganic composite scaffolds for bone tissue engi- neering, *Biomaterials*, 27, 3413–3431 (2006).

117. H. Yoshimotoa, Y. M. Shina, H. Teraia, and J. P. Vacanti, A biodegradable nano- fiber scaffold by electrospinning and its potential for bone tissue engineering, *Biomaterials*, 24, 2077–2082 (2003).

118. B. Sitharaman, X. Shi, G. J. Meijer, H. Liao, F. Walboomers, J. J. Jansen, L. J. Wilson, and A. G. Mikos, In vivo biocompatibility of ultra-short single walled carbon nanotube/biodegradable polymer nanocomposites for bone tissue engi- neering, *Bone*, 43, 362–370 (2008).

119. C. Vitale-Brovarone, F. Baino, O. Bretcanu, and E. Verné, Foam-like scaffolds for bone tissue engineering based on a novel couple of silicate-phosphate spec- ular glasses: Synthesis and properties, *Journal of Materials Science: Materials in Medicine*, 20, 2197–2205 (2009).

120. V. Salih, A. Patel, and J. C. Knowles, Zinc-containing phosphate-based glasses for tissue engineering, *Biomedical Materials*, 2, 11–20 (2007).

121. Q. Yuan, Ectopic bone formation in vivo induced by a novel synthetic peptide derived from BMP-2 using porous collagen scaffolds, *Journal of Wuhan University of Technology-Materials Science Education*, 22, 701–705 (2007).

122. T. Hayashibara, T. Hiraga, B. Yi, M. Nomizu, Y. Kumagai, R. Nishimura, and T. Yoneda, A synthetic peptide fragment of human MEPE stimulates new bone formation in vitro and in vivo, *Journal of Bone and Mineral Research*, 19, 455–462 (2004).

123. A. J. García and C. D. Reyes, Bio-adhesive surfaces to promote osteoblast differentiation and bone formation, *Journal of Dental Research*, 84, 407–413 (2005).

124. F. Quintero, J. Pou, R. Comesaña, F. Lusquiños, A. Riveiro, A. B. Mann, R. G. Hill, Z. Y. Wu, and J. R. Jones, Laser spinning of bioactive glass nanofibers, *Advanced Functional Materials*, 19, 3084–3090 (2009).

125. G. E. Poinern, R. K. Brundavanam, N. Mondinos, and Z.-T. Jiang, Synthesis and characterisation of nanohydroxyapatite using an ultrasound assisted method, *Ultrasonics Sonochemistry*, 16, 469–474 (2009).

126. A. G. Mikos, S. W. Herring, P. Ochareon, J. Elisseeff, H. H. Lu, R. Kandel, F. J. Schoen et al., Engineering complex tissues, *Tissue Engineering*, 12, 3307–3339 (2006).

127. J. D. Kretlow, S. Young, L. Klouda, M. Wong, and A. G. Mikos, Injectable biomaterials for regenerating complex craniofacial tissues, *Advanced Materials*, 21, 3368–3393 (2009).

128. T. J. Webster, R. W. Siegel and R. Bizios, Enhanced functions of osteoblasts on nanophase ceramics, *Biomaterials*, 21, 1803–1810 (2000).

129. G. Balasundaram and T. J. Webster, Nano-structured biodegradable ceramics for the treatment of osteoporosis, *Nanotech 2006*, 2, 133–135 (2002).

130. A. A. Pillar, Low-intensity electromagnetic and mechanical modulation of bone growth and repair: Are they equivalent? *Journal of Orthopaedic Science*, 7, 420–428 (2002).

131. R. K. Aaron, B. D. Boyan, D. McKciombor, Z. Schwartz, and B. J. Simon, Stimulation of growth factor synthesis by electric and electromagnetic fields, *Clinical Orthopaedics and Related Research*, 419, 30–37 (2004).

132. R. C. Shetty, Benefits of nanotechnology in cardiovascular surgery—A review of potential applications, *US Cardiovascular Disease*, 2006, 1–3 (2006).

133. B. Thierry, F. M. Winnik, Y. Merhi, J. Silver, and M. Tabrizian, Bioactive coatings of endovascular stents based on polyelectrolyte multilayers, *Biomacromolecules*, 4, 1564–1571 (2003).

134. A. Mahapatro, D. M. Johnson, D. N. Patel, M. D. Feldman, A. A. Ayon, and C. M. Agrawal, The use of alkanethiol self-assembled monolayers on 316L stainless steel for coronary artery stent nanomedicine applications: An oxidative and in vitro stability study, *Nanomedicine: Nanotechnology, Biology, and Medicine*, 2, 182–190 (2006).

135. I. Tsujino, J. Ako, Y. Honda, and P. J. Fitzgerald, Drug delivery via nano-, micro and macroporous coronary stent surfaces, *Expert Opinion on Drug Delivery*, 3, 287–295 (2007).

136. J. M. Caves and E. L. Chaikof, The evolving impact of microfabrication and nanotechnology on stent design, *Journal of Vascular Surgery*, 44, 1363–1368 (2006).

137. A. P. Beltrami, K. Urbanek, J. Kajstura, S.-M. Yan, N. Finato, R. Bussani, B. Nadal-Ginard et al., Evidence that human cardiac myocytes divide after myocardial infarction, *New England Journal of Medicine*, 344, 1750–1757 (2001).

138. O. Bergmann, R. D. Bhardwaj, S. Bernard, S. Zdunek, F. Barnabé-Heider, S. Walsh, J. Zupicich et al., Evidence for cardiomyocyte renewal in humans, *Science*, 324, 98–102 (2009).

139. S. Rajanayagam, Intervention: Growing new heart muscle cells, *Nature Reviews Cardiology*, 6, 388 (2009).

140. J. Zhang, G. F. Wilson, A. G. Soerens, C. H. Koonce, J. Yu, S. P. Palecek, J. A., Thomson, and T. J. Kamp, Functional cardiomyocytes derived from human induced pluripotent stem cells, *Circulation Research*, 104, e30-e41 (2009).

141. T. J. Kamp and G. E. Lyons, On the road to iPS cell cardiovascular applications, *Circulation Research*, 105, 617–619 (2009).

142. H. Nakajima, Y. Sakakibara, K. Tambara, A. Iwakura, K. Doi, A. Marui, K. Ueyama, T. Ikeda, Y. Tabata, and M. Komeda, Therapeutic angiogenesis by the controlled release of basic fibroblast growth factor for ischemic limb and heart injury: Toward safety and minimal invasiveness, *Journal of Artificial Organs*, 7, 58–61 (2004).

143. K. Doi, T. Ikeda, A. Marui, T. Kushibiki, Y. Arai, K. Hirose, Y. Soga et al., Enhanced angiogenesis by gelatin hydrogels incorporating basic fibroblast growth factor in rabbit model of hind limb ischemia, *Heart Vessels*, 22, 104–108 (2007).

144. Y.-T. Kim, R. Hitchcock, K. W. Broadhead, D. J. Messina, and P. A. Tresco, A cell encapsulation device for studying soluble factor release from cells transplanted in the rat brain, *Journal of Controlled Release*, 102, 101–111 (2005).

145. T. M. S. Chang, 50th anniversary of artificial cells: Their role in biotechnology, nanomedicine, regenerative medicine, blood substitutes, bioencapsulation, cell/stem cell therapy and nanorobotics, *Artificial Cells, Blood Substitutes, and Immobilization Biotechnology*, 35, 545–554 (2007).

146. C. Smith, R. Kirk, T. West, M. Bratzel, M. Cohen, F. Martin, A. Boiarski, and A. A. Rampersaud, Diffusion characteristics of microfabricated silicon nano-pore membranes as immunoisolation membranes for use in cellular therapeutics, *Diabetes Technology and Therapeutics*, 7, 151–162 (2005).

147. P. A. Tresco, R, Biran, and M. D. Noble, Cellular transplants as sources for therapeutic agents, *Advanced Drug Delivery Reviews*, 42, 3–27 (2000).

148. J. T. Wilson and E. L. Chaikof, Challenges and emerging technologies in the immunoisolation of cells and tissues, *Advanced Drug Delivery Reviews*, 60, 124–145 (2008).

149. G. Orive, A. R. Gascón, R. M. Hernández, M. Igartua, and J. L. Pedraz, Cell microencapsulation technology for biomedical purposes: Novel insights and challenges, *Trends in Pharmacological Sciences*, 24, 207–210 (2003).

150. F. J. Martin and C. Grove, Microfabricated drug delivery systems: Concepts to improve clinical benefit, *Biomedical Microdevices*, 3, 97–108 (2001).

151. P. de Vos, A. F. Hamel, and K. Tatarkiewicz, Considerations for successful transplantation of encapsulated pancreatic islets, *Diabetologia*, 45, 159–173 (2002).

152. P. de Vos and P. Marchetti, Encapsulation of pancreatic islets for transplantation in diabetes: The untouchable islets, *Trends in Molecular Medicine*, 8, 363–366 (2002).

153. T. A. Desai, W. H. Chu, J. K. Tu, G. M. Beattie, A. Hayek, and M. Ferrari, Mircofabricated immunoisolating biocapsules, *Biotechnology and Bioengineering*, 57, 118–120 (1998).

154. B. Gimi, T. Leong, Z. Gu, M. Yang, D. Artemov, Z. M. Bhujwalla, and D. H. Gracias, Self-assembled three dimensional radio frequency (RF) shielded containers for cell encapsulation, *Biomedical Microdevices*, 7, 341–345 (2005).

155. E. J. A. Pope, K. Braun, and C. M. Peterson, Bioartificial organs I: Silica gel encapsulated pancreatic islets for the treatment of diabetes mellitus, *Journal of Sol-Gel Science and Technology*, 8, 635–639 (1997).

156. P. de Vos, J. L. Hillebrands, B. J. De Haan, J. H. Strubbe, and R. Van Schilfgaarde, Efficacy of a prevascularized expanded polytetrafluoroethylene solid support system as a transplantation site for pancreatic islets, *Transplantation*, 63, 824–830 (1997).

157. G. Erdodi, J. Kang, B. Yalcin, M. Cakmak, K. S. Rosenthal, S. Grundfest-Broniatowski, and J. P. Kennedy, A novel macroencapsulating immunoisolatory device: The preparation and properties of nanomat-reinforced amphiphilic conetworks deposited on perforated metal scaffold, *Biomedical Microdevices*, 11, 297–312 (2009).

158. K. E. La Flamme, K. C. Popat, L. Leoni, E. Markiewicz, T. J. La Tempa, B. B. Roman, C. A. Grimes, and T. A. Desai, Biocompatibility of nanoporous alumina membranes for immunoisolation, *Biomaterials*, 28, 2638–2645 (2007).

159. F. Lim and A. M. Sun, Microencapsulated islets as bioartificial endocrine pancreas, *Science*, 210, 908–910 (1980).

160. A. I. Silva, A. N. de Matos, I. G. Brons, and M. Mateus, An overview on the development of a bio-artificial pancreas as a treatment of insulin-dependent diabetes mellitus, *Medicinal Research Reviews*, 26, 181–222 (2006).

161. R. Calafiore and G. Basta, Artificial pancreas to treat type 1 diabetes mellitus, in H. Hauser and M. Fussenegger (eds.), *Methods in Molecular Medicine: Tissue Engineering*, Vol. 140, 2nd edn., Chap. 12, Humana Press, Totowa, NJ, 2007, pp. 197–236.

162. S. Schneider, P. J. Feilen, F. Brunnenmeier, T. Minnemann, H. Zimmermann, U. Zimmermann, and M. M. Weber, Long-term graft function of adult rat and human islets encapsulated in novel alginate-based microcapsules after transplantation in immunocompetent diabetic mice, *Diabetes*, 54, 687–693 (2005).

163. S. F. Grundfest-Broniatowski, G. Tellioglu, K. S. Rosenthal, J. Kang, G. Erdodi, B. Yalcin, M. Cakmak et al., A new bioartificial pancreas utilizing amphiphilic membranes for the immunoisolation of porcine islets: A pilot study in the canine, *ASAIO Journal*, 55, 400–405 (2009).

164. T. Yuasa, J. D. Rivas-Carrillo, N. Navarro-Alvarez, A. Soto-Gutierrez, Y. Kubota, Y. Tabata, T. Okitsu et al., Neovascularization induced around an artificial device implanted in the abdomen by the use of gelatinized fibroblast growth factor 2, *Cell Transplantation*, 18, 683–688 (2009).

165. J. I. Lee, R. Nishimura, H. Sakai, N. Sasaki, and T. Kenmochi, A newly developed immunoisolated bioartificial pancreas with cell sheet engineering, *Cell Transplantation*, 17, 51–59 (2008).

166. J. Z. Hilt and N. A. Peppas, Microfabricated drug delivery devices, *International Journal of Pharmaceutics*, 306, 15–23 (2005).

167. STMicroelectronics and Debiotech announce first prototypes of disposable insulin nanopump, June 23,2008, http://www.st.com/stonline/stappl/cms/press/news/year2008/t2301.htm (2008).

168. Insulet Corporation, http://www.myomnipod.com/ (2009).

169. K. A. Ellenbogen and M. A. Wood, *Cardiac Pacing and ICDs*, 4th edn., Blackwell, Malden, MA, 2005.
170. R. E. Klabunde, *Cardiovascular Physiology Concepts*, 4th edn., Lippincott Williams & Wilkins, Philadelphia, PA, 2005.
171. P. J. Rosch and M. S. Markov, *Bioelectromagnetic Medicine*, Informa Health Care, London, U.K., 2004.
172. R. J. Vetter, J. C. Williams, J. F. Hetke, F. A. Nunamaker, and D. R. Kipke, Chronic neural recording using silicon-substrate microelectrode arrays implanted in cerebral cortex, *IEEE Transactions on Biomedical Engineering*, 51, 896–904 (2004).
173. M. Glikson and P. Friedman, The implantable cardioverter defibrillator, *Lancet*, 357, 1107–1117 (2001).
174. R. Kötz and M. Carlen, Principles and applications of electrochemical capacitors, *Electrochimica Acta*, 45, 2483–2498 (2000).
175. W. E. Finn and P. G. LoPresti, *Handbook of Neuroprosthetic Methods*, CRC Press, Boca Raton, FL, 2002.
176. K. W Horch and G. S Dhillon (eds.), *Neuroprosthetics, Theory and Practice*, World Scientific Publishing, Singapore, 2004.
177. D. H. Delgado, V. Rao, H. J. Ross, S. Verma, and N. G. Smedira, Mechanical circulatory assistance: State of art, *Circulation*, 106, 2046–2050 (2002).
178. H. H. Hu, P. Jia, T. Lu, and K. Yuan, Head gesture recognition for hands-free control of an intelligent wheelchair, *Industrial Robot: An International Journal*, 34, 60–68 (2007).
179. H.-N. Teodorescu and L. C. Jain, *Intelligent Systems and Technologies in Rehabilitation Engineering*, CRC Press, Boca Raton, FL, 2001.
180. D. Taylor, *Neural Control of Assistive Technology*, in M. Akay (ed.), Wiley Encyclopedia of Biomedical Engineering, John Wiley & Sons, New York, 2006.
181. G. M. Friehs, V. A. Zerris, C. L. Ojakangas, M. R. Fellows, and J. P. Donoghue, Brain–machine and brain–computer interfaces, *Stroke*, 35, 2702–2705 (2004).
182. R. Gailey, Rehabilitation of a traumatic lower limb amputee, *Physiotherapy Research International*, 3, 239–243 (2006).
183. B. Beckwith, Medicine meets virtual reality 2001, *Clinical Chemistry*, 47, 2190-a (2001)
184. S. Canright (ed.), Amy Ross, Space suit designer, NASA Education Home, STS-118, Resources for Educators (2007), Webpage at: http://www.nasa.gov/audience/foreducators/stseducation/stories/Amy_Ross_Profile.html
185. P. Danaher, K. Tanaka, and A. R. Hargens, Mechanical counter-pressure vs. gas-pressurized spacesuit gloves: Grip and sensitivity, *Aviation, Space and Environmental Medicine*, 76, 381–384 (2005).
186. S. E. Lyshevski, *Nano- And Micro-Electromechanical Systems: Fundamentals of Nano- and Microengineering*, CRC Press, Boca Raton, FL, 2005.
187. R. Zurawski, *Embedded Systems Handbook*, CRC Press, Boca Raton, FL, 2006.
188. M. Gad-el-Hak, *The MEMS Handbook*, CRC Press, Boca Raton, FL, 2002.
189. B. G. Lipták, *Instrument Engineers' Handbook: Process Control and Optimization*, CRC Press, Boca Raton, FL, 2005.
190. Y. Osada and D. E. De Rossi, *Polymer Sensors and Actuators (Macromolecular Systems—Materials Approach)*, Springer Verlag, Berlin, Germany, 1999.
191. M. Shahinpoor, K. J. Kim, and M. Mojarrad, *Artificial Muscles: Applications of Advanced Polymeric Nanocomposites*, Taylor & Francis, New York, 2007.

192. K. Bullis, Ultrastrong carbon-nanotube muscles: Artificial muscles made from carbon nanotubes are 100 times stronger than human muscles, *MIT Technology Review*, online at: http://www.technologyreview.com/biomedicine/17872/page1/ (December 8, 2006).

193. K. M. Tsui and H. A. Yanco, Assistive, rehabilitation, and surgical robots from the perspective of medical and healthcare professionals, in *Workshop at the 22nd AAAI Conference on Artificial Intelligence (AAAI-07)*, Vancouver, Canada, WS-07-07, 2007, pp. 34–39.

194. *The New York Times, Electronic Brain in an Artificial Foot*, NYT October 3 (2006), web animation at: http://www.nytimes.com/packages/html/science/20061003_FOOT_GRAPHIC/index.html

195. G. Lundborg, Tomorrow's artificial hand, *Scandinavian Journal of Plastic and Reconstructive Surgery and Hand Surgery*, 34, 97–100 (2000).

196. F. L. Lewis, D. M. Dawson, and C. T. Abdallah, *Robot Manipulator Control: Theory and Practice*, 2nd edn., CRC Press, Boca Raton, FL, 2003.

197. T. R. Kurfess, *Robotics and Automation Handbook*, CRC Press, Boca Raton, FL, 2004.

198. A. Poulton, P. J. Kyberd, and D. Gow, Progress of a modular prosthetic arm, in S. Keates, P. Langdon, P. J. Clarkson, and P. Robinson (eds.), *Universal Access and Assistive Technology*, Springer Verlag, Berlin, Germany, 2002.

199. R. Rupp and H. J. Gerner, Neuroprosthetics of the upper extremity-clinical application in spinal cord injury and future perspectives, *Biomedical Technology*, 49, 93–98 (2004).

200. F. W. J. Cody (ed.), *Neural Control of Skilled Human Movement*, Portland Press, Colchester, U.K., 1995.

201. J. M. Winters and P. E. Crago (eds.), *Biomechanics and Neural Control of Movement*, Springer Verlag, New York, 2000.

202. C. Castellini, E. Gruppioni, A. Davalli, and G. Sandini, Fine detection of grasp force and posture by amputees via surface electromyography, *Journal of Physiology, Paris*, 103, 255–262 (2009).

203. Touch Bionics, Livingston, U.K., website at: www.touchbionics.com/ (2009).

204. C. Connolly, Prosthetic hands from Touch Bionics, *Industrial Robot: An International Journal*, 35, 290–293 (2008).

205. T. Nef, M. Mihelj, and R. Riener, ARMin: A robot for patient-cooperative arm therapy, *Medical and Biological Engineering and Computing*, 45, 887–900 (2007).

206. P. Staubli, T. Nef, V. Klamroth-Marganska, and R. Riener, Effects of intensive arm training with the rehabilitation robot ARMin II in chronic stroke patients: Four single cases, *Journal of NeuroEngineering and Rehabilitation*, 6, 46 (2009).

207. D. Pope, DARPA Prosthetics programs seek natural upper limb, Neurotech Business Report, San Francisco, CA, online at: http://www.neurotechreports.com/pages/darpaprosthetics.html (2009).

208. M. Zecca, S. Micera, M. C. Carrozza, and P. Dario, Control of multifunctional prosthetic hands by processing the electromyographic signal, *Critical Reviews in Biomedical Engineering*, 30, 459–485 (2002).

209. Editorial, Is this the bionic man? *Nature*, 442, 164–171 (2006).

210. W Craelius, The bionic man: Restoring mobility, *Science*, 295, 1018–1021 (2002).

211. S. H. Scott, Neuroscience: Converting thoughts into action, *Nature*, 442, 164–171 (2006).

212. M. A. Lebedev and M. A. L. Nicolelis, Brain–machine interfaces: Past, present and future, *Trends in Neurosciences*, 29, 536–546 (2006).

213. P. D. Cheney, J. Hill-Karrer, A. Belhaj-Saïf, B. J. McKiernan, M. C. Park, and J. K. Marcario, Cortical motor areas and their properties: Implications for neuroprosthetics, *Progress in Brain Research*, 1, 135–160 (2000).

214. L. G. Cohen and N. Birbaumer, The physiology of brain-computer interfaces, *The Journal of Physiology*, 579, 570 (2009).

215. A. B. Schwartz, Useful signals from motor cortex, *The Journal of Physiology*, 579, 581–601 (2007).

216. J. P. Donoghue, Connecting cortex to machines: Recent advances in brain interfaces, *Nature Neuroscience*, 5, 1085–1088 (2002).

217. J. R. Wolpaw, N. Birbaumer, D. J. McFarland, G. Pfurtscheller, and T. M. Vaughan, Brain-computer interfaces for communication and control, *Clinical Neurophysiology*, 113, 767–791 (2002).

218. A. Pascual-Leone, N. Davey, J. C. Rothwell, E. M. Wassermann, and B. K. Puri, *Handbook of Transcranial Magnetic Stimulation*, CRC Press, Boca Raton, FL, 2002.

219. V. Walsh and A. Pascual-Leone, *Transcranial Magnetic Stimulation*, MIT Press, Cambridge, MA, 2003.

220. P. B. Fitzgerald, S. Fountain, and Z. J. Daskalakis, A comprehensive review of the effects of rTMS on motor cortical excitability and inhibition, *Clinical Neurophysiology*, 117, 2584–2596 (2006).

221. A. T. Barker, R. Jalinous, and I. L. Freeston, Non-invasive magnetic stimulation of human motor cortex, *Lancet*, 1, 1106–1107 (1985).

222. T. Kujirai, Corticocortical inhibition of the motor cortex, *Journal of Physiology*, 471, 501–509 (1993).

223. A. Pascual-Leone, D. Bartres-Faz, and J. P. Keenan, Transcranial magnetic stimulation: Studying the brain-behaviour relationship by induction of 'virtual lesions', *Philosophical Transactions of the Royal Society London B. Biological Sciences*, 354, 1229–1238 (1999).

224. S. Tumanski, *Thin Film Magnotoresistive Sensors*, CRC Press, Boca Raton, FL, 2001.

225. J. R. Brauer, *Magnetic Actuators and Sensors*, IEEE/Wiley Interscience, New York, 2006.

226. S. L. Mouaziz, Micro and nano tools for magnetic field imaging, in P. A. Besse, J. Brugger, M. Gijs, R. S. Popovic, and P. Renaud (eds.) *Series in Microsystems*, Vol. 21, Hartung-Gorre Verlag, Konstanz, Germany, 2007.

227. D. King, A resonant MEMS magnetometer, in *IEE Seminar and Exhibition on MEMS Sensor Technologies*, London, U.K., 2005, pp. 1–12.

228. C. Schott, F. Burger, H. Blanchard, and L. Chiesi, Modern integrated silicon Hall sensors, *Sensor Reviews*, 18, 252–257 (1998).

229. A. P. Ramirez, Colossal magnetoresistance, *Journal of Physics*: *Condensed Matter*, 9, 8171–8199 (1997).

230. J. Clarke, Principles and applications of SQUIDs, *Proceedings of the IEEE*, 77, 1208–1223 (1989).

231. Y. Okada, K. Pratt, C. Atwood, A. Mascarenas, R. Reineman, J. Nurminen, and D. Paulson, BabySQUID: A mobile, high-resolution multichannel magnetoencephalography system for neonatal brain assessment, *Review of Scientific Instruments*, 77, 024301 (2006).

232. L. A. Bradshaw, A. Irinia, J. A. Sims, M. R. Gallucci, R. L. Palmer, and W. O. Richards, Biomagnetic characterization of spatiotemporal parameters of the gastric slow wave, *Neurogastroenterology and Motility*, 18, 619–631 (2006).

233. V. Shah, S. Knappe, P. D. D. Schwindt, and J. Kitching, Subpicotesla atomic magnetometry with a microfabricated vapour cell, *Nature Photonics*, 1, 649–652 (2007).

234. S. Xu, M. H. Donaldson, A. Pinesb, S. M. Rochester, D. Budkerc, and V. V. Yashchuk, Application of atomic magnetometry in magnetic particle detection, *Applied Physics Letters*, 89, 224105 (2006).

235. I. K. Kominis, T. W. Kornack, J. C. Allred, and M. V. Romalis, A subfemtotesla multichannel atomic magnetometer, *Nature*, 442, 596–599 (2003).

236. D. S. Greywall, Sensitive magnetometer incorporating a high-Q nonlinear mechanical resonator, *Measurement in Science and Technology*, 16, 2473–2482 (2005).

237. H. Xia, A. B.-A. Baranga, D. Hoffman, and M. V. Romalis, Magnetoencephalography with an atomic magnetometer, *Applied Physics Letters*, 89, 211104 (2006).

238. Z. Li, R. T. Wakai, and T. G. Walker, Parametric modulation of an atomic magnetometer, *Applied Physics Letters*, 89, 134105 (2006).

239. L. Balcells, E. Calvo, and J. Fontcuberta, Room-temperature anisotropic magnetoresistive sensor based on manganese perovskite thick films, *Journal of Magnetism and Magnetic Materials*, 242–245, 1166–1168 (2002).

240. M. M. Raja, R. J. Gambino, S. Sampath, and R. Greenlaw, Thermal sprayed thick-film anisotropic magnetoresistive sensors, *IEEE Transactions on Magnetics*, 40, 2685–2687 (2004).

241. G. B. Donaldson, SQUIDs—Ultimate magnetic sensors, *Physica Status Solidi*, 2, 1463–1467 (2005).

242. A. Candini, G. C. Gazzadi, A. di Bona, M. Affronte, D. Ercolani, G. Biasio, and L Sorba, Hall nano-probes fabricated by focused ion beam, *Nanotechnology*, 17, 2105–2109 (2006).

243. J. Vrba and S. E. Robinson, Signal processing in magnetoencephalography, *Methods*, 25, 249–271 (2001).

244. A. A. Fife, J. Vrba, S. E. Robinson, G. Anderson, K. Betts, M. B. Burbank, D. Cheyne et al., Synthetic gradiometer systems for MEG, *IEEE Transactions in Applied Superconductivity*, 9, 4063–4068 (1999).

245. J. Vrba and S. E. Robinson, Linearly constrained minimum variance beamformers, synthetic aperture magnetometry, and MUSIC in MEG applications, in *34th Asilomar Conference on Signals, Systems and Computers*, Vol. 1, 2000, Pacific Grove, CA, 2000, pp. 313–317.

246. R. Frostig (ed.), *In Vivo Optical Imaging of Brain Function* (*Methods and New Frontiers in Neuroscience*), CRC Press, Boca Raton, FL, 2002.

247. J. Wells, C. Kao, K. Mariappan, J. Albea, E. D. Jansen, P. Konrad, and A. Mahadevan-Jansen, Optical stimulation of neural tissue in vivo, *Optics Letters*, 30, 504–506 (2005).

248. J. Wells, C. Kao, P. Konrad, T. Milner, J. Kim, A. Mahadevan-Jansen, and E. D. Jansen, Biophysical mechanisms of transient optical stimulation of peripheral nerve, *Biophysics Journal*, 93, 2567–2580 (2007).

249. G. Caetano and V. Jousmäki, Evidence of vibrotactile input to human auditory cortex, *NeuroImage*, 29, 15–28 (2005).

250. T. N. Lal, M. Schröder, J. Hill, H. Preissl, T. Hinterberger, J. Mellinger, M. Bogdan et al., A brain computer interface with online feedback based on magnetoencephalography, in L. De Raedt and S. Wrobel (eds.), *Proceedings of the 22nd International Conference on Machine Learning*, Bonn, Germany, 2005, pp. 465–472, ACM Press, Washington, DC.

251. D. Hecht and M. Reiner, Field dependency and the sense of object-presence in haptic virtual environments, *CyberPsychology & Behavior*, 10, 243–251 (2007).

252. C. R. Wagner and R. D. Howe, Mechanisms of performance enhancement with force feedback, in *First Joint Eurohaptics Conference and Symposium on Haptic Interfaces for Virtual Environment and Teleoperator Systems* (*WHC05*), Pisa, Italy, 2005, pp. 21–29.

253. A. M. Okamura, Methods for haptic feedback in teleoperated robot-assisted surgery, *Industrial Robot: An International Journal*, 31, 499–508 (2004).

254. G. A. Calvert, C. Spence, and B. E. Stein, *The Handbook of Multisensory Processes*, MIT Press, Cambridge MA, 2004.

255. L. Hochberg and D. Taylor, Intuitive prosthetic limb control, *The Lancet*, 369, 345–346 (2007).

256. J. Arnott, N. Alm, and A. Waller, Cognitive prostheses: Communication, rehabilitation and beyond, in *IEEE International Conference on Systems Man & Cybernetics* (*IEEE SMC 1999*) Vol.6, 1999, pp. 346–351.

257. W. Barfield and T. Caudell, *Fundamentals of Wearable Computers and Augmented Reality*, Lawrence Erlbaum Associates/CRC Press, Boca Raton, FL, 2001.

258. US NIDCD: National Institute on Deafness and Other Communication Disorders, Cochlear implants, MD, NIH Publication No. 00–4798, NIDCD, Bethesda, MD, 2007, Website at: http://www.nidcd.nih.gov/

259. US NIDCD: National Institute on Deafness and Other Communication Disorders, Statistics about hearing disorders, ear infections, and deafness, NIDCD, Bethesda, MD, 2009, Website at: http://www.nidcd.nih.gov/health/statistics/hearing.asp

260. R. D. Kent, *The MIT Encyclopedia of Communication Disorders*, MIT Press, Cambridge MA, 2004.

261. D. E. Ingber, Cellular mechanotransduction: Putting all the pieces together again, *FASEB Journal*, 20, 811–827 (2006).

262. D. I. Margolin, *Cognitive Neuropsychology in Clinical Practice*, Oxford University Press, New York, 1992.

263. P. R. Cook, Music, *Cognition, and Computerized Sound: An Introduction to Psychoacoustics*, MIT Press, Cambridge, MA, 2001.

264. V. K. Madisetti and D. Williams, *The Digital Signal Processing Handbook*, CRC Press, Boca Raton, FL, 1997.

265. M. Kahrs and K. Brandenburg, *Applications of Digital Signal Processing to Audio and Acoustics*, Springer Verlag, Berlin, Germany, 1998.

266. B. Wilson, Digital signal processing applications for hearing accessibility, *IEEE Signal Processing Magazine*, 20, 14–18 (2003).

267. J. Tierny, M. A. Zissman, and D. K. Eddington, Digital signal processing applications in cochlear-implant research, *Lincoln Laboratory Journal*, 7, 31–62 (1994).

268. G. J. M. Krijnen, M. Dijkstra, J. J. van Baar, S. S. Shankar, W. J. Kuipers, R. J. H. de Boer, D. Altpeter, and T. S. J. Lammerink, R. Wiegerink, MEMS based hair flow-sensors as model systems for acoustic perception studies, *Nanotechnology*, 17, S84–S89 (2006).

269. G. Clark, *Cochlear Implants: Fundamentals and Applications*, Springer Verlag, Berlin, Germany, 2003.

270. US FDA: Food and Drug Administration, Cochlear implants, FDA, Silver Spring, MD, Website at: http://www.fda.gov/cdrh/cochlear/index.html (2009).

271. M. Valente, H. Hosford-Dunn, and R. J. Roeser, *Audiology: Treatment*, Thieme Medical Publishers, New York, 2000.
272. J. W. Hall, *New Handbook for Auditory Evoked Responses*, Allyn & Bacon, Boston, MA, 2006.
273. G. Miller, *Sensory Organ Replacement and Repair*, Morgan & Claypool Publishers, San Rafael, CA, 2006.
274. A. R. Moller, *Cochlear and Brainstem Implants (Advances in Otorhinolaryngology)*, Karger, Basel, Switzerland, 2006.
275. K. S. Pawlowski, Anatomy and physiology of the cochlea, in P. S. Roland and J. A. Rutka (eds.), *Ototoxicity*, BC Decker, London, U.K., 2004.
276. K. S. Pawlowski, D. Wawro, and P. S. Roland, Bacterial biofilm formation on a human cochlear implant, *Otology and Neurotology*, 26, 972–975 (2005).
277. T. A. Johnson, K. A. Loeffler, R. A. Burne, C. N. Jolly, and P. J. Antonelli, Biofilm formation in cochlear implants with cochlear drug delivery channels in an in vitro model, *Otolaryngology-Head and Neck Surgery*, 136, 577–582 (2007).
278. R. Cristobal, C. E. Edmiston Jr., C. L. Runge-Samuelson, H. A. Owen, J. B. Firszt, and P. A. Wackym, Fungal biofilm formation on cochlear implant hardware after antibiotic-induced fungal overgrowth within the middle ear, *Pediatric Infectious Disease Journal*, 23, 774–777 (2004).
279. B. Gold and N. Morgan, *Speech and Audio Signal Processing: Processing and Perception of Speech and Music*, John Wiley & Sons, New York, 1999.
280. G. P. Jacobson, C. W. Newman, and J. M. Kartush, *Handbook of Balance Function Testing*, Springer Verlag, Berlin, Germany, 1997.
281. J. M. Goldberg and C. Fernandez, Vestibular mechanisms, *Annual Review of Physiology*, 37, 129–162 (1975).
282. K. W. Lindsay, T. D. Roberts, and J. R. Rosenberg, Asymmetric tonic labyrinth reflexes and their interaction with neck reflexes in the decerebrate cat, *Journal of Physiology*, 261, 583–601 (1976).
283. M. F. Reschke, J. M. Krnavek, J. T. Somers, and G. Ford, A Brief history of space flight with a comprehensive compendium of vestibular and sensorimotor research conducted across the various flight programs, NASA/ SP–2007–560, National Center for AeroSpace Information, Hanover, MD, 2007.
284. A. M. Shkel and F.-G. Zeng, An electronic prosthesis mimicking the dynamic vestibular function, *Audiology and Neurotology*, 11, 113 (2006).
285. A. A. Maltan and T. K. Whitehurst, Stimulation using a microstimulator to treat tinnitus, U.S. Patent 20,070,021,804, Advanced Bionics Corporation, Valencia, CA, 2007.
286. S. A. Gelfand, *Essentials of Audiology*, 2nd edn., Thieme, New York, 2001.
287. V. P. Eroschenko and M. S. H. di Fiore, *Di Fiore's Atlas of Histology*, 10th edn., Lippincott Williams & Wilkins, Philadelphia, PA, 2004.
288. S. S. Corbett III, J. W. Swanson, J. Martyniuk, T. A. Clary, F. A. Spelman, B. Clopton, A. H. Voie, and C. N. Jolly, Multi-electrode cochlear implant and method of manufacturing the same, U.S. Patent 5,630,839, PI Medical Corporation, Portland, OR/University of Washington, Seattle, WA, 1997.
289. C.-P. Richter and S. Ho, Cochlear implant including a modiolar return electrode, U.S. Patent 7194314, Northwestern University, 2007.
290. D. Rejalia, V. A. Leec, K. A. Abrashkina, N. Humayuna, D. L. Swiderskia, and Y. Raphaela, Cochlear implants and ex vivo BDNF gene therapy protect spiral ganglion neurons, *Hearing Research*, 228, 180–187 (2007).

291. W. Lee and V. Parpura, Wiring neurons with carbon nanotubes, *Frontiers in Neuroengineering*, 2, 8 (2009).
292. D. Seybold, The psychosocial impact of acquired vision loss, in *Vision 2005— Proceedings of the International Congress*, Vol. 1282, London, U.K., 2005, pp. 298–301.
293. S. H. Schwartz, *Visual Perception*, 3rd edn., McGraw-Hill, New York, 2004.
294. P. G. Simos, *Vision in the Brain*, CRC Press, Boca Raton, FL, 2001.
295. P. L. Kaufman and A. Alm, *Adler's Physiology of the Eye*, 10th edn., Harcourt/ Mosby, London, U.K., 2002.
296. S. E. Palmer, *Vision Science: Photons to Phenomenology*, MIT Press, Cambridge, MA, 1999.
297. J. E. Dowling, *The Retina: An Approachable Part of the Brain*, Belknap Harvard Press, Cambridge, MA, 1987.
298. A. M. P. Hamilton, R. Gregson, and G. E. Fish, *Text Atlas of the Retina*, Informa Healthcare, London, U.K., 1998.
299. M. E. Brezinski, *Optical Coherence Tomography: Principles and Applications*, Academic Press, Boston, MA, 2006.
300. D. T. Hartong, E. L. Berson, and T. P. Dryja, Retinitis pigmentosa, *Lancet*, 386, 1795–1809 (2006).
301. T. Suzuki, M. Akimoto, H. Imai, Y. Ueda, M. Mandai, N. Yoshimura, A. Swaroop, and M. Takahashi, Chondroitinase ABC treatment enhances synaptogenesis between transplant and host neurons in a mouse model of retinal degeneration, *Cell Transplantation*, 16, 493–503, (2007).
302. W. Roush, Envisioning an artificial retina, *Science*, 268, 637–8 (1995).
303. R. R. Lakhanpal, D. Yanai, J. D. Weiland, G. Y. Fujii, S. Caffey, R. J. Greenberg, E. de Juan Jr., and M. S. Humayun, Advances in the development of visual prostheses, *Current Opinion in Ophthalmology*, 14, 122–127 (2003).
304. J. D. Weiland, W. T. Liu, and M. S. Humayun, Retinal prosthesis, *Annual Review of Biomedical Engineering*, 7, 361–401 (2005).
305. P. Hossain, I. W. Seetho, A. C. Browning, and W. M. Amoaku, Science, medicine, and the future—Artificial means for restoring vision, *British Medical Journal*, 330, 30–33 (2005).
306. M. Javaheri, D. S. Hahn, R. R. Lakhanpal, J. D. Weiland, and M. S. Humayun, Retinal prostheses for the blind, *Annals of the Academy of Medicine of Singapore*, 35, 137–144 (2006).
307. G. Dagnelie, Visual prosthetics 2006: Assessment and expectations, *Expert Reviews of Medical Devices*, 3, 315–326 (2006).
308. D. E. Casey (ed.), Envisioning sight for the blind: The DOE artificial retina project, *Artificial Retina News*, 1, 1–3 (2006).
309. J. D. Weiland and M. S. Humayun, A biomimetic retinal stimulating array, IEEE *Engineering in Medicine and Biology Magazine*, 24, 14–21 (2005).
310. J. D. Weiland and M. S. Humayun, Intraocular retinal prosthesis—Big steps to sight restoration, *IEEE Engineering in Medicine and Biology Magazine*, 25, 60–66 (2006).
311. C.-Y. Wu, F. Cheng, C.-T. Chiang, and P.-K. Lin, A low-power implantable pseudo-BJT-based silicon retina with solar cells for artificial retinal prostheses, in *Proceedings of the 2004 International Symposium on Circuits Systems (ISCAS 04)*, Vol. 4, Vancouver, Canada, 2004, pp. 37–40.
312. G. J. Suaning and N. H. Lovell, CMOS Neurostimulation system with 100 electrodes and radio frequency telemetry, in *Conference of IEEE EMBS, Melbourne*, Australia, 1999.

313. D. C. Rodger and Y.-C. Tai, Microelectronic packaging for retinal prostheses, *IEEE Engineering in Medicine and Biology Magazine*, 24, 52–57 (2005).

314. F. Paillet, D. Mercier, and T. M. Bernard, Second generation programmable artificial retina, in *Proceedings of the 12th Annual IEEE International ASIC/SOC Conference 1999*, Washington, DC, 304–309 (1999).

315. F. Gekeler and E. Zrenner, Status of the subretinal implant project: An overview, *Ophthalmologe*, 102, 941–52 (2005).

316. E. Funatsu, Y. Nitta, Y. Miyake, T. Toyoda, J. Ohta, and K. Kyuma, An artificial retina chip with current-mode focal plane imageprocessing functions, *IEEE Transactions in Electronic Devices*, 44, 1777–1782 (1997).

317. J. Ohta, T. Tokuda, K. Kagawa, T. Furumiya, A. Uehara, Y. Terasawa, M. Ozawa, T. Fujikado, and Y. Tano, Silicon LSI-based smart stimulators for retinal prosthesis—A flexible and extendable microchip-based stimulator, *IEEE Engineering in Medicine and Biology Magazine*, 25, 47–59 (2006).

318. A. Stett, A. Mai, and T. Herrmann, Retinal charge sensitivity and spatial discrimination obtainable by subretinal implants: Key lessons learned from isolated chicken retina, *Journal of Neural Engineering*, 4, S7–S16 (2007).

319. T. Schanze, H. G. Sachs, C. Wiesenack, U. Brunner, and H. Sailer, Implantation and testing of subretinal film electrodes in domestic pigs, *Experimental Eye Research*, 82, 332–340 (2006).

320. M. T. Pardue, M. J. Phillips, H. Yin, B. D. Sippy, S. Webb-Wood, A. Y. Chow, and S. L. Ball, Neuroprotective effect of subretinal implants in the RCS rat, *Investigative Ophthalmology and Visual Science*, 46, 674–682 (2005).

321. M. T. Pardue, M. J. Phillips, B. Hanzlicek, H. Yin, A. Y. Chow, and S. L. Ball, Neuroprotection of photoreceptors in the RCS rat after implantation of a subretinal implant in the superior or inferior retina, *Advances in Experimental Medicine and Biology*, 572, 321–326 (2006).

322. M. T. Pardue, S. L. Ball, M. J. Phillips, A. E. Faulkner, T. A. Walker, and A. Y. Chow, Status of the feline retina 5 years after subretinal implantation, *Journal of Rehabilitation Research and Development*, 43, 723–732 (2006).

323. A. P Fornos, J. Sommerhalder, B. Rappaz, A. B. Safran, and M. Pelizzone, Simulation of artificial vision, III: Do the spatial or temporal characteristics of stimulus pixelization really matter? *Investigative Ophthalmology and Visual Science*, 46, 3906–3912 (2005).

324. S. I. Fried, H. A. Hsueh, and F. S. Werblin, A method for generating precise temporal patterns of retinal spiking using prosthetic stimulation, *Journal of Neurophysiology*, 95, 970–978 (2006).

325. L. Johnson, D. Scribner, P. Skeath, R. Klein, D. Ilg, K. Perkins, M. Helfgott, R. Sanders, and D. Panigrahi, Impedance-based retinal contact imaging as an aid for the placement of high resolution epiretinal prostheses, *Journal of Neural Engineering*, 4, S17–S23 (2007).

326. E. Margalit and W. B. Thoreson, Inner retinal mechanisms engaged by retinal electrical stimulation, *Investigative Ophthalmology and Visual Science*, 47, 2606–2612 (2006).

327. T. Yagi and Y. Hayashida, Artificial retina implantation, *Nippon Rinsho*, 57, 1208–1215 (1999).

328. W. H. Dobelle, Artificial vision for the blind by connecting a television camera to the visual cortex: State of the art, *American Society for Artificial Internal Organs Journal*, 46, 3–9 (2000).

329. J. F. Doorish, A wireless photovoltaic mini epi-retinal prosthesis (MeRP) 1: Concept and design, *Journal of Modern Optics*, 53, 1267–1285 (2006).
330. A. Y. Chow, V. Y. Chow, K. H. Packo, J. S. Pollack, G. A. Peyman, and R. Schuchard, The artificial silicon retina microchip for the treatment of vision loss from retinitis pigmentosa, *Archives of Ophthalmology*, 122, 460–469 (2004).
331. K. Hungar, M. Gortz, E. Slavcheva, G. Spanier, W. C. Weidig, and W. Mokwa, Production processes for a flexible retina implant (Eurosensors XVIII, Session C6.6), *Sensors and Actuators A: Physical*, 123, 172–178 (2005).
332. P. Walter, Z. F. Kisvárday, M. Görtz, N. Alteheld, G. Rossler, T. Stieglitz, and U. T. Eysel, Cortical activation via an implanted wireless retinal prosthesis, *Investigative Ophthalmology and Visual Science*, 46, 1780–1785 (2005).
333. J. Ohta, T. Tokuda, K. Kagawa, S. Sugitani, M. Taniyama, A. Uehara, Y. Terasawa, K. Nakauchi, T. Fujikado, and Y. Tano, Laboratory investigation of microelectronics-based stimulators for large-scale suprachoroidal transretinal stimulation (STS), *Journal of Neural Engineering*, 4, S85–S91 (2007).
334. J. S. Pezaris and R. C. Reid, Demonstration of artificial visual percepts generated through thalamic microstimulation, *Proceedings of the National Academy of Sciences*, 104, 7670–7675 (2007).
335. R. J. Jensen, O. R. Ziv, and J. F. Rizzo, Thresholds for activation of rabbit retinal ganglion cells with relatively large, extracellular microelectrodes, *Investigative Ophthalmology and Visual Science*, 46, 1486–1496 (2005).
336. L. B. Merabet, J. F. Rizzo, A. D. Amedi, D. C. Somers, and A. Pascual-Leone, What blindness can tell us about seeing again: Merging neuroplasticity and neuroprostheses, *Nature Reviews Neuroscience*, 6, 71–77 (2005).
337. D. W. Chun, J. S. Heier, M. B. Raizman, and B. Michael, Visual prosthetic device for bilateral end-stage macular degeneration, *Expert Review of Medical Devices*, 6, 657–665 (2005).
338. J. O. Winter, S. F. Cogan, and J. F. Rizzo, Retinal prostheses: Current challenges and future outlook, *Journal of Biomaterials Science Polymer Edition*, 18, 1031–1055 (2007).
339. J. Sommerhalder, ARVO annual meeting 2008: Visual prostheses research, *Expert Review of Ophthalmology*, 3, 389–391 (2008).
340. P. Walter, Implants for artificial vision, *Expert Review of Ophthalmology*, 4, 515–523 (2009).
341. H. A. Hassan, S. R. Montezuma, and J. F. Rizzo, In vivo electrical stimulation of rabbit retina: Effect of stimulus duration and electrical field orientation, *Experimental Eye Research*, 83, 247–254 (2006).
342. H. L. Hudson, S. S. Lane, J. S. Heier, R. D. Stulting, L. Singerman, P. R. Lichter, P. Sternberg, and D. F. Chang, Implantable miniature telescope for the treatment of visual acuity loss resulting from end-stage age-related macular degeneration: 1-year results, *Ophthalmology*, 113, 1987–2001 (2006).
343. S. J. Fliesler and O. G. Kisselev (eds.), *Signal Transduction in the Retina*, CRC Press, Boca Raton, FL, 2007.
344. T. V. Chirila (ed.), *Biomaterials and Regenerative Medicine in Ophthalmology*, CRC Press, Boca Raton, FL, 2010.
345. M. C. Peterman, D. M. Bloom, C. Lee, S. F. Bent, M. F. Marmor, M. S. Blumenkranz, and H. A. Fishman, Localized neurotransmitter release for use in a prototype retinal interface, *Investigative Ophthalmology and Visual Science*, 44, 3144–3149 (2003).

346. D. Johnston and S. M.-S. Wu, *Foundations of Cellular Neurophysiology*, Bradford Books/MIT Press, Cambridge, MA, 1994.

347. Structure of protein collagen seen at unprecedented level of detail, U.S. Department of Energy, Argonne National Laboratory, *Science Daily*, Science News, online at: http://www.anl.gov/Media_Center/News/2008/APS080222. html (2008).

348. C. Chen et al., Nanoparticle-templated assembly of viral protein cages, *Nano Letters*, 6, 611–615 (2006).

9

Diagnosis: Nanosensors in Diagnosis and Medical Monitoring

The advent of 21st century medicine will be based on a comprehensive approach to achieving the highly sensitive and specific detection of diseases, as well as the development of novel materials and devices based on biotic-abiotic interfacing as interventional modalities. Novel technologies that enable early identification of physiological changes will serve as a gateway tool for the proper treatment of these disorders. [1]

9.1 Introduction

In this chapter, we conclude Part II with a look at how nanotechnology makes feasible and affordable sensors for single molecule detection, the monitoring of disease, personal DNA analysis, personal monitoring, and other new capabilities for diagnosis, monitoring, and care management.

9.2 Overview

Diagnosis is based on observation and reasoning. Nanotechnology gives us the ability to observe in great detail on the scale of cells and biological molecules. Thus, it opens new possibilities for diagnostic sensing and analysis for medicine. These possibilities are rapidly being realized in the form of smaller sensors with new capabilities [2–5]. Nanotechnology has produced a new generation of sensors with advanced characteristics:

1. Smaller
2. Require less power
3. More sensitive
4. More selective
5. Wireless operation
6. Integration with microelectronics and microfluidics
7. Biocompatible

In the first section of this chapter, we will review the nanotechnology upon which these sensor capabilities are based. We will see how designers are taking advantage of the special properties of matter and energy at the nanoscale to build these capabilities. In the next sections, we will give an overview of how these sensors are being used in medicine for

1. Diagnosis and monitoring of diseases and disorders: in the research and clinical laboratory, in vivo, and in the field for epidemiology and public health.

2. Genetic analysis and screening based on rapid and inexpensive DNA sequencing capabilities, which, when combined with systems biology and targeted nanomedicines, are opening new possibilities for personalized therapies.

3. Personal health monitoring based on adaptable wearable and implantable wireless devices for clinical and ambulatory use, providing improved patient health management everywhere from the intensive care unit to the patients home, work, and recreation environment.

These medical uses of nanosensors are rapidly being translated from research and development into clinical practice. The time line of this translation begins with clinical laboratory instruments, as advanced research analysis is integrated into new types of standardized, high-throughput instruments for the clinical lab bench. Personalized medicine for cancer and other complex multigenic diseases is translating into clinical practice, led by genomic testing and systems biology approaches emerging from the NIH and other research institutions. Personal mobile health monitoring is gradually coalescing into an integrated concept, starting from numerous incompatible monitors for separate types of physiological sensors and disease indicators, and moving toward compatible standards based on mass-produced devices such as cell phones, which will enable widespread adoption. These and other new sensor technologies, such as smart fabrics containing physiological sensors and communication capabilities, are fast becoming reality.

9.3 Sensors: Nanotechnology-Driven Advances in Diagnostic and Monitoring Technology

Nanotechnology is the ability to observe, measure, and control matter on the nanoscale. Nanotechnology makes possible extremely subtle and precise measurements of very small quantities of matter, and it makes such measurements fast and cheap.

Here is an example: the traditional way to find and identify a harmful bacterium is to sample its environment, and transfer the sample to a friendly culture environment where it can multiply. If you have caught a few bacteria in your sample, and if the culture dish into which you put them meets the needs for nutrients and chemicals and other environmental conditions for growth, the bacteria will multiply. After a few score doublings by cell division, a colony will be formed large enough to be seen under the microscope, or even with the naked eye. You can then observe distinctive colors and shapes of the colony to begin to identify the bacteria. You can refine the identification by placing samples in several different cultures, if you know that some bacteria will grow where others will not. And once you have enough bacteria to form a colony so that you can find them, you can prepare a slide and look at their shape and other distinguishing characteristics under the microscope, perhaps with the aid of stains. All of this takes time—perhaps a few days.

Now this is a slow, expensive, and messy process—perhaps dangerous if the bacteria are really virulent. It has been, until recently, the gold standard for identifying harmful disease bacteria such as those that cause tuberculosis. This method is analogous to the way that chemical analysis had to be done before spectroscopic and other physical methods were developed—it is slow, wet, messy, risky, and unreliable. It is predicated on the fact that we are too big to see the individual molecules or bacteria, so we had to manipulate them into making large scale effects that we could find. Over the past few decades, more and more alternatives were devised for identifying bacteria and molecules quickly and reliably using nanotechnology. We will explore a few of them and their implications.

9.3.1 Examples of Nanosensors

We will take two examples of nanosensors to illustrate how things are different on the nanoscale. The first is based on the nanoscale cantilever, and the second on photon resonance.

9.3.1.1 Cantilever Sensors

A diving board is a good example of a cantilever. You could use a diving board as a kind of scale—the heavier you were, the more it would bend when you stand out on the end of it—and the greater the extent of the vibration when you jump off. We can make very tiny cantilevers out of silicon, or use a carbon nanotube as an equivalent to measure very small amounts of matter (think of hanging off a horizontal flagpole).

Tiny cantilevers do not bend under the weight of tiny amounts of matter, because as you approach the nanoscale, mass is so small that gravity becomes negligible. But other forces become relatively much more important, and we can and do use them to make measurements. We can measure

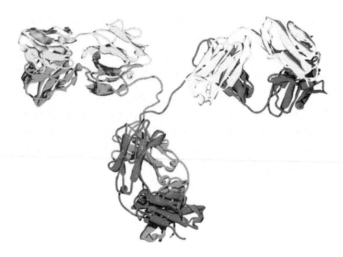

FIGURE 9.1
Antibody structure—antibodies produced by vertebrate immune systems represent a highly developed form of molecular recognition that is exploitable in nanosensors. (Image courtesy of Tim Vickers at the Wikepedia Project: http://en.wikipedia.org/wiki/File:Antibody_IgG2.png)

the frequency of the vibration of nanocantilevers by using them as charged oscillators in electric circuits, or we can magnify the effect of a slight deflection by the displacement of reflected light at a distance. Both ways of measurement amplify a slight deflection, and can be interfaced into an electronic measurement system, such as a computer.

To measure a small number of molecules, or a bacterium, we need to find a force that affects the deflection or vibration of the cantilever, and we need to have some means of making the interaction with the cantilever selective and specific. Fortunately, we know about highly specific selective mechanisms in biology—between antibodies and antigens, between complementary nucleotide sequences, and the lock and key interactions of all types of macromolecules (Figure 9.1). We can take advantage of active vibration forces or passive deflection forces in combination with selective surface interactions to make very powerful detectors.

9.3.1.2 Active Cantilever Sensors

9.3.1.2.1 Active Cantilever Sensing: Vibration Resonance

A tiny cantilever etched from silicon or other single crystalline material will have a characteristic resonant vibration frequency, like the tine of a microscopic tuning fork. The physics that describes vibrations of bulk materials applies well to submicroscopic cantilevers provided that their composition is uniform, without defects that lead to loss of elasticity. A carbon nanotube or fiber is composed of bonded atoms, so it can be used as a cantilever that is more perfectly elastic than a deflecting or resonating structure etched from even the best single-crystal silicon, but nonlinear effects at the nanoscale must be taken into account.

Nanoscale cantilevers can be used to measure density and viscosity of fluids, because their rate of vibration is damped by collisions with molecules in the fluid. The rate of vibration of a cantilever can be forced and monitored electronically by an electronic circuit designed with the cantilever as a capacitive plate element. The deflection of a cantilever can also be measured optically, by changes in the angle of reflection or by interferometry. Cantilevers can be used to detect and determine the mass of molecules that are absorbed or bonded to their surface, since the resonant frequency of the oscillation of a vibrating object depends on its inertial mass as well as its elasticity. At the nanoscale, the difference in mass made by the addition of just a few large molecules such as proteins or DNA is large enough in relation to the mass of the cantilever to make it possible to detect minute quantities of biological substances [2,3].

9.3.1.3 Passive Cantilever Sensors

9.3.1.3.1 Passive Cantilever Sensing: Measuring Deformation

Nanoscale cantilevers can be distorted passively, without vibrating, due to differences in the amount and strength of absorption on opposite sides of the sliver of material. This is perhaps the most striking example of how things are different at the nanoscale with regard to cantilevers. This phenomenon follows the same laws of surface chemistry and physics as for larger-scale bulk materials, but at the nanoscale, the surface forces dominate over the internal properties of the material.

For a cantilever on the order of 500 μm length, 100 μm width, and 0.5 μm thickness, the free energy differences between a surface covered with absorbed molecules and a clean surface, although small, are enough to force a displacement in the shape of the cantilever, which can be detected when one side is coated with an agent that binds with an absorbate. The absorption of the analyte may be highly specific, as between an antibody and an antigen, or may be merely weakly selective. In the latter case, the combinations of coatings on groups of cantilevers can be used to obtain patterns for recognition, as in the artificial nose device.

9.3.1.4 Surface Effects on Nanocantilevers

9.3.1.4.1 Absorption Strength and Surface Crowding: Absorption Affinity

To envisage the effect of absorbed molecules on the cantilever, consider that as bonds are formed with the absorbate on one specially coated or prepared side of the sliver of material, the absorbed molecules will tend to push their way into the matrix of molecules that make up the surface of the cantilever. This crowding into the surface will tend to distend the surface ever so slightly. The stronger the affinity or attractive force that binds the absorbed molecules to the substrate, the greater the crowding force will be and the more it will tend to push the molecules apart near the surface of the cantilever. If no absorption takes place on the other side, there will be a slight differential expansion on the absorption side, and this expansion will cause a deflection, with a convex curvature on the absorption side, and a concave curvature on the opposite side.

9.3.1.5 Steric Effects

9.3.1.5.1 Surface Crowding: Steric Effects

An additional force for expansion on the absorption side will occur if the absorbed molecules repel each other or push against each other; in that case, they will tend to pull apart the molecules in the cantilever to which they are bonded. These two forces are sufficient to produce a measurable deflection if the cantilever is small enough that the effects on the surface overpower the forces holding the internal molecules in their preferred places relative to each other in the bulk material matrix.

9.3.1.6 Micro- and Nanosensors and Applications

Many cantilever and similar devices for detecting molecules have been described and developed. Carbon nanotubes or other fibers of nano-dimensions can be used in a similar way, provided that a means of inducing and measuring vibrations, or coating selectively, is devised. A number of books and reviews are available on the subject of nanoscale cantilever molecular sensors, which will give a mathematical treatment if one needs more details [2–6].

9.3.1.7 Biomedical Cantilever Applications

To make a cantilever sensor with a medical application, one may coat one surface with a reactant such as an antibody specific for an antigen. When the surface is exposed to solutions of the antigen, it becomes coated with molecules of the antigen, producing a small but detectable deformation of the cantilever due to surface forces. This deformation can be detected by optical reflection. Only for devices of nanoscale proportions are the intermolecular nanomechanics at the surface sufficient to produce a detectable deflection usable as a sensor (Figure 9.2).

9.3.1.7.1 Cantilever Sensor for Cancer Screening

An interdisciplinary team of coworkers at the University of California Berkeley, University of Southern California, and Oak Ridge National Laboratories developed an application of this technique to detect prostate cancer antigen (PSA). Using 600-μm-long and 0.65-μm-thick silicon nitride

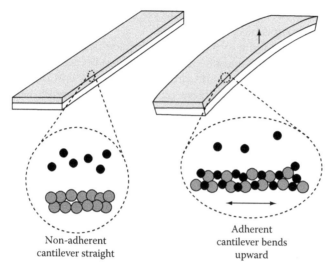

FIGURE 9.2

Absorption and steric crowding on an antibody-coated cantilever. (From Hornyak, G.L. et al., *Introduction to Nanoscience and Nanotechnology*, CRC Press, Boca Raton, FL, 2009. With permission.)

cantilevers, it was feasible with their technique to detect fPSA concentrations of 0.2 ng/mL. Since this antigen is produced by the body in response to cancer cells, this sensor could be useful in a blood screening test for the early detection of cancer in humans. This example of the cantilever sensor technique could lead to devices for high-throughput label-free analysis of protein—protein binding, DNA hybridization, and DNA—protein interactions, as well as drug discovery [2].

9.3.1.8 Surface Plasmon Nanosensors

A surface plasmon is a charge density wave that is induced by light striking an interface between a thin film and another medium. Surface plasmon resonance (SPR) is the coupling of energy from incident light with the charge density in the surface, resulting in energy being transferred into a thin layer on the surface instead of being reflected. Resonance occurs only when the energy of the incident light is of the right frequency and angle of incidence for coupling with the specific materials and dimensions of the surface and thin film.

SPR is the phenomenon that gives rise to intense colors in butterfly wings, diatoms, nanodots, and other materials with thin layers on the nanoscale, corresponding to resonant frequencies with incident light. It is a useful phenomenon for optical detection and measurement of thin films that can vary in composition and thickness. The waveform and intensity of the plasmon depend strongly on the thickness of the film and the type of material on which the film is deposited. So if an analyte is absorbed on the surface, it will alter the thin film and be detectable.

SPR is used to study the formation of self-assembled layers and structures of organic molecules formed on surfaces. SPR can be used to detect biological substances, such as DNA and proteins. A surface can be coated in patterns with different specific antigens or DNA complementary test strands to make an array in which a combination of biological target molecules can be detected [2].

9.3.2 Nanosensor Technologies

In addition to cantilevers with antigens or DNA markers, and SPR detectors, there are a number of other effects that can be magnified electrically or optically from the nanoscale to make a measurable difference in an electrical circuit for detection and analysis. These include electrochemical potentials, electronic frequency effects, surface acoustic and magnetoacoustic effects, effects of absorbed materials on fluorescence, molecular templating, and other modalities, including combinations of the above [2–6].

9.3.2.1 Nanosensor Fabrication

A number of fabrication techniques integrate sensors directly into materials, which can be used to make arrays of sensors, microfluidic devices for sampling and delivering analytes, wearable patches, and other biochip, lab-on-a-chip, and smart material applications [2–12]. Sensor materials, like other nanomaterials and MEMS, are fabricated by top-down lithography approaches, bottom-up self-assembly, nanoskiving, templating, and combinations of these techniques [13–19].

The ability to fabricate materials on the nanoscale opens up new possibilities for sensor design. Engineers and analytical scientists can make smaller, lower power sensors by shrinking devices based on familiar principles to measure electromagnetic potentials, impedances, magnetic fields, optical absorption and diffraction, and other effects used to detect and analyze biochemical materials. But in addition, working at the nanoscale involves effects that are very sensitive to the small forces and interactions of small numbers of atoms and molecules, making it possible to create new classes of extremely sensitive and specific sensors, as we saw in the two examples above.

9.3.2.2 An Example of Sensor Protection by Nanofabrication

Let us look at how sensors can be improved by nanotechnology simply by size of features. Enzymes are potentially a good basis for making nanosensors extremely selective and sensitive as they react with substrates without being consumed themselves. Enzyme sensors are especially good for measuring small molecules such as glucose. But biosensors to which enzymes are immobilized tend to lose activity and sensitivity. One cause of the loss is attachment of large molecular weight proteins onto the sensor, blocking the enzyme function. Nanofabrication of protective nanoporous membranes or needles with nanopore openings is one way to filter out large molecular weight compounds while maintaining sensitivity to small biochemicals such as glucose. A sensor of this design has been developed for glucose monitoring [20].

9.3.2.2.1 Piezoelectric Nanofiber Sensors

Sophisticated cantilever nanosensors include piezoelectric fibers whose vibrational resonance in an electrical circuit is very sensitive to absorbed macromolecules or viruses, which can be selectively attached to the resonator element by treatment with antibodies or complementary nucleotides as biological templates. Sensors based on this principle have been designed to monitor for the hepatitis C virus, and for DNA analysis [21–23]. Piezoelectric sensors are a useful technique for measuring protein interactions and bond rupture, along with surface acoustic wave sensors, for studies in affinities, immunology, protein structure, and protein misfolding diseases [24–26].

9.3.2.2.2 Electrochemical Nanosensors

Electrochemical nanosensors detect and analyze proteins, viruses, and cell membranes by measuring minute changes in potential or impedance, taking advantage of the sampling geometries and high surface area electrodes that can be fabricated with nanotechnology [27–29]. Electrochemical sensors are readily fabricated and integrated by top-down lithography techniques into arrays [30–33]. Electrochemical sensors that measure potential or impedance are useful for the development of label-free detection protocols for DNA, proteins, and viruses [34,35]. Being label-free and readily integrated into electronics, electrochemical sensors lend themselves to devices for continuous monitoring [36]. Functionalized carbon nanotubes have been integrated with field-effect transistors to detect selected biomolecules and microorganisms [37,38]. Carbon nanofibers, nanotubes, and diamond films have been found particularly useful in fabricating sensitive nanoelectrodes for biological measurements [39–43].

9.3.2.2.3 Optical Nanosensors

In Chapter 5, we discussed many types of nanoparticles that can be functionalized to provide specifically targeted drug and phototherapy delivery. Nanoparticles with fluorescence, SPR, or other optical activity combined with biomolecular specificity can be used to analyze biomedical samples [44,45]. These types of nanoparticle optical reporters can be used as probes for biochemical activity and structure within cells. A wide variety of optical probes have been introduced into a range of cell types for research investigations, including PEBBLEs (photonic explorers for bioanalysis with biologically localized embedding) and multifunctional dumbbells [46–51]. Methods for introducing optical probes into cells include surface functionalization with cell-penetrating peptides, pinocytosis, lipid transfection agents, cytochalasin D, picoinjection, and gene gun bombardment [52,53].

9.3.2.2.4 *Surface Plasmon Resonance Nanosensors*

Optical measurements at the nanoscale can utilize SPR effects, which are extremely sensitive to absorbed layers of molecules, and can even detect single molecules if the quantum resonance well is suitably designed. In earlier chapters, we have seen how surface resonance is used in quantum-dot nanoparticles to enhance medical imaging and diagnosis. Quantum dots are also being used as intracellular probes for medical research, clinical laboratory diagnostic tests, and pathology examinations [54–56]. To provide analytical selectivity, the same principles of functionalization apply, as discussed in Chapter 5 on nanoparticles for medical imaging and drug delivery, to target specific types of molecules with molecular affinity and template matching by means of enzyme activity, immunity, protein interactions, nucleic acid pairing, or other types of templating. Gold nanodots are particularly useful because they are readily functionalized by way of thiol linkages with a variety of analyte-specific ligands, they can be fabricated in a number of controlled sizes and forms, and they are relatively non-toxic [57–59]. SPR is being used in a number of in vitro and in vivo biosensing applications for clinical and pathological diagnostics [56,60–63].

9.3.2.2.5 *Surface-Enhanced Raman Scattering*

Surface-enhanced Raman scattering (SERS) is a complex phenomenon, which is observed when molecules are absorbed on nano-roughened metal surfaces, resulting in the enhancement of Raman scattering by factors as high as 10^{14}–10^{15}, making it an extremely sensitive technique capable of detecting individual biomolecules. SERS is due to the interaction of chemical bonds with nanosurface features that are much smaller than the wavelength of the infrared radiation associated with Raman scattering by the absorbed molecules, resulting in the amplification of electromagnetic fields and localized surface plasmon effects [64–66]. SERS detectors depend on special nanosurface preparation of metals such as gold in which the SPR frequencies can be made to fall within the visible and infrared frequency ranges that excite Raman scattering modes in the analyte molecules [67,68]. Biomolecules that have no Raman excitation modes can be detected by use of hybridization with Raman labels such as rhodamine B [69]. SERS detectors can be fabricated as arrays on metallized substrates for the detection of DNA and proteins [70,71]. SERS detectors can be prepared as nanoparticles for use with microscopy or on specially prepared tips of optical fibers for use as probes [72–74].

9.3.2.2.6 *Magnetic Nanosensors*

Magnetic nanoparticles can be combined with SPR or the fluorescence of nanoporous silicon or silica to create multifunctional diagnostic sensors that combine magnetic separation and concentration with optical reporting [76,77]. Nanoscale magnetic effects also can be used to trap and manipulate biomolecules for study or analysis [78]. In Chapter 8, we discussed the use of magnetoresistive sensors for sensing electromagnetic activity in nerves. Magnetoresistive sensor technology has been pushed to new limits by the demands for higher density, higher-capacity computer memory storage devices, as well as other nonbiological applications. Anyone who is familiar with computer technology knows how rapidly the capacity (and corresponding speed) of computer disk drives has risen over the past 20 years. The magnetoresistive sensors that make these advances possible can be harnessed to design bionanosensors that are extremely sensitive to the presence of selected proteins, and insensitive to the biological matrix in the background [79].

9.3.2.3 Making Sensors Bio-Specific: Antibodies, Antigens, Templates, and Aptamers

Useful nanosensors must have a way to make them selective for specific biomolecules or surfaces, even in the presence of potentially interfering substances. There are two general approaches to selective analyzers: one is to precede the detector step with a discriminating separation process, so that only molecules with specific sets of properties reach the detector. This can be achieved with electromagnetic fields (mass spectrometry or dielectrophoresis) or by physical and chemical separation (chromatography, molecular sieves, ion-selective electrodes, etc.), or other means such as affinity chromatography and electrochemical bioaffinity sensors [80,81]. Semipermeable membranes can be very useful for selecting small molecules from the presence of a complex mixture, but for biomedical applications, we also frequently need to detect large biological macromolecules. For large biomolecules, the most natural and readily available means of selection are those that emulate natural biological selectivity, utilizing lock-and-key template mechanisms for selective affinity [2].

The immune systems of vertebrates produce antibodies that bind tightly to molecules and surfaces that are recognized as antigens. Oligonucleotides such as DNA and RNA segments bind to their complementary strands. Enzymes and other proteins can bind and self-assemble with high specificity and affinity to selected ligands. These affinities are the basis of techniques such as enzyme-linked immunosorbent assay (ELISA), Southern blotting, western blotting, using monoclonal antibodies, DNA, RNA, and proteins [82–89]. All of these mechanisms can be, and are, exploited to make selective biosensors. Each has its own advantages and drawbacks with regard to stability, degree of selectivity, availability, and difficulty of synthesis and purification. To avoid these drawbacks and to provide a direct means of generating desired selectivity, a number of synthetic techniques have been devised.

There are a number of approaches to the design of synthetic macromolecular selectivity for biosensors and similar applications. Two of the most important are molecular templating and aptamer selection.

Molecular templating simulates the templating effect of the natural lock-and-key mechanism by nanoimprinting target molecules on the surface of polymers made from small-molecule monomers. This technique has been especially useful with drug delivery systems, and has also found application in detection systems such as SERS sensors [7,73,90,91].

Another technique for highly specific recognition of biological macromolecules is the generation of *aptamers* through the process of Systematic Evolution of Ligands by Exponential Enrichment (SELEX). The term *aptamer* (from Latin, *aptus*, "to fit") was coined by A. D. Ellington and J. W. Szostak, who published the technique in 1990, at the same time that L. Gold and his research group independently published the SELEX method [92]. The principle of SELEX was elucidated in 1990; its practical application since that time has been enabled by advances in miniaturization and automation made possible by nanotechnology [92–95]. Aptamers are developed by a reiterative process of in vitro selection and the amplification of oligonucleotides, resulting in the isolation of progressively more targeted sequences, obtaining exponential optimization through screening large combinatorial libraries of oligonucleotides. The technique can also be applied to generate peptide aptamers; it has the potential for generating ligands to recognize virtually any class of target molecules with high affinity and specificity [96–99].

In addition to having very high affinity and selectivity, many synthetic aptamers are more stable than natural peptide and nucleotide sequences, and less prone to activating immune responses. These properties add to the utility of aptamers for highly specific fiber optics, electrochemical, and nanoparticle biosensors [100–103]. One of their main applications is in proteomics, as aptamer arrays for the high-throughput identification of multiple proteins [103–106].

9.3.2.3.1 Intracellular Sensing

New generations of nanosensors have made possible the direct measurement of biochemical processes within living cells [107–111]. PEBBLE, SPR, SERS, combined with aptamers, fiber optics, cell-penetrating peptides, nano-dumbbells, and nanowire electrodes are being used to map subtle details of cellular metabolic processes in compartmentalized structures [46–55,103–105]. Nanoparticle and nanoprobe methods are being used in conjunction with new fluorescence proteins and dyes, and powerful microscopy techniques made possible by advanced computerized digital optics [112–114]. These include the "F" techniques: Förster resonance energy transfer, fluorescence correlation spectroscopy, and fluorescence lifetime imaging [115–117], along with multispectral confocal microscopy [118,119]. The proteomic databases that result will have significant diagnostic and therapeutic applications [120].

9.3.2.3.2 Single Molecule Sensing

Sophisticated design of devices to exploit quantum resonance, magnetoresistive effects, aptamers, and other nanoscale imaging and sensing modalities are making it possible to detect and characterize single molecules, opening unprecedented opportunities for medical diagnosis through accessible analysis of proteins, RNA, DNA, and other biomolecules [121–125]. As one example, DNA can be threaded through a suitably functionalized tunneling gap of a scanning tunneling microscope to give signals that can distinguish the four bases (A, C, T, G) of the genetic code [126]. Although currently only an experiment, this capability may eventually be developed so that strands of DNA could be read like tape in a tape recorder. (We will review some other advanced sensor methods for DNA sequencing in Section 9.4.)

9.3.2.3.3 Biomolecular Nanosensors

Nanosensors and nanoactuators can be synthesized by the self-assembly of macromolecules. This area is on the boundary between nanotechnology, molecular biology, and synthetic macromolecular chemistry—an artificial boundary that disappears when one works at the nanoscale [127–130]. For example, nanopore proteins are being explored as highly sensitive sensors for the detection and rapid sequencing of single molecules of DNA [131,132], and glutamate receptors have been nano-engineered to allow photonic control of activation [133]. This convergence of molecular biology and nanotechnology promises new modes and levels of therapy and diagnostics for a truly integrated nanomedicine. In the meantime, work continues on micro- and nano-engineered sensors and devices fabricated for medical application by more conventional means.

9.3.2.4 Sensors for Physiological Parameters

Physical and physiological parameters such as temperature, pressure, pH, potential, and electromagnetic activity are also useful and important to medical diagnosis and monitoring. MEMS and nanosensors are used for pressure, impedance, pH, membrane potentials and other vital signs. Examples include the sensors used in ingestible and implantable capsules for gastric measurements and imaging (Chapter 6, Section 6.6.4.1) [134,135].

9.3.2.4.1 Pressure

Pressure is an especially important physiological indicator for which many MEMS devices have been developed. A wireless MEMS blood pressure monitor has been developed and approved for use in monitoring for aneurysms [136]. Other pressure MEMS have been developed for intraperitoneal, bladder, and detrusor pressures [137] and for hydrocephalus [138]. A number of MEMS have been developed for intraocular pressure measurement, including wireless devices [139,140]. Pressure-monitoring MEMS are used in the measurement of function and pain in arthritis, and in monitoring to prevent bedsores [141,142]. An intraoperative plantar pressure device has been developed to be used as a guide in surgery [143]. New and improved designs for wireless pressure MEMS continue to be developed for physiological applications [144].

9.3.2.5 Sensors for Nerve Activity

In Chapter 8, we discussed sensors and monitors for neural activity in connection with the design and use of prostheses, and briefly mentioned the importance of the interface between nerves and electrodes. Magnetic nanosensors are being developed, as discussed in Chapter 8, which may one day enable the monitoring of nerve activity noninvasively with portable devices, and magnetic neurostimulation is also advancing. But for the present, there is still a need to interface bioelectrodes to nerves for prostheses, relief of pain, support of cardiac pacing, and suppression of tremors and seizures, as well as a large number of applications of neural monitoring and stimulation in biomedical research, both in vitro and in vivo [145,146].

Research areas for neural interfaces include the gathering and analysis of patterns of neural activity associated with movement, for the design of improved prosthetics, and the monitoring of spontaneous firing in growing neural networks, to understand problems in development [147–152]. Neural networks in culture can be used as sensitive monitors for drug testing certain types of drug candidates, reducing or even eliminating the need for animal tests [153,154].

Clinical applications for neural interfaces include cardiac pacemakers, neuromodulation for pain relief, monitoring for incipient seizures and applying preventive stimulation, suppression of tremor, neuromuscular prosthetics, brain-computer interfaces, cochlear implants, and retinal prostheses [155,156].

The nanoengineering of surfaces is a key technology for electrodes used in neural monitoring and stimulation [157–159]. Research in nanoengineering of surfaces is yielding better understanding of factors that cause the deterioration of nerves experiencing chronic stimulation in contact with electrodes [159,160]. Electrode arrays for neural monitoring and stimulation have been microfabricated on a variety of substrates, including silicon, using both surface and bulk micromachining techniques, and more recently, polymers. Biocompatible materials that can be applied to the fabrication of microelectrode arrays include indium tinoxide and iridium oxide [161]. Effective surface areas on these materials can be increased by electroactivation, resulting in lowered interface impedances. Coatings and surface treatments are being investigated with promising results, including use of nanofibers such as carbon nanotubes to increase surface area [160–164] and electroconductive polymers [165,166]. Current approaches to achieving stable long-term neural interfaces focus on engineering surface properties to control protein adsorption, and on the release of bioactive molecules to guide and maintain the activity of interfaced neurons [167–169].

We will review more types and uses of physiological sensors when we discuss real-time patient-monitoring applications of medical nanotechnologies later in this chapter. But first, we will look at the role of laboratory diagnostics, genomics, and proteomics, which are gaining increasing clinical relevance with the advance of technologies that provide extremely detailed information in great volume, in a timely and useful form for diagnosis.

9.3.3 Integrated Nanosensor Technologies

Nanotechnology-based materials and devices have unique interactions at the biotic–abiotic interface, giving information about the specific nanobiology of cells, proteins, and DNA. These novel advanced sensors have the potential to provide early identification of physiological changes for diagnosis and effective treatment. The realization of that potential in clinical practice requires implementation in a clinically usable form [170].

While the advanced capabilities of individual nanosensors are remarkable and useful, the use of micro- and nano-fabrication technologies to create integrated arrays of sensors with other functionalities has resulted in even greater advances in single molecule diagnostics, sensitive detection, amplification, and analysis of DNA and RNA, cell counting and measuring, in vivo monitoring, and other areas. We will review some examples to illustrate how integrated nanosensor devices are enabling new diagnostic capabilities, including in vitro clinical tests, in vivo tests, portable diagnostics for personal testing and screening, bedside monitoring, and personal monitoring with portable and implanted sensors. Biochips are also being used in biomedical research for sensitive and accurate assays, which evaluate selected responses of cell receptors and cellular physiology to drugs, without having to use living cell cultures or animals. The technologies on which these advances are based include microarrays, microfluidics, MEMS, and advanced robotics, automation, and information systems for collecting, managing, and analyzing large amounts of data that are derive from new test modalities [2–6,171–173].

In some cases, nanoscience has revealed new sensing and detecting modalities. In other cases, the biological, chemical, and physical principles behind novel diagnostic technologies were known many years ago, but available methods to implement them were labor intensive and unreliable. The principles underlying current new bioanalytical methods were conceived decades ago (e.g., aptamer generation), but they did not become widely useful until nanotechnology-driven advances provided high-quality systems and sensors with precision robotics for handling and reading, resulting in high-throughput with reproducible results. New sensors are being integrated onto biochips and arrays, with fiber optics, wireless communications, and microfluidics for convenient and fast analysis in clinical and home settings [174–178].

9.3.3.1 Integration of Nanosensors with Fiber Optics

Fiber optics provides a very useful means of extending individual sensor probes and fabricating addressable arrays of nanosensors. The tip of a fiber waveguide provides ample area for surface treatments to fabricate nanosensors based on electroluminescence, fluorescence, SERS, plasmon resonance, and other sensing modalities. Communicating along the fiber with light is an efficient and fast way of collecting information; both electrochemical and optical nanosensors are readily interfaced to electronics for analysis and storage of data [179–182].

9.3.3.2 BioMEMS for Integration with Sensors

A wide variety of MEMS and NEMS devices have been designed for integration with biochips to perform useful functions. These include pumps, energy harvestors, and actuators, which can be utilized to activate a sensor or act as fluidic switches or gates for analytes or cells [2–6,183–185]. MEMS micropumps are used mainly for drug delivery, but they also have applications in microchips for monitoring and analysis [186]. Besides pumps, other types of MEMS actuators can be used to control valves and gates on biochips for sample collection and handling [187–189]. MEMS for harvesting mechanical, radio frequency, or heat energy have been designed to provide low-power needs of nanosensors, and to trickle charge batteries in implanted devices [190–193].

9.3.3.3 Microfluidics and Nanofluidics

One of the most important ways in which sensors are integrated into complete systems is by incorporation as components of microfluidic biochips. These "labs on a chip" have many forms and uses, and can be fabricated or molded from a variety of materials [194–203]. Microfluidic devices for biochemical analysis channel fluids and/or cells through microscale channels for analysis by micro- and nanosensors. While nanotechnology may not have shrunken the surgeon, it has miniaturized the clinical laboratory (Figure 9.3).

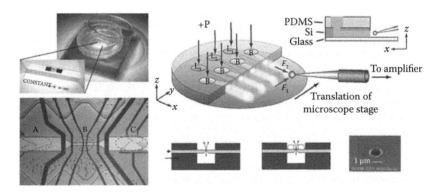

FIGURE 9.3
Different microfluidic devices applied to analysis of cells. (From Bao, N. et al., *Anal. Bioanal. Chem.*, 391, 933, 2008, Abstract figure from http://www.springerlink.com/content/a52nl4668q431748/. With permission.)

Microfluidics is used in flow cytometry to stream cells past an analysis point for counting and classification [204–206]. In addition to cell analysis or cellomics, microfluidic methods of flow cytometry can also be used to sample and analyze streams of quantum dot–encoded mesoporous beads functionalized to detect specific proteins, antibodies, or DNA sequences [207–209]. Capillary electrophoresis and dielectrophoresis techniques can be used for electrokinetic separation, focusing, and selection of cells and particles in microfluidic chips [210–212].

9.3.3.4 Manipulation and Imaging of Cells, Particles, and Fluids

In microfluidic chips, MEMS micropumps and microvalves have been used to drive and control the flow of analytes and reagents. Since the channels are capillary sized, samples can be kept separated within the microscopic flow channels by air bubbles. Alternatively, aqueous microsample alliquoits, labeled beads, or cells can be separated by suspension as droplets or particles in a stream of oil [213]. But newer microfluidic technology is obviating the need for micropumps and valves, and is instead controlling the movement of droplets by optical and electromagnetic forces. This newer version of microfluidics is called *electrokinetics*, or *digital microfluidics* [214–216].

9.3.3.5 Dielectrophoresis

Cells and polarizable particles can be moved and manipulated by the application of electromagnetic fields, either static (*electrophoresis*) or dynamic (*dielectrophoresis*) [216–218]. Electrophoresis is a relatively straightforward technique compared to generating and applying more complex variable fields needed for dielectrophoresis, whose development has only come about with the availability of sophisticated digital electronics. The forces on cells produced by dielectrophoresis depend on the polarizability as well as size; dynamic electromagnetic fields focused by electrodes surrounding a fluid can be used to separate different types of cells, including normal and cancer cells [219–221]. Nonlinear effects produced by high localized field strengths and spatial variation of the field densities can produce eddys, traps, and nonlinear effects [222,223]. Electromagnetic fields can be used for electroosmotic mixing in microfluidics. Dielectrophoresis and electroosmotic mixing can be applied by means of noncontact electrodes, eliminating contamination and electrochemical reactions at the electrode surface, and facilitating reusable designs [224,225]. Electrodes surrounding or incorporating microfluidic channels and chambers can be made by coatings of biocompatible conductive materials, machined out of metals, or printed on circuit boards [226–228]. Various related means of forming traps with electromagnetic fields have been developed and applied to microfluidic analysis [228,229].

9.3.3.6 Optical Tweezers and Photonic Vortex Traps

Tightly focused laser beams can form optical traps on the micro- to nanoscale, which can be used to manipulate cells and microparticles, as *optical tweezers* [230,231]. Polarized laser beams can be used to form optical vortex traps, where the central region of the trap has a lower optical intensity than the surrounding ring; this type of trap is superior for the manipulation of cells and other materials that are vulnerable to photochemical reactions or photo-thermal effects [232–235]. Optical vortex traps are a useful way of manipulating droplet samples in microfluidics [236,237].

9.3.3.7 Electrokinetics on Hydrophobic Surfaces

Certain types of nanostructured surfaces create a superhydrophobic effect—the well-known Lotus Effect®, which has been used to make water- and stain-resistant fabrics, coatings, and materials [2,238–241]. The water-repellent properties of the lotus leaf are due not simply to its chemical composition, but also depend critically upon its nanostructure. Nanoscale posts on the surface reduce the available contact area for water, so that the surface tension causes the formation of droplets suspended on top of the posts. The low contact area makes the droplets free to roll over the surface, absorbing and carrying away particles of dirt, thus cleaning the surface as well as keeping it dry. The same effect is found in many insect bodies, bird feathers, and other natural biomaterials [2].

The contact angle of a droplet of solution on a surface is a measure of the surface tension of the liquid and the affinity between the molecules of the liquid and the surface. This affinity can be biased by the application of an electric potential difference between a surface and a droplet, a phenomenon known as electrowetting. When a droplet of electrolyte is in contact with a hydrophobic polarizable material, applying an electronic potential can switch the surface from hydrophobic to hydrophilic and back [242–244]. This phenomenon can be used to manipulate droplets and control fluid flow electronically or optically on surfaces, giving a way to design microfluidic devices with electrodes beneath a layer of hydrophobic conducting material to define channels and holding areas for droplets. With suitable droplet formation devices, no material confinement of the fluid is necessary—the entire fluid flow is controlled on the surface by electronics. This opens the way for greatly simplified and cheaper reusable or disposable microfludic devices. All of the electrokinetic dielectrophoretic and electroosmotic mixing techniques are applicable to surface-suspended droplet microfluidics.

The droplet electrokinetic approach is being used to fabricate a number of devices with programmable and reconfigurable fluidics. Controlled and rapid mixing and reaction of fluids in droplets results in fast reaction time. Droplet digital fluidics is an ideal platform for high-throughput analysis and screening. Techniques have also been developed using digital microfluidics for the synthesis and encapsulation of nanoparticles for medical and biotechnology uses [245–247].

9.3.3.8 Microfluidics and Nanotechnology in Mass Spectrometry

Microfluidics and nanoscale technology for the formation of ions from large biomoledules have played an important role in adapting mass spectrometry (MS) for protein analysis, one of the key enabling factors for the field of proteomics [249–252]. Microfluidic chips interfaced to the sample inlet systems of mass spectrometers are excellent tools for performing complex analytical steps in the analysis of proteins, such as sample purification, digestion, and separations. They provide the ability to handle small sample quantities accurately and are adaptable to the high-throughput automation and parallel analysis from microwell plates required for the field of proteomics. Microfluidic devices for proteomic analysis can be interfaced efficiently to mass spectrometer ionization systems such as electrospray ionization and matrix-assisted laser desorption/ionization (MALDI) [253–257].

The manipulation of polarizable microdroplets over hydrophobic surfaces by electric fields bears some resemblances to the focusing of ions and charged macromolecules in mass spectrometer ion sources and quadrupole analyzers. The preparation of ions for mass analysis is a kind of three-dimensional gas-phase nanotechnology—for macromolecules the techniques are not purely chemical or electrophysical, but involve electronic and physical manipulations on the nanoscale. For example, the thermospray, electrospray, and nanospray ion sources prepare ions for mass analysis by creating tiny droplets of solution. As the droplets evaporate, the process is accelerated by charge, leading to loss of all of the solvent and leaving a bare macromolecule holding the charge that was on the droplet [258–262].

MALDI—matrix assisted laser desorption ionization—is a complex process that depends on interactions between an energy-absorbing matrix surrounding the macromolecule, which is targeted for laser photoionization, and the excited macromolecular ion. The matrix absorbs excess energy following ionization and prevents the decomposition of the macromolecule into small fragments [263–266].

Electrospray and MALDI have turned mass spectroscopy into a powerful tool for analyzing large molecules, especially proteins and DNA [267,268]. Mobilizing large biomolecules in a form suitable for mass analysis has been described as "giving wings to molecular elephants." So great was the impact of these techniques that their inventors, John Fenn and Koichi Tanaka, were recognized by a Nobel Prize award in 2002, along with Kurt Wüthrich, who developed nuclear magnetic resonance techniques for application to large biomolecules [269–272].

Since electrospray is a microfluidic technique, it is readily integrated into monolithic chips with multiple channels and sample-preparation operations, including fiber-optic UV detectors to monitor samples separated by chromatographic or electrophoretic methods. The microfluidic electrospray sources are simplified by the design of miniaturized pneumatic nebulizers driven by electroosmotic pumps, integrated directly into the chip [273–284].

MALDI is essentially a method for surface desorption with ionization by laser irradiation. The laser targets can be on thin films, microdroplets, or even tissue slices or three-dimensional gels. MALDI is adaptable with microfluidics and/or microarrays with multiple laser targets, which can be prepared on a microplate or a CD for high-throughput sampling [285–292].

Biomolecules are separated prior to mass spectral analysis by physical techniques such as two-dimensional gel electrophoresis, high-performance liquid chromatography (HPLC), capillary electrophoresis, or other advanced separations, including dielectrophoretic methods on microchips integrated with electrospray injection, or inkjet printing for the preparation of MALDI sampling plates [293–299]. Integrated microfluidic systems have been designed for interfacing with thin-film MALDI flat-surface target plates, and for sampling from microwell titer plates for automated high-throughput analysis [300–302].

9.3.3.9 Mass Spectrometry Imaging

With precise microscopic computer controls and registration with microscopy images, laser ionization techniques used with mass spectroscopy, such as MALDI, SELDI-TOF (surface-enhanced laser desorption ionization time-of-flight) MS, and laser ablation inductively coupled plasma ionization for inorganic elements, can be used to create biochemical maps of suitably prepared tissue slices (Figure 9.4). These techniques have been used to map the distribution of pharmaceuticals and to create images with quantitative biochemical information from brain slices and other tissues—powerful tools for pathology, histology, diagnosis, and basic research [303–309].

9.3.3.10 Imaging with Functional MRI

A complementary imaging technology to MS is nuclear magnetic resonance (NMR) spectroscopy, upon which medical magnetic resonance imaging (MRI) is based. Whereas MS yields information about structural units of large molecules as building blocks, NMR gives subtle information about the shape and interrelationships of atoms within the molecule. NMR and MRI are only obtainable by observing the interaction of atoms with radio frequency electromagnetic signals in the presence of strong magnetic fields, which require large and powerful magnets and sensitive electromagnetic detectors [310,311].

A number of nanotechnology-driven improvements in materials science, computer systems, and image-enhancement agents have advanced the

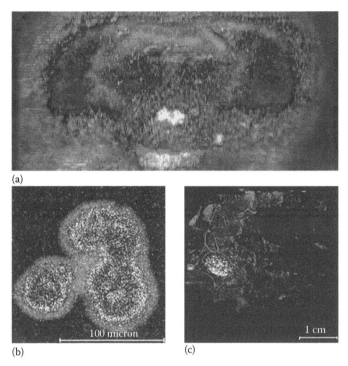

(a)

(b) 100 micron

(c) 1 cm

FIGURE 9.4
Laser microscanning mass spectrometry can be used for chemically specific imaging of tissue to give information on (a) proteomics, (b) lipidomics, and (c) drugs and metabolites. (Reprinted from Heeren, R.M. et al., *J. Am. Soc. Mass Spectrom.*, 20(6), 1006, 2008. With permission.)

capabilities of NMR and MRI. These include new high-temperature super-conducting materials for magnets, faster and higher-capacity computer system, more efficient radio frequency generators and detectors, and a number of macromolecular and nanoparticle signal–enhancement agents. MRI has advanced to the point that it can be used to distinguish molecular states and compositions in living tissues and cells, with a resolution that approaches the dimensions of tissue microstructures. This capability, called *functional MRI,* can be used to map images of electrochemical activity in the brain, observe metabolic changes in tissues, and distinguish healthy tissue from cancerous and diseased tissues [312–314].

This revolutionary capability has become well known for its use to observe physical changes in the brain in real time during mental and neuro-muscular tasks and states. It is producing new insights into the physiological and biochemical correlates of thought, emotion, memory, and learning processes. These capabilities, coupled with advances in imaging MS, take biomedical science a step closer to the ultimate goal of complete temporal and spatial information on all the species present in a heterogeneous, living biological system.

9.3.4 Summary: From Separate Sensors to Labs on Chips

The growing capabilities for miniaturization of every kind of chemical and physical measurement and manipulation have created enormous opportunities for exploring the chemical basis of life and expanding the monitoring and diagnosis of health and disease. Biochips and labs on chips are being designed and utilized for measurements, which once required large instruments and significant work time at the laboratory bench. Measurements of bodily fluids and tissues can now be done affordably and conveniently at the point of care, in the doctor's office or the local clinic. The integration of sensors on monolithic chips compresses measurement, analysis, and communication of results to deliver multiple streams of converging information [315–317].

The capability for high-throughput measurements provided by highly parallel and massively integrated measurements is needed in order to deal with the enormous amount of simultaneous complex information presented by biological networks. For the first time, highly integrated sensors give at least a start toward being able to analyze living systems. Whether we look at genes, proteins, or physiology, we find that only by measuring and analyzing large numbers of parallel inputs, interacting with each other, can we obtain a realistic picture of the symbiotic networks that support health and whose malfunctions create diseases and disorders [318–321].

9.4 Technologies for Genomics and Proteomics

In this section, we will look at how integrated sensors are being used to create new fields of genomics and proteomics. These fields have emerged as the capabilities provided by high-throughput analysis of genes and proteins are laying the foundations for personalized medicine.

9.4.1 Genomics, Proteomics, and Personalized Medicine

One of the most important measurements that we can make in biology is to determine a sequence for DNA. Whether for a human or a disease bacterium, the DNA sequence holds a great deal of information about the organism—including its strengths and weaknesses with regard to certain diseases. We know that DNA does not tell us everything. There are epigenetic and environmental factors that play important roles in our makeup and health. But DNA and the genome are very important in telling some unique things about how our bodies are programmed [322–324].

DNA can tell whether we are vulnerable to certain kinds of diseases, and not just congenital diseases. The onset and progression of cancer is related to the genetic programming of our cells in subtle and complex ways that interact with environmental factors. We are learning how vulnerabilities to certain cancers are related to our genetic makeup, and why some treatments can be expected to depend on that makeup [325–327].

If we are fighting a disease like cancer, which involves a problem in the programming of some of our cells, it could be important to know more about that specific program. That turns out to be the case—there are many kinds of cancer, each characterized by different programming disorders that turn genes on or off, or up- or down-regulate certain genes, turning a normal cell into a wildly multiplying cancer cell. Depending on the type of cancer and the genes of the individual, some types of chemotherapy or radiation treatments will work well on that individual, and not work at all on another with different genetic makeup, because the therapy is targeting certain pathways in the metabolism of the cell. Whether the therapy can effectively block the growth of cancer cells may depend on whether a particular version of a gene can be up- or down-regulated by the therapy. Research in these areas is termed *genomics*, with particular focus on the interaction between drugs, disease, and genes in the area called *pharmocogenomics* [328–333].

Because of the importance of genetic makeup to the outcome of serious diseases like cancer, the concept of personalized medicine has been developed. Personalized medicine takes the approach that therapy should be specifically designed for each patient based on knowledge of their genetic profile. Progress in characterizing the human genome, with efforts like the Human Genome Project and the HapMap Consortium, has provided the knowledge and tools to make personalized medicine a possibility. Based on some important demonstrations of effectiveness, this emerging concept is beginning to gain ground. Efforts are continuing to gather and manage extensive representative data on human genomic and phenotypic variability, for a necessary knowledge base on which personalized nutrition and medicine can be built [334–340].

To be meaningful in practice, personalized medicine must have two capabilities: the ability to read the genetic code of an individual and the ability to formulate customized therapies. It is in providing these capabilities that nanotechnology comes into the clinical picture.

9.4.1.1 Gene Amplification—A Basic Technique for DNA Measurement

The standard way of amplifying a small amount of DNA so that a sequence can be made is by a cyclical reaction technique, the polymerase chain reaction (PCR). A single strand of DNA can serve as a template for the reproduction of its complementary copy, with the aid of an enzyme (DNA polymerase) and suitable base components as building blocks (nucleoside triphosphates).

In the thermocycled PCR reaction, a single strand of primer DNA is allowed to replicate repeatedly in a medium of base components and replication enzymes. The reaction is repeated through temperature cycles that cause the DNA chains to be replicated and separate, doubling the amount of DNA on each cycle [341,342].

New DNA-amplification techniques have been developed and refined in recent years to permit faster amplification without the necessity of repeated heating and cooling cycles. These isothermal gene-amplification methods (loop mediated, rolling circle, ramification amplification, etc.) have become faster and less expensive than standard PCR [343–348]. One of the first isothermal replication methods to be discovered uses a DNA repair enzyme from bacteria to drive the replication process by cleaving the primer DNA in a manner that lets the DNA polymerase initiate the addition of nucleotides to create a complementary strand [349].

Both thermocycling and isothermal DNA-replication techniques have been refined by implementation on biochips, including chips with picoliter droplet–sized reaction samples [350–352].

Another refinement is the incorporation of real-time fluorescent or other indicators to monitor the reaction. This makes PCR a useful technique for detecting selected DNA markers [353,354]. It is very desirable to have an optical indicator that gives an intensity reading to quantitatively identify the amplified DNA. So-called *real-time PCR* techniques use optical indicators that are amplified along with the DNA to give a direct measure of DNA amplification. The color or light signal is specific and quantitative to the extent that the indicators are linked to the DNA strand being amplified. Optical indication systems designed for use with thermocycling PCR are, in general, not suitable for isothermal DNA amplification. Optical indicators used in thermocycling include systems known as TaqMan® and molecular beacons, which are molecularly engineered nucleic acids [355].

Special optical amplifiers have to be designed for isothermal amplification for specificity, sensitivity, cost effectiveness, and ease of use. A system called "Molecular Zipper" amplifies a fluorescent probe along with DNA in isothermal systems. This system uses a fluorometer with an optical excitation source in order to observe and measure the amplified signal [356]. Other optical probes for measuring isothermal amplification have been developed, including nanoparticle quantum dots. One approach to quantifying amplified DNA would be to amplify a chemiluminescent indicator that could be measured with a luminometer instead of a fluorometer.

Other methods for quantifying isothermal DNA amplification include measuring the buildup of by-product pyrophosphate ions, which react with $Mg2+$ ions to form the insoluble product magnesium pyrophosphate. A measure of DNA amplification can be obtained by measuring the $Mg2+$ ion concentration electrochemically or by measuring turbidity due to the insoluble precipitate. A simple colorimetric assay complexes the $Mg2+$ ion with calcein, which gives a fluorescent complex with magnesium ion. A similar but improved assay uses hydroxy naphthol blue, which is less likely to interfere with the replication or give a fluorescent signal with by-products [357].

9.4.1.2 Technology for DNA Sequencing

The technology for determining DNA sequences has progressed rapidly, aided by the application of advances in miniaturized automation. A few decades ago, determining a DNA sequence required many months of painstaking work at the lab bench. Within the past few years, the process has been accelerated as the cost has fallen drastically. High-throughput single-molecule analysis based on nanosensors packed into microarrays for parallel sensing and reporting have brought the cost down toward the goal of three dollars or less per base pair.

A number of innovative nanoscale technologies have been applied to the sequencing of DNA, during the push to decode the human genome that began in the 1990s. These include capillary electrophoresis with polyacrylamide solutions, by means of which rapid sequencing of more than 1000 bases per run was demonstrated [358]. Also, capillary electrophoresis microchips were fabricated for DNA sequencing [359].

Another approach developed during the 1990s used DNA sequencing chips for combinatoric matching based on thousands of sequences, fabricated by light-directed synthesis. This technique enables massively parallel gene expression and gene discovery studies. In this method, arrays of immobilized DNA or oligonucleotides are fabricated by high-speed robotics on glass or nylon substrates; then labeled probes are used to determine complementary bindings. Sample DNA is amplified by PCR, and a fluorescent label is inserted and hybridized to the microarray. This technology was widely applied to the simultaneous expression of many thousands of genes for large-scale gene discovery, as well as polymorphism screening and mapping of genomic DNA clones [360–362].

The reconstruction of a complete genome by combinatoric matching of short peptide sequences is known as *shotgun sequencing by hybridization*. The basic approach is to match an array of short DNA fragment strings with complementary strings of the same length on an unknown DNA fragment. Combinatorial algorithms can then reconstruct the sequence of the unknown fragment by finding consistent matches from overlapping strings [363–366].

Using these approaches, advances have continued with miniaturization, faster processing, fewer errors, and lower costs for DNA sequencing, based on microfabrication of devices and improvements in strategies and algorithms [367–371]. Sequencing can be performed using MALDI MS; the sequence read lengths attainable by mass spectral methods are not sufficient for large-scale sequencing of unknown DNA, but the technique is ideal for re-sequencing to verify results from other methods. Compared to most conventional methods, MS can produce high resolution of sequence fragments and rapid separations on microsecond time scales. For this reason, MS sequencing has been used to screen for mutations and single nucleotide polymorphisms (SNPs). Assays have also been developed to indirectly sequence DNA by first generating

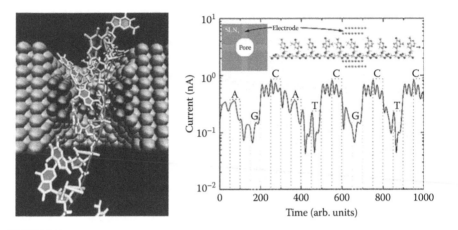

FIGURE 9.5
A new technique for DNA sequencing threads a strand of DNA through a carbon nanopore, measuring differences in electronic affinity among the four DNA bases. (From Lagerqvist, J. et al., *Nano Lett.*, 6(4), 779. With permission.)

the corresponding RNA, to take advantage of the increased resolution and detection ability of MALDI time of flight MS for RNA [372,373].

More recently, a new generation of DNA sequencing approaches has been developed, including single-molecule methods. One method uses functionalized carbon nanowires; as the DNA strand is passed over the nanowires, conductivity differences between different bases can be measured, allowing an intact strand to be decoded sequentially [374]. Another technique passes the DNA strand through a functionalized carbon nanopore of precise dimensions, so that the differences in electrical potential created by interactions with the four different DNA bases can be distinguished (Figure 9.5) [375]. New methods and refinements continue to be developed, with improvements in both devices and computational methods [121–126,376–378].

Development of these new high-throughput sequencing instruments is a very active area, marked by a flurry of start-up companies with mergers and acquisitions by major players with some of the most innovative technology solutions. Examples of a few highlights of this activity are as follows: In 2007, Roche acquired the NimbleGen Systems, Inc.; Invitrogen acquired VisiGen Biotechnologies, Inc. in 2008; more than 30 major mergers and acquisitions involving sequencing and proteomics companies took place in recent years (through 2009) [379]. As usual in the early stages, having an innovative technology was not the only criteria for survival in the marketplace [380].

From among the more than 30 large and small companies developing gene sequencing instrumentation, here are a few examples. Founded in 2000, the company 454 Life Sciences has developed an innovative Genome Sequencer™ system for ultra-high- throughput DNA sequencing that uses chemiluminescence in gene array chips to generate 400 million high-quality base results per 10 hr instrument run.

Raindance Technologies, founded in 2004, uses a combination of micro-droplets and microfluidic systems to create digital packets of chemical information called NanoReactors™. Like a computer manipulating bits of information, the PLS enables the programmable handling of cells and fluid samples for innovative assay and screening applications.

Ion Torrent Systems is another new company that is developing disruptive massively parallel technology for high-throughput, low-cost, rapid DNA sequencing. Pacific Biosciences of California is developing a DNA sequencer chip called SMRT (single-molecule, real-time) with the goal of sequencing an entire human genome in 15 min by 2013, using a shotgun process with libraries of very long strings.

Larger established companies such as GE Medical, Packard Biosciences, Siemens, and others are also developing and acquiring competitive DNA-sequencing methods. In general, sequencing technologies have been exhibiting a Moore's law trajectory, reducing the time and cost of genome decoding by about half every 18 months.

As the speed and cost of DNA sequencing fall, personalized medicine is becoming a reality. The NIH and many academic centers are developing the concept and tools, compiling data, and studying how best to implement personalized medicine and validate the efficiency of any given procedure.

9.4.1.3 Genetic Screening and Genomic Medicine

As libraries of completed human genomes and polymorphisms are accumulating, the knowledge about relationships between genes, diseases, and therapies is being gathered as well. It is not necessary to completely sequence an individual genome to obtain much information that is relevant to health and disease—panels of sample DNA sequences can provide selected information focused on diseases or conditions. Many variations found in the human genome involve a single base substitution—single gene microchips with complementary DNA sequences that have been found to have significance can be used to screen for matches in samples taken from healthy and diseased tissues. This creates a huge potential for medical applications, in diagnostics, the development of drugs, and personalized medicine [330–334,366–369,381–383]. Gene array chips can be mass produced to screen for disease markers and SNPs. MALDI MS and capillary or microdrop electrophoresis can be used in laboratories to read and characterize extremely small samples separated and selected on chip targets for diagnoses.

Major pharmaceutical companies and start-ups are assessing and preparing for opportunities in custom personalized therapies; a Personalized Medicine Coalition has been formed. Clinics like Brigham and Women's Hospital in Boston, and the Mary Crowley Medical Center in Dallas pioneered personalized medicine for cancer patients in translating the protocols into practice. At these and other centers, DNA sequencing is performed at the beginning of every cancer patient's care. The sequencing of normal as well as cancer cells provides information on what genetic pathways are deregulated and helps to target therapies. A number of new customized therapies are being produced, based on the new genetic knowledge, by both start-up and established pharmaceutical and biotechnology companies [384–386]. The genomics-based personalized medicine paradigm is being applied to many other complex multifactor diseases besides cancer. At the same time, the proteome—information about the proteins that are produced by genetic programming—is proving valuable for diagnosis and therapy along with the genome.

As more understanding of genomics and proteomics is gained, increasing attention is being paid to *epigenetics*, the study of the factors through which genetic information is expressed across the varied developmental stages, tissue types, and disease states. Epigenetics deals with chemical modifications to DNA and their supporting histone proteins, which form a complex regulatory network that modulates genome functions. The complete description of these potentially heritable changes across the genome is called the *epigenome* [387].

Growing evidence from studies based on molecular biosensing and systematic genomics and proteomics suggests that acquired epigenetic abnormalities participate with genetic alterations to cause complex diseases such as cancer. Advances in knowledge of epigenetics should contribute toward the development of new strategies to control many types of cancer as well as autoimmune and degenerative diseases [388].

9.4.2 Analyzing the Proteome

The proteins, which are produced by RNA transcribed from the genetic code in DNA, are a much more direct indicator of the status of a cell's metabolism than the genes themselves. The same nanotechnologies that allow the detection and characterization of the genome are equally applicable to the analysis of proteins. Proteomics, the knowledge of the proteins and their status in the organism, and genomics, the knowledge of the DNA and genes, are complementary—each is much more meaningful and valuable when used in conjunction with the other [318,389–391].

The emergence of proteomics comes from the growing base of DNA sequence information and new analysis technologies. The proteomics field has been fed by a range of new methods for determining protein localization, protein–protein interactions, posttranslational modifications, and the alteration of protein composition (e.g., differential expression) in tissues and body fluids. Protein analysis is used to characterize gene function, to understand functional relationships between protein molecules, and to provide insight into the mechanisms of complex biological process networks. High throughput techniques such as yeast two-hybrid analysis and affinity tag purification are used to build protein–protein interaction maps. Large-scale protein tagging with subcellular-specific localization provides information about protein function in the cell, and for intercell signaling. MS has emerged as a powerful tool for the analysis of protein complexes. Recent developments in protein microarray technology provide versatile tools for analysis of protein–protein, protein–nucleic acid, protein–lipid, enzyme–substrate, and protein–drug interactions [392–395].

Proteomics is potentially much more complex than genomics—and certainly involves many more types of biomolecules and molecular structures and interactions. The volume of information obtainable with protein analysis requires sophisticated attention to data management and informatics analysis to extract the most useful information [396–398].

Other types of microarrays and portable instruments are being developed for diagnostics, protein profiling, and drug identification and validation [399–401]. Protein profiling of easily obtainable body fluids such as saliva can potentially lead to the discovery of disease markers and health indicators for diagnosis and prognosis—for example, indicators of likelihood of cancers or preterm births [402–405].

9.4.2.1 Protein Analysis by Mass Spectrometry

Following on the early work and insights of pioneers like Klaus Biemann and Fred MacLafferty, MS has been developed into a leading method for protein analysis by a number of research groups, notably those of Mattias Mann and colleagues [406–409]. MS is currently the most powerful method for protein identification, due largely to rapid advances in instrumentation capability and automation, and the exponential increase in computing power over past decades.

MS is used in proteomics for the identification of individual proteins from a mixture, the quantification of proteins in a cell or organism and the characterization of proteins' composition and structure. The identification of all the proteins in a cell or organism is often a daunting task and poses a challenge even in the case of simple bacteria. Tandem mass analysis is especially effective in distinguishing mixtures of many proteins of similar mass. Ion-trap mass spectrometers represent the state of the art in protein identification research, with techniques such as ion storage for accumulating ions from low-intensity samples prior to mass analysis. Modern instruments have sophisticated digitally controlled radio frequency and magnetic scanning to ionize biomolecules and accumulate them into the ion trap before selecting specific masses for analysis and detection. MALDI or other laser-desorption methods are the most effective for ionization [410–413].

Extensive high-throughput studies are being carried out with the aid of mass spectrometers, to characterize proteins at all levels, starting from their primary structure through studying protein–protein interactions, for basic biomedical research, drug discovery, and clinical diagnostics [414–416].

9.4.2.2 Protein Analysis Array BioChips

Microarray technology has come into applications for proteins as well as DNA and RNA, and is key to the implementation of a number of large-scale and high-throughput characterizations. Although automation for the production and reading of protein microchips is not as far developed as it is for genomics, many automated systems exist. Some systems produce protein microarrays by microprinting as the output of separation methods, and the array media are designed for interrogation by MS or laser spectroscopy, which can utilize extremely small samples with excellent detection limits [292,417–419].

Because they allow easy and parallel detection of thousands of addressable elements in a single experiment, they are an essential tool to meet the demands of high-volume analysis of antibody–antigen, protein–protein, protein–nucleic acid, protein–lipid, and protein–small-molecule interactions, as well as enzyme–substrate interactions. Protein analysis biochips have been developed for testing unknown samples of serum, body fluids, or other biological materials against panels of known protein antibodies, and similar types of protein–protein interaction analysis [420–422].

The essential technologies that underlie protein biochips are being aided by nanotechnology, including surface chemistry, capture molecule attachment, protein labeling and detection methods, high throughput protein/antibody production, and computerized robotic automation to analyze entire proteomes. Bottlenecks that are recognized in protein microarray development include protein instability, nonspecific interactions, lack of amplification techniques for lower abundance proteins, and the availability of purified high-affinity probes. Promising approaches for high-volume fabrication of probes include single-chain antibodies displayed on phage protein coats, protein–oligonucleotide conjugates, and aptamers. Widespread and routine biomedical and diagnostic applications will depend upon technological developments to increase sensitivity, improve specificity, and reduce costs [423–426].

Protein arrays have been of high interest recently for use in verifying the results of mRNA expression studies, in serum profiling, in the discovery of biomarkers, and in cell physiology studies. In cancer applications, antibody arrays have been developed for oncoproteomic profiling, and protein microarrays of cloned tumor antigens have been developed for the discovery of tumor antibody biomarkers [427–429].

9.4.3 The Metabolome: The Emerging Concept of Metabolomics

High-throughput MS and array technologies provide a powerful means to analyze diverse mixtures of complex biomolecules with high sensitivity and selectivity. These methods make it possible to characterize a biological system by means of global and nontargeted metabolite profiling. As a result, the concept of the *metabolome*—the comprehensive set of all molecular products of cell metabolism present in an organism—can become a concrete measurable entity, rather than an abstraction. This introduces a new level of chemical information in addition to the genome and proteome. In general, the metabolome is made up of smaller and simpler molecules than the macromolecules that produce and regulate it: metabolites, metabolic intermediates, hormones, signaling molecules, and by-products of metabolism. The variability in forms and concentrations is immense. The accurate measurement of the complete metabolome varying over time is attainable only within limited scopes, but new high-throughput analysis technologies at least allow an approach to that goal [430].

The metabolome is important because it is the most definitive characterization of the individual phenotype; at any given time, metabolites are an ultimate product of the actions of genes, mRNA, and proteins. There are a growing number of metabolomics research efforts aimed at finding biomarkers, which could assist diagnosis, provide therapy guidance, and evaluate response to therapy for particular diseases. Metabolics is emerging as a powerful concept and tool for the fields of drug discovery, drug toxicology, and personalized pharmacology. In pharmacology, metabalomic studies extend the concepts of pharmacokinetics and pharmacodynamics to include the effects of drugs on metabolism as well as the fate of the drugs themselves. In diagnostics, metabolomic biomarkers have been found related to neurological, cardiovascular, and cancer diseases [431].

It is not possible to characterize a complete metabolome by means of a single analytical method, but MS, because of its sensitivity and selectivity, has become the major method for characterizing the human metabolome. Mass spectroscopy–based metabolomics is being used to characterize the complex metabolic effects of nutrients and food components, as well as the effects of drugs and diseases on the body. Recently, a team of scientists at the University of Alberta and the University of Calgary released a comprehensive human metabolomic database [432].

The same analytical and informatics capabilities that make it possible to realize the genome, proteome, and metabolome have also led to the concepts of the *transcriptome, signalosome,* and other constructs for the systematic study of the complexities of biology.

9.5 Applied Genomics and Proteomics: From Personalized Medicine to Global Epidemiology

The availability of immense new volumes of information about the genome, proteome, and metabolome—the new *biodata*—is having an impact on medicine, as seen with the emerging concept of personalized medicine. Translating the new knowledge to useful medical practice is a challenge. The disciplined organization, integration, and analysis of the large volume of information coming from the new analytical capabilities has been taken on by the field of *systems biology*. Systems biology utilizes the mathematical and organizational tools of informatics to analyze the patterns of complex regulatory pathways revealed in the *biodata* to obtain meaningful information that guides the diagnoses and therapies that implement personalized medicine [433,434].

9.5.1 Systems Biology

Systems biology seeks to elucidate how biological function arises from the interactions of biological macromolecules: "Its main focus is to understand in quantitative, predictable ways the regulation of complex cellular pathways and of intercellular communication so as to shed light on complex biological functions (e.g., metabolism, cell signaling, cell cycle, apoptosis, differentiation, and transformation.) It is for lack of achieving this understanding of living systems that the existing paradigms for biomedical research fail for the majority of diseases on the Northern Hemisphere. Systems Biology appears appropriate for these complex and multifunctional diseases" [435].

In practice, systems biology involves database management, the orderly and accurate management of what would appear to be unmanageable volumes of information, constantly being updated and growing in volume and detail. To accomplish this, mastery of the disciplines of computing science and informatics is required. Computation techniques for pattern matching, correlations from array matches, the extraction of significance from data, data mining, and data representation, and information presentation for human comprehension are all significant aspects of systems biology. But most important is the comprehension of the biology itself—understanding the patterns and pathways behind the data. These patterns are the biological circuits and networks by which health is regulated, and whose malfunctions represent disease [436–438].

Systems biology integrates and analyzes information from genomics, proteomics, and metabolomics to find discriminating signals that will be useful in predicting the course of diseases, managing health, and discovering therapies [439–441].

9.5.2 Genomics, Proteomics, and Cancer

Cancer, as one of the most complex, frequent, and intractable diseases, has been a focus for the application of systems biology. In practice, systems biology compares large amounts of data obtained from genetic, protein, and metabolite profiles obtained with high-throughput analysis techniques such as biochips and MS. Correlations and patterns are sought, to identify which genes, expression networks, or metabolic pathways are amplified or suppressed (up-regulated, down-regulated, or turned off, etc.) in diseased and normal states of cells. These correlations can be recognized by the human eye and brain as patterns in gene chips with color-coded readouts, and confirmed by mathematical pattern recognition and statistical correlations [442–445].

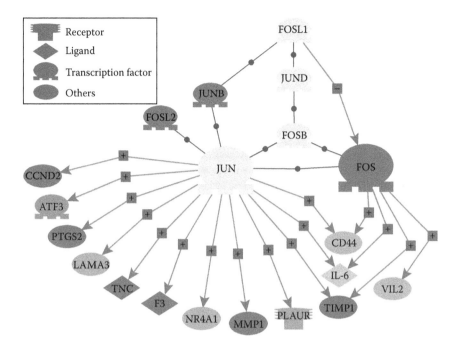

FIGURE 9.6

Gene networks of activator protein 1 (AP-1) transcription factors in the progenitor signature hepatocellular carcinoma (HCC) liver cells. Lines with boxes and arrows represent the direction of transcriptional regulation, and the plus and minus signs indicate positive and negative regulations of gene expression. Purple lines represent known physical interactions between connected genes [442]. (Adapted from Lee J.-S. and Thorgeirsson, S. S., Application of integrative functional genomics to decode cancer signatures, NIH/CCR Web site at: http://ccr.cancer.gov/news/frontiers/september2006/thorgeirsson_fig2.asp. With permission.)

Based on the knowledge of the biochemistry involved in the pathways, therapies can be designed to counteract the mis-regulation associated with the disease. The pathways involved are complex, as shown by the example of gene regulation in a partial pathway involved in a particular type of cancer of the liver (Figure 9.6).

Data used to search for tumor markers is gathered using the MS and biochip techniques reviewed earlier [446–450]. Chips are used to measure gene expression, proteins, and metabolites and design patient-tailored therapy based on the findings [331,445,451–455].

9.5.3 Genomics, Proteomics, and Immunology

Another important application for genomics and proteomics is the matching of tissues for transplantation. The better the match between donor and recipient tissues, the lower will be the immune rejection activity. The methods discussed earlier for comparing genes and protein expression between tissues provide the means for the detailed evaluation of transplant candidate tissues to a degree previously not available [456]. Metabolomic comparison for transplantation evaluations is a newly emerging area [457].

9.5.4 Personalized Medicine for Complex Multigenomic Disorders

Genomic, proteomic, and metabolomic profiling are being translated from research into clinical practice for cancer and a number of other complex diseases and disorders [458–460]. Studies are being conducted to improve human nutrition, and understand the susceptibilities of different human genotypes to various disorders, which could be avoided with nutrition better adapted to the individual metabolism. MS techniques, because of their sensitivity and selectivity, have become methods of choice to characterize the human metabolome, and MS-based metabolomics is increasingly used to characterize the complex metabolic effects of nutrients as well as drugs and disease agents. The understanding of the interactions of metabolome, proteome, and genome could have implications for the prevention of heart and vascular diseases, asthma, diabetes, arthritis, certain dermalogical conditions, and other degenerative and autoimmune diseases, as well as their treatment [461–470].

A rapidly expanding list of noninvasive diagnostic tests is being produced from genomic and proteomic biomarker research, for conditions including inflammatory bowel disease, chronic kidney disease, wound healing and inflammation, and macular degeneration [471–474]. These diagnostic tests provide new means of objective assessments of disease activity, early diagnosis, prognosis evaluation, surveillance, and management.

Protein glycosylation regulates protein function and cellular distribution, and aberrant protein glycosylations play a role in many human disorders, including neurodegenerative diseases. Using proteomics to systematically characterize the complex mixture of glycopeptides and glycoproteins in body fluids has great potential for finding diagnostic and prognostic markers. The application of MS-based profiling to the study of neurodegenerative disorders (e.g., Alzheimer's disease and Parkinson's disease) could discover biomarkers and provide insight into the biochemical pathogenesis of neurodegeneration [475].

Systems biology is being applied to a number of mental and developmental disorders. Genomic and proteomic profiling and pharmacogenomics are being used to develop personalized medical treatment for schizophrenia [476]. Systems biology has revealed associations between GABA receptor genes and anxiety spectrum disorders [477]. Translational systems biology is being applied to the understanding and treatment of voice pathophysiology [478], and metabolomics is being analyzed for small molecule signatures of motor neuron diseases such as ALS [479].

A number of studies are being conducted to identify and evaluate potential biomarkers for preterm birth, from the analysis of body fluids of mother and fetus [480–482]. These could have a significant medical impact in preventing and managing the occurrence of spontaneous preterm birth and its associated health and economic liabilities [483].

Another major area of impact for systems biology is in the development of vaccines [484]. Systems biology has the potential for producing effective personalized vaccines against cancers. A number of research tests and trials are underway for vaccines against renal cell carcinoma, advanced gastric and colorectal carcinoma, and pancreatic cancer [485–487].

9.5.5 Monitoring for Disease

Complex degenerative conditions are not the only diseases for which the new ability to monitor changes in DNA can prove vital. More effective vaccines and drugs against disease pathogens can be produced more quickly by profiling the systems biology of the disease-causing organisms, as well as their potential hosts [488,489]. Around the world, bacteria such as the pathogen for tuberculosis and pathogens such as the malaria parasite are evolving and adapting to overwhelm the antibiotics and drugs, which we have come to depend upon. It is becoming a matter of great importance to monitor the genomes of these disease organisms in order to be aware of the nature and extent of their threat, and to prepare research to develop new antibiotics and other countermeasures.

The new field of *metagenomics* is the study of bacteria and other microorganisms by the analysis of their genomes. This field is producing more effective vaccines, diagnostics, and is discovering new antibiotics and enzymes through the screening and analysis of the genomes of organisms that cannot be cultured [490–492].

New, simple, inexpensive, rugged, and fast methods for rapidly identifying and characterizing massively antibiotic resistant disease organisms are needed, and are being developed to stave off the return of once prevalent contagions. Advances have been made in MEMS and nanosensors based on molecular recognition and surface plasmon detection, using molecular biomarkers developed from genomic and proteomic analysis [493–495]. Easy to use microfluidic diagnostics based on molecular markers can provide highly sensitive and selective diagnoses [496,497]. Inexpensive, disposable microfluidic devices are especially useful in disease monitoring, which must be conducted away from well-equipped clinical laboratories [498,499]. Another key technology for fighting global disease is isothermal gene amplification, which is simpler than traditional PCR and more appropriate for use in developing countries [500–502].

9.6 Real-Time and In Vivo Medical Monitoring

In addition to monitoring the traditional vital signs, new nanosensor technology makes possible patient monitoring by genomics, proteomics, and metabolomics.

9.6.1 Patient Monitoring in Clinic and Hospital

Microfluidics is reducing the cost and complexity of many clinical monitoring tests, and allowing testing to be brought closer to the point of care [503–506]. A number of minimally invasive glucose sensors are being developed based on MEMS [506–511]. Advanced wireless biosensors are beginning to replace wired monitors for critical care and hospital recovery monitoring [512–514]. Current sensor capabilities have the potential to reduce the number of wires attached to the patient, reducing clutter in critical care areas, eliminating accidental catching and disconnecting of wires from patients to monitors, and reducing the risk of infection and mis-attachments. The minimization of wiring also makes it easier for the patient to move or be moved by attendants. Obstacles remaining are the standardization of wireless communication frequencies and protocols to enable multiple types of devices to be monitored by a single simple controller and data-collection system. These interoperability issues are being worked out by the FDA and a number of other organizations and developers. Attention is being given to reducing risks of wireless interference with critical devices; one strategy is to utilize advanced agile frequency and error-correction protocols for assured and secure data communication. These protocol technologies are available for transfer from other fields in data communication.

9.6.2 Personal Monitoring

Cancer and virulent diseases are high priorities for personalized medicine based on DNA. But simpler forms of personal monitoring could also have a huge impact on health. The shrinking costs and exponentially growing capabilities of microelectronics are placing highly sophisticated personal devices—augmented cell phones and digital assistants—within reach of people all over the world. The same technology drivers are bringing high-speed wireless communications with further and deeper coverage [515,516].

Personal wireless electronic devices have the potential to become highly capable medical monitors, tracking physiological and chemical parameters such as pulse, temperature, blood sugar, adherence to medications and/or exercise and routine. The level of monitoring and the degree of communication with a healthcare base such as a clinic or a hospital would vary depending on the health situation of the individual. It is a matter of time, and of the establishment of intercommunicating standards for interfacing mass-produced sensors to cell phones and personal digital devices, before the spread of health monitoring, and healthcare, goes beyond any one location, and becomes mobile with the patient.

Such monitoring could reduce healthcare risks and costs by catching health disorders in vulnerable persons before the status reaches a critical stage, by reducing the risks of leaving the hospital early after treatment, by reducing the number and frequency of follow-up visits for testing and monitoring recovery, and by smarter and more efficient scheduling and staging of hospital visits for noncritical care, such as childbirth, checkups, and preventive therapies.

The technologies for building these mobile monitoring capabilities already exist. It is a matter of economics and implementation for mobile medical monitoring to come into widespread use. Military projects are currently developing sensors that will report on the condition of soldiers in response to fatigue or wounds.

A number of advanced research projects are developing wearable sensors and smart fabric clothing to provide various types of continuous monitoring. Several such systems include communication capabilities to alert the wearer to reduce strenuous activity, for example, or to automatically alert healthcare givers of a serious change or trend in physiological signs. Some of the most sophisticated nano-engineered smart fabrics include combinations of hydrophobic and hydrophilic surfaces in channels to guide perspiration passively toward sensors without the need for an active pump mechanism. This biomimetic design is borrowed from the capabilities found in a number of insects with the ability to harvest water from the atmosphere.

9.7 Conclusion

Nanotechnology-based biosensors in many forms are impacting medicine both directly and indirectly by providing advances in diagnosis, and by underlying the advance of personalized medicine and home-based patient-centered monitoring. As a result, the advance of sensor technology, including DNA analysis, could have the most profound effects on medicine of any of the medical nanotechnologies that we have reviewed.

References

1. D. Ho, A. O. Fung, and C. D. Montemagno, Engineering novel diagnostic modalities and implantable cytomimetic nanomaterials for next-generation medicine, *Biology of Blood and Marrow Transplantation*, 12, 92–99 (2006).
2. G. L. Hornyak, H. F. Tibbals, J. Dutta, and J. J. Moore, *Introduction to Nanoscience and Nanotechnology*, CRC Press, Boca Raton, FL, 2009.
3. H. G. Craighead, Nanoelectromechanical systems, *Science*, 290, 1532–1535 (2000).
4. R. S. Greco, F. B. Prinz, and R. L. Smith (eds.), *Nanoscale Technology in Biological Systems*, CRC Press, Boca Raton FL, 2004.

5. M. Ferrari, A. P. Lee, and L. J. Lee, *BioMEMS and Biomedical Nanotechnology: Volume I Biological and Biomedical Nanotechnology*, Springer, New York, 2006.

6. W. Wang and S. Soper, *Bio-MEMS: Technologies and Applications*, CRC Press, Boca Raton, FL, 2007.

7. N. A. Peppas and M. E. Byrne, New biomaterials for intelligent biosensing, recognitive drug delivery and therapeutics, *Bulletin Technique Gattefossé*, 96, 23–35 (2003).

8. T. Vo-Dinh (ed.), *Nanotechnology in Biology and Medicine: Methods, Devices and Applications*, CRC Press, Boca Raton, FL, 2007.

9. A. N. Reshetilov and A. M. Bezborodov, Nanobiotechnology and biosensor research—in Russian, *Prikladnaia Biokhimiia Mikrobiologiia*, 44, 3–8 (2008).

10. K. K. Jain, Current status of molecular biosensors, *Medical Device Technology*, 14, 10–15 (2003).

11. S. Kurkela and D. W. G. Brown, Molecular diagnostic techniques, *Medicine*, 37, 535–540 (2009).

12. G. P. Patrinos and W. J. Ansorge, *Molecular Diagnostics*, 2nd. edn., Elsevier, Amsterdam, the Netherlands, 2010.

13. R. Cao, R. Villalonga, and A. Fragoso, Towards nanomedicine with a supramolecular approach: A review, *IEEE Proceedings—Nanobiotechnology*, 152, 159–164 (2005).

14. M. J. Schulz, A. D. Kelkar, and M. J. Sundaresan, *Nanoengineering of Structural, Functional and Smart Materials*, CRC Press, Boca Raton, FL, 2005.

15. C. Alexander, H. S. Andersson, L. I. Andersson, R. J. Ansell, N. Kirsch, I. A. Nicholls, J. O'Mahony, and M. J. Whitcombe, Molecular imprinting science and technology: A survey of the literature for the years up to and including 2003, *Journal of Molecular Recognition*, 19, 106–180 (2006).

16. G. A. Ozin, A. C. Arsenault, and L. Cademartiri, *Nanochemistry: A Chemical Approach to Nanomaterials*, RSC Publishing, Cambridge, U.K., 2008.

17. X. Wang, L. H. Liu, O. Ramström, and M. Yan, Engineering nanomaterial surfaces for biomedical applications, *Experimental Biology and Medicine*, 234, 1128–1139 (2009).

18. Q. Xu, R. M. Rioux, and G. M. Whitesides, Fabrication of complex metallic nanostructures by nanoskiving, *ACS Nano*, 1, 215–227 (2007).

19. A. R. Tao, J. Huang, and P. Yang, Langmuir–Blodgettry of nanocrystals and nanowires, *Accounts of Chemical Research*, 41, 1662–1673 (2008).

20. J. D. Zahn, D. Trebotich, and D. Liepmann, Microdialysis microneedles for continuous medical monitoring, *Biomedical Microdevices*, 7, 59–69 (2005).

21. P. Skládal, C. dos Santos Riccardi, H. Yamanaka, and P. I. da Costa, Piezoelectric biosensors for real-time monitoring of hybridization and detection of hepatitis C virus, *Journal of Virological Methods*, 117, 145–151 (2004).

22. S. Tombelli, M. Minunni, and M. Mascini, Piezoelectric biosensors: Strategies for coupling nucleic acids to piezoelectric devices, *Methods*, 37, 48–56 (2005).

23. R. Fogel, P. Mashazi, T. Nyokong, and J. Limson, Critical assessment of the Quartz Crystal Microbalance with Dissipation as an analytical tool for biosensor development and fundamental studies: Metallophthalocyanine-glucose oxidase biocomposite sensors, *Biosensors and Bioelectronics*, 23, 95–101 (2007).

24. S. Tombelli, A. Bini, M. Minunni, and M. Mascini, Piezoelectric biosensors for aptamer-protein interaction, *Methods in Molecular Biology*, 504, 23–36 (2009).

25. E. R. Hirst, Y. J. Yuan, W. L. Xu, and J. E. Bronlund, Bond-rupture immunosensors—A review, *Biosensors and Bioelectronics*, 23, 1759–1768 (2008).

26. P. Skládal, Piezoelectric quartz crystal resonators applied for immunosensing and affinity interaction studies, *Methods in Molecular Biology*, 504, 37–50 (2009).
27. H. Shi and J. I. Yeh, Part I: Recent developments in nanoelectrodes for biological measurements, *Nanomedicine*, 2, 587–598 (2007).
28. H. Shi, T. Xia, A. E. Nel, and J. I. Yeh, Part II: Coordinated biosensors—Development of enhanced nanobiosensors for biological and medical applications, *Nanomedicine*, 2, 599–614 (2007).
29. J. Guo and E. Lindner, Cyclic voltammograms at coplanar and shallow recessed microdisk electrode arrays: Guidelines for design and experiment, *Analytical Chemistry*, 81, 130–138 (2009).
30. A. Fang, H. T. Ng, and S. F. Li, A high-performance glucose biosensor based on monomolecular layer of glucose oxidase covalently immobilised on indium-tin oxide surface. *Biosensors and Bioelectronics*, 19, 43–49 (2003).
31. Z. Lin, Y. Takahashi, Y. Kitagawa, T. Umemura, H. Shiku, and T. Matsue, An addressable microelectrode array for electrochemical detection, *Analytical Chemistry*, 80, 6830–6833 (2008).
32. X. J. Huang, R. M. O'Mahony, and R. G. Compton, Microelectrode arrays for electrochemistry: Approaches to fabrication, *Small*, 5, 776–788 (2009).
33. X. Xu, S. Zhang, H. Chen, and J. Kong, Integration of electrochemistry in micro-total analysis systems for biochemical assays: Recent developments, *Talanta*, 80, 8–18 (2009).
34. B. Fang, S. Jiao, M. Li, Y. Qu, and X. Jiang, Label-free electrochemical detection of DNA using ferrocene-containing cationic polythiophene and PNA probes on nanogold modified electrodes, *Biosensors and Bioelectronics*, 23, 1175–1179 (2008).
35. Y. Wang, M. Rafailovich, Z. Zhang, B. Rigas, K. Levon, S. Mueller, V. Jain, J. Yi, and J. Sokolov, A potentiometric sensor for the detection of proteins or viruses built with surface molecular imprinting method, *International Symposium on Spectral Sensing Research, Steven Institute of Technology*, Hoboken, NJ, 2008.
36. J. Albers, T. Grunwald, E. Nebling, G. Piechotta, and R. Hintsche, Electrical biochip technology—A tool for microarrays and continuous monitoring, *Analytical and Bioanalytical Chemistry*, 377, 521–527 (2003).
37. R. A. Villamizar, A. Maroto, and F. X. Rius, Improved detection of Candida albicans with carbon nanotube field-effect transistors, *Sensors and Actuators B: Chemical*, 136, 451–457 (2009).
38. B. L. Allen, P. D. Kichambare, and A. Star, Carbon nanotube field-effect-transistor-based biosensors, *Advanced Materials*, 19, 1439–1451 (2007).
39. Y. Cui, Q. Wei, H. Park, and C. M. Lieber, Nanowire nanosensors for highly sensitive and selective detection of biological and chemical species, *Science*, 293, 1289–1292 (2001).
40. T. E. McKnight, A. V. Melechko, D. W. Austin, T. Sims, M. A. Guillorn, and M. L. Simpson, Microarrays of vertically-aligned carbon nanofiber electrodes in an open fluidic channel, *Journal of Physical Chemistry B*, 108, 7115–7125 (2004).
41. M. J. Schulz, Y. Yun, A. Bange, W. R. Heineman, H. B. Halsall, V. N. Shanov, Z. Dong et al., An impedance biosensor based on carbon nanotubes, *Nanomedicine: Nanotechnology, Biology and Medicine*, 2, 280 (2006).
42. A. Qureshi, W. P. Kang, J. L. Davidson, and Y. Gurbuz, Review on carbon-derived, solid-state, micro and nano sensors for electrochemical sensing applications, *Diamond and Related Materials*, 18, 1401–1420 (2009).

43. J. Huang, Y. Liu, and T. You, Carbon nanofiber based electrochemical biosensors: A review, *Analytical Methods*, 2, 202–211 (2010).
44. K. C. P. Li, S. D. Pandit, S. Guccione, and M. D. Bednarski, Molecular imaging applications in nanomedicine, *Biomedical Microdevices*, 6, 113–116 (2004).
45. T. Vo-Dinh (ed.), *Biomedical Photonics Handbook*, 2nd edn., CRC Press, Boca Raton, FL, 2003.
46. H. A. Clark, M. Hoyer, M. A. Philbert, and R. Kopelman, Optical nanosensors for chemical analysis inside single living cells. 1. Fabrication, characterization, and methods for intracellular delivery of PEBBLE sensors, *Analytical Chemistry*, 71, 4831–4836 (1999).
47. J. Lu and Z. Rosenzweig, Nanoscale fluorescent sensors for intracellular analysis, *Fresenius' Journal of Analytical Chemistry*, 366, 569–575 (2000).
48. S. M. Buck, Y. E. L. Koo, E. Park, H. Xu, M. A. Philbert, M. A. Brasuel, and R. Kopelman, Optochemical nanosensor PEBBLEs: Photonic explorers for bioanalysis with biologically localized embedding, *Current Opinion in Chemical Biology*, 8, 540–546 (2004).
49. C. Xu, D. Ho, J. Xie, C. Wang, N. Kohler, E. G. Walsh, J. R. Morgan, Y. E. Chin, and S. Sun, Au-Fe$_3$O$_4$ dumbbell nanoparticles as dual-functional probes, *Angewandte Chemie International Edition*, 47, 173–176, (2008).
50. J. Kneipp, H. Kneipp, M. McLaughlin, D. Brown, and K. Kneipp, In vivo molecular probing of cellular compartments with gold nanoparticles and nanoaggregates, *Nano Letters*, 6, 2225–2231 (2006).
51. A. Myc, I. J. Majoros, T. P. Thomas, and J. R. Baker, Dendrimer-based targeted delivery of an apoptotic sensor in cancer cells, *Biomacromolecules*, 8, 13–18 (2007).
52. A. Webster, P. Coupland, F. D. Houghton, H. J. Leese, and J. W. Aylott, The delivery of PEBBLE nanosensors to measure the intracellular environment, *Biochemical Society Transactions*, 35, 538–543 (2007).
53. J. A. O'Brien and S. C. Lummis, Diolistics: Incorporating fluorescent dyes into biological samples using a gene gun, *Trends in Biotechnology*, 25, 530–534 (2007).
54. D. A. Stuart, A. J. Haes, C. R. Yonzon, E. M. Hicks, and R. P. Van Duyne, Biological applications of localised surface plasmonic phenomenae, *IEEE Proceedings—Nanobiotechnology*, 152, 13–32 (2005).
55. H. Matoussia, Use of quantum dot-bioconjugates for sensing and probing cellular processes, *Nanomedicine: Nanotechnology, Biology and Medicine*, 2, 282 (2006).
56. X. D. Hoa, A. G. Kirk, and M. Tabrizian, Towards integrated and sensitive surface plasmon resonance biosensors: A review of recent progress, *Biosensors and Bioelectronics*, 23, 151–160 (2007).
57. P. K. Jain, X. Huang, I. H. El-Sayed, and M. A. El-Sayed, Noble metals on the nanoscale: Optical and photothermal properties and some applications in imaging, sensing, biology, and medicine, *Accounts of Chemical Research*, 41, 1578–1586 (2008).
58. S. E. Skrabalak, J. Chen, Y. Sun, X. Lu, L. Au, C. M. Cobley, and Y. Xia, Gold nanocages: Synthesis, properties, and applications, *Accounts of Chemical Research*, 41, 1587–1595 (2008).
59. J. C. Sharpe, J. S. Mitchell, L. Lin, N. Sedoglavich, and R. J. Blaikie, Gold nanohole array substrates as immunobiosensors, *Analytical Chemistry*, 80, 2244–2249 (2008).

60. M. Willander and S. Al-Hilli, Analysis of biomolecules using surface plasmons, *Methods in Molecular Biology*, 544, 201–229 (2009).
61. K. S. Phillips and Q. Cheng, Recent advances in surface plasmon resonance based techniques for bioanalysis, *Analytical and Bioanalytical Chemistry*, 387, 1831–1840 (2007).
62. R. Gordon, D. Sinton, K. L. Kavanagh, and A. G. Brolo, A new generation of sensors based on extraordinary optical transmission, *Accounts of Chemical Research*, 41, 1049–1057 (2008).
63. M. Piliarik, H. Vaisocherová, and J. Homola, Surface plasmon resonance biosensing, *Methods in Molecular Biology*, 503, 65–88 (2009).
64. X. M. Qian and S. M. Nie, Single-molecule and single-nanoparticle SERS: From fundamental mechanisms to biomedical applications, *Chemical Society Reviews*, 37, 912–920 (2008).
65. W. E. Smith, Practical understanding and use of surface enhanced Raman scattering/surface enhanced resonance Raman scattering in chemical and biological analysis, *Chemical Society Reviews*, 37, 955–964 (2008).
66. J. Kneipp, H. Kneipp, and K. Kneipp, SERS—A single-molecule and nanoscale tool for bioanalytics, *Chemical Society Reviews*, 37, 1052–1060 (2008).
67. X. M. Lin, Y. Cui, Y. H. Xu, B. Ren, and Z. Q. Tian, Surface-enhanced Raman spectroscopy: Substrate-related issues, *Analytical and Bioanalytical Chemistry*, 394, 1729–1745 (2009).
68. M. K. Hossain, Y. Kitahama, G. C. Huang, X. Han, and Y. Ozaki, Surface-enhanced Raman scattering: Realization of localized surface plasmon resonance using unique substrates and methods, *Analytical and Bioanalytical Chemistry*, 394, 1747–1760 (2009).
69. C. Fang, A. Agarwal, K. D. Buddharaju, N. M. Khalid, S. M. Salim, E. Widjaja, M. V. Garland, N. Balasubramanian, and D. L. Kwong, DNA detection using nanostructured SERS substrates with Rhodamine B as Raman label, *Biosensors and Bioelectronics*, 24, 216–221 (2008).
70. D. R. Chamberlin, Z. Wang, K. A. Sultana, E. K. Chow, M. M. Sigalas, M. Liu, A. C. Grot, and S. Fan, SERS and plasmon resonance of engineered nanoparticle arrays, *Plasmonics: Metallic nanostructures and their optical properties III*, *Plasmonics Conference No. 3*, 31st July–3rd August, 2005, San Diego, CA, 5927, 592708.1–592708.8, 2005.
71. X. X. Han, B. Zhao, and Y. Ozaki, Surface-enhanced Raman scattering for protein detection, *Analytical and Bioanalytical Chemistry*, 394, 1719–1727 (2009).
72. S. Schlücker, SERS microscopy: Nanoparticle probes and biomedical applications, *ChemPhysChem*, 10, 1344–1354 (2009).
73. G. Kostovski, D. J. White, A. Mitchell, M. W. Austin, and P. R. Stoddart, Nanoimprinted optical fibres: Biotemplated nanostructures for SERS sensing, *Biosensors and Bioelectronics*, 24, 1531–1535 (2009).
74. C. Shi, Y. Zhang, C. Gu, B. Chen, L. Seballos, T. Olson, and J. Z. Zhang, Molecular fiber sensors based on surface enhanced Raman scattering (SERS), *Journal of Nanoscience and Nanotechnology*, 9, 2234–2246 (2009).
75. P. R. Stoddart and D. J. White, Optical fibre SERS sensors, *Analytical and Bioanalytical Chemistry*, 394, 1761–1774 (2009).
76. W. Zhao, J. Gu, L. Zhang, H. Chen, and J. Shi, Fabrication of uniform magnetic nanocomposite spheres with a magnetic core/mesoporous silica shell structure, *Journal of the American Chemical Society*, 127, 8916–8917 (2005).

77. T. R. Sathe, A. Agrawal, and S. Nie, Mesoporous silica beads embedded with semiconductor quantum dots and iron oxide nanocrystals: Dual-function micro-carriers for optical encoding and magnetic separation, *Analytical Chemistry*, 78, 5627–5632 (2006).

78. E. Mirowski, J. Moreland, S. Russek, M. Donahue, and K. Hsieh, Manipulation of magnetic particles by patterned arrays of magnetic spin-valve traps, *Journal of Magnetism and Magnetic Materials*, 311, 401–404 (2007).

79. R. S. Gaster, D. A. Hall, C. H. Nielsen, S. J. Osterfeld, H. Yu, K. E. Mach, R. J. Wilson et al., Matrix-insensitive protein assays push the limits of biosensors in medicine, *Nature Medicine*, 15, 1327–1332 (2009).

80. O. A. Sadik, A. O. Aluoch, and A. Zhou, Status of biomolecular recognition using electrochemical techniques, *Biosensors and Bioelectronics*, 24, 2749–2765 (2009).

81. D. Wei, M. J. Bailey, P. Andrew, and T. Ryhänen, Electrochemical biosensors at the nanoscale, *Lab on a Chip*, 9, 2123–2131 (2009).

82. W. J. Payne Jr., D. L. Marshall, R. K. Shockley, and W. J. Martin, Clinical laboratory applications of monoclonal antibodies, *Clinical Microbiology Reviews*, 1, 313–329 (1988).

83. S. Matzku and R. A. Stahel (eds.), Antibodies *in Diagnosis and Therapy: Technologies, Mechanisms, and Clinical Data*, Harwood Academic Publishers/OPA, Amsterdam, the Netherlands, 1999.

84. S. Madersbacher and P. Berger, Antibodies and immunoassays, *Methods*, 21, 41–50 (2000).

85. J. Ince and A. McNally, Development of rapid, automated diagnostics for infectious disease: Advances and challenges, *Expert Review of Medical Devices*, 6, 641–651 (2009).

86. N. E. Thompson, K. M. Foley, E. S. Stalder and R. R. Burgess, Identification, production, and use of polyol-responsive monoclonal antibodies for immunoaffinity chromatography, *Methods in Enzymology*, 463, 475–494 (2009)

87. A. Alegria-Schaffer, A. Lodge, and K. Vattem, Performing and optimizing western blots with an emphasis on chemiluminescent detection, *Methods in Enzymology*, 463, 573–599 (2009).

88. M. L. Landry, Developments in immunologic assays for respiratory viruses, *Clinics in Laboratory Medicine*, 29, 635–647 (2009).

89. D. Romanazzo, F. Ricci, S. Vesco, S. Piermarini, G. Volpe, D. Moscone, and G. Palleschi, ELIME (enzyme linked immuno magnetic electrochemical) method for mycotoxin detection, *Journal of Visualized Experiments*, 2009 Oct 23; pii: 1588. doi: 10.3791/1588 (2009).

90. N. Bergmann and N. A. Peppas, Biomimetic imprinted microparticles for the recognition and capture of serum proteins, *Transactions, Society for Biomaterials*, 30, 62–63 (2005).

91. E. Oral and N. A. Peppas, Hydrophilic molecularly imprinted PHEMA-polymers, *Journal of Biomedical Materials Research*, 78A, 205–210 (2006).

92. S. D. Jayasena, Aptamers: An emerging class of molecules that rival antibodies in diagnostics, *Clinical Chemistry*, 45, 1628–1650 (1999).

93. R. Stoltenburg, C. Reinemann, and B. Strehlitz, SELEX—A revolutionary method to generate high-affinity nucleic acid ligands, *Biomolecular Engineering*, 24, 381–403 (2007).

94. S. C. Gopinath, Methods developed for SELEX, *Analytical and Bioanalytical Chemistry*, 387, 171–182 (2007).

95. S. M. Shamah, J. M. Healy, and S. T. Cload, Complex target SELEX, *Accounts of Chemical Research*, 41, 130–138 (2008).
96. E. J. Cho, J. W. Lee, and A. D. Ellington, Applications of aptamers as sensors, *Annual Review of Analytical Chemistry*, 2, 241–264 (2009).
97. S. Tombelli, M. Minunni, and M. Mascini, Analytical applications of aptamers, *Biosensors and Bioelectronics*, 20, 2424–2434 (2005).
98. T. Mairal, V. C. Ozalp, P. L. Sánchez, M. Mir, I. Katakis, and C. K. O'Sullivan, Aptamers: Molecular tools for analytical applications, *Analytical and Bioanalytical Chemistry*, 390, 989–1007 (2008).
99. J. Qian, X. Lou, Y. Zhang, Y. Xiao, and H. T. Soh, Generation of highly specific aptamers via micromagnetic selection, *Analytical Chemistry*, 81, 5490–5495 (2009).
100. M. Lee and D. R. Walt, A fiber-optic microarray biosensor using aptamers as receptors, *Analytical Biochemistry*, 282, 142–146 (2000).
101. R. J. White, N. Phares, A. A. Lubin, Y. Xiao, and K. W. Plaxco, Optimization of electrochemical aptamer-based sensors via optimization of probe packing density and surface chemistry, *Langmuir*, 24, 10513–10518 (2008).
102. A. K. Cheng, D. Sen, and H. Z. Yu, Design and testing of aptamer-based electrochemical biosensors for proteins and small molecules, *Bioelectrochemistry*, 77, 1–12 (2009).
103. W. Wang, C. Chen, M. Qian, and X. S. Zhao, Aptamer biosensor for protein detection using gold nanoparticles, *Analytical Biochemistry*, 373, 213–219 (2008).
104. D. H. Burke and D. G. Nickens, Expressing RNA aptamers inside cells to reveal proteome and ribonome function, *Briefings in Functional Genomics*, 1, 169–188 (2002).
105. S. P. Radko, S. Yu. Rakhmetova, N. V. Bodoev, and A. I. Archakov, Aptamers as affinity reagents for clinical proteomics, *Biochemistry* (Moscow), 1, 198–209 (2007).
106. J. R. Collett, E. J. Cho, J. F. Lee, M. Levy, A. J. Hood, C. Wan, and A. D. Ellington, Functional RNA microarrays for high-throughput screening of antiprotein aptamers, *Analytical Biochemistry*, 338, 113–123 (2005).
107. T. Vo-Dinh, Nanobiosensors: Probing the sanctuary of individual living cells, *Journal of Cellular Biochemistry, Supplement*, 39, 154–161 (2002).
108. H. Andersson and A. van den Berg, Microtechnologies and nanotechnologies for single-cell analysis, *Current Opinion in Biotechnology*, 15, 44–49 (2004).
109. T. Vo-Dinh (ed.), *Protein Nanotechnology: Protocols, Instrumentation, and Applications*, Humana Press, Totwa, NJ, 2005.
110. T. Vo-Dinh, P. Kasili, and M. Wabuyele, Nanoprobes and nanobiosensors for monitoring and imaging individual living cells, *Nanomedicine*, 2, 22–30 (2006).
111. T. Vo-Dinh, Nanosensing at the single cell level, *Spectrochimica Acta Part B: Atomic Spectroscopy*, 63, 95–103 (2008).
112. R. N. Day and F. Schaufele, Imaging molecular interactions in living cells, *Molecular Endocrinology*, 19, 1675–1686 (2005).
113. Y. Wang, J. Y. Shyy, and S. Chien, Fluorescence proteins, live-cell imaging, and mechanobiology: Seeing is believing, *Annual Review of Biomedical Engineering*, 10, 1–38 (2008).
114. M. N. Velasco-Garcia, Optical biosensors for probing at the cellular level: A review of recent progress and future prospects, *Seminars in Cell & Developmental Biology*, 20, 27–33 (2009).

115. Y. Chen, J. D. Mills, and A. Periasamy, Protein localization in living cells and tissues using FRET and FLIM, *Differentiation*, 71, 528–541 (2003).

116. G. Bunt and F. S. Wouters, Visualization of molecular activities inside living cells with fluorescent labels, *International Review of Cytology*, 237, 205–278 (2004).

117. P. Liu, S. Ahmed, and T. Wohland, The F-techniques: Advances in receptor protein studies, *Trends in Endocrinology and Metabolism*, 19, 181–190 (2008).

118. T. Zimmermann, J. Rietdorf, and R. Pepperkok, Spectral imaging and its applications in live cell microscopy, *FEBS Letters*, 546, 87–92 (2003).

119. L. Gao, R. T. Kester, and T. S. Tkaczyk, Compact Image Slicing Spectrometer (ISS) for hyperspectral fluorescence microscopy, *Optics Express*, 17, 12293–12308 (2009).

120. V. V. Demidov, Nanobiosensors and molecular diagnostics: A promising partnership, *Expert Review of Molecular Diagnostics*, 4, 267–268 (2004).

121. I. Braslavsky, B. Hebert, E. Kartalov, and S. R. Quake, Sequence information can be obtained from single DNA molecules, *Proceedings of the National Academy of Sciences*, 100, 3960–3964 (2003).

122. J. Nakane, M. Wiggin, and A. Marziali, A nanosensor for transmembrane capture and identification of single nucleic acid molecules, *Biophysical Journal*, 87, 615–621 (2004).

123. M. P. Elenko, J. W. Szostak, and A. M. van Oijen, Single-molecule imaging of an in vitro-evolved RNA aptamer reveals homogeneous ligand binding kinetics, *Journal of the American Chemical Society*, 131, 9866–9867 (2009).

124. S. Wilk, S. Aboud, L. Petrossian, M. Goryll, J. Tang, R. S. Eisenberg, M. Saraniti, S. Goodnick, and T. J. Thornton, Ion channel conductance measurements on a silicon-based platform, *Journal of Physics: Conference Series*, 38, 21–24 (2006).

125. G. W. Li and J. Elf, Single molecule approaches to transcription factor kinetics in living cells, *FEBS Letters*, 583, 3979–3983 (2009).

126. S. Chang, S. Huang, J. He, F. Liang, P. Zhang, S. Li, X. Chen, O. Sankey, and S. Lindsay, Electronic signatures of all four DNA nucleosides in a tunneling gap, *Nano Letters*, 10, 1070–1075 (2010).

127. S. S. Smith, Nucleoprotein assemblies at the nanoscale: Medical implications, *Nanomedicine*, 1, 427–436 (2006).

128. F. C. Simmel, Towards biomedical applications for nucleic acid nanodevices, *Nanomedicine*, 2, 817–830 (2007).

129. H. Bayley and P. S. Cremer, Stochastic sensors inspired by biology, *Nature*, 413, 226–230 (2001).

130. A. D. Hibbs and G. A. Barrall, *Engineered Bio-Molecular Nano-Devices/Systems*, USDOD Final rept. 22 Oct 2005–30 Sep 2008, Storming Media, Pentagon Reports (2009). Online at: http://www.stormingmedia.us/34/3458/A345894.html (Jan 2010).

131. D. Stoddart, A. J. Heron, E. Mikhailova, G. Maglia, and H. Bayley, Single-nucleotide discrimination in immobilized DNA oligonucleotides with a biological nanopore, *Proceedings of the National Academy of Sciences*, 106, 7702–7707 (2009).

132. R. F. Purnell and J. J. Schmidt, Discrimination of single base substitutions in a DNA strand immobilized in a biological nanopore, *ACS Nano*, 3, 2533–2538 (2009).

133. R. Numano, S. Szobota, A. Y. Lau, P. Gorostiza, M. Volgraf, B. Roux, D. Trauner, and E. Y. Isacoff, Nanosculpting reversed wavelength sensitivity into a photoswitchable iGluR, *Proceedings of the National Academy of Sciences*, 106, 6814–6819 (2009).

134. T. Ativanichayaphong, S. J. Tang, J. Wang, W. D. Huang, H. F. Tibbals, S. J. Spechler, and J. C. Chiao, An implantable, wireless and batteryless impedance sensor capsule for detecting acidic and non-acidic reflux, *Gastroenterology*, 134, A-63 (2008).

135. J. M. Pritchett, M. Aslam, J. C. Slaughter, R. M. Ness, C. G. Garrett, and M. F. Vaezi, Efficacy of esophageal impedance/pH monitoring in patients with refractory gastroesophageal reflux disease, on and off therapy, *Clinical Gastroenterology and Hepatology*, 7, 743–748 (2009).

136. T. Ohki, D. Stern, M. Allen, and J. Yada, Wireless pressure sensing of aneurysms, *Endovascular Today*, 52, 47–52 (2004).

137. T. D. McClure, R. Tan, A. Breda, C. K. Lin, J. Schmidt, and P. Schulam, Development of a microelectromechanical system (MEMS) pressure sensor for monitoring intraperitoneal, bladder, and detrusor pressures, *Journal of Endourology*, 22, 2583–2640 (2008).

138. Y. Tardy Y, A. Ginggen, T. Pipoz, R. Crivelli, P. Renaud, R. Holzer, and P. A. Neukomm, Development of a new implantable pressure sensor for the optimization of the treatment of hydrocephalus, *16th International Symposium on Biotelemetry*, May 6–11, 2001, Vienna, Austria (2001).

139. P. Walter, U. Schnakenberg, G. vom Bögel, P. Ruokonen, C. Krüger, S. Dinslage, H. C. L. Handjery et al., Development of a completely encapsulated intraocular pressure sensor, *Ophthalmic Research*, 32, 278–284 (2000).

140. P.-J. Chen, D. C. Rodger, S. Saati, M. S. Humayun, and Y.-C. Tai, Implantable parylene-based wireless intraocular pressure sensor, *IEEE MEMS 2008*, January 13–17, 2008, Tucson, AZ, 58–61 (2008).

141. M. van der Leeden, M. P. Steultjens, C. B. Terwee, D. Rosenbaum, D. Turner, J. Woodburn, and J. Dekker, A systematic review of instruments measuring foot function, foot pain, and foot-related disability in patients with rheumatoid arthritis, *Arthritis and Rheumatism*, 59, 1257–1269 (2008).

142. A. Heyneman, K. Vanderwee, M. Grypdonck, and T. Defloor, Effectiveness of two cushions in the prevention of heel pressure ulcers, *Evidence Based Nursing*, 6, 114–120 (2009).

143. S. J. Ellis, H. Hillstrom, R. Cheng, J. Lipman, G. Garrison, and J. T. Deland, The development of an intraoperative plantar pressure assessment device, *Foot and Ankle International*, 30, 333–340 (2009).

144. P. S. Cottler, W. R. Karpen, D. A. Morrow, and K. R. Kaufman, Performance characteristics of a new generation pressure microsensor for physiologic applications, *Annals of Biomedical Engineering*, 37, 1638–1645 (2009).

145. K. C. Cheung, Implantable microscale neural interfaces, *Biomedical Microdevices*, 9, 923–938 (2007).

146. N. G. Hatsopoulos and J. P. Donoghue, The science of neural interface systems, *Annual Review of Neuroscience*, 32, 249–266 (2009).

147. M. A. L. Nicolelis (ed.), *Methods for Neural Ensemble Recordings*, 2nd edn., CRC Press, Boca Raton, FL, 2007.

148. T. Stieglitz, B. Rubehn, C. Henle, S. Kisban, S. Herwik, P. Ruther, and M. Schuettler, Brain-computer interfaces: An overview of the hardware to record neural signals from the cortex, *Progress in Brain Research*, 175, 297–315 (2009).

149. Q. R. Quian and S. Panzeri, Extracting information from neuronal populations: Information theory and decoding approaches, *Nature Reviews Neuroscience*, 10, 173–185 (2009).

150. K. Josić, E. Shea-Brown, B. Doiron, and J. de la Rocha, Stimulus-dependent correlations and population codes, *Neural Computation*, 21, 2774–2804 (2009).
151. E. K. Miller and M. A. Wilson, All my circuits: Using multiple electrodes to understand functioning neural networks, *Neuron*, 60, 483–488 (2008).
152. F. Hofmann and H. Bading, Long term recordings with microelectrode arrays: Studies of transcription-dependent neuronal plasticity and axonal regeneration, *Journal of Physiology* (Paris), 99, 125–132 (2006).
153. S. Hafizovic, F. Heer, T. Ugniwenko, U. Frey, A. Blau, C. Ziegler, and A. Hierlemann, A CMOS-based microelectrode array for interaction with neuronal cultures, *Journal of Neuroscience Methods*, 164, 93–106 (2007).
154. A. Stett, U. Egert, E. Guenther, F. Hofmann, T. Meyer, W. Nisch, and H. Haemmerle, Biological application of microelectrode arrays in drug discovery and basic research, *Analytical and Bioanalytical Chemistry*, 377, 486–495 (2003).
155. J. K. Chapin and K. A. Moxon (eds.), *Neural Prostheses for Restoration of Sensory and Motor Function*, CRC Press, Boca Raton, FL, 2000.
156. D. E. Sakas, B. A. Simpson and E. S. Krames (eds.), *Neural Prostheses in Clinical Practice: Biomedical Microsystems in Neurological Rehabilitation*, Springer Vienna, Vienna, Austria, 2007.
157. S. F. Cogan, Neural stimulation and recording electrodes, *Annual Review of Biomedical Engineering*, 10, 275–309 (2008).
158. J. J. Pancrazio, Neural interfaces at the nanoscale, *Nanomedicine*, 3, 823–830 (2008).
159. W. M. Reichert (ed.), *Indwelling Neural Implants: Strategies for Contending with the In Vivo Environment*, CRC Press, Boca Raton, FL, 2007.
160. S. Negi, R. Bhandari, L. Rieth, R. Van Wagenen, and F. Solzbacher, Neural electrode degradation from continuous electrical stimulation: Comparison of sputtered and activated iridium oxide, *Journal of Neuroscience Methods*, 186, 8–17 (2010).
161. S. Gawad, M. Giugliano, M. Heuschkel, B. Wessling, H. Markram, U. Schnakenberg, P. Renaud, and H. Morgan, Substrate arrays of iridium oxide microelectrodes for in vitro neuronal interfacing, *Frontiers in Neuroengineering*, 2, 1, doi:10.3389/neuro.16.001.2009 (2009).
162. E. B. Malarkey and V. Parpura, Applications of carbon nanotubes in neurobiology, *Neurodegenerative Diseases*, 4, 292–299 (2007).
163. E. W. Keefer, B. R. Botterman, M. I. Romero, A. F. Rossi, and G. W. Gross, Carbon nanotube coating improves neuronal recordings, *Nature Nanotechnology*, 3, 434–439 (2008).
164. A. Sucapane, G. Cellot, M. Prato, M. Giugliano, V. Parpura, and L. Ballerini, Interactions between cultured neurons and carbon nanotubes: A nanoneuroscience vignette, *Journal of Nanoneuroscience*, 1, 10–16 (2009).
165. S. M. Richardson-Burns, J. L. Hendricks, and D. C. Martin, Electrochemical polymerization of conducting polymers in living neural tissue, *Journal of Neural Engineering*, 4, L6–L13 (2007).
166. R. A. Green, N. H. Lovell, G. G. Wallace, and L. A. Poole-Warren, Conducting polymers for neural interfaces: Challenges in developing an effective long-term implant, *Biomaterials*, 29, 3393–3399 (2008).
167. J. Noel, W. Teizer, and W. Hwang, Antifouling self-assembled monolayers on microelectrodes for patterning biomolecules, *Journal of Visualized Experiments*, 2009 Aug 25;(30). pii: 1390. doi: 10.3791/1390 (2009).

168. T. Lee, S. U. Kim, J. H. Lee, J. Min, and J. W. Choi, Fabrication of nano scaled protein monolayer consisting of cytochrome c on self-assembled 11-MUA layer for bioelectronic device, *Journal of Nanoscience and Nanotechnology*, 9, 7136–7140 (2009).

169. S. K. Arya, P. R. Solanki, M. Datta, and B. D. Malhotra, Recent advances in self-assembled monolayers based biomolecular electronic devices, *Biosensors and Bioelectronics*, 24, 2810–2817 (2009).

170. J. Durner, Clinical chemistry: Challenges for analytical chemistry and the nanosciences from medicine, *Angewandte Chemie International Edition*, 49, 1026–1051 (2010).

171. G. Leegsma-Vogt, M. M. Rhemrev-Boom, R. G. Tiessen, K. Venema, and Jakob Korf, The potential of biosensor technology in clinical monitoring and experimental research, *Bio-Medical Materials and Engineering*, 14, 455–464 (2004).

172. T. Laurell, J. Nilsson, and G. Marko-Varga, The quest for high-speed and low volume bioanalysis, *Analytical Chemistry A*, 77, 264A–272A (2005).

173. B. A. Parviza, Integrated electronic detection of biomolecules, *Trends in Microbiology*, 14, 373–375 (2006).

174. M. J. Madou, *Fundamentals of Microfabrication: The Science of Miniaturization*, 2nd edn., CRC Press, Boca Raton, FL, 2002.

175. B. H. Weigl, R. L. Bardell, and C. R. Cabrera, Lab-on-a-chip for drug development, *Advanced Drug Delivery Reviews*, 55, 349–377 (2003).

176. G. Hardiman (ed.), *Biochips as Pathways to Drug Discovery*, CRC Press, Boca Raton, FL, 2006.

177. M. Gad-el-Hak (ed.), *The MEMS Handbook*, 2nd edn. *MEMS Applications*, CRC Press, Boca Raton, FL, 2006.

178. R. R. Sathuluri, S. Yamamura, and E. Tamiya, Microsystems technology and biosensing, *Advances in Biochemical Engineering—Biotechnology*, 109, 285–350 (2008).

179. S. Szunerits and D. R. Walt, The use of optical fiber bundles combined with electrochemistry for chemical imaging, *ChemPhysChem*, 4, 186–192 (2003).

180. J. R. Epstein and D. R. Walt, Fluorescence-based fibre optic arrays: A universal platform for sensing, *Chemical Society Reviews*, 32, 203–214 (2003).

181. L. D. Lavis and R. T. Raines, Bright ideas for chemical biology, *ACS Chemical Biology*, 3, 142–155 (2008).

182. O. S. Wolfbeis, Fiber-optic chemical sensors and biosensors, *Analytical Chemistry*, 80, 4269–4283 (2008).

183. A. Lee and R. B. Fair, Special issue on biomedical applications for MEMS and microfluidics, *Proceedings of the IEEE*, 92, 3–189 (2004).

184. M. Ryo, S. Yasuhiko, S. Hiroshi, I. Hisao, and O. Toshio, MEMS for biomedical applications, *Hitachi Hyoron*, 86, 517–520 (2004).

185. M. B. Fox, D. C. Esveld, A. Valero, R. Luttge, H. C. Mastwijk, P. V. Bartels, A. Berg, and R. M. Boom, Electroporation of cells in microfluidic devices: A review, *Analytical and Bioanalytical Chemistry*, 385, 474 (2006).

186. A. Nisar, N. Afzulpurkar, B. Mahaisavariya, and A. Tuantranont, MEMS-based micropumps in drug delivery and biomedical applications, *Sensors and Actuators B: Chemical*, 130, 917–942 (2008).

187. E. Smela, Conjugated polymer actuators for biomedical applications, *Advanced Materials*, 15, 481–494 (2003).

188. J. Bergkvist, T. Lilliehorn, J. Nilsson, S. Johansson, and T. Laurell, Miniaturized flow-through micro-dispenser with piezoceramic tripodactuation, *Journal of Microelectromechanical Systems*, 14, 134–140 (2005).

189. W. D. Niles and P. J. Coassin, Piezo- and solenoid valve-based liquid dispensing for miniaturized assays, *Assay and Drug Development Technologies*, 3,189–202 (2005).

190. P. Miao, P. D. Mitcheson, A. S. Holmes, E. M. Yeatman, T. C. Green, and B. H. Stark, Mems inertial power generators for biomedical applications, *Microsystem Technologies*, 12, 1079–1083 (2006).

191. Z. L. Wang, Towards self-powered nanosystems: From nanogenerators to nanopiezotronics, *Advanced Functional Materials*, 18, 1–15 (2008).

192. S. Priya and D. J. Inman (eds.), *Energy Harvesting Technologies*, Springer, New York, 2008.

193. R. Yang, Y. Qin, C. Li, G. Zhu, and Z. L. Wang, Converting biomechanical energy into electricity by a muscle-movement-driven nanogenerator, *Nano Letters*, 9, 1201–1205 (2009).

194. M. A. Northrup, Microfluidics: A few good tricks, *Nature Materials*, 3, 282–283 (2004).

195. P. B. Allen, B. R. Doepker, and D. T. Chiu, Introduction to photolithography, soft lithography, and microfluidics, *Chemical Education*, 14, 61–63 (2009).

196. P. Tabeling, *Introduction to Microfluidics*, Oxford University Press, Oxford, U.K., 2005.

197. N.-T. Nguyen and S. Wereley, *Fundamentals and Applications of Microfluidics*, 2nd edn., Integrated Microsystems, Artech House, Norwood, MA, 2006.

198. F. A. Gomez (ed.), *Biological Applications of Microfluidics*, John Wiley & Sons, Inc., Hoboken, NJ, 2008.

199. J. Berthier and P. Silberzan, *Microfluidics for Biotechnology*, Artech House Publishers, Norwood, MA, 2005.

200. T. Thorsen, S. J. Maerkl, and S. R. Quake, Microfluidic large-scale integration, *Science*, 298, 580–584 (2002).

201. G. M. Whitesides, The origins and the future of microfluidics, *Nature*, 442, 368–373 (2006).

202. M. L. Kovarik and S. C. Jacobson, Nanofluidics in lab-on-a-chip devices, *Analytical Chemistry* 81, 7133–7140 (2009).

203. B. Weigl, G. Domingo, P. Labarre, and J. Gerlach, Towards non- and minimally instrumented, microfluidics-based diagnostic devices, *Lab on a Chip*, 8, 1999–2014 (2008).

204. T. S. Hawley and R. G. Hawley (eds.), *Flow Cytometry Protocols*, 2nd edn., Humana Press, Totowa, NJ (2004).

205. H. Andersson and A. van den Berg, Microfluidic devices for cellomics: A review, *Sensors and Actuators B: Chemical*, 92, 315–325 (2003).

206. C. Yi, C.-W. Li, S. Ji, and M. Yang, Microfluidics technology for manipulation and analysis of biological cells, *Analytica Chimica Acta*, 560, 1–23 (2006).

207. X. Gao and S. Nie, Quantum dot-encoded mesoporous beads with high brightness and uniformity: Rapid readout using flow cytometry, *Analytical Chemistry*, 76, 2406–2410 (2004).

208. D. Huh, W. Gu, Y. Kamotani, J. B. Grotberg, and S. Takayama, Microfluidics for flow cytometric analysis of cells and particles, *Physiological Measurement*, 26, R73–R98 (2005).

209. C. Simonnet and A. Groisman, High-throughput and high-resolution flow cytometry in molded microfluidic devices, *Analytical Chemistry*, 78, 5653–5663 (2006).

210. W.-H. Huang, F. Ai, Z.-L. Wang, and J.-K. Cheng, Recent advances in single-cell analysis using capillary electrophoresis and microfluidic devices, *Journal of Chromatography B*, 866, 104–122 (2008).

211. D. P. Schrum, C. T. Culbertson, S. C. Jacobson, and J. M. Ramsey, Microchip flow cytometry using electrokinetic focusing, *Analytical Chemistry*, 71, 4173–4177 (1999).

212. G. Velve-Casquillas, M. Le Berre, M. Piel, and P. T. Tran, Microfluidic tools for cell biological research, *Nano Today*, 5, 28–47 (2010).

213. A. Huebner, S. Sharma, M. Srisa-Art, F. Hollfelder, J. B. Edel, and A. J. deMello, Microdroplets: A sea of applications? *Lab on a Chip*, 8, 1244–1254 (2008).

214. K. Chakrabarty, *Digital Microfluidic Biochips: Synthesis, Testing, and Reconfiguration Techniques*, CRC Press, Boca Raton, FL, 2006.

215. J. Berthier, *Microdrops and Digital Microfluidics*, William Andrew, Norwich, NY, 2008.

216. J. Voldman, Electrical forces for microscale cell manipulation, *Annual Review of Biomedical Engineering*, 8, 425–454 (2006).

217. J. Wu, Interactions of electrical fields with fluids: Laboratory-on-a-chip applications, *IET Nanobiotechnology*, 2, 14–27 (2008).

218. D. Chugh and K. V. Kaler, Leveraging liquid dielectrophoresis for microfluidic applications, *Biomedical Materials*, 3, 034009 (2008).

219. J. Vykoukal and P. R. C. Gascoyne, Particle separation by dielectrophoresis, *Electrophoresis*, 23, 1973–1983 (2002).

220. Y. Kang, D. Li, S. A. Kalams, and J. E. Eid, DC-dielectrophoretic separation of biological cells by size, *Biomedical Microdevices*, 10, 243–249 (2008).

221. L. Wang, J. Lu, S. A. Marchenko, E. S. Monuki, L. A. Flanagan, and A. P. Lee, Dual frequency dielectrophoresis with interdigitated sidewall electrodes for microfluidic flow-through separation of beads and cells, *Electrophoresis*, 30, 782–791 (2009).

222. L. S. Jang, P. H. Huang, and K. C. Lan, Single-cell trapping utilizing negative dielectrophoretic quadrupole and microwell electrodes, *Biosensors and Bioelectronics*, 24, 3637–3644 (2009).

223. S. Barany, Electrophoresis in strong electric fields, *Advances in Colloid and Interface Science*, 147–148, 36–43 (2008).

224. I. Glasgow, J. Batton, and N. Aubry, Electroosmotic mixing in microchannels, *Lab on a Chip*, 4, 558–562 (2004).

225. S. C. Wang, H. P. Chen, C. Y. Lee, C. C. Yu, and H. C. Chang, AC electro-osmotic mixing induced by non-contact external electrodes, *Biosensors and Bioelectronics*, 22, 563–567 (2006).

226. Y. T. Zhang, F. Bottausci, M. P. Rao, E. R. Parker, I. Mezic, and N. C. Macdonald, Titanium-based dielectrophoresis devices for microfluidic applications, *Biomedical Microdevices*, 10, 509–517 (2008).

227. K. Park, H. J. Suk, D. Akin, and R. Bashir, Dielectrophoresis-based cell manipulation using electrodes on a reusable printed circuit board, *Lab on a Chip*, 9, 2224–2229 (2009).

228. J. P. Desai, A. Pillarisetti, and A. D. Brooks, Engineering approaches to biomanipulation, *Annual Review of Biomedical Engineering*, 9, 35–53 (2007).

229. M. Willander, K. Risveden, B. Danielsson, and O. Nur, Trapping and detection of single molecules in water, *Methods in Molecular Biology*, 544, 163–186 (2009).

230. D. G. Grier, A revolution in optical manipulation, *Nature*, 424, 810–816 (2003).
231. K. T. Gahagan and G. A. Swartzlander Jr., Optical vortex trapping of particles, *Optics Letters*, 21, 827–829 (1996).
232. H. Zhang and K. K. Liu, Optical tweezers for single cells, *Journal of the Royal Society Interface*, 5, 671–690 (2008).
233. K. F. Lei, W. C. Law, Y. K. Suen, W. J. Li, Y. Yam, H. P. Ho, and S. K. Kong, A vortex pump-based optically-transparent microfluidic platform for biotech and medical applications, *Proceedings of the Institution of Mechanical Engineers H*, 221, 129–141 (2007).
234. G. D. M. Jeffries, J. S. Kuo, and D. T. Chiu, Controlled shrinkage and re-expansion of a single aqueous droplet inside an optical vortex trap, *Journal of Physical Chemistry B*, 111, 2806–2812 (2007).
235. G. D. M. Jeffries, G. Milne, Y. Zhao, C. Lopez-Mariscal, and D. T. Chiu, Optofluidic generation of Laguerre-Gaussian beams, *Optics Express*, 17, 17555–17562 (2009).
236. D. T. Chiu and R. M. Lorenz, Chemistry and biology in femtoliter and picoliter volume droplets, *Accounts of Chemical Research*, 42, 649–658 (2009).
237. J. Nilsson, M. Evander, B. Hammarström, and T. Laurell, Review of cell and particle trapping in microfluidic systems, *Analytica Chimica Acta*, 649, 141–157 (2009).
238. W. Barthlott and C. Neinhuis, Purity of the sacred lotus, or escape from contamination in biological surfaces, *Planta*, 202, 1–8 (1997).
239. L. Gao and T. J. McCarthy, The "lotus effect" explained: Two reasons why two length scales of topography are important, *Langmuir*, 22, 2966–2967 (2006).
240. Y. T. Cheng, D. E. Rodak, C. A. Wong, and C. A. Hayden, Effects of micro- and nano-structures on the self-cleaning behaviour of lotus leaves, *Nanotechnology*, 17, 1359–1362 (2006).
241. R. D. Anandjiwala, L. Hunter, R. Kozlowski, and G. Zaikov (eds.), *Textiles for Sustainable Development*, Nova Science Publishers, New York, 2007.
242. R. Shamai, D. Andelman, B. Berge, and R. Hayes, Water, electricity, and between ... On electrowetting and its applications, *Soft Matter*, 4, 38–45 (2008).
243. J.-T. Feng, F.-C. Wang, and Y.-P. Zhao, Electrowetting on a lotus leaf, *Biomicrofluidics*, 3, 022406 (2009).
244. N. Verplanck, Y. Coffinier, V. Thomy, and R. Boukherroub, Wettability switching techniques on superhydrophobic surfaces, *Nanoscale Research Letters*, 2, 577–596 (2007).
245. S.-Y. Teh, R. Lin, L.-H. Hung, and A. P. Lee, Droplet microfluidics, *Lab on a Chip*, 8, 198–220 (2008).
246. C. T. Kuo and C. H. Liu, A novel microfluidic driver via AC electrokinetics, *Lab on a Chip*, 8, 725–733 (2008).
247. J. R. Dorvee, M. J. Sailor, and G. M. Miskelly, Digital microfluidics and delivery of molecular payloads with magnetic porous silicon chaperones, *Dalton Transactions*, 2008, 721–730 (2008).
248. S. Aghdaei, M. E. Sandison, M. Zagnoni, N. G. Green, and H. Morgan, Formation of artificial lipid bilayers using droplet dielectrophoresis, *Lab on a Chip*, 8, 1617–1620 (2008).
249. J. S. Becker and N. Jakubowski, The synergy of elemental and biomolecular mass spectrometry: New analytical strategies in life sciences, *Chemical Society Reviews*, 38, 1969–1983 (2009).

250. I. M. Lazar, J. Grym, and F. Foret, Microfabricated devices: A new sample introduction approach to mass spectrometry, *Mass Spectrometry Reviews*, 25, 573–594 (2008).

251. I. M. Lazar, Recent advances in capillary and microfluidic platforms with MS detection for the analysis of phosphoproteins, *Electrophoresis*, 30, 262–275 (2009).

252. J. Lee, S. A. Soper, and K. K. Murray, Microfluidic chips for mass spectrometry-based proteomics, *Journal of Mass Spectrometry*, 44, 579–593 (2010).

253. A. L. Burlingame (ed.), *Biological Mass Spectrometry*, Elsevier Academic Press, San Diego, CA, 2005.

254. D. S. Sem (ed.), *Spectral Techniques in Proteomics*, CRC Press, Boca Raton, FL, 2007.

255. D. J. Bell, Mass spectrometry, *Methods in Molecular Biology*, 244, 447–454 (2004).

256. M. Mann, R. C. Hendrickson, and A. Pandley, Analysis of proteomes by mass spectrometry, *Annual Review of Biochemistry*, 70, 437–473 (2001).

257. N. Mano and J. Goto, Biomedical and biological mass spectrometry, *Analytical Sciences*, 19, 3–14 (2003).

258. M. L. Vestal, Thermospray liquid chromatographic interface for magnetic mass spectrometers, *Analytical Chemistry*, 56, 2590–2592 (1984).

259. J. B. Fenn, M. Mann, C. K. Meng, S. F. Wong, and C. M. Whitehouse, Electrospray ionization—Principles and practice, *Mass Spectrometry Reviews*, 9, 37–70 (1990).

260. R. D. Smith, J. A. Loo, C. G. Edmonds, C. J. Barinaga, and H. R. Udseth, New developments in biochemical mass spectrometry: Electrospray ionization, *Analytical Chemistry*, 62, 882–899 (1990).

261. M. Wilm and M. Mann, Analytical properties of the nanoelectrospray ion source, *Analytical Chemistry*, 68, 1–8 (1996).

262. W. J. Griffiths, A. P. Jonsson, S. Liu, D. K. Rai, and Y. Wang, Electrospray and tandem mass spectrometry in biochemistry, *Biochemical Journal*, 355, 545–561 (2001).

263. Shimadzu Corporation, MALDI-TOF/MS principle, Online at: www.shimadzu. com/about/nobel/noblesoul/tec.html (2010).

264. F. Hillenkamp and J. P. Katalinic, *MALDI-MS: A Practical Guide to Instrumentation, Methods, and Applications*, Wiley-VCH, Weinheim, Germany, 2007.

265. M. Karas, U. Bahr, and U. Gießmann, Matrix-assisted laser desorption ionization mass spectrometry, *Mass Spectrometry Reviews*, 10, 335–357 (1991).

266. R. C. Beavis, Matrix-assisted ultraviolet laser desorption: Evolution and principles, *Organic Mass Spectrometry*, 27, 653–659 (1992).

267. U. Bahr, M. Karas, and F. Hillenkamp, Analysis of biopolymers by matrix-assisted laser desorption ionization (MALDI) mass-spectrometry, *Fresenius' Journal of Analytical Chemistry*, 348, 783–791 (1994).

268. J. Kast, C. E. Parker, K. van der Drift, J. M. Dial, S. L. Milgram, M. Wilm, M. Howell, and C. H. Borchers, Matrix-assisted laser desorption/ionization directed nano-electrospray ionization tandem mass spectrometric analysis for protein identification, *Rapid Communications in Mass Spectrometry*, 17, 1825–1834 (2003).

269. J. B. Fenn, *Electrospray Wings for Molecular Elephants*, Nobel Lecture, 2002, online at: http://nobelprize.virtual.museum/nobel_prizes/chemistry/laureates/2002/fenn-lecture.pdf (2010).

270. K. Tanaka, *The Origin of Macromolecule Ionization by Laser Irradiation*, Nobel Lecture, 2002, online at: http://nobelprize.org/nobel_prizes/chemistry/laureates/2002/tanaka-lecture.pdf (2010).

271. A. Cho and D. Normile, Nobel Prize in Chemistry: Mastering macromolecules, *Science*, 298, 527–528 (2002).
272. J. R. Yates, III, Mass spectral analysis in proteomics, *Annual Review of Biophysics and Biomolecular Structure*, 33, 297–316 (2004).
273. Q. Xue, F. Foret, Y. M. Dunayevskiy, P. M. Zavracky, N. E. McGruer, and B. L. Karger, Multichannel microchip electrospray mass spectrometry, *Analytical Chemistry*, 69, 426–430 (1997).
274. R. S. Ramsey and J. M. Ramsey, Generating electrospray from microchip devices using electroosmotic pumping, *Analytical Chemistry*, 69, 1174–1178 (1997).
275. B. Zhang, H. Liu, B. L. Karger, and F. Foret, Microfabricated devices for capillary electrophoresis—Electrospray mass spectrometry, *Analytical Chemistry*, 71, 3258–3264 (1999).
276. I. M. Lazar, R. S. Ramsey, S. Sundberg, and J. M. Ramsey, Subattomole-sensitivity microchip nanoelectrospray source with time-of-flight mass spectrometry detection, *Analytical Chemistry*, 71, 3627–3631 (1999).
277. G. A. Schultz, T. N. Corso, S. J. Prosser, and S. Zhang, A fully integrated monolithic microchip electrospray device for mass spectrometry, *Analytical Chemistry*, 72, 4058–4063 (2000).
278. L. Licklider, X.-Q. Wang, A. Desai, Y.-C. Tai, and T. D. Lee, A micromachined chip-based electrospray source for mass spectrometry, *Analytical Chemistry*, 72, 367–375 (2000).
279. T. Wachs and J. Henion, Electrospray device for coupling microscale separations and other miniaturized devices with electrospray mass spectrometry, *Analytical Chemistry*, 73, 632–638 (2001).
280. S. Zhang and C. K. Van Pelt, Chip-based nanoelectrospray mass spectrometry for protein characterization, *Expert Review of Proteomics*, 1, 449–468 (2004).
281. P. V. Balimane, E. Pace, S. Chong, M. Zhu, M. Jemal, and C. K. Pelt, A novel high-throughput automated chip-based nanoelectrospray tandem mass spectrometric method for PAMPA sample analysis, *Journal of Pharmaceutical and Biomedical Analysis*, 39, 8–16 (2005).
282. W. C. Sung, H. Makamba, and S. H. Chen, Chip-based microfluidic devices coupled with electrospray ionization-mass spectrometry, *Electrophoresis*, 26, 1783–1791 (2005).
283. A. G. Pereira-Medrano, A. Sterling, A. P. Snijders, K. F. Reardon, and P. C. Wright, A systematic evaluation of chip-based nanoelectrospray parameters for rapid identification of proteins from a complex mixture, *Journal of the American Society for Mass Spectrometry*, 18, 1714–1725 (2007).
284. S. Koster and E. Verpoorte, A decade of microfluidic analysis coupled with electrospray mass spectrometry: An overview, *Lab on a Chip*, 7, 1394–1412 (2007).
285. D. L. DeVoe and C. S. Lee, Microfluidic technologies for MALDI-MS in proteomics, *Electrophoresis*, 27, 3559–3568 (2006).
286. J. Lee, S. A. Soper, and K. K. Murray, Microfluidics with MALDI analysis for proteomics—A review, *Analytica Chimica Acta*, 649, 180–190 (2009).
287. P. Önnerfjord, J. Nilsson, L. Wallman, T. Laurell, and G. Marko-Varga, Picoliter sample preparation in MALDI-TOF MS using a micromachined silicon flow-through dispenser, *Analytical Chemistry*, 70, 4755–4760 (1998).
288. J.-O. Koopmann and J. Blackburn, High affinity capture surface for matrix-assisted laser desorption/ionisation compatible protein microarrays, *Rapid Communications in Mass Spectrometry*, 17, 455–462 (2003).

289. R. Frank, High-density synthetic peptide microarrays: Emerging tools for functional genomics and proteomics, *Combinatorial Chemistry and High Throughput Screening*, 5, 429–440 (2002).

290. O. Brandt, J. Feldner, A. Stephan, M. Schröder, M. Schnölzer, H. F. Arlinghaus, J. D. Hoheisel, and A. Jacob, PNA microarrays for hybridisation of unlabelled DNA samples, *Nucleic Acids Research*, 31, e119 (2003).

291. M. F. Lopez and M. G. Pluskal, Protein micro- and macroarrays: Digitizing the proteome, *Journal of Chromatography B Analytical Technologies in the Biomedical and Life Sciences*, 787, 19–27 (2003).

292. I. M. Gavin, A. Kukhtin, D. Glesne, D. Schabacker, and D. P. Chandler, Analysis of protein interaction and function with a 3-dimensional MALDI-MS protein array, *BioTechniques*, 39, 99–107 (2005).

293. G. B. Smejkal and A. Lazarev, *Separation Methods In Proteomics*, CRC Press, Boca Raton, FL, 2005.

294. M. Moini, Capillary electrophoresis mass spectrometry and its application to the analysis of biological mixtures, *Analytical and Bioanalytical Chemistry*, 373, 466–480 (2002).

295. S. Zhang, C. K. Van Pelt, and J. D. Henion, Automated chip-based nanoelectrospray-mass spectrometry for rapid identification of proteins separated by two-dimensional gel electrophoresis, *Electrophoresis*, 24, 3620–3362 (2003).

296. M. Moini, Capillary electrophoresis-electrospray ionization mass spectrometry of amino acids, peptides, and proteins, *Methods in Molecular Biology*, 276, 253–290 (2004).

297. H. Stutz, Advances in the analysis of proteins and peptides by capillary electrophoresis with matrix-assisted laser desorption/ionization and electrospray-mass spectrometry detection, *Electrophoresis*, 26, 1254–1290. (2005).

298. R. Haselberg, G. J. de Jong, and G. W. Somsen, Capillary electrophoresis-mass spectrometry for the analysis of intact proteins, *Journal of Chromatography A*, 1159, 81–109 (2007).

299. R. S. Matson, *Applying Genomic and Proteomic Microarray Technology in Drug Discovery*, CRC Press, Boca Raton, FL, 2005.

300. T. Miliotis, G. Marko-Varga, J. Nilsson, and T. Laurell, Development of silicon microstructures and thin-film MALDI-target plates for automated proteomic sample identification, *Journal of Neuroscience Methods*, 109, 41–46 (2001).

301. C. Felten, F. Foret, M. Minarik, W. Goetzinger, and B. L. Karger, Automated high-throughput infusion ESI-MS with direct coupling to a microtiter plate, *Analytical Chemistry*, 73, 1449–1454 (2001).

302. B. Zhang, F. Foret, and B. L. Karger, High-throughput microfabricated CE/ESI-MS: Automated sampling from a microwell plate, *Analytical Chemistry*, 73, 2675–2681 (2001).

303. P. Chaurand, S. A. Schwartz, and R. M. Caprioli, Imaging mass spectrometry: A new tool to investigate the spatial organization of peptides and proteins in mammalian tissue sections, *Current Opinion in Chemical Biology*, 6, 676–681 (2002).

304. R. M. A. Heeren and J. V. Sweedler, Imaging mass spectrometry imaging, *International Journal of Mass Spectrometry*, 260, 89 (2007).

305. Y. Hsieh, J. Chen, and W. A. Korfmacher, Mapping pharmaceuticals in tissues using MALDI imaging mass spectrometry, *Journal of Pharmacological and Toxicological Methods*, 55, 193–200 (2007).

306. N. Liu, F. Liu, B. Xu, Y.-B. Gao, X.-H. Li, K.-H. Wei, X. Zhang, and S. Yang, Establishment of imaging mass spectrometry for biological tissues and its application on the proteome analysis of microwave radiated rat hippocampus, *Chinese Journal of Analytical Chemistry*, 36, 421–425 (2008).

307. J. S. Becker, M. V. Zoriy, J. Dobrowolska, and A. Matucsh, Imaging mass spectrometry in biological tissues by laser ablation inductively coupled plasma mass spectrometry, *European Journal of Mass Spectrometry*, 13, 1–6 (2007).

308. J. Dobrowolska, M. Dehnhardt, A. Matusch, M. Zoriy, N. Palomero-Gallagher, P. Koscielniak, K. Zilles, and J. S. Becker, Quantitative imaging of zinc, copper and lead in three distinct regions of the human brain by laser ablation inductively coupled plasma mass spectrometry, *Talanta*, 74, 717–723 (2007).

309. R. M. A. Heeren, D. F. Smith, J. Stauber, B. Kükrer-Kaletas, and L. MacAleese, Imaging mass spectrometry: Hype or hope? *Journal of the American Society for Mass Spectrometry*, 20, 1006–1014 (2009).

310. D. W. McRobbie, E. A. Moore, M. J. Graves, and M. R. Prince, *MRI from Picture to Proton*, Cambridge University Press, Cambridge, U.K., 2007.

311. M. M. J. Modo and J. W. M. Bulte (eds.), *Molecular and Cellular MR Imaging*, CRC Press, Boca Raton, FL, 2007.

312. C. T. W. Moonen and P. A. Bandettini (eds.), *Functional MRI*, Springer Verlag, Berlin, 2000.

313. P. Jezzard, P. M. Matthews, and S. M. Smith (eds.), *Functional MRI: An Introduction to Methods*, Oxford University Press, Oxford, U.K., 2001.

314. S. H. Faro and F. B. Mohamed (eds.), *Functional MRI: Basic Principles and Clinical Applications*, Springer Science and Business Media, New York, 2006.

315. S. Haeberle and R. Zengerle, Microfluidic platforms for lab-on-a-chip applications, *Lab on a Chip*, 7, 1094–1110 (2007).

316. A. A. Ewis, Z. Zhelev, R. Bakalova, S. Fukuoka, Y. Shinohara, M. Ishikawa, and Y. Baba, A history of microarrays in biomedicine, *Expert Review of Molecular Diagnostics*, 5, 315–328 (2005).

317. G. M. Whitesides, The 'right' size in nanobiotechnology, *Nature Biotechnology*, 21, 1161–1165 (2003).

318. J. S. Albala and I. Humphery-Smith (eds.), *Protein Arrays, Biochips and Proteomics: The Next Phase of Genomic Discovery*, CRC Press, Boca Raton, FL, 2003.

319. J. H. Ng and L. L. Ilag, Biochips beyond DNA: Technologies and applications, *Biotechnology Annual Reviews*, 9, 1–149 (2003).

320. M. West, G. S. Ginsburg, A. T. Huang, and J. R. Nevins, Embracing the complexity of genomic data for personalized medicine, *Genome Research*, 16, 559–566 (2006).

321. P. Bernini et al., Individual human phenotypes in metabolic space and time, *Journal of Proteome Research*, 8, 4264–4271 (2009).

322. T. D. Gelehrter, F. S. Collins, and D. Ginsburg, *Principles of Medical Genetics*, 2nd. edn., Williams and Wilkins, Baltimore, MD, 1998.

323. Interview with NIH Director Elias A. Zerhouni, The promise of personalized medicine, *NIH Medline Plus*, Winter 2007, 2–3 (2007) online at: http://www.nih.gov/about/director/interviews/NLMmagazinewinter2007.pdf (January 2010).

324. NIH Fact Sheet, From Genes to Personalized Medicine, online at: http://www.nih.gov/about/researchresultsforthepublic/Genes_PersonalizedMed.pdf (January 2010).

325. A. E. Guttmacher and F. S. Collins, Realizing the promise of genomics in biomedical research, *Journal of the American Medical Association*, 294, 1399–1402 (2005).
326. D. Christensen, Targeted therapies: Will gene screens usher in personalized medicine? *Science News*, 162, 171–172 (2002).
327. C. Brownlee, Me and my metabolism: Personalized medicine takes new direction, *Science News*, 169, 244–245 (2006).
328. J. F. Hocquette, Where are we in genomics? *Journal of Physiology and Pharmacology*, 56(S3) 37–70 (2005).
329. R. March, Pharmacogenomics: The genomics of drug response, *Yeast*, 17, 16–21 (2000).
330. W. Kalow, Pharmacogenetics and personalised medicine, *Fundamental and Clinical Pharmacology*, 16, 337–342 (2002).
331. K. M. Carr, K. Rosenblatt, E. F. Petricoin, and L. A. Liotta, Genomic and proteomic approaches for studying human cancer: Prospects for true patient-tailored therapy, *Human Genomics*, 1, 134–140 (2004).
332. K.-V. Chin et al., Application of expression genomics in drug development and genomic medicine, *Drug Development Research*, 62, 124–133 (2004).
333. J. Yang, Exploring the molecular basis of tumor metastasis by microarray analysis, *Assay and Drug Development Technologies*, 4, 483–488 (2006).
334. S. A. Waldman, W. K. Kraft, T. J. Nelson, and A. Terzic, Experimental therapeutics: A paradigm for personalized medicine, *Clinical and Translational Science*, 2, 436–438 (2009).
335. E. P. Bottinger, Foundations, promises and uncertainties of personalized medicine, *Mount Sinai Journal of Medicine: A Journal of Translational and Personalized Medicine*, 74, 15–21 (2007).
336. M. Janitz (ed.), *Next-Generation Genome Sequencing: Towards Personalized Medicine*, Wiley Interscience, Hoboken, NJ, 2008.
337. W. G. Feero, A. E. Guttmacher, and F. S. Collins, The genome gets personal—Almost, *Journal of the American Medical Association*, 299, 1351–1352 (2008).
338. M. J. Khoury et al., The scientific foundation for personal genomics: Recommendations from a National Institutes of Health-Centers for Disease Control and Prevention multidisciplinary workshop, *Genetics in Medicine*, 11, 559–567 (2009).
339. J. Kaput et al., Planning the Human Variome Project: The Spain Report, *Human Mutation*, 30, 496–510 (2009).
340. D. Levenson, Personalized medicine presents challenges and opportunities, *American Journal of Medical Genetics Part A*, 152, fm vii–fm viii (2010).
341. J. M. S. Bartlett and D. Stirling, *A Short History of the Polymerase Chain Reaction, in PCR Protocols*, 2nd edn., *Methods in Molecular Biology*, Vol. 226, Humana Press, Totowa, NJ, 2003.
342. M. Altwegg, General problems associated with diagnostic applications of amplification methods, *Journal of Microbiological Methods*, 23, 21–30 (1995).
343. V. V. Demidov, Rolling-circle amplification in DNA diagnostics: The power of simplicity, *Expert Review of Molecular Diagnostics*, 2, 542–548 (2002).
344. P. Gill and A. Ghaemi, Nucleic acid isothermal amplification technologies: A review, *Nucleosides, Nucleotides and Nucleic Acids*, 27, 224–243 (2008).
345. T. Notomi, H. Okayama, H. Masubuchi, T. Yonekawa, K. Watanabe, N. Amino, and T. Hase, Loop-mediated isothermal amplification of DNA, *Nucleic Acids Research*, 28, E63–E63 (2000).

346. D. Y. Zhang, M. Brandwein, T. Hsuih, and H. B. Li, Ramification amplification: A novel isothermal DNA amplification method, *Molecular Diagnosis*, 6, 141–150 (2001).

347. M. Vincent, Y. Xu, and H. Kong, Helicase-dependent isothermal DNA amplification, *EMBO Reports*, 5, 795–800 (2004).

348. H. Mukai, T. Uemori, O. Takeda, E. Kobayashi, J. Yamamoto, K. Nishiwaki, T. Enoki, H. Sagawa, K. Asada, and I. Kato, Highly efficient isothermal DNA amplification system using three elements of 5′-DNA-RNA-3′ chimeric primers, RNaseH and strand-displacing DNA polymerase, *Journal of Biochemistry*, 142, 273–281 (2007).

349. Y.-J. Jeong, K. Park, and D.-E. Kim, Isothermal DNA amplification in vitro: The helicase-dependent amplification system, *Cellular and Molecular Life Sciences*, 66, 3325–3336 (2009).

350. C. Zhang and D. Xing, Miniaturized PCR chips for nucleic acid amplification and analysis: Latest advances and future trends, *Nucleic Acids Research*, 35, 4223–4237 (2007).

351. Y. Zhang and P. Ozdemir, Microfluidic DNA amplification—A review, *Analytica Chimica Acta*, 638, 115–125 (2009).

352. M. M. Kiss, L. Ortoleva-Donnelly, N. R. Beer, J. Warner, C. G. Bailey, B. W. Colston, J. M. Rothberg, D. R. Link, and J. H. Leamon, High-throughput quantitative polymerase chain reaction in picoliter droplets, *Analytical Chemistry*, 80, 8975–8981 (2008).

353. E. Tan, J. Wong, D. Nguyen, Y. Zhang, B. Erwin, L. K. Van Ness, S. M. Baker, D. J. Galas, and A. Niemz, Isothermal DNA amplification coupled with DNA nanosphere-based colorimetric detection, *Analytical Chemistry*, 77, 7984–7992 (2005).

354. N. C. Cady, S. Stelick, M. V. Kunnavakkam, Y. Liu, and C. A. Batt, A microchip-based DNA purification and real-time PCR biosensor for bacterial detection, *Sensors 2004: Proceedings of the IEEE*, 3, 1191–1194 (2004).

355. W. Tan, K. Wang, and T. J. Drake, Molecular beacons, *Current Opinion in Chemical Biology*, 8, 547–553 (2004).

356. J. Yi, W. Zhang, and D. Y. Zhang, Molecular zipper: A fluorescent probe for real-time isothermal DNA amplification, *Nucleic Acids Research*, 34, e81 (2006).

357. M. Goto, E. Honda, A. Ogura, A. Nomoto, and K.-I. Hanaki, Colorimetric detection of loop-mediated isothermal amplification reaction by using hydroxy naphthol blue, *BioTechniques*, 46, 167–172 (2009).

358. E. Carrilho, M. C. Ruiz-Martinez, J. Berka, I. Smirnov, W. Goetzinger, A. W. Miller, D. Brady, and B. L. Karger, Rapid DNA sequencing of more than 1000 bases per run by capillary electrophoresis using replaceable linear polyacrylamide solutions, *Analytical Chemistry*, 68, 3305–3313 (1996).

359. D. Schmalzing, A. Adourian, L. Koutny, L. Ziaugra, P. Matsudaira, and D. Ehrlich, DNA sequencing on microfabricated electrophoretic devices, *Analytical Chemistry*, 70, 2303–2310 (1998).

360. P. A. Pevzner and R. J. Lipshutz, Towards DNA sequencing chips, *Mathematical Foundations of Computer Science 1994 (Springer Lecture Notes in Computer Science)*, 841, 143–158 (1994).

361. J. Weber and H. Meyers, Human whole-genome shotgun sequencing, *Genome Research*, 7, 401–409 (1997).

362. G. Ramsay, DNA chips: State-of-the art, *Nature Biotechnology*, 16, 40–44 (1998).

363. A. Tefferi, M. E. Bolander, S. M. Ansell, E. D. Wieben, and T. C. Spelsberg, Primer on medical genomics. Part III: Microarray experiments and data analysis, *Mayo Clinic Proceedings*, 77, 927–940 (2002).
364. P. M. Lizardi, Next-generation sequencing-by-hybridization, *Nature Biotechnology*, 26, 649–650 (2008).
365. A. Pihlak, G. Baurén, E. Hersoug, P. Lönnerberg, A. Metsis, and S. Linnarsson, Rapid genome sequencing with short universal tiling probes, *Nature Biotechnology*, 26, 676–684 (2008).
366. G. Gibson and S. V. Muse, *A Primer of Genome Science*, 3rd edn., Sinauer Associates, Inc., Sunderland, MA, 2009.
367. D. Schmalzing, L. Koutny, A. Adourian, P. Belgrader, P. Matsudaira, and D. Ehrlich, DNA typing in thirty seconds with a microfabricated device, *Proceedings of the National Academy of Sciences*, 94, 10273–10278 (1997).
368. P. A. Auroux, Y. Koc, A. deMello, A. Manz, and P. J. Day, Miniaturised nucleic acid analysis, *Lab on a Chip*, 4, 534–546 (2004).
369. P. Jaluria, K. Konstantopoulos, M. Betenbaugh, and J. Shiloach, A perspective on microarrays: Current applications, pitfalls, and potential uses, *Microbial Cell Factories*, 6, (2007) online as: doi:10.1186/1475-2859-6-4 (2007).
370. A. Marziali and M. Akeson, New DNA sequencing methods, *Annual Review of Biomedical Engineering*, 3, 195–223 (2001).
371. M. Q. Yang, B. D. Athey, H. R. Arabnia, A. H. Sung, Q. Liu, J. Y. Yang, J. Mao, and Y. Deng, High-throughput next-generation sequencing technologies foster new cutting-edge computing techniques in bioinformatics, *BMC Genomics*, 10(S1), I1 (2009).
372. J. R. Edwards and H. Ju.-J. Ruparel, Mass-spectrometry DNA sequencing, *Mutation Research*, 573, 3–12 (2005).
373. F. Kirpekar, E. Nordhoff, L. K. Larsen, K. Kristiansen, P. Roepstorff, and F. Hillenkamp, DNA sequence analysis by MALDI mass spectrometry, *Nucleic Acids Research*, 26, 2554–2559 (1998).
374. J. Hahm and C. M. Lieber, Direct ultrasensitive electrical detection of DNA and DNA sequence variations using nanowire nanosensors, *Nano Letters*, 4, 51–54 (2004).
375. J. Lagerqvist, M. Zwolak, and M. Di Ventra, Fast DNA sequencing via transverse electronic transport, *Nano Letters*, 6, 779–782 (2006).
376. E. R. Mardis, Next-generation DNA sequencing methods, *Annual Review of Genomics and Human Genetics*, 9, 387–402 (2008).
377. J. Ragoussis, Genotyping technologies for genetic research, *Annual Review of Genomics and Human Genetics*, 10, 117–133, (2009).
378. F. McCaughan and P. H. Dear, Single-molecule genomics, *The Journal of Pathology*, 220, 297–306 (2010).
379. MarketResearch.com, The DNA sequencing business, Web site at: http://www.marketresearch.com/map/prod/1195362.html (accessed February 8, 2010).
380. J. Hodgson, Hyseq–Variagenics merger signals end of the line, *Nature Biotechnology*, 21, 5 (2003).
381. R. Molidor, A. Sturn, M. Maurer, and Z. Trajanoski, New trends in bioinformatics: From genome sequence to personalized medicine, *Experimental Gerontology*, 38, 1031–1036 (2003).
382. P. Jares, DNA microarray applications in functional genomics, *Ultrastructural Pathology*, 30, 209–219 (2006).

383. V. Trevino, F. Falciani, and H. A. Barrera-Saldaña, DNA microarrays: A powerful genomic tool for biomedical and clinical research, *Molecular Medicine*, 13, 527–541 (2007).

384. C. Brownlee, Faster, cheaper, better: Easier genetic sequencing could make personalized medicine a reality, *Science News*, 171, 235–236 (2007).

385. E. Abrahams, Right drug—Right patient—Right time: Personalized Medicine Coalition, *Clinical and Translational Science*, 1, 11–12 (2008).

386. GEN MarketWire, DNA sequencing at your doctor's office? Not impossible, says report, *Genetic Engineering and Biotechnology News*, online at: http://www.genengnews.com/news/bnitem.aspx?name=64183240 (September 30, 2009).

387. B. Bernstein, A. Meissner, and E. Lander, The mammalian epigenome, *Cell*, 128, 669–681 (2007).

388. P. A. Jones and S. B. Baylin, The epigenomics of cancer, *Cell*, 128, 683–692 (2007).

389. D. Figeys, Proteomics: The basic overview, *Methods of Biochemical Analysis*, 45, 1–62 (2005).

390. K. Cottingham, Meeting news: NIH Standards in Proteomics Workshop, *Journal of Proteome Research*, 4, 220 (2005).

391. R. Groleau, H. Steen, P. Recinos, and J. Testa, *Introduction to Proteomics*, Children's Hospital, Boston, MA, Web site at: http://www.childrenshospital.org/cfapps/research/data_admin/Site602/mainpageS602P0.html (February 8, 2010).

392. H. Zhu, M. Bilgin, and M. Snyder, Proteomics, *Annual Review of Biochemistry*, 72, 783–812 (2003).

393. X. Han, A. Aslanian, and J. R. Yates 3rd, Mass spectrometry for proteomics, *Current Opinion in Chemical Biology*, 12, 483–490 (2008).

394. H. Mischak, J. J. Coon, J. Novak, E. M. Weissinger, J. P. Schanstra, and A. F. Dominiczak, Capillary electrophoresis-mass spectrometry as a powerful tool in biomarker discovery and clinical diagnosis: An update of recent developments, *Mass Spectrometry Reviews*, 28, 703–724 (2009).

395. S. Mouradian, Lab-on-a-chip: Applications in proteomics, *Current Opinion in Chemical Biology*, 6, 51–56 (2002).

396. M. Hamady, T. H. Cheung, K. Resing, K. J. Cios, and R. Knight, Key challenges in proteomics and proteoinformatics, *IEEE Engineering in Medicine and Biology Magazine*, 24, 34–40 (2005).

397. R. Falk, M. Ramström, S. Ståhl, and S. Hober, Approaches for systematic proteome exploration, *Biomolecular Engineering*, 24, 155–168 (2007).

398. S. Srivastava (ed.), *Informatics In Proteomics*, CRC Press, Boca Raton, FL, 2005.

399. W. Kolch, H. Mischak, M. J. Chalmers, A. Pitt, and A. G. Marshall, Clinical proteomics: A question of technology, *Rapid Communications in Mass Spectrometry*, 18, 2365–2366 (2004).

400. D. H. Geho, N. Lahar, M. Ferrari, E. F. Petricoin, and L. A. Liotta, Opportunities for nanotechnology-based innovation in tissue proteomics, *Biomedical Microdevices*, 6, 231–239 (2004).

401. P. A. Binz, M. Müller, C. Hoogland, C. Zimmermann, C. Pasquarello, G. Corthals, J. C. Sanchez, H. F. Hochstrasser, and R. D. Appel, The molecular scanner: Concept and developments, *Current Opinion in Biotechnology*, 15, 17–23 (2004).

402. K. R. Coombes, J. S. Morris, J. Hu, S. R. Edmonson, and K. A. Baggerly, Serum proteomics profiling—A young technology begins to mature, *Nature Biotechnology*, 23, 291–292 (2005).

403. S. Hu, J. A. Loo, and D. T. Wong, Human body fluid proteome analysis, *Proteomics*, 6, 6326–6353 (2006).

404. S. Hu, J. A. Loo, and D. T. Wong, Human saliva proteome analysis, *Annals of the New York Academy of Sciences*, 1098, 323–329 (2007).

405. G. Zegels, G. A. Van Raemdonck, E. P. Coen, W. A. Tjalma, and X. W. Van Ostade, Comprehensive proteomic analysis of human cervical-vaginal fluid using colposcopy samples, *Proteome Science*, 7, 17 (2009), Online at doi: 10.1186/1477-5956-7-17.

406. M. Wilm, A. Shevchenko, T. Houthaeve, S. Breit, L. Schweigerer, T. Fotsis, and M. Mann, Femtomole sequencing of proteins from polyacrylamide gels by nano-electrospray mass spectrometry, *Nature*, 379, 466–469 (1996).

407. S. D. Patterson, Mass spectrometry and proteomics, *Physiological Genomics*, 2, 59–65 (2000).

408. R. Aebersold and M. Mann, Mass spectrometry-based proteomics, *Nature*, 422, 198–207 (2003).

409. K. Breuker, M. Jin, X. Han, H. Jiang, and F. W. McLafferty, Top-down identification and characterization of biomolecules by mass spectrometry, *Journal of the American Society for Mass Spectrometry*, 19, 1045–1053 (2008).

410. M. Tyers and M. Mann, From genomics to proteomics, *Nature*, 422, 193–197 (2003).

411. G. G. Pedrioli et al., A common open representation of mass spectrometry data and its application to proteomics research, *Nature Biotechnology*, 22, 1459–1466 (2004).

412. G. Cagney and A. Emili, Proteogest: A tool for facilitating proteomics using mass spectrometry, *Drug Discovery Today: TARGETS*, 3(Sup. 1), 63–65 (2004).

413. J. J. Coon, Collisions or electrons? Protein sequence analysis in the 21st century, *Analytical Chemistry*, 81, 3208–3215 (2009).

414. J. R. Yates, C. I. Ruse, and A. Nakorchevsky, Proteomics by mass spectrometry: Approaches, advances, and applications, *Annual Review of Biomedical Engineering*, 11, 49–79 (2009).

415. W. J. Qian, J. M. Jacobs, T. Liu, D. G. Camp 2nd, and R. D. Smith, Advances and challenges in liquid chromatography-mass spectrometry-based proteomics profiling for clinical applications, *Molecular and Cellular Proteomics*, 5, 1727–1744 (2006).

416. P. Findeisen and M. Neumaier, Mass spectrometry based proteomics profiling as diagnostic tool in oncology: Current status and future perspective, *Clinical Chemistry and Laboratory Medicine*, 47, 666–684 (2009).

417. L. Moulédous and H. B. Gutstein, Gene arrays and proteomics. A primer, *Methods in Molecular Medicine*, 84, 141–154 (2003).

418. H. Zhu and M. Snyder, Protein chip technology, *Current Opinion in Chemical Biology*, 7, 55–63 (2003).

419. D. A. Hall, J. Ptacek, and M. Snyder, Protein microarray technology, *Mechanisms of Aging and Development*, 128, 161–167 (2007).

420. W. Kusnezow and J. D. Hoheisel, Antibody microarrays: Promises and problems, *Biotechniques*, 2002, S14–S23 (2002).

421. L. L. Lv and B. C. Liu, High-throughput antibody microarrays for quantitative proteomic analysis, *Expert Review of Proteomics*, 4, 505–513 (2007).

422. M. A. Coleman, P. T. Beernink, J. A. Camarero, and J. S. Albala, Applications of functional protein microarrays: Identifying protein–protein interactions in an array format, *Methods in Molecular Biology*, 385, 121–130 (2007).

423. W. Liao, S. Guo, and X. S. Zhao, Novel probes for protein chip applications, *Frontiers in Bioscience*, 11, 186–197 (2006).
424. S. L. Seurynck-Servoss, C. L. Baird, K. D. Rodland, and R. C. Zangar, Surface chemistries for antibody microarrays, *Frontiers in Bioscience*, 12, 3956–3964 (2007).
425. S. Spisak, Z. Tulassay, B. Molnar, and A. Guttman, Protein microchips in biomedicine and biomarker discovery, *Electrophoresis*, 28, 4261–4273 (2007).
426. O. Stoevesandt, M. J. Taussig, and M. He, Protein microarrays: High-throughput tools for proteomics, *Expert Review of Proteomics*, 6, 145–157 (2009).
427. S. Spisák and A. Guttman, Biomedical applications of protein microarrays, *Current Medicinal Chemistry*, 16, 2806–2815 (2009).
428. M. S. Alhamdani, C. Schröder, and J. D. Hoheisel, Oncoproteomic profiling with antibody microarrays, *Genome Medicine*, 1, 68 (2009).
429. M. Chatterjee, J. Wojciechowski, and M. A. Tainsky, Discovery of antibody biomarkers using protein microarrays of tumor antigens cloned in high throughput, *Methods in Molecular Biology*, 520, 21–38 (2009).
430. R. Goodacre, S. Vaidyanathan, W. B. Dunn, G. G. Harrigan, and D. B. Kell, Metabolomics by numbers: Acquiring and understanding global metabolite data, *Trends in Biotechnology*, 22, 245–252 (2004).
431. A. Scalbert, L. Brennan, O. Fiehn, T. Hankemeier, B. S. Kristal, B. van Ommen, E. Pujos-Guillot, E. Verheij, D. Wishart, and S. Wopereis, Mass-spectrometry-based metabolomics: Limitations and recommendations for future progress with particular focus on nutrition research, *Metabolomics*, 5, 435–458 (2009).
432. D. S. Wishart, C. Knox, A. C. Guo, R. Eisner, N. Young, B. Gautam, D. D. Hau et al., HMDB: A knowledgebase for the human metabolome, *Nucleic Acids Research*, 37(Database issue), D603–610 (2009).
433. U. Alon, *An Introduction to Systems Biology: Design Principles of Biological Circuits*, Chapman and Hall/CRC Press, Boca Raton, FL, 2007.
434. I. V. Maly (ed.), *Systems Biology*, Humana Press, New York, 2009.
435. L. Alberghina and H. V. Westerhoff, Systems biology: Did we know it all along? in *Systems Biology: Definitions and Perspectives*, Springer Verlag, Berlin, Germany (2005).
436. E. Klipp, R. Herwig, A. Kowald, C. Wierling, and H. Lehrach, *Systems Biology in Practice: Concepts, Implementation and Application*, Wiley-VCH, Weinheim, Germany, 2005.
437. A. Kriete and R. Eils (eds.), *Computational Systems Biology*, Elsevier Academic Press, Burlington, MA, 2006.
438. K. Najarian, C. N. Eichelberger, S. Najarian, and S. Gharibzadeh, *Systems Biology and Bioinformatics*, CRC Press, Boca Raton, FL, 2009.
439. D. K. Slonim, From patterns to pathways: Gene expression data analysis comes of age, *Nature Genetics*, 32,S502–S508 (2002).
440. R. S. Matson, *Applying Genomic and Proteomic Microarray Technology in Drug Discovery*, CRC Press, Boca Raton, FL, 2004.
441. E. Werner, J. F. Heilier, C. Ducruix, E. Ezan, C. Junot, and J. C. Tabet, Mass spectrometry for the identification of the discriminating signals from metabolomics: Current status and future trends, *Journal of Chromatography B Analytical Technologies in the Biomedical and Life Sciences*, 2008 Aug 15; 871(2), 143–163 (2008).
442. J.-S. Lee, I.-S.Chu, A. Mikaelyan, D. F. Calvisi, J. Heo, J. K. Reddy, and S. S. Thorgeirsson, Application of comparative functional genomics to identify best-fit mouse models to study human cancer, *Nature Genetics*, 36, 1306–1311 (2004).

443. J. K. Habermann, U. J. Roblick, M. Upender, T. Ried, and G. Auer, From genome to proteome in tumor profiling: Molecular events in colorectal cancer genesis, *Advances in Experimental Medicine and Biology*, 587, 161–177 (2006).
444. M. C. Gast, J. H. Schellens, and J. H. Beijnen, Clinical proteomics in breast cancer: A review, *Breast Cancer Research and Treatment*, 116, 17–29 (2009).
445. S. M. McHugh, J. O'Donnell, and P. Gillen, Genomic and oncoproteomic advances in detection and treatment of colorectal cancer, *World Journal of Surgical Oncology*, 1(7), 36 (2009).
446. J. Y. Engwegen, M. C. Gast, J. H. Schellens, and J. H. Beijnen, Clinical proteomics: Searching for better tumour markers with SELDI-TOF mass spectrometry, *Trends in Pharmacological Science*, 27, 251–259 (2006).
447. S. Mohr, G. D. Leikauf, G. Keith, and B. H. Rihn, Microarrays as cancer keys: An array of possibilities, *Journal of Clinical Oncology*, 20, 3165–3175 (2002).
448. S. Ramaswamy and T. R. Golub, DNA microarrays in clinical oncology, *Journal of Clinical Oncology*, 20, 1932–1941 (2002).
449. U. Schmidt and C. G. Begley, Cancer diagnosis and microarrays, *International Journal of Biochemistry and Cell Biology*, 35, 119–124 (2003).
450. G. Russo, C. Zegar, and A. Giordano, Advantages and limitations of microarray technology in human cancer, *Oncogene*, 22, 6497–6507 (2003).
451. G. Bucca, G. Carruba, A. Saetta, P. Muti, L. Castagnetta, and C. P. Smith, Gene expression profiling of human cancers, *Annals of the New York Academy of Sciences*, 1028, 28–37 (2004).
452. R. Wadlow and S. Ramaswamy, DNA microarrays in clinical cancer research, *Current Molecular Medicine*, 5, 111–120 (2005).
453. K.-V. Chin, L. Alabanza, K. Fuji, K. Kudoh, T. Kita, Y. Kikuchi, Z. E. Selvanayagam, Y. F. Wong, Y. Lin, and W. C. Shih, Application of expression genomics for predicting treatment response in cancer, *Annals of the New York Academy of Sciences*, 1058, 186–195 (2005).
454. P. Jares and E. Campo, Genomic platforms for cancer research: Potential diagnostic and prognostic applications in clinical oncology, *Clinical and Translational Oncology*, 8, 161–172 (2006).
455. W. C. Cho, Contribution of oncoproteomics to cancer biomarker discovery, *Molecular Cancer*, 6, 25 (2007).
456. L. Ying and M. Sarwal, In praise of arrays, *Pediatric Nephrology*, 24, 1643–1659 (2009).
457. A. Nordström and R. Lewensohn, Metabolomics: Moving to the Clinic, *Journal of Neuroimmune Pharmacology*, 5, 4–17 (2010).
458. D. W. Bell, Our changing view of the genomic landscape of cancer, *The Journal of Pathology*, 220, 231–243 (2010).
459. C. D. Berdanier and N. Moustaid-Moussa, *Genomics and Proteomics in Nutrition*, CRC Press, Boca Raton, FL, 2004.
460. B. van Ommen, J. Keijer, S. G. Heil, and J. Kaput, Challenging homeostasis to define biomarkers for nutrition related health, *Molecular Nutrition and Food Research*, 53, 795–804 (2009).
461. L. C. Manace, T. N. Godiwala, and M. W. Babyatsky, Genomics of cardiovascular disease, *Mount Sinai Journal of Medicine*, 76, 613–623 (2009).
462. R. Roberts and A. F. R. Stewart, Personalized genomic medicine: A future prerequisite for the prevention of coronary artery disease, *The American Heart Hospital Journal*, 4, 222–227 (2006).

463. K. C. P. Li, S. Guccione, and M. D. Bednarski, Combined vascular targeted imaging and therapy: A paradigm for personalized treatment, *Journal of Cellular Biochemistry*, 87, 65–71 (2009).

464. F. E. Hargreave and P. Nair, The definition and diagnosis of asthma, *Clinical and Experimental Allergy*, 39, 1652–1658 (2009).

465. Z. Wei, K. Wang, H.-Q. Qu, H. Zhang, J. Bradfield, C. Kim, E. Frackleton et al., From disease association to risk assessment: An optimistic view from genome-wide association studies on type 1 diabetes, *PLoS Genetics*, Published online October 09, 2009, doi:10.1371/journal.pgen.1000678 (2009).

466. R. Dankner, A. Danoff, and J. Roth, Can personalized diagnostics promote earlier intervention for dysglycaemia? Hypothesis ready for testing, *Diabetes/ Metabolism Research and Reviews*, 26, 7–9 (2010).

467. M. O. Glocker, R. Guthke, J. Kekow, and H.-J. Thiesen, Rheumatoid arthritis, a complex multifactorial disease: On the way toward individualized medicine, *Medicinal Research Reviews*, 26, 63–87 (2006).

468. A. J. Silman and J. E. Pearson, Epidemiology and genetics of rheumatoid arthritis, *Arthritis Research*, 4, S265–S272 (2002).

469. C. S. Haas, C. J. Creighton, X. Pi, I. Maine, A. E. Koch, G. K. Haines, S. Ling, A. M. Chinnaiyan, and J. Holoshitz, Joseph, Identification of genes modulated in rheumatoid arthritis using complementary DNA microarray analysis of lymphoblastoid B cell lines from disease-discordant monozygotic twins, *Arthritis and Rheumatism*, 54, 2047–2060 (2006).

470. K. Sellheyer and T. J. Belbin, DNA microarrays: From structural genomics to functional genomics. The applications of gene chips in dermatology and dermatopathology, *Journal of the American Academy of Dermatology*, 51, 681–692 (2004).

471. X. Li and A. P. Conklin, New serological biomarkers of inflammatory bowel disease, *World Journal of Gastroenterology*, 14, 5115–5124 (2008).

472. K. Luttropp, B. Lindholm, J. J. Carrero, G. Glorieux, E. Schepers, R. Vanholder, M. Schalling, P. Stenvinkel, and L. Nordfors, Genetics/genomics in chronic kidney disease—Towards personalized medicine? *Seminars in Dialysis*, 22, 417–422 (2009).

473. Y. Vodovotz, Translational systems biology of inflammation and healing, *Wound Repair and Regeneration*, 18, 3–7 (2010).

474. P. N. Baird, G. S. Hageman, and R. H. Guymer, New era for personalized medicine: The diagnosis and management of age-related macular degeneration, *Clinical and Experimental Ophthalmology*, 37, 814–821 (2009).

475. H. Hwang et al., Glycoproteomics in neurodegenerative diseases, *Mass Spectrometry Reviews*, 29, 79–125 (2010).

476. D. Gurwitz, Pharmacogenomics of schizophrenia: Towards personalized psychiatry, *Drug Development Research*, 60, 71–74 (2003).

477. X. Pham, C. Sun, X. Chen, E. J. C. G. van den Oord, M. C. Neale, K. S. Kendler, and J. M. Hettema, Association study between GABA receptor genes and anxiety spectrum disorders, *Depression and Anxiety*, 26, 998–1003 (2009).

478. N. Y. K. Li, K. V. Abbott, C. Rosen, G. An, P. A. Hebda, and Y. Vodovotz, Translational systems biology and voice pathophysiology, *The Laryngoscope*, 511–515 (2009).

479. S. Rozen et al., Metabolomic analysis and signatures in motor neuron disease, *Metabolomics*, 1, 101–108 (2005).

480. L. Pereira, A. P. Reddy, T. Jacob, A. Thomas, K. A. Schneider, S. Dasari, J. A. Lapidus et al., Identification of novel protein biomarkers of preterm birth in human cervical-vaginal fluid, *Journal of Proteome Research*, 6, 1269–1276 (2007).

481. R. L. Goldenberg, A. R. Goepfert, and P. S. Ramsey, Biochemical markers for the prediction of preterm birth, *American Journal of Obstetrics and Gynecology*, 192, S36–46 (2005).

482. V. Berghella, E. J. Hayes, J. Visintine, and J. K. Baxter, Fetal fibronectin testing for reducing the risk of preterm birth, *Cochrane Database Systematic Reviews*, 2008, CD006843 (2008).

483. H. Honest, C. A. Forbes, K. H. Durée, G. Norman, S. B. Duffy, A. Tsourapas, T. E. Roberts et al., Screening to prevent spontaneous preterm birth: Systematic reviews of accuracy and effectiveness literature with economic modeling, *Health Technology Assessment*, 13, 1–627 (2009).

484. C. D. Rinaudo, J. L. Telford, R. Rappuoli, and K. L. Seib, Vaccinology in the genome era, *Journal of Clinical Investigation*, 119, 2515–2525 (2009).

485. S. Suekane, M. Nishitani, M. Noguchi, Y. Komohara, T. Kokubu, M. Naitoh, S. Honma et al., Phase I trial of personalized peptide vaccination for cytokine-refractory metastatic renal cell carcinoma patients, *Cancer Science*, 98, 1965–1968 (2007).

486. Y. Sato et al., Immunological evaluation of personalized peptide vaccination in combination with a 5-fluorouracil derivative (TS-1) for advanced gastric or colorectal carcinoma patients, *Cancer Science*, 98, 1113–1119 (2007).

487. H. Yanagimoto et al., Immunological evaluation of personalized peptide vaccination with gemcitabine for pancreatic cancer, *Cancer Science*, 98, 605–611 (2007).

488. K. L. Seib, G. Dougan, and R. Rappuoli, The key role of genomics in modern vaccine and drug design for emerging infectious diseases, *PLoS Genetics*, 5, e1000612 (2009) doi:10.1371/journal.pgen.1000612.

489. R. Moxon and R. Rappuoli, Bacterial pathogen genomics and vaccines, *British Medical Bulletin*, 62, 45–58 (2002).

490. J. Singh, A. Behal, N. Singla, A. Joshi, N. Birbian, S. Singh, V. Bali, and N. Batra, Metagenomics: Concept, methodology, ecological inference and recent advances, *Biotechnology Journal*, 4, 480–494 (2009).

491. P. D. Schloss and J. Handelsman, Biotechnological prospects from metagenomics *Current Opinion in Biotechnology*, 14, 303–310 (2003).

492. J. Xu, Microbial ecology in the age of genomics and metagenomics: Concepts, tools, and recent advances, *Molecular Ecology*, 15, 1713–1731 (2006).

493. M. H. Wilcox and W. N. Fawley, Molecular diagnostic techniques, *Surgery*, 21, iii–vi (2003).

494. F. C. Dudak and I. H. Boyaci, Rapid and label-free bacteria detection by surface plasmon resonance (SPR) biosensors, *Biotechnology Journal*, 4, 1003–1011 (2009).

495. A. A. Bergwerff and F. van Knapen, Surface plasmon resonance biosensors for detection of pathogenic microorganisms: Strategies to secure food and environmental safety, *Journal of the Association of Official Analytical Chemists International*, 89, 826–831 (2006).

496. D. Bravo, B. Muñoz-Cobo, E. Costa, M. A. Clari, N. Tormo, and D. Navarro, Evaluation of an immunofiltration assay that detects immunoglobulin M antibodies against the ZEBRA protein for the diagnosis of Epstein-Barr virus infectious mononucleosis in immunocompetent patients, *Clinical and Vaccine Immunology*, 16, 885–888 (2009).

497. P. Yager, T. Edwards, E. Fu, K. Helton, K. Nelson, M. R. Tam, and B. H. Weigl, Microfluidic diagnostic technologies for global public health, *Nature*, 442, 412–418 (2006).

498. A. W. Martinez, S. T. Phillips, B. J. Wiley, M. Gupta, and G. M. Whitesides, FLASH: A rapid method for prototyping paper-based microfluidic devices, *Lab on a Chip*, 8, 2146–2150 (2008).

499. G. S. Fiorini and D. T. Chiu, Disposable microfluidic devices: Fabrication, function, and application, *Biotechniques*, 38, 429–446 (2005).

500. E. K. Binga, R. S. Lasken, and J. D. Neufeld, Something from (almost) nothing: The impact of multiple displacement amplification on microbial ecology, *ISME Journal*, 2, 233–241 (2008).

501. C. C. Ginocchio, Life beyond PCR: Alternative target amplification technologies for the diagnosis of infectious diseases, part I, *Clinical Microbiology Newsletter*, 26, 121–128 (2004).

502. C. C. Ginocchio, Life beyond PCR: Alternative target amplification technologies for the diagnosis of infectious diseases, part II, *Clinical Microbiology Newsletter*, 26, 129–136 (2004).

503. T. H. Schulte, R. L. Bardell, and B. H. Weigl, Microfluidic technologies in clinical diagnostics, *Clinica Chimica Acta*, 321, 1–10 (2002).

504. S. Derveaux, B. G. Stubbe, K. Braeckmans, C. Roelant, K. Sato, J. Demeester, and S. C. De Smedt, Synergism between particle-based multiplexing and microfluidics technologies may bring diagnostics closer to the patient, *Analytical and Bioanalytical Chemistry*, 391, 2453–2467 (2008).

505. C. G. J. Schabmueller, D. Loppow, G. Piechotta, B. Schütze, J. Albers, and R. Hintsche, Micromachined sensor for lactate monitoring in saliva, *Biosensors and Bioelectronics*, 21, 1770–1776 (2006).

506. D. M. Porterfield, E. S. McLamore, and M. K. Banks, Microsensor technology for measuring H+ flux in buffered media, *Sensors and Actuators B: Chemical*, 136, 383–387 (2009).

507. E. Diessel, P. Kamphaus, K. Grothe, R. Kurte, U. Damm, and H. M. Heise, Nanoliter serum sample analysis by mid-infrared spectroscopy for minimally invasive blood glucose monitoring, *Applied Spectroscopy*, 59, 442–451 (2005).

508. H. M. Heise, U. Damm, M. Bodenlenz, V. R. Kondepati, G. Köhler, and M. Ellmerer, Bedside monitoring of subcutaneous interstitial glucose in healthy individuals using microdialysis and infrared spectrometry, *Journal of Biomedical Optics*, 12, 024004 (2007), doi:10.1117/1.2714907.

509. X. Li, Q. Zhu, S. Tong, W. Wang, and W. Song, Self-assembled microstructure of carbon nanotubes for enzymeless glucose sensor, *Sensors and Actuators B: Chemical*, 136, 444–450 (2009).

510. N. J. Forrow and S. W. Bayliff, A commercial whole blood glucose biosensor with a low sensitivity to hematocrit, *Biosensors and Bioelectronics*, 21, 581–587 (2005).

511. G. Piechotta, J. Albers, and R. Hintsche, Novel micromachined silicon sensor for continuous glucose monitoring, *Biosensors and Bioelectronics*, 21, 802–808 (2005).

512. D. Brennan, J. Justice, B. Corbett, T. McCarthy, and P. Galvin, Emerging optofluidic technologies for point-of-care genetic analysis systems: A review, *Analytical and Bioanalytical Chemistry*, 395, 621–636 (2009).

513. F. B. Myers and L. P. Lee, Innovations in optical microfluidic technologies for point-of-care diagnostics, *Lab on a Chip*, 8, 2015–2031 (2008).

514. P. von Lode, Point-of-care immunotesting: Approaching the analytical performance of central laboratory methods, *Clinical Biochemistry*, 38, 591–606 (2005).

515. N. M. Jokerst, M. A. Brooke, S.-Y. Cho, and A. B. Shang, Chip-scale sensor system integration for portable health monitoring, *Anesthesia and Analgesia*, 105, S42–S47 (2007).

516. G. S. Wilson and R. Gifford, Biosensors for real-time in vivo measurements, *Biosensors and Bioelectronics*, 20, 2388–2403 (2005).

517. N. Bao, J. Wu, and C. Lu, Recent advances in electric analysis of cells in microfluidic systems, *Analytical and Bioanalytical Chemistry*, 391, 933–942, (2008).

518. J.-S. Lee and S. S. Thorgeirsson, Application of integrative functional genomics to decode cancer signatures, NIH/CCR Website at: http://ccr.cancer.gov/news/frontiers/september2006/thorgeirsson_fig2.asp (2009).

Part III

Future Directions and Transformations

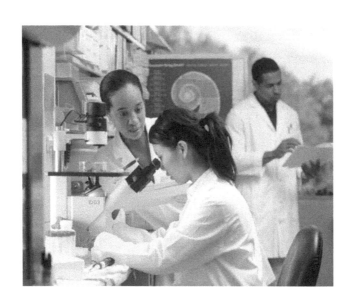

10

Thesis, Antithesis, Synthesis: Integrated Biomolecular Nanoscience

> ... it is apparent that nanoscience and nanotechnology-based approaches are poised to revolutionize research in biology and medicine
>
> **NIH: "Nanoscience and Nanotechnology in Biology and Medicine"** [1]

10.1 Maturation of Medical Nanotechnologies

Medical nanotechnology and nanomedicine are now generally established as having key roles to play in medical research and increasingly in medical practice. Nanoscience and nanotechnology subject papers are published in leading medical journals, including traditional prestige publications like *The Lancet*, *The New England Journal of Medicine*, and the *Journal of the American Medical Society*. In addition, leading publishing houses, societies, and reporting channels for scientific research now have specialist publications devoted to nano subjects [2–4].

It is no longer necessary to debate whether nanotechnology has a place in medicine; now the open questions relate to the nature and impact of its role in different aspects of medicine. Nanotechnology is being used pragmatically by medicine because it is yielding results in drug delivery, imaging, surgery, tissue repair, and other areas. Medicine, much more than many fields, is buffered against taking up new technologies merely because they are seductively promising, exciting, or in popular demand [5–8].

10.2 Continued Impacts of Nanotechnology-Driven Capabilities

The direct application of nanotechnology tends to start first in biomedical research, and then progress to applications through stages of development, evaluation, validation, adoption, and standardization. But medicine is also impacted indirectly by applications of nanotechnology that start in other areas such as computers, imaging, and communications, and then rapidly pervade in all directions.

10.3 Nanotechnologies in Translation from Research

Nanotechnology, the ability to observe and manipulate matter at the nanoscale, arose independently from several lines of research. One line was developed as researchers devised ways to study smaller and smaller aspects of living and physical systems. Some of the first nanotechnologies were research tools for biology, chemistry, and physics. Practical application of nanotechnology came out of research labs into widespread application with the development of microelectronics. As integrated microelectronics expanded rapidly to meet the demands of its various markets, a virtuous cycle evolved—each generation of miniaturization provided capabilities that enabled further improvements in size, speed, and power consumption. Moore's law was the prescient observation and tidy description of this expansion.

Microelectronics and related technologies such as displays and communications provided powerful capabilities that spilled out from their originally intended applications. (When the first digital computers were being developed, it was estimated that the total world market would be 10 machines.) Innovations such as the atomic force microscope were developed in the research laboratories of computer companies to help analyze and design shrinking solid state electronic chips. But their usefulness for biology was appreciated and seized upon even by the original developers. It was the same with other developments that were the key to nanotechnology, such as quantum dots and ultrafast lasers—technology cannot be kept in the bag.

Independently, another aspect of nanotechnology was developed in the pharmaceutical industry, deliberately to meet the requirement of encapsulating drugs to protect them, make them more soluble, and provide a means for slow release. Other key techniques for nano-observation and manipulation came from the study of viruses, and from electrophysiology of cell membranes, proteins, colloids, catalysts, and surface interactions of materials with all of their practical applications.

These developments of tools for specialized disciplines went on fairly independently, until the genesis of nanotechnology as a concept and a challenge. This brought about focus, definition of concepts and goals, communication across disciplines, competition, and wider realization of potential capabilities and benefits. With communication came the spread of knowledge to fresh sources of talent and energy, where the challenges were taken up, sometimes in the face of skepticism. As always, much of the skepticism was directed at overblown or overenthusiastic claims, but neither the overreaching nor the resistance slowed progress as lively discussions ensued.

In medicine, the initial vision of nano-robots tended to discredit the idea of nanotechnology for medical applications. But the definition of nanoscience and its proper integration with the ongoing nanoscale aspects of physics, chemistry, and biology, with their evident medical applications, has refocused medical nanotechnologies on areas where they are even more powerful.

The current leading areas of medical nanotechnology that are emerging from research laboratories are as follows:

1. Theranostic nanomedicines (diagnosis, therapy targeting, and therapy delivery in multifunctional nanoparticles)
2. Personalized medicine (based on nanotechnology-derived methods for rapid and inexpensive genome profiling, coupled with the nanofabrication of customized therapies)
3. Tissue regeneration (based on cell programming by generation and application of cell penetrating peptides for iPSC, coupled with the nanofabrication of tissue engineering scaffolding with coded cell signaling and release of bioactive agents)
4. Advanced diagnostics (based on nanotechnology-enabled advanced imaging, chemical analysis, and physiology measurement modalities, coupled with microelectronics and data processing)

In addition, other nanotechnologies are of significance in biomedical research, such as laser nanosurgery and microdissection, quantum resonance single molecule detection, etc. These nanotechnologies may lead to clinical applications soon, but for now they are useful mainly in research.

10.4 Indirect Impacts of Nanotechnology-Enabled Systems on Practice

Currently, the major impacts on medical practice of systems whose capabilities are driven by nanotechnology are as follows:

1. Personalized patient monitoring (based on microelectronics with medical sensing integrated into inexpensive and widely used personal digital accessories and global connectivity to extend care and communication from the hospital to wherever the patient goes, supplemented by ingestible, insertable, or implantable wireless sensors and actuators)
2. Advanced robotic-assisted minimally invasive surgery (based on microelectronics, wireless endoscopic tools, advanced controls, and

user interfaces, integrated with diagnostic imaging and surgery planning and treatment staging systems)

3. Advanced personalized patient health management (based on digital patient records; integrated with personal monitoring and diagnostic imaging and laboratory databases, coupled with advanced data management, visualization, and interaction user interfaces; and advanced analysis and review aids in an integrated practice system)

In addition, a number of other new capabilities for work and lifestyle are being enabled indirectly by advances in nanotechnology, such as increasing wireless and Internet connectivity; these are having a strong impact for healthcare.

The above technology-based capabilities exist; although they are not yet universally diffused into practice, it is a matter of time and economics before they become part of the standard of care in the most advanced societies. If this does not happen soon, you may find yourself falling behind China, India, or other parts of the world that were once considered the developing nations.

10.5 Translation of Medical Nanotechnologies into Clinical Practice

The translation of a new technology from an experimental stage to hospital or clinical practice is always challenging and risky. The many steps and procedures required for this process are intended to minimize risks and manage the risks that remain. The situation is summed up for surgical robotics in neurosurgery as follows:

> Obviously, the results presented here still need to be extensively validated. Clinical reality is far from laboratory experiments. Human surgical targets—be it deep tumors or functional nuclei—are not steel balls, and the radiographic coordinates may indeed differ from anatomical or physiological "sweet spots," and that's why the robots of future will be equipped with "smart guidance" systems that will include haptic, optical, electrophysiological, or chemical feedback. Sooner we embrace the idea of robotization, the more prepared we will be when the technology catches up with our demands. It is quite possible that opening our mind is just as difficult as teaching a robot to drill through the skull! [9]

This quotation is generally applicable. The final step in the translation of new technologies to clinical practice is one that takes place in the mind—when we are satisfied that the technology actually provides benefit and is safe.

References

1. NIH, PA-08-052, Nanoscience and nanotechnology in biology and medicine, NIH, Bethesda, MD, http://grants.nih.gov/grants/guide/pa-files/pa-08-052.html (2008).
2. M. C. Roco, Nanotechnology: Convergence with modern biology and medicine, *Current Opinion in Biotechnology*, 14, 337–346 (2003).
3. V. Wagner, A. Dullaart, A.-K. Bock, and A. Zweck, The emerging nanomedicine landscape, *Nature Biotechnology*, 24, 1211–1217 (2006).
4. Editorial, Nanomedicine: A matter of rhetoric? *Nature materials*, 5, 243 (2006).
5. K. J. Morrow, R. Bawa, and C. Wei, Recent advances in basic and clinical nanomedicine, *Medical clinics of North America*, 91, 805–843 (2007).
6. K. K. Jain, Nanomedicine: Application of nanobiotechnology in medical practice, *Medical Principles and Practice*, 17, 89–101 (2008).
7. J. S. Murday, R. W. Siegel, J. Stein, and J. F. Wright, Translational nanomedicine: Status assessment and opportunities, *Nanomedicine: Nanotechnology, Biology and Medicine*, 5, 251–273 (2009).
8. K. Riehemann, S. W. Schneider, T. A. Luger, B. Godin, M. Ferrari, and H. Fuchs, Nanomedicine-challenge and perspectives, *Angewandte Chemie International Edition*, 48, 872–897 (2009).
9. K. V. Slavin, Commentary, *Surgical Neurology*, 71, 647–648 (2009).

11

Challenging Boundaries: Life and Material, Self and Environment

> The nano-scale is the interface between the weird quantum world and our own more classical world, and tapping into that weirdness may lead to technologies that transform not only materials but also biologies—and, as material, biological entities, ourselves as well.

> **David H. Guston, Center for Nanotechnology in Society,**
> *Consortium for Science, Policy, and Outcomes,*
> *Arizona State University.*

11.1 Nanotechnology and Medicine: A Powerful Confluence

Medicine is as old as humanity if not older. Nanotechnology and nanoscience are new on the scene. Medicine has a record of adopting and using revolutionary new technologies, and changing them to serve its needs, and being changed in turn. It is worth remembering that medicine may be considered a technology as well as an art.

Both medicine and technology are potentially powerful disruptive forces in societies—in the positive economic sense. They can and have brought about fundamental changes in the way people live and the assumptions they have about their lives—the way they see themselves and think of themselves. Changes in security, longevity, well-being, life span, and expectation of survival for infants and children are all changed by technology [1–6].

If nanotechnology is adopted fully by medicine, it will make medicine even more effective and powerful in saving and altering lives than it has already become by adopting other innovations of science and technology. This will bring more choices and more responsibilities. If we do not think about these choices beforehand, the choices may be made for us. These issues have been the subject of a number of seminars, reports, articles, and books in recent years [7–18].

11.2 Historical Origins of Medical Traditions

In order to make meaningful choices about the future direction of human nature and society, it is necessary to have an understanding of the historical origins of our current standards. The rich and strong history of medical science originates with empirical observations of outcomes of surgical and pharmaceutical applications. Prior to development of written records and a system of critical evaluation of outcomes, primeval societies had oral traditions regarding herbs and other remedies. Archeological evidence for primitive surgical operations has been found. The development of written records accelerated the communication of medical remedies and the development of a long-term body of experience and outcomes. Stone Age sites in Baluchistan have revealed evidence of dental drilling with flint tools in an early farming culture [3,19]. Some of the oldest known medical writings are Egyptian papyri from 1600 to 1700 BCE, which record surgical cases and outcomes, and document established practices that may predate the papyri by several thousand years [20].

Early civilizations held healers in high esteem; their reputations became legendary and they were elevated to godlike status. In ancient Egypt, Imhotep (meaning "one who comes in peace") was a historical figure who rose from common beginnings to become the vizier to the Pharaoh Djoser (reigned 2630–2611 BCE). In ancient cultures, the roles of doctor, priest, scribe, sage, poet, astrologer, architect, vizier, and chief minister were all intertwined. There was a degree of interaction between the Egyptian culture and the civilizations of the Tigris and Euphrates valley, such as the Persians. After his death, Imhotep (or Greek: Imouthes) was elevated to demigod status and became a cult figure for healing and a focal point for collections of writings and medical practices in temples and courts in many cultures [21–23]. He became identified with the Greek god of healing, Aslepius, and the Greek and Arabian civilizations continued the medical heritage of the Egyptians and Asians.

The most famous Greek doctor was Hippocrates, who also was elevated to cult status, with an attributed genealogy descending from Aslepius. Modern Western science–based medicine reveres Hippocrates as a physician who applied philosophical enquiry to medicine and encoded ethical standards for practice. The admonition in the Hippocratic oath: "First, do no harm," is still the foundation of medical practice.

In the Indus civilization, the Ayurvedic tradition of medicine (meaning "life knowledge") is documented by the works of Agnivesha, whose writings were later revised by Charaka, about 300 BCE. Charaka held that health is not predetermined and life may be prolonged by human effort. This was a major development in outlook for prescientific societies. He defined the goals of medicine as follows: to cure the diseases of the sick, protect the healthy, and to prolong life. Medical students in the Charaka tradition were given a code of practice with parallels to the Hippocratic oath, including honesty, devotion to learning, sober living, and respect for patient confidentiality. The Indus tradition was very systematic with division of medicine into categories such as toxicology, obstetrics, etc., and a rigorous qualifying exam for practitioners.

In China, medical knowledge was documented in the classical period in texts with parallels to the other ancient traditions, basing illness on a balance of the primary elements and astrological influences. A unique aspect of Chinese medicine was the practice of acupuncture, which is systematically treated in the early treatises, with highly developed anatomical descriptions.

In large part, because of the care to avoid doing harm, the practice of medicine has traditionally been experience based and very conservative when adopting new practices and theories. The germ theory of disease was famously resisted by medical practitioners in the nineteenth century until the evidence gained from actual practice became overwhelming, notably due to the work of Louis Pasteur, Claude Bernard, and Robert Koch [3,24,25]. At least as much harm has been done in the history of medicine by adherence to theories as doctrines as by rational experimentation with new techniques. That said, the goal of minimizing harm is best served by a skeptical approach to new developments.

Modern medicine has its roots in many ancient cultures, and is today transnational and transcultural, forming its own special fraternity into which individuals from all over the world earn their place to work, communicate, and serve cooperatively across boundaries.

Nanotechnology is a new transnational and transcultural development that is here to stay and is growing rapidly and pervasively. Medicine has many choices to make about how it is to be harnessed. Because medicine deals with life, death, and the quality of life, such choices are always measured against the standards of medical ethics. Nanotechnology in itself does not create any new ethical questions, but like other technologies, its application raises old and fundamental ethical questions in new forms.

Technologies give humans more power over their lives and the lives of others. Technologies give humans more choices over how to shape the world around them, and ultimately, the power to alter their own bodies and minds. With new and powerful technologies, old boundaries and assumptions are being called into question, not as a theoretical philosophical question, but as an immediate choice to be made.

Boundaries that limited our control over longevity, physical powers, mental capacity, reproduction, and other fundamental aspects of our lives are being challenged by new technologies, including those being driven by nanotechnology. New technologies may remove some immediate ethical dilemma with technical fixes that avoid the need to make hard choices, but in many other areas the dilemmas are exacerbated.

Here is a summary of some of the questions and issues being raised by nanomedicine and related technologies.

11.3 Knowledge of the Genome

As knowledge of each individual's genome becomes easier to obtain, and becomes a part of personalized medicine, who will own that knowledge? This issue needs to be thoroughly discussed and decided in order to avoid the kinds of problems now arising over human cell cultures. In the information age, the information content of the cell will be as great a commodity as the cell itself.

11.3.1 Should an Individual Have the Right Not to Know Their Genome: The "Right to Ignorance"?

Should an individual have the right to keep others from knowing their genome, even their healthcare provider, or those responsible for public health—or their relatives or children? This question raises issues of public good and even public protection versus rights to privacy. It is faced in older forms in questions of quarantine and vaccination [25–37].

11.3.2 Cultural Diversity in Attitudes toward Personal Control

One of the challenges faced in considering issues of privacy is that different cultures and ethnicities may have subtle or even quite marked differences in attitude toward privacy and the relationship between the individual, the family, and the caregiver [38–46].

11.4 Replacement Parts for the Body

As replacement parts for the body become more readily available, how will their distribution be allocated? Will there be a technological fix based on superabundance, or will there be some form of economic rationing? Are xenotransplants, which may become feasible with nanoengineered encapsulation, unethical? Issues of medical and moral benefits and risks raised by the greater feasibility and wider types of transplantation through nanotechnologies include boundaries for research, allocation, patient selection, organ donation, artificial organs, and xenografts. Most of these issues are not fundamentally new for nanomedicine, but are made more relevant by the enabling of new capabilities for replacement and regeneration [47–51].

11.5 Augmentation of Human Characteristics and Abilities

Medicine already has the ability to augment human performance and ability. At what point does such augmentation change our humanity? Do we inevitably lose something when we take on artificial enhancements? Are we on the way to becoming automatons, merging with our machines? How much of our body can we replace without losing our identity? Do we weaken our bodies and minds through over-reliance on artificial aids for protection and enhancement? These are questions that are brought to the fore with potential nanotechnology-based augmentations of human capabilities, but they are questions that have been discussed for a long time in relation to athletic equipment, and drugs for enhancement of performance, mental alertness, memory, and "expansion of consciousness" [52–56].

These issues are faced with brain–machine interfaces and neuroprosthetics. Typically, neuroprosthetics are resorted to only after pharmacologic and neurosurgical options have been exhausted. Bioengineers and other designers of systems to augment human capabilities are cognizant that their role should be to assist the body's adaptation and compensation for a deficit, rather than replace any remaining function. Systems that surpass natural capabilities can be intimately interfaced to the human body, in "bionic human" or cyborg scenarios. Nanotechnology is making such capabilities more feasible and affordable, obliging us to confront the social, medical, and ethical consequences [57–59].

The extent to which a person can project their personality into a virtual reality environment is growing ever more complete. At what point if any could a virtual reality avatar reach a sustainable existence without its creator? Can part or all of our consciousness eventually be extendable into machine intelligence? Could a sufficiently capable autonomous entity have something like consciousness? These are very deep questions that deal with issues of the nature of personality and consciousness, the relationship between mind and matter, self and body [60,61].

The immediate practical implications are whether there should be limits imposed upon such embellishment, and if so, in what circumstances, and how such limits should be enforced, and whether they are inherently unenforceable. When we consider that the use of mind-altering drugs is an example of this category, the difficulty of the issue comes starkly into focus [62–65].

11.6 Extension of Life

If medicine achieves the ability to extend life well beyond current limits of longevity, what would be the economic consequences? What choices would have to be made? New technologies such as regeneration of tissues and regulatory peptides are showing how life could be extended. One question that is being considered is whether new medical capabilities should be aimed at intervening into the process of aging itself rather than at diseases associated with aging—toward compression of morbidity to the final period of life. Bioethicists, social scientists, and antiaging proponents frame anti-aging goals differently. Some proponents hold the medical construction of immortality as their explicit aim. An alternative is that the goal should be alleviation of the painful, physiological decline of aging rather than elimination of ultimate death [66,67].

11.7 Issues with Transplanted Cells for Regeneration

Nanotechnology and biotechnology appear to have provided a technological fix to the vexed ethical questions surrounding the use of human embryonic stem cells. If the current promising research on methods to create autologous induced pluripotent stem cells reaches the application stage, it will no longer be necessary to use embryonic stem cells for tissue regeneration. Cell transposing peptides, semiochemical reprogramming, and other epigenetic technologies are beginning to show results that promise the practical ability to reprogram an individual's cells into regenerative stem cells for all types of tissues, without cloning, viral transfection, oncogenes, or genetic modification of any kind. Focus is now turning to the issues of artificial cells and xenotransplantation [68,69].

11.8 Medicalization of Normal Conditions

The ethical questions raised about eliminating aging and augmenting human capabilities by medicine have given rise to broader questions about the sphere of medicine [70–73]. To what extent are we "medicalizing" conditions that are not diseases, but either normal courses of life or social adjustments or variations within the normal range of genetic and phenotypic diversity? If a trend toward medicalization is adopted by society to minimize human differences, what are the implications? Could the trend be leading toward a new type of eugenics?

11.9 Other Boundaries Yet More Weird

Another example of a direction in which the capability for virtual reality is going is the FeTouch project [74]. Three dimensional virtual reality interfaces with haptics can now be implemented to a very high standard, using stereo-visual feedback and haptic devices. Computing and interactive communication capacity now permit such systems to support virtual interaction with three-dimensional images produced in real time from medical imaging of the interior of the human body. This capability is potentially useful for telesurgery and medical diagnosis and training, and those applications are being developed, as we saw in Chapter 6.

A rather different use is being made of this capability with the FeTouch project, whose aim is to allow mothers to interact with the fetus that they are carrying. The authors of the project take pains to point out that the FeTouch system has not been designed with medical diagnosis in gynecology and obstetrics as a prime focus. It is not clear what benefit or harm could come from opening windows of this nature in the natural barriers inherent in our bodies. The project illustrates how quickly such barriers are being breached in unexpected places, and how the technological capabilities may be outpacing considerations of efficacy, safety, ethics, and social values.

11.10 Summary

These are just a few of the questions that nanotechnology is raising in new forms. It is important that scientists and medical caregivers give thought and discussion to the ethical and social implications of their work, or else, without the attention of the individuals who engage in the social activity of science, "science does not think," but follows its own inevitable course [75–78]. Today, with the capabilities of nanoengineered biomaterials and genetics, we are being asked the old question: "How dare you sport thus with life?" [78] Hopefully, we are not playing thoughtlessly, but carefully and responsibly.

References

1. D. O. Weber, Nanomedicine, *Health Forum Journal*, 42, 32–37 (1999).
2. P. McCray, Will small be beautiful? Making policies for our nanotech future, *History and Technology*, 21, 177–203 (2005).
3. G. L. Hornyak, H. F. Tibbals, J. Dutta, and J. J. Moore, Medical nanotechnology, in *Introduction to Nanoscience and Nanotechnology*, CRC Press, Boca Raton, FL, 2009.
4. F. Allhoff, The coming era of nanomedicine, *American Journal of Bioethics*, 9, 3–11 (2009).
5. V. Gewin, Big opportunities in a small world, *Nature*, 460, 540–541 (2009).
6. C. Groves, Nanotechnology, contingency and finitude, *NanoEthics*, 3, 1–16 (2009).
7. J. Bird, B. Curtis, M. Mash, T. Putnam, G. Robertson, and L. Tickner (eds.), *Futurenatural - Nature, Science, Culture*, Routledge, NY, 1996.

8. R. M. Satava, Biomedical, ethical, and moral issues being forced by advanced medical technologies, *Proceedings of the American Philosophical Society*, 147, 246–258 (2003).

9. C. M. Kelty (ed.), *The Ethics and Politics of Nanotechnology*, UNESCO, Paris, France, 2006, Online at: http:// unesdoc.unesco.org/images/0014/001459/145951e.pdf (2010).

10. M. Ebbesen and T. G. Jensen, Nanomedicine: Techniques, potentials, and ethical implications, *Journal of Biomedicine and Biotechnology*, 2006, 1–11 (2006).

11. M. Ebbesen, S. Andersen, and F. Besenbacher, Ethics in nanotechnology: Starting from scratch? *Bulletin of Science, Technology and Society*, 26, 451–462 (2006).

12. Johann Ach and Ludwig Siep (eds.), *Nano-Bio-Ethics: Ethical Dimensions of Nanobiotechnology (Münsteraner Bioethik-Studien, 6)*, Lit Verlag, Berlin-Münster-Wien-Zürich-London, 2007.

13. F. Allhoff, P. Lin, J. Moor, and J. Weckert, *Nanoethics: The Ethical and Societal Implications of Nanotechnology*, John Wiley & Sons, Hoboken, NJ, 2007.

14. D. Bennett-Woods, *Nanotechnology: Ethics and Society*, CRC Press, Boca Raton, FL, 2008.

15. Nuffield Council on Bioethics, Topic 1. Nanotechnology, *Forward Look Seminar*, London May 8, 2008, Nuffield Council on Bioethics, London, U.K., website at: http:// www.nuffieldbioethics.org/ (2009).

16. F. Allhoff and P. Lin (eds.), *Nanotechnology & Society: Current and Emerging Ethical Issues*, Springer Science and Business Media, New York, 2009.

17. J. Jaeger, M. Marcin, and P. Wolpe, Ethical issues in nano-medicine, Chap. 10, in V. Ravitsky, A. Fiester and A. L. Caplan (eds.), *The Penn Center Guide to Bioethics*, Springer Publishing Company, New York, 2009.

18. I. F. Purchase, Ethical issues for bioscientists in the new millennium, *Toxicology Letters*, 127, 307–313 (2009).

19. A. Coppa, L. Bondioli, A. Cucina, D. W. Frayer, C. Jarrige, J.-F. Jarrige, G. Quivron et al., Palaeontology: Early neolithic tradition of dentistry, *Nature*, 440, 755–756 (2006).

20. B. Morris, Surgery on papyrus, *Student BMJ*, 12, 309–348 (2004).

21. M. Kennedy, *A Brief History of Disease, Science, and Medicine*, Asklepiad Press, Mission Viejo, CA, 2004.

22. I. Shaw, *The Oxford History of Ancient Egypt*, Oxford University Press, Oxford, U.K., 2000.

23. J. F. Nunn, *Ancient Egyptian Medicine*, University of Oklahoma Press, Norman, OK, 1996.

24. R. Porter, *The Greatest Benefit to Mankind: A Medical History of Humanity from Antiquity to the Present*, HarperCollins, New York, 1997.

25. J. H. Moor, Towards a theory of privacy in the information age, *ACM SIGCAS Computers and Society*, 27, 27–32 (1997).

26. G. T. Marx, Murky conceptual waters: The public and the private, *Ethics and Information Technology*, 3, 157–169 (2001).

27. C. A. Tauer, Genetics and the common good, *Second Opinion*, 8, 14–35 (2001).

28. T. Takala and H. A. Gylling, Who should know about our genetic makeup and why? *The Western Journal of Medicine*, 175, 260–263 (2001).

29. M. Häyry and T. Takala, Genetic information, rights, and autonomy, *Theoretical Medicine and Bioethics*, 22, 403–414 (2001).

30. J. Harris and K. Keywood, Ignorance, information and autonomy, *Theoretical Medicine and Bioethics*, 22, 415–436 (2001).
31. D. A. Fleming, Ethical considerations of genetic testing, *Journal of Clinical Ethics*, 13, 316–323 (2002).
32. L. Beckman, Are genetic self-tests dangerous? Assessing the commercialization of genetic testing in terms of personal autonomy, *Theoretical Medicine and Bioethics*, 25, 387–398 (2004).
33. R. McDougall, Rethinking the 'right not to know', *Monash Bioethics Review*, 23, 22–36 (2004).
34. J. Wilson, To know or not to know? Genetic ignorance, autonomy and paternalism, *Bioethics*, 19, 492–504 (2005).
35. L. Floridi, The ontological interpretation of informational privacy, *Ethics and Information Technology*, 7, 185–200 (2005).
36. L. Marx-Stölting, Pharmacogenetics and ethical considerations: why care? *Pharmacogenomics Journal*, 7, 293–296 (2007)
37. P. J. Malpas, Is genetic information relevantly different from other kinds of non-genetic information in the life insurance context? *Journal of Medical Ethics*, 34, 548–551 (2008).
38. S. R. Benatar, Just healthcare beyond individualism: Challenges for North American bioethics, *Cambridge Quarterly of Healthcare Ethics*, 6, 397–415 (1997).
39. T. Takala, The right to genetic ignorance confirmed, *Bioethics*, 13, 288–293 (1999).
40. D. Lamb and S. M. Easton, Philosophy of medicine in the United Kingdom, *Metamedicine*, 3, 3–34 (1982).
41. H. T. Engelhardt Jr., Critical care: Why there is no global bioethics, *Current Opinion in Critical Care*, 11, 605–609 (2005).
42. M. A. Horton and A. Khan, Medical nanotechnology in the UK: A perspective from the London Centre for Nanotechnology, *Nanomedicine*, 2, 42–48 (2006).
43. A. Saniotis, Changing ethics in medical practice: A Thai perspective, *Indian Journal of Medical Ethics*, 4, 24–25 (2007).
44. T. Metz, African and Western moral theories in a bioethical context, *Developing World Bioethics*, 8, 192–196 (2008).
45. B. Larijani and F. Zahedi, Contemporary medical ethics: An overview from Iran, *Developing World Bioethics*, 8, 192–196 (2008).
46. S. Chattopadhyay and R. De Vries, Bioethical concerns are global, bioethics is Western, *Eubios Journal of Asian and International Bioethics*, 18, 106–109 (2008).
47. R. Kielstein and H.-M. Sass, From wooden limbs to biomaterial organs: The ethics of organ replacement and artificial organs, *Artificial Organs*, 19, 475–480 (1995).
48. P. S. Malchesky, Artificial organs and vanishing boundaries, *Artificial Organs*, 25, 5–88 (2001).
49. B. H. Scribner, Medical dilemmas: The old is new, *Nature Medicine*, 8, 1066–1067 (2002).
50. M. Sykes, A. d'Apice, M. Sandrin, and the IXA Ethics Committee, Position paper of the ethics committee of the international xenotransplantation association, *Transplantation*, 78, 1101–1107 (2004).
51. J. P. Kahn, Listening to the Tin Man, *Ethics Matters Website*, July 9, 2001 Posted: 12:30 p.m. EDT (1630 GMT), Online at: http://archives.cnn.com/2001/HEALTH/07/09/ethics.matters/index.html (2009).

52. J. S. Donath, Identity and deception in the virtual community, in M. A. Smith, and P. Kollock (eds.), *Communities in Cyberspace*, Routledge, London, U.K., 1999.

53. C. N. Milburn, Nanotechnology in the age of posthuman engineering: Science fiction as science, *Configurations*, 10, 261–295 (2002).

54. M. J. Sandel, The case against perfection: What's wrong with designer children, bionic athletes, and genetic engineering, *Atlantic Monthly*, 292, 50–54, 56–60, 62 (2004).

55. A. Chatterjee, Cosmetic neurology: The controversy over enhancing movement, mentation, and mood, *Neurology*, 63, 968–974 (2004).

56. S. O. Hansson, The ethics of enabling technology, *Cambridge Quarterly of Healthcare Ethics, Cambridge Quarterly of Healthcare Ethics*, 16, 257–267 (2007).

57. M. E. Clynes and N. S. Kline, Cyborgs and space, *Astronautics*, September, 26–27 (1960).

58. R. Clarke, Human-artefact hybridisation: Forms and consequences, *Ars Electronica 2005 Symposium on Hybrid—Living in Paradox*, Linz, Austria, September 2–3, 2005.

59. J. Bohn, V. Coroama, M. Langheinrich, F. Mattern, and M. Rohs, Living in a world of smart everyday objects—Social, economic, and ethical implications, *Human and Ecological Risk Assessment*, 10, 763–785 (2004).

60. P. Wolpe, Is my mind mine? Neuroethics and brain imaging, Chap. 8, in V. Ravitsky, A. Fiester, and A. L. Caplan (eds.), *The Penn Center Guide to Bioethics*, Springer Publishing Company, New York, 2009.

61. G. Stock, From regenerative medicine to human design: What are we really afraid of? *Free Inquiry*, 24, 27–30 (2004).

62. A. Chatterjee, The promise and predicament of cosmetic neurology, *Journal of Medical Ethics*, 32, 110–113 (2006).

63. S. K. Rosahl, Neuroprosthetics and neuroenhancement: Can we draw a line? *Virtual Mentor*, 9, 132–139 (2007).

64. C. Lanni, S. C. Lenzken, A. Pascale, I. Del Vecchio, M. Racchi, F. Pistoia, and S. Govoni, Cognition enhancers between treating and doping the mind, *Pharmacological Research*, 57, 196–213 (2008).

65. S. Schneider, Future minds: Transhumanism, cognitive enhancement and the nature of persons, Chap. 9, in V. Ravitsky, A. Fiester, and A. L. Caplan (eds.), *The Penn Center Guide to Bioethics*, Springer Publishing Company, New York, 2009.

66. D. MacDonald, Unlimited claims on limited resources: Entropy, health care, and a hospice world view. Third in a series, *American Journal of Hospice and Palliative Medicine*, 8, 27–34. (1991).

67. C. E. Mykytyn, Anti-aging is not necessarily anti-death: Bioethics and the front lines of practice, *Medicine Studies*, 1, 209–228 (2009).

68. R. Sherlock and J. D. Morrey, Ethical issues in transgenics, *Cloning*, 2, 137–144 (2000).

69. H. W. Grosse, Xenotransplantation aus christlich-ethischer Sicht [Xenotransplantation from a Christian-ethical perspective], *ALTEX*, 20, 259–269 (2003).

70. M. J. Trappenburg, Defining the medical sphere, *Cambridge Quarterly of Healthcare Ethics*, 6, 416–434 (1997).

71. R. M. Satava, Disruptive visions, *Surgical Endoscopy*, 16, 1403–1408 (2002).

72. L. R. Kass and P. McHugh, *Exchange of Letters on Medicalization between Leon R. Kass, M.D. and Paul McHugh, M.D., I. Paul McHugh to Leon Kass*—May 27, 2003, Online at: http://www.bioethics.gov/background/kass_mchugh.html (2009).

73. P. Conrad, *The Medicalization of Society: On the Transformation of Human Conditions into Treatable Disorders*, Johns Hopkins University Press, Baltimore, MD, 2007.
74. D. Prattichizzo, B. la Torre, F. Barbagli, A. Vicino, F. M. Severi, and F. Petraglia, The FeTouch Project: An application of haptic technologies to obstetrics and gynaecology, *The International Journal of Medical Robotics & Computer Assisted Surgery*, 1, 1–5 (2004).
75. T. Glazebrook, *Heidegger's Philosophy of Science*, Fordham University Press, New York, 2000.
76. A. De Vries, Reflections on a medical ethics for the future, *Metamedicine*, 3, 115–120 (1982).
77. R. W. Berne, *Nanotalk: Conversations with Scientists and Engineers about Ethics, Meaning, and Belief in the Development of Nanotechnology*, Lawrence Erlbaum Associates, Mahwah, NJ, 2006.
78. R. C. Goldbort, "How dare you sport thus with life?": Frankensteinian fictions as case studies in scientific ethics, *Journal of Medical Humanities*, 16, 79–91 (1995).

12

Sustainability and Future
Choices for Societies

Nano optimists see nanotechnology delivering … environmentally
benign material abundance for all …

Nano sceptics suggest that nanotechnology will simply exacerbate problems stemming from existing socio-economic inequity and unequal dis-
tributions of power … [1]

12.1 Nanotechnology and Medicine
as a Socioeconomic Activity

In this chapter, we discuss the social and economic implications of medical
nanotechnology and nanomedicine. With any technology, changes in tools
and techniques bring changes in the way work is organized; and therefore
in economic and social relationships. Nanotechnology has been described
as a disruptive technology in the economic sense. Its potential is frequently
described as revolutionary: turning the world upside down, bringing a tsu-
nami, etc. On the whole, nanomedicine has been welcomed as providing economic opportunities on a new frontier, with some cautions about possible
negative impacts [2–9].

12.2 Questions of Change

Granted that nanotechnology involves a change in the way work is being
done, including procedures, operations, and techniques in medicine, to what
extent will it change the practice and perhaps even the conceptual base of
medicine? What directions will any such changes take? [10,11].

Will new technologies lead to greater expense, and more inequities in provision of medical services, or lower costs and wider availability of healthcare? [12,13].

What will be the impact on health and healthcare of other nonmedical
changes driven by application of nanotechnology, which produce major

changes in other areas such as manufacturing, transportation, consumer, communications, education, agricultural, energy, military, leisure, and entertainment? [14,15].

What will be the timescale of any changes brought about by application of nanotechnology—how rapid and over what period? Specifically, when will emerging nanotechnologies actually reach clinical practice—what is the time line? [7,16].

Will nanomedicine and medical nanotechnology create a divide between developed economies and those struggling to emerge into the world economy, or will they provide low-cost alternatives to the existing investment in medical infrastructure? [17].

Will nanotechnology produce unforeseen consequences—side effects that result in long-term health problems and/or environmental harm? [18–20].

Answers to these questions cannot be offered here; it is difficult to predict the future. However, it is important to consider these types of questions, especially when we do not have answers. As Eisenhower said, "Plans are worthless, but planning is everything." So some speculative considerations are offered here on just a few of the above questions.

12.2.1 Disruptive Technology

Industrial revolutions are marked not merely by technological innovation, but also by the social and economic changes brought about by new human capabilities. It is widely observed that nanotechnology is a disruptive technological development, opening vast new possibilities for economic growth and human control over health, the environment, and efficiency and precision of production of goods and services [21,22].

Societies have different ways of reacting to new technological developments. Innovation can be resisted and suppressed, it can be ignored, or it can be harnessed. Suppressing or ignoring innovation has historically led to stagnation, leaving nations behind as innovation flows to other outlets. History provides ample examples. Attempting to harness innovation by rigid controls typically has led to either complete failure or short-term results followed by decline. Innovation and its applications seem to thrive best with a subtle combination of social support and freedom to follow the pursuits directed by human creativity [23,24].

It has also been noted with some concern that developments made possible by nanotechnology provide greater capability for monitoring and control of the daily life of individuals. Whether this technical capability is used to increase the power of states or the influence of corporations and political entities over people, or to improve health and education and increased freedom of individuals, is a matter to be decided [25–27].

We have already experienced sweeping changes brought about by continually accelerating progress in scientific and technological research. Changes made by application of nanotechnology will be a continuation of the changes made by previous technological advances, but may be expected to be more rapid. Exploration of space has brought many changes, including those resulting from satellites for communications and environmental monitoring. The frontier looking out into extraterrestrial space, despite its remoteness, opened many new changes in our lives. The frontier opened by nanotechnology—control over the very small and subtle mechanisms of matter—is much closer to our lives and activities, and therefore may open more immediate and profound changes.

It has been often noted that the pace of change brought about by technology is increasing. Nanotechnology is no different, and simply adds a new driver and new directions to the exponential growth and change that has characterized the industrial revolution [28].

12.2.2 Impacts on Medical Practice

Every new technology brings impacts by changing the details and efficacy of procedures and introducing new methods of diagnosis and treatment. Indirectly, new technologies create changes in the organization and provision of healthcare. Doctors no longer make house calls; TB sanatoria and iron lungs are memories. Laboratory tests, imaging, and pharmaceuticals have changed medical practice. New technologies have shifted the economics of cost and demand for whole specializations—for example, the effect of cardiac catheterization procedures on open-heart surgeries. New technologies made possible by nanotechnology will produce similar translations and shifts in emphasis within medical care [29–31]:

> These nanostructured medicines will eventually turn the world of drug delivery upside down [32].

Every revolution goes through a radical stage, followed by a period of consolidation, accommodation, and integration into the mainstream. Nanotechnology is beyond the far-out fringe stage and is now on its way to being integrated into the mainstream. Nanotechnology is being used directly and/or indirectly in every discipline and speciality of medicine. It is relatively easy to see where nanotechnology is producing direct impacts, as in nanomedicines and tissue engineering. Another level of impact is indirect, as in surgical robotics, created with new capabilities in computing, communications, sensing, and automation, and in personalized medicine, in the sense of diagnosis and therapies based on knowledge of the patient's genome. A third level is social and economic, as new technologies influence the way healthcare is being delivered, organized, and perceived by providers and the public.

12.2.3 Impact of Technological Developments on Personal Healthcare

To the extent that nanotechnology (and, more broadly, genomic and systematic medicine) leads to personalization of healthcare, they will be in concert with other economic influences that have led to greater specialization of healthcare services. Tailoring healthcare to the patient's individual genome is different in that the knowledge of the patient is so fundamental. The patient has no choice over their genome, nor can they change it, but it can have profound implications for their life. This creates a new depth to the relationship between doctor and patient, and new attention is being given to the management of the information and the relationship. It also could lead to more focus on the patient information record than on the patient as a person [33–35].

There is another way in which technology is tending to personalize healthcare. Increased individual choice is a general trend driven by flexible manufacturing and instant and global communications. Consumers have more choices than 100 years ago in everything from automobiles to cell phones to breakfast cereals. The popularity of personalized medicine as a label is due in part to this general trend in which people expect to have more choices and at least the illusion of more control over goods and services. The greater variety in consumer offerings is increasingly based on more detailed information gathered about individuals and their preferences, habits, and spending. Individual consumers may not always be in proactive control of the choices generated, but it is now much less expensive to have a product built to one's own specifications, within the framework of a system of flexible mass production. The technology is in place to provide consumers with enormous amounts of information (or misinformation) and access to pharmaceuticals over the Internet and wireless networks. Increasingly, patients want to be active coproducers of their healthcare. The medical profession will be called upon increasingly to provide quality information through these new channels, as educating and informing patients is becoming more important to healthcare outcomes [36,37].

12.2.3.1 Evolution of Choice in Healthcare

In primitive societies, health services such as they were, were provided by a village, or tribal shaman or priest, who typically held a monopoly for service over everyone in his or her group. Family and comrades might offer succor and aid for wounds and injuries, help with childbirth, and basic maintenance of hygiene, but to the extent that there was such a thing as medicine outside of normal maintenance of life, food, and shelter, it was typically provided by individuals who held secret monopolies on healing techniques passed down to their apprentices only.

In early civilizations, ordinary medicine was practiced by special slaves or servants to those wealthy or powerful enough to afford them, with special interventions reserved for priesthoods or practitioners of magic—the latter feared and shunned to the outskirts of society, but tolerated and called upon in desperation if one dared. Development of richer civilizations saw the rise of independent practitioners able to offer medical services and knowledge in a free market and establish independent schools in which medical knowledge could be developed and propagated.

In the European Middle Ages and in other feudal societies, legitimate healthcare knowledge, and to a large extent, provision of medical services, was claimed as the monopoly of the church and its institutions, including the monastery and hospital. Any practice of healing outside of the auspices of the established religion, even provision of herbal remedies, was suspect at best [38].

The enlightenment and the industrial revolution opened healthcare based on scientific knowledge to all in principle. Beginning in the eighteenth century, the traditional loyalty toward the individual patient (or patron) was challenged by a greater social orientation in the physician's ethos. Medical care, like so much else, gradually became available as a service on the market rather than as a service owed and rendered to one's overlords, and to society in general; but in practice, the fruits of developing, though still terribly primitive, medical science were available to a small number of the educated and elite. Through all this time, medicine was personal, and variable from region to region and doctor to doctor. Treatment and remedies were prescribed and compounded specifically for each patient and each illness. If choices were limited, it was because of paucity of knowledge and alternatives rather than lack of attention and care in attempting to meet the needs of the individual patient (lack of knowledge of both the patient's internal condition and genetics as well as of alternative remedies) [39].

12.2.3.2 Standardization of Care and Mass Production of Drugs

Industrialization, standardization of education, and the mass production of drugs tended to diminish personalized care. On the whole, the benefits of scientifically designed chemical remedies and hygienic proscriptions with wide general applicability far outweighed any drawbacks from lack of personalization. Mass-produced antibiotics, vaccines, and other drugs along with public health measures made enormous progress in overcoming infectious disease. The paradigm for treatment became diagnosis of a pathogen or condition, and treatment with a drug that had been developed to target some aspect of the pathogen or disease. Having few drugs in the armatorium was adequate; therapy needed to be customized only in case of allergies in the patient or resistance in the pathogen. All kinds of epidemics, from cholera to tuberculosis to polio, became less common and less severe, at least in the developed world, and medicine changed—sanatoria and asylums ceased to be major landmarks on the landscape [40].

12.2.3.3 New Needs of Personalized Medicine in Cancer and Infectious Disease

But cancer, along with some degenerative and autoimmune diseases, did not yield to therapies based on targeted drug strategies aimed broadly at the disease. Only after it became possible to know the detailed genome of an individual, plus an understanding of the network of oncologic cell signaling pathways was it possible to realize personalized medicine in the new sense of therapeutics, which targeted specific regulatory paths based on the specific proteomic metabolism of the individual and the disorder [10].

As disease organisms claw their way back against our onslaught of antibiotics, personalized medicine strategies will also be required—targeted in this case against the specific genome and signaling pathways by which the pathogens evade and defeat normal antibiotic drugs. And in some cases, these pathways interact with and exploit the human cells' defense mechanisms in diabolically intricate and subtle ways, giving a new twist to the development of personalized therapies for infectious diseases. Nanotechnology for improved diagnosis and nanomedicines for effective therapies will be needed to meet these emerging threats [41].

12.2.4 Distribution and Extension of Healthcare by Telecommunications and Nanosensors

In addition to the capability of knowing the patient's genome, healthcare providers and patients are being given the potential to monitor the status of health-related indicators taken directly from the body continually and globally in the patient's daily life and routine. Personal monitoring devices and systems are falling in price along with ways to communicate their data. This leads to the need for systems to manage the process. Decisions about when and what to measure need to be agreed upon by patient and caregivers; improved information handling, processing, and analysis systems and capabilities are needed to filter useful information from streams of data, which are increasingly easier to generate and transmit. The feedback and decision loops fed by monitoring data will inevitably have to be distributed out toward the patient, or any central focal point will be overwhelmed. With the expansion of cell phones over geographical and economic spaces, affordable telemedicine will increasingly become an option for millions of people. Healthcare practice, insurance, and regulation will restructure and take new forms to accommodate these new options. Doctors may advise patients via cell phone with the aid of portable imaging and testing. Referring patients to, and teaming with, remote specialists may become a standard practice, along with consulting and mentoring via telerobotics [42–46].

12.2.5 Synergistic Economic Impact of Nanomedicines with Biotechnology and Genomics

Since the emergence of the biotechnology industry beginning in the 1970s, technology has been available to make a large number of entirely new pharmaceuticals. With the elucidation of the human genome, the targeting of diseases by biotechnology-engineered drugs has become accelerated and focused. And the availability of widespread and low-cost decoding of individual genomes has opened even more opportunities of targeted bioengineered therapeutics. Much research effort has been directed toward identifying and producing small molecule therapeutics, which could be delivered by traditional means. At first, peptide therapeutics, the most natural outcome of the biotechnology and genome revolution, had been accumulating on the shelf. But as nanomedicines provide effective protection and targeted release mechanisms, the huge backlog of biotechnology-generated peptide therapeutics is beginning to move toward clinical applications. This movement will have large health and economic impacts. It could hold the promise of defeat of intractable scourges such as malaria and cholera, with enormous economic consequences [47].

12.2.6 Restorative and Regenerative Medicine

To the extent that nanomedicines and medical nanotechnology provide affordable and effective replacement for degenerative and diseased organs, they will extend the length and quality of life for millions of people. This could affect the demographics and economics of whole societies, possibly prolonging active and productive working lives. The basis for economic models of healthcare and life insurance and social welfare and retirement programs might have to be altered, especially if neurodegenerative diseases are conquered by induced stem cell therapies. The changes would be as great as those brought about through the conquest of infectious diseases by antibiotics. In addition, any medication that halted or reversed the aging process would introduce thorny social, economic, and ethical dilemmas [48,49].

12.2.7 Global Divide

The prospect of nanotechnology and nanomedicine raises concerns that their development will create global divides in access to these technologies between rich and poor populations. This is unlikely, as people in developing nations have shown great agility in adopting new technologies that offer greater personal flexibility, ways around bureaucracy and regulation, and inexpensive alternatives to centralized established ways of providing services. Examples are abundant in telecommunications, banking, transportation, and other areas. If nanotechnology can offer cost savings, flexibility, and greater individual choice, it will give people in developing areas opportunities to leapfrog economies where adoption of new alternatives are slowed by established ways of doing things.

These opportunities will be facilitated and accelerated by a number of innovative nonprofit organizations supporting change in the developing world, as well as by companies who see profitable opportunities to supply low-cost flexible technology to meet new needs. Emerging economies such as China and India, as well as countries such as Korea, Singapore, Japan,

Israel, Iran, Brazil, and Argentina are leading the way in adopting many new medical nanotechnologies to meet the needs of their populations and to serve the needs of less developed markets. For corporations today, national and regional boundaries are largely irrelevant. If nanomedicine creates a divide, it will be more along economic lines within countries than between north and south, or older and emerging economies. Public education and awareness is needed, since perception that new technologies will bring harmful social and environmental effects can create a public backlash that will prevent the benefits from reaching those most in need [50].

12.2.8 The Threat of Grey Goo

There is still some concern about the possibility of self-replicating autonomous nanomachines causing environmental and economic havoc. These concerns, as usually expressed, are based on misconceptions of the nature of nanomachinery. Compared with the natural reproduction of the biological carbon-based nanomachinery of living organisms, including viruses and prions, self-reproduction of hard silicon and metal nanobots is expensive in terms of energy and readily available raw materials. It is difficult to envision how these hard nanobots could be as adaptable to our natural defenses and random physical disorder as the virtuoso nanomachinery that is the basis of living creatures.

If we have concerns about runaway self-replicating machines, they would be better directed at microorganisms, which have demonstrated over many eons their capacity for catastrophic interventions in human history. Currently, mycobacteria and other organisms are adapting to bypass the drugs and other mechanisms that have come to be taken for granted after many decades of successful use. Ironically, it is nanotechnology-based diagnostics and medicines that offer the best hope of countering this age-old, well-demonstrated threat of self-replicating aggressive and destructive hordes of wet micromachinery [51–55].

Concerns about man-made nanobots getting out of control and wrecking unforeseen environmental and human damage may have a more valid basis if we consider not MEMS and NEMS nanobots but artificial life forms created by manipulation of novel genetics and exotic amino acid building blocks. But then these concerns merely merge with the existing vigilance against natural disease organisms, which have every opportunity to take on novel forms through the many natural mechanisms creating genetic variation, and are continually demonstrating their propensities and abilities in this regard. Of course, we should take precautions and seek reasoned restraints on release of random materials, devices, and organisms into the environment—it is simply good housekeeping, one of the basic prerequisites to hygiene for humans as well as planets [56–58].

12.3 Conclusion

It would be a poor science indeed that was unable to change itself. Chemistry, whose name comes from an old Arabic word meaning roughly "the art of change", like astronomy and most sciences, has its roots in concepts of nature held in awe and ruled by supernatural forces. Medicine, as a healing art, emerged from this background with the growth of a pragmatic and results-based focus. And, it was in part, the demands of and interactions with medicine that helped to draw alchemy and astrology out of darkness. Nanotechnology began as a rather self-confident assertion of almost limitless technical capabilities; its interaction with the more mature sciences and with the demands and disciplines of medicine have helped tame and harness its concepts and develop more techniques for useful ends.

Thus, nanoscience, nanotechnology, and nanomedicine have changed a great deal since their launch a few decades ago as concepts and disciplines. As these concepts, techniques, and ways of describing and manipulating matter by exploiting phenomena on the nanoscale are developed and applied, they are evolving and converging with older disciplines and technologies. This is only what we must expect if we believe that all of nature is unified. It is a sign of the validity and usefulness of nanotechnology that it is being adopted and integrated into medicine and other disciplines, and a sign of the health and vitality of medicine that it is carefully and judiciously adapting nanotechnology to is own uses.

References

1. Nanotechnology Citizen Engagement Organization, *Latest Nanonews*, October 19, 2007, on website at: http://www.nanoceo.net/nanonews_10_19_07 (retrieved December 1, 2009).
2. D. O. Weber, The next little thing, *Health Forum Journal*, 45, 10–15 (2002).
3. S. Vinogradov, The second annual symposium on nanomedicine and drug delivery: Exploring recent developments and assessing major advances, August 19–20, 2004, Polytechnic University, Brooklyn, NY, *Expert Opinion on Drug Delivery*, 1, 181–184 (2004).
4. K. Donaldson, Resolving the nanoparticles paradox, *Nanomedicine*, 1, 229–234 (2006).
5. K. J. Morrow, R. Bawa, and C. Wei, Recent advances in basic and clinical nanomedicine, *Medical Clinics of North America*, 91, 805–843 (2007).
6. B. Walker and C. P. Mouton, Nanotechnology and nanomedicine: A primer, *Journal of the National Medical Association*, 98, 1985–1988 (2007).

7. S. D. Caruthers, S. A. Wickline, and G. M. Lanza, Nanotechnological applications in medicine, *Current Opinion in Biotechnology*, 18, 26–30 (2007).

8. V. Gewin, Big opportunities in a small world, *Nature*, 460, 540–541 (2009).

9. F. Allhoff, The coming era of nanomedicine, *American Journal of Bioethics*, 9, 3–11, (2009).

10. K. K. Jain, Role of nanobiotechnology in developing personalized medicine for cancer, *Technology in Cancer Research and Treatment*, 4, 645–650 (2006).

11. F. Jotterand, Nanomedicine: How it could reshape clinical practice, *Nanomedicine*, 2, 401–405 (2007).

12. E. Lahelma Eero and O. Lundberg, Health inequalities in European welfare states, *European Journal of Public Health*, 19, 445–446 (2009).

13. M. Ebbesen, The principle of justice and access to nanomedicine in national healthcare systems, *Studies in Ethics, Law, and Technology*, 3, 5 (2009). doi: 10.2202/1941-6008.1121, Online at: http://www.bepress.com/selt/vol3/iss3/art5/ (2009).

14. R. N. Kostoff, R. Boylan, and G. R. Simons, Roadmapping: From sustainable to disruptive technologies, *Technological Forecasting and Social Change*, 71, 141–159 (2004).

15. J. S. Patton, A historical perspective on convergence technology, *Nature Biotechnology*, 24, 280–281 (2006).

16. B. Wintle, M. Burgman, and F. Fidler, How fast should nanotechnology advance? *Nature Nanotechnology*, 2, 327 (2007).

17. N. Kondo, G. Sembajwe, I. Kawachi, R. M. van Dam, S. V. Subramanian, and Z. Yamagata, Income inequality, mortality, and self rated health: Meta-analysis of multilevel studies, *British Medical Journal*, 339, b4471 (2009).

18. P. Hoet, B. Legiest, J. Geys, and B. Nemery, Do nanomedicines require novel safety assessments to ensure their safety for long-term human use? *Drug Safety*, 32, 625–636 (2009).

19. G. H. Reynolds, Nanotechnology and regulatory policy: Three futures, *Harvard Journal of Law and Technology*, 17, 179–205 (2003).

20. A. Anderson, S. Allan, A. Petersen, and C. Wilkinson, The framing of nanotechnologies in the British newspaper press, *Science Communication*, 27, 200–220 (2005).

21. R. M. Satava, Disruptive visions, *Surgical Endoscopy*, 16, 1403–1408 (2002).

22. D. Bennett-Woods, Nanotechnology in medicine: Implications of converging technologies on the human community, *Development*, 49, 54–59 (2006).

23. J. Needham, G.-W. Lu, and N. Sivin (eds.), *Science and Civilisation in China: Vol. 6, Biology and Biological Technology; Part 6, Medicine*, Cambridge University Press, Cambridge, U.K., 2000.

24. P. Starr, *The Social Transformation of American Medicine: The Rise of a Sovereign Profession and the Making of a Vast Industry*, Basic Books, New York, 1984.

25. K. Häyrinen, K. Saranto, and P. Nykänen, Definition, structure, content, use and impacts of electronic health records: A review of the research literature, *International Journal of Medical Informatics*, 77, 291–304 (2008).

26. A. R. Kovner and J. R. Knickman (eds.), *Jonas and Kovner's Health Care Delivery in the United States*, 9th edn., Springer Publishing Company, Inc., New York, 2008.

27. R. S. Jones, Medicine, government, and capitalism, *Journal of the American College of Surgeons*, 194, 111–120 (2002).

28. L. Laurent and J.-C. Petit, Nanosciences and its convergence with other technologies: New golden age or apocalypse? *HYLE–International Journal for Philosophy of Chemistry*, 11, 45–76 (2005).

29. D. Miller, 50 years of health-care delivery: A personal perspective, 1956–2006, *Connecticut Medicine*, 70, 101–104 (2006).
30. A. Solovy, Creating health: The history of health care enters a new era, *Hospitals and Health Networks*, 81, 26 (2007).
31. M. J. Zinner and K. R. Loughlin, The evolution of health care in America, *Urology Clinics of North America*, 36, 1–10 (2009).
32. S. Parveen and S. K. Sahoo, Nanomedicine: Clinical applications of polyethylene glycol conjugated proteins and drugs, *Clinical Pharmacokinetics*, 45, 965–988 (2006).
33. R. M. Satava, Biomedical, ethical, and moral issues being forced by advanced medical technologies, *Proceedings of the American Philosophical Society*, 147, 246–258 (2003).
34. G. Khushf, Health as intra-systemic integrity: Rethinking the foundations of systems biology and nanomedicine, *Perspectives in Biology and Medicine*, 51, 432–449 (2008).
35. V. Maizes, D. Rakel, and C. Niemiec, Integrative medicine and patient-centered care, *Explore*, 5, 277–289 (2009).
36. H. S. Wald, C. E. Dube, and D. C. Anthony, Untangling the web—The impact of internet use on health care and the physician–patient relationship, *Patient Education and Counseling*, 68, 218–224 (2007).
37. M. Swan, Emerging patient-driven health care models: An examination of health social networks, consumer personalized medicine and quantified self-tracking, *International Journal of Environmental Research and Public Health*, 6, 492–525 (2009).
38. R. Porter, *The Greatest Benefit to Mankind: A Medical History of Humanity from Antiquity to the Present*, Harper Collins, New York, 1997.
39. J. Vollmann and A. Dörries, Dem Einzelnen oder dem Ganzen verpflichtet? Ethische Überlegungen zur ärztlichen Verantwortung [Responsibility for the individual or the whole? Ethical considerations on medical responsibility], *Zeitschrift für ärztliche Fortbildung*, 90, 527–532 (1996).
40. M. Kennedy, *A Brief History of Disease, Science, and Medicine*, Asklepiad Press, Mission Viejo, CA, 2004.
41. W. C. Hellinger, Confronting the problem of increasing antibiotic resistance, *Southern Medical Journal*, 93, 842–848 (2000).
42. R. Agarwala, A. W. Levinsona, M. Allafa, D. V. Makarova, A. Nasonb, and L.-M. Su, The RoboConsultant: Telementoring and remote presence in the operating room during minimally invasive urologic surgeries using a novel mobile robotic interface, *Urology*, 70, 970–974 (2007).
43. Y. Granot, A. Ivorra, and B. Rubinsky, A new concept for medical imaging centered on cellular phone technology, *PLoS ONE*, 3, e2075. doi:10.1371/journal.pone.0002075 (2008).
44. R. Bellazzi, Telemedicine and diabetes management: Current challenges and future research directions, *Journal of Diabetes Science and Technology*, 2, 98–104 (2008).
45. T. R. McLean, Will India set the price for teleradiology? *International Journal of Medical Robotics and Computer Assisted Surgery*, 5, 178–183 (2009).
46. M. McKinney, Decision support for docs, *Hospitals and Health Networks*, 83, 42–44 (2009).
47. H. Onyüksel, F. Séjourné, H. Suzuki, and I. Rubinstein, Human VIP-alpha: A long-acting, biocompatible and biodegradable peptide nanomedicine for essential hypertension, *Peptides*, 27, 2271–2275 (2006).

48. C. E. Mykytyn, Medicalizing the optimal: Anti-aging medicine and the quandary of intervention, *Journal of Aging Studies*, 22, 313–321 (2008).
49. A. Petersen and K. Seear, In search of immortality: The political economy of anti-aging medicine, *Medicine Studies*, 1, 267–279 (2009).
50. T. Sheetz, J. Vidal, T. D. Pearson, and K. Lozano, Nanotechnology: Awareness and societal concerns, *Technology in Society*, 27, 329–345 (2005).
51. J. N. Hays, *The Burdens of Disease: Epidemics and Human Response in Western History*, Rutgers University Press, New Brunswick, NJ, 2003.
52. E. Barnes, *Diseases and Human Evolution*, University of New Mexico Press, Albuquerque, NM, 2005.
53. J. N. Hays, *Epidemics and Pandemics: Their Impact on Human History*, ABC-CLIO, Inc., Santa Barbara, CA, 2005.
54. J. Aberth, *The First Horseman: Disease in Human History*, Pearson Prentice Hall, Upper Saddle River, NJ, 2007.
55. H. Zinsser, *Rats, Lice, and History*, with a New Introduction by Gerald N. Grob, Transactions Publishers, New Brunswick, NH, 2008.
56. O. Renn and M. C. Roco, Nanotechnology and the need for risk governance, *Journal of Nanoparticle Research*, 8, 153–191 (2006).
57. K. Sellers, C. Mackay, L. L. Bergeson, S. R. Clough, M. Hoyt, J. Chen, K. Henry, and J. Hamblen, *Nanotechnology and the Environment*, CRC Press, Boca Raton, FL (2008).
58. J. A. Shatkin, *Nanotechnology: Health and Environmental Risks*, CRC Press, Boca Raton, FL (2008).

Index